The Surgical Rehabilitation of Vision

An Integrated Approach to Anterior Segment Surgery

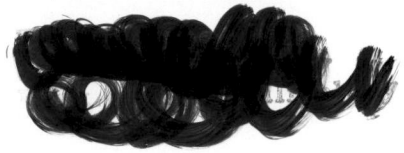

The Surgical Rehabilitation of Vision

An Integrated Approach to Anterior Segment Surgery

edited by

LEE T. NORDAN, M.D.
Assistant Clinical Professor
Jules Stein Eye Institute
University of California at
  Los Angeles
Los Angeles, California

W. ANDREW MAXWELL, M.D., Ph.D.
Assistant Clinical Professor
Department of Ophthalmology
University of California at San Francisco
San Francisco, California

JAMES A. DAVISON, M.D.
Wolfe Clinic
Marshalltown, Iowa

forewords by

James H. Little, M.D.   R. Bruce Grene, M.D.

Gower Medical Publishing • London • New York

Distributed in USA and Canada by:
JB Lippincott Company
East Washington Square
Philadelphia, PA 19105
USA

Distributed in the UK and Continental Europe by:
Gower Medical Publishing
Middlesex House
34-42 Cleveland Street
London W1P 5FB, UK

Distributed in Australia and New Zealand by:
HarperEducational (Australia)Pty Ltd.
P.O. Box 226
Artarmon
NSW 2064 Australia

Distributed in Southeast Asia, Hong Kong, India and Pakistan by:
APAC Publishers Services
30 Jalan Bahasa
Singapore 1129

Distributed in Japan by:
Nankodo Co. Ltd.
42-6, Hongo 3-chome
Bunkyo-Ku
Tokyo 113, Japan

Distributed in South America by:
Harper Collins Publishers Latin America
701 Brickell Avenue - Suite 1750
Miami, FL 33131
USA

Library of Congress Cataloging-in-Publication Data
The Surgical rehabilitation of vision: an integrated approach to anterior segment surgery / [edited by] Lee T. Nordan, W. Andrew Maxwell, James A. Davison.
p.   cm.
Includes bibliographical references.
ISBN 0-397-44693-4
  1. Eye—Surgery. I. Nordan, Lee T. II. Maxwell, W. Andrew,
   1942– .   III. Davison, James A.
   [DNLM: 1. Anterior Eye Segment—surgery. 2. Eye—surgery.
   3. Vision Disorders—rehabilitation. WW 140 S961]
   RE80.S853   1991
   617.7'1—dc20
                                                91-9860

Editor/Project Manager: **Elizabeth Greenspan**
Illustration Director/Illustrator: **Laura Pardi Duprey**
Art Director: **Jill Feltham**
Interior and Cover Designer: **Thomas Tedesco**
Editorial Assistant: **Jean Unger**

Printed in Hong Kong
Produced by Mandarin Offset

10   9   8   7   6   5   4   3   2   1

© Copyright 1992 by Gower Medical Publishing, 101 Fifth Avenue, New York, NY 10003, USA. The right of [the authors] to be identified as the authors of this work has been asserted by them in accordance with the Copyright, Designs and Patents Act 1988. All rights reserved. No part of this publication may be reproduced, stored in a retrieval system, transmitted in any form or by any means, electronic, mechanical, photocopying, recording or otherwise, without prior written permission of the publisher.

DEDICATION

The editors of *The Surgical Rehabilitation of Vision* feel honored to have the opportunity to present many aspects of anterior segment surgery. Ophthalmic surgery continues to advance because new ideas and technology are added to pre-existing methods. We salute our colleagues who have provided the foundation for current techniques and those who are contributing to continue this dynamic process.

Lee Nordan, Andy Maxwell, and Jim Davison
dedicate
The Surgical Rehabilitation of Vision
especially to our
Families and Friends

They make us feel that…

No goal is too far,
No challenge too great,
Success is within our power, and
Excellence is a virtue within our grasp

ACKNOWLEDGMENTS

The editors and authors wish to express their most profound personal thanks and admiration to the Gower Medical Publishing staff who have labored long and hard so that this project could come into fruition. Specifically, Abe Krieger believed in the concept of a medical book dedicated to excellence; Elizabeth Greenspan, the project editor, provided us with exceptional editing, a refreshing perspective, and constant reassurance; Laura Pardi Duprey, the artist, adroitly and magically converted our thoughts into pictures; Tom Tedesco skillfully laid out the pages and designed the cover; Randy Rodriguez reproduced the beautiful color photographs, and Terri Painter and Walkyria de Mello smoothly maintained the communication between editors and authors.

Members of our own staffs deserve recognition for their contributions, which are too numerous to recall. Special thanks to Karen Iovin, Kathy Orlando-Ploszaj, and Kayla Danielson, as well as to Dr. Gayle Amemiya.

To all those who have contributed in any way, we thank you for helping us on our one and one half year journey from concept to publication.

PREFACE

Knowledge enlightens, excellence rewards.

The process of learning often creates a thrill as the genius of our predecessors is revealed. For most of us in medicine, however, any hope of leisurely intellectual pursuits is soon shattered by the practical need to apply learning to patients who demand effective therapy. Eventually, we encounter someone who commands our respect not only because of accumulated knowledge but also by the manner of its application. Perhaps, our attention has been drawn to excellence.

What is excellence? How is excellence achieved?

Although an all-encompassing definition of excellence is difficult, certain characteristics are identifiable:

• Universality—excellence can be exhibited in any field of human endeavor.

• Essential knowledge—excellence requires an extensive working knowledge of the subject at hand.

• Desire—excellence requires the burning desire to be the best.

• Courage—excellence requires the courage to apply the best solutions, despite previous failures.

• Benevolence—the efforts of excellence must benefit society.

In ophthalmic surgery, good results alone do not define excellence. Excellence demands that basic medical and surgical principles be applied to the patient with both skill and compassion. Excellence is a human achievement, not a statistic. A problem is solved but then another boundary must be pushed aside so other patients can benefit.

Excellence requires taking the responsibility to do the best that can be done, all the time. Excellence should not be confused with an accumulation of knowledge, money, adulation, or volume of surgical cases. Good technical surgeons abound, but excellence does not deal only with the surgical act.

Excellence is the highest goal of human endeavor. Aristotle called excellence "all that is virtuous." This book is offered as a tribute to those in eye surgery who quest for excellence. Attempting to be the best is the essence of excellence because it elevates performance and instills personal pride.

Excellence is like a fire on a distant hill. From afar the light is a guide; up close the glow keeps you warm.

Lee T. Nordan
W. Andrew Maxwell
James A. Davison

FOREWORDS

Lee Nordan, Andy Maxwell, and Jim Davison are bright, innovative, and curious. From this triumvirate has emerged *The Surgical Rehabilitation of Vision: An Integrated Approach to Anterior Segment Surgery*.

Twenty-seven years ago, when the authors were in high school, I was introduced to ocular surgery as a first-year resident in ophthalmology. I'll never forget the movie I was shown—a fairly large scalpel made a 180-degree corneal groove incision just anterior to the limbus with three sutures of 6-0 black silk preplaced into the groove, looped out, and laid aside. The anterior chamber was entered by a scratch incision in the groove and the incision was enlarged to 180 degrees using scissors. A capsule forceps appeared, grasped the anterior lens capsule, and while a muscle hook gouged and mashed at the inferior aspect of the limbus, the forceps holding the lens was pulled upward and superiorly across the endothelium, creating a tumbling action of the cataract, thereby dragging the lens out of the eye (feet first, so to speak). "This is the way to remove cataracts," our lecturer said.

Why vitreous didn't follow the lens out of the eye, I've often wondered. Of course, if vitreous had presented, the prescribed procedure would have been a sector iridectomy, then suturing the wound closed, entrapping the vitreous. Everyone knew it was better to lose only a "bead" of vitreous than to further manipulate the vitreous body.

Later in the same decade (the 1960s), it was discovered that, at times, vitreous could and should be gently removed. A young man named Kelman began to work feverishly on a method to remove a cataract through a much smaller incision than had ever been imagined. Indeed, in 1968, Charlie Kelman presented twelve cases in which he had performed "phacoemulsification."

In the 1970s, Binkhorst's iridocapsular lens implants were seen to be weathering the test of time reasonably well. Fyodorov presented the techniques and results of radial keratotomy. Machamer presented automated vitrectomy and Wise presented laser trabeculoplasty. Shearing placed some old Danheim anterior chamber IOLs in the posterior chamber and off we sailed into the 1980s.

Radial keratotomy boomed and scores of IOL modifications were made with each new IOL renamed. A few ophthalmologists, as in every period of change and achievement, became known as "super surgeons," because they exhibited exceptional skills and judgment and had innovative ideas.

I first heard about Lee when I was asking around the ophthalmic industry seeking "the best guy to consult about the surgical correction of astigmatism." The name Nordan came up so frequently I decided to make the trip from Oklahoma City to La Jolla ... what a day! I was fortunate to find that Lee's sidekick and talented coworker, Andy Maxwell, was also visiting. Three corneal transplants, three keratomileuses, three or four phaco/IOL cases, and a dozen or so patients later, I was dazzled by the combination of surgical skill, knowledge, and compassion. In between all this activity, I was able to extract from Lee and Andy the information I needed to help complete a study on the surgical correction of astigmatism.

I have been performing phaco/IOL surgery since the early 1970s, when Charlie Kelman and a small group of "renegades" would meet around the country to observe surgery in an attempt to improve phacoemulsification and IOL implantation techniques. I appreciate that few surgeons, if any, have been as capable as Jim Davison in analyzing, performing, and writing about phacoemulsification and IOL design. Jim is able to recount his surgical experiences with the accuracy and honesty that befit a confident, concerned, masterful surgeon.

Believe me when I say that these fellows have a lot of information to share with you. They are on top of anterior segment advances and are directly responsible for some of these advances. But more importantly, Lee, Andy, and Jim strive for excellence as both physicians and surgeons. They are willing to make clear decisions about achieving surgical objectives, yet they continually seek better solutions, without regard to ego or preconceived ideas. Their job is to help the patient by performing the best surgery possible, and they are proud to present their concepts. The techniques described in this book present anterior segment surgery as an art form of the highest level.

I am proud to have Lee, Andy, and Jim as friends and colleagues. They are contributing to improvement and excellence by welcoming, rather than fearing, the accelerated rate of change and progress that confronts us all. It's nice to know that there are still a few wholesome, concerned renegades around. Without them, we might get too comfortable and actually believe that there's no better way to perform anterior segment surgery than the way it was learned when we were residents. I am honored that Lee, Andy, and Jim chose me to write a foreword for their book.

James H. Little

CHANGE IN OPHTHALMOLOGY: INTEGRATION AND INNOVATION

I found that the entrepreneurial spirit producing innovation is associated with a particular way of approaching problems that I call integrative: the willingness to move beyond received wisdom, to combine ideas from unconnected sources, to embrace change as an opportunity to test limits. To see problems integratively is to see them as wholes, related to larger wholes, and thus challenging established practices—rather than walling off a piece of experience and preventing it from being touched or affected by any new experiences.
Rosabeth Moss Kanter
The Change Masters

This book, *The Surgical Rehabilitation of Vision: An Integrated Approach to Anterior Segment Surgery*, has a unique perspective on the disparate components of anterior segment ophthalmic surgery. Rather than perpetuate the increasingly artificial boundaries that fragment the field, the authors are guided by an entrepreneurial spirit and a willingness to embrace change and combine techniques from many different schools of thought. These are the characteristics of a model surgeon; that is, one who integrates the best innovations for the patient's benefit. To achieve this requires an understanding of, and a commitment to, change.

Few areas of medicine, or of any other profession, have undergone as much change during the past two decades as ophthalmology. It is a challenge to comprehend the scope of this change, and it is even more difficult to explain the forces behind it. Why does change occur? What governs rate of change? *How* and *why* did we move so quickly?

Only two decades ago, the standard cataract surgery was intracapsular cataract extraction using a 14 mm to 15 mm arc incision. The patient generally remained aphakic and recovery of visual acuity and full mobility was slow and uncertain. In contrast, in-the-bag phacoemulsification with implantation of a foldable multifocal intraocular lens (IOL) through a 4.00-mm incision with transverse corneal incisions, used as necessary, to reduce preoperative astigmatism, results in complete visual recovery in less than one week. This example reflects the dramatic changes in the technology, surgical technique, and fundamental goals that have shaped anterior segment surgery during the last decades.

A widely held view is that change, even change of this magnitude and speed, occurs in a series of small, orderly steps. Each change in this supposedly smooth, continuous curve is based on refinements of previous work. This view is based on the premise that everyone is working toward a shared goal. In fact, change rarely occurs in this way. The forces that initiate, perpetuate, and resist change in ophthalmology are probably similar to those that affect other technological revolutions. The ophthalmic literature provides few insights into this area. To explain these events, three models from the fields of business and philosophy of science will be examined.

Model 1: The S-Curve
The literature of business offers us a rich source of material with which to better understand innovation and change within ophthalmology. In *Innovation: The Attackers Advantage*, Richard M. Foster maintains that competitive strength depends upon the recognition of new, promising technologies and knowing when to adopt them. "Whenever technological discontinuities occur, companies' [substitute "ophthalmologists" for "companies"] fortunes change dramatically. The leaders in the current technology rarely survive to become leaders in the new technology...even when top managers [ophthalmologists] understand what is necessary to stay ahead, only a handful have the conviction and discipline to act on that understanding." What an apt analogy for ophthalmologists. Many of today's most successful cataract practices are the direct outgrowth of their leaders' early transition to phacoemulsification, and later, posterior chamber IOLs. But how does one know when the next technological train will be leaving and avoid being left standing at the station once again?

Foster offers the model of the S-curve (Fig. 1), a graph of the relationship between the effort put into improving a product or process and the results one gets back for that investment. The S-curve illustrates the "infancy, explosion, and then gradual maturation of technological progress. Initially, as funds are put into developing a new product or process, progress is very slow. Then all hell breaks loose as the key knowledge necessary to make advances is put in place. Finally, as more dollars are put into development of a product or process, it becomes more and more difficult and expensive to make technical progress."

This second, flat portion of the S-curve represents the mature stages of technology during which growth is limited. Foster describes the downfall of dozens of businesses and technologies due to their preoccupation with perfecting mature technologies—the commercial sailing ship, the electromechanical typewriter, and bias ply tires are all excellent examples. It is more comfortable to persist in an area that has reached its innovative limit rather than move to a new technology (and a new curve). To shift from a mature technology to a new revolutionary one is termed "discontinuity." To stop doing what we do well and adopt an imperfect, new technique that we do poorly requires not only insight but a tremendous amount of courage. Nonetheless, this is the essence of healthy change.

The move from intracapsular cataract extraction to extracapsular cataract extraction was a tremendous leap forward. The discontinuity was great and effectively ended the careers of many ophthalmologists who were unable to change. At present, we are faced with another discontinuity, the move from extracapsular cataract extraction to phacoemulsification small incision surgery. It is valuable for the surgeon to place on a personal S-curve entities such as intracapsular cataract extraction, PMMA IOLs, multifocal IOLs, YAG laser posterior capsulotomy, excimer laser refractive surgery, and aphakic spectacles.

Most of us have an intellectual understanding of the technologies and techniques of cataract surgery that are moving steadily along the S-curve. The transition to the steep ascending part of the curve is occurring right now. Armed with this understanding, why do the majority of ophthalmologists cling to the flattening slope of the previous decades' S-curve (extracapsular cataract extraction with rigid PMMA IOL)? It seems unlikely that marked improvement in performance will be possible in either extracapsular cataract extraction technique or in the technology of rigid PMMA lenses.

It would be acceptable to acknowledge and take responsibility for our inability to change. Unfortunately, when faced with the challenge of change, this "opportunity" is more often interpreted as a threat. Feeling threatened, ophthalmologists have a history of devoting significant amounts of time and energy to attacking emerging technologies. An alternative is offered by the editor of *Harvard Business Review*, Alan M. Kantrow, who states that companies (ophthalmologists) must "face the rather unpalatable reality that there may have to be fundamental changes in who they are, what they do and how they do it, as wrenching and dislocating as it may be."

Our view of our own identity colors our response to change. Railroads dominated transportation of freight in the previous century. Had these industrial giants viewed themselves as being in the "transportation business" rather than in the "train business" they might have used their considerable resources to develop and dominate commercial trucking, their principle competitor today. Our view of ourselves as "extracapsular cataract surgeons" limits our ability to change. The extent to which we see our identity as *physicians committed to maximizing our patients' uncorrected visual acuity* allows us to integrate whatever new skills and technologies serve our needs.

Model 2: The Theory of Paradigms

Thomas S. Kuhn's *The Structure of Scientific Revolutions* was originally published in 1962. Kuhn proposed a model very much at odds with the pre-

Figure 1

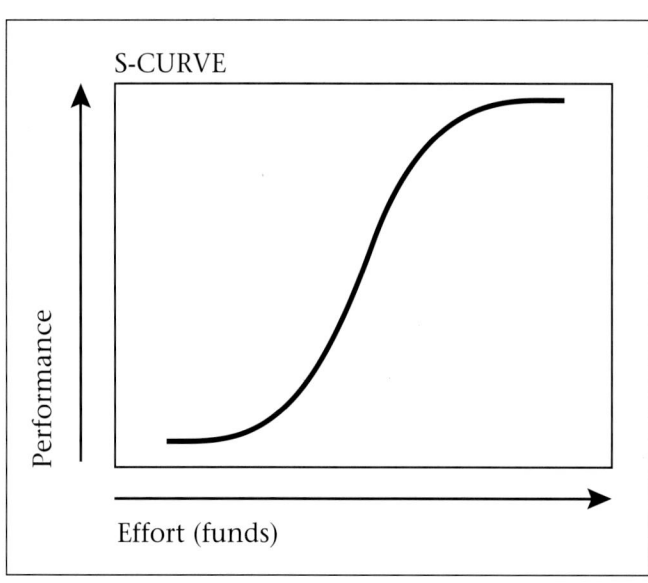

vailing view that science is a logical process towards common goals. He describes the birth, establishment, domination, and decline of a given set of scientific beliefs as a "paradigm" (examples of which include Copernican astronomy and Newtonian physics). This view of change was the genesis of Foster's S-curve. Anterior segment surgery has functioned under two dominant sets of beliefs or paradigms over the past decade and is currently in transition to a third paradigm. The first six decades of this century were shaped by our commitment to preventing blindness. The second paradigm emerged as a result of the development of the IOL. This fundamental change moved us from the prevention of blindness to the goal of maximum corrected visual acuity. This caused dramatic change in the indications for and timing of cataract surgery. The third and emerging paradigm is represented by the work of the authors of this book: a belief in the value of maximal uncorrected visual acuity.

Meeting the demand for maximal uncorrected visual acuity requires that we redefine the rules of the game. Kuhn notes that "As with many emerging paradigms, the majority question the very existence of a defect in the old school. Indeed, during the transition period, there will be a large but never complete overlap between the problems that can be solved by the old and by the new paradigm. But there will also be a decisive difference in the modes of solution. When the transition is complete, the profession will have changed its view of the field, its methods, its goals." The most fundamental change described in this text is not the change of technique or technology. It is the change on the part of a growing number of ophthalmologists in the way they view their identity and purpose. The common thread among those of us who endorse phacoemulsification, foldable and multifocal IOLs, and the many techniques of refractive surgery is the belief that patients' lives are significantly improved through our success in maximizing uncorrected visual acuity.

Note the ages of the authors of this text, most of whom made the leap to refractive surgery a decade ago. A final view by Kuhn is of interest. "Almost always the men who achieve these fundamental inventions of a new paradigm have been either very young or very new to the field whose paradigm they change. And perhaps that point need not have been made explicit, for obviously these are the men who, being little committed by prior practice to the traditional rules of normal science, are particularly likely to see that those rules no longer define a playable game and to conceive another set that can replace them."

Model 3: Competition, Change and the Defense of Vested Interest

The role of the authors as champions of the new S-curve or the new paradigm is certainly laudable. The third model introduces a cautionary note, however. In *Science As a Process*, David L. Hull points out that the young innovator and attacker of the status quo, if successful, defines the next status quo. Each component of the techniques and technologies discussed in this text has its own S-curve and rate of maturation. The young innovator, if successful, lives long enough to fight tooth and nail to crush the subsequent paradigm, which will threaten the authority snatched from his predecessors. If today's innovators follow the pattern of centuries of scientists, they will develop a vested interest in perpetuating their own paradigm (today's champions of change become tomorrow's tenured professors and acknowledged experts).

This description of ophthalmology suggests that bias, self interest, and conflict are fundamental to the process of change. Hull argues that science evolves precisely because of these forces, not because of a rational and orderly progression of discovery. Substitute ophthalmologists for scientists and ophthalmology for science in the following paragraph.

"After reading about the fighting and personal vendettas that have occupied so much of the time of the scientists I have studied, the reader is likely to conclude that these scientists are really not behaving in the way scientists should behave. To the contrary, I argue not only that these scientists are behaving in the way that all innovative scientists behave but also that this sort of behavior actually facilitates scientific development. One of the chief messages of the book is that factionalism, social cohesion, and professional interests need not frustrate the traditional goals of knowledge acquisition." This "survival of the fittest" preserves dominant paradigms until a hardy and fit successor emerges. The winnowing of new, weak challenges to the status quo is usually performed with ruthless efficiency by these ophthalmologists in power.

Reflect for a moment on the response of incumbent ophthalmic leaders to the threat of refractive surgery. Discontinuities between S-curves and shifts between paradigms are usually accompanied by intense fighting on both sides. Hull notes "Although objective knowledge through bias and commitment sounds as paradoxical as bombs for peace, I agree that the existence and ultimate rationality of science can be explained in terms of bias, jealousy, and irrationality. As it turns out, the least productive scientists tend to behave the most admirably, while those who make the greatest contributions just as frequently behave the most deplorably."

Summary
I have sought to describe the dynamics of change within ophthalmology, using three major business and philosophy of science works. Foster has given us the S-curve in order to illustrate change within ophthalmology; both anterior segment surgical techniques and technologies can be analyzed according to this model. Kuhn uses the paradigm to help us define ourselves and our profession; as our traditional rules and beliefs fail to meet our changing needs, it may help to recognize that our discipline is in a state of flux, moving from old paradigm to new. As we observe, and perhaps participate in, the battle between the old and new, Hull assures us that our actions, although not always honorable, are the part of the very essence of change. Change is a battle, a contest, and those that fight hardest and longest generally win. He also points out that those of us fighting hardest for change today will in turn fight hardest to protect the status quo that we create.

The editors of *The Surgical Rehabilitation of Vision: An Integrated Approach to Anterior Segment Surgery* are to be commended for several reasons. They have collected and presented a group of advanced surgical techniques while emphasizing that the basic skills of anterior segment surgery, including knowledge of needles, sutures, instruments, and machines, are a necessary foundation for achieving excellent surgical results. Perhaps, more importantly, the editors are unabashedly willing to present the concept that an eye surgeon should strive to provide a patient with the *best uncorrected vision possible*, understanding the limitations imposed by specific medical problems and appropriate consideration of the risk/benefit ratio.

The application of ophthalmic surgical techniques should, and must, be a dynamic process. The surgeon needs to successfully integrate ideas that may have been learned in training or only recently. Some ocular surgical techniques have changed little in the past century, while others are emerging. Most importantly, the truly accomplished eye surgeon must have a desire and an ability to constantly consider new ideas and techniques and to then be committed to employ those, old or new, that offer the best chance of success for a patient.

This remarkable text shows us that anterior segment ophthalmic surgery is full of excitement, opportunity and change. Our ability to understand and manage this change affects our individual level of anxiety, anger, fulfillment, economic prosperity, and, most importantly, our patients' vision.

R. Bruce Grene

TABLE OF CONTENTS

Chapter 1 The Philosophy of Eye Surgery   1.1
*Lee T. Nordan, M.D. W. Andrew Maxwell, M.D., Ph.D.
James A. Davison, M.D.*
The Art of Anterior Segment Surgery   1.1
The Best Unaided Vision   1.3
The Goal: Excellence   1.3

SECTION I: RECENT DEVELOPMENTS
Chapter 2 New Optics for the Eye Surgeon   2.1
Lee T. Nordan, M.D.
Optical Mechanics   2.1
Clinical Experience   2.4
Topography   2.9
Additional Clinical Considerations   2.17
    Visual Function Index/Surgical Efficacy Index   2.17
Conclusion   2.20

Chapter 3 Viscoelastics   3.1
D.A. Benedetto, M.D.
Principles and Concepts   3.2
Space Maintenance   3.4
    Intraocular Pressure   3.4
    Aspiration   3.4
    Ease of Injection and Tissue Manipulation   3.4
    Shock Absorption   3.5
    Surface Coating   3.5

Chapter 4 Computers and Ophthalmic Surgery   4.1
Jeffrey Hightower
Computer-Designed Cataract and Refractive Surgery   4.2
    Cataract/IOL Module   4.2
    Refractive Surgery Module   4.4
    Evaluation Module   4.4
Conclusion   4.4

Chapter 5 Ocular Surgery Anesthesiology   5.1
Edward Kane, M.D.
Preoperative Considerations   5.1
    NPO Policy   5.1
    Topical Medications   5.1
    Intravenous Line   5.2
    Analgesia/Sedation/Amnesia   5.2
    Ocular Pressure Device   5.5
    Blood Pressure   5.5
Intraoperative Considerations   5.5
    Patient Position and Draping   5.5
    Blood Pressure Cuff   5.6
    Sedation/Coughing   5.6
Postoperative Considerations   5.7
Conclusion   5.7

SECTION II: ANTERIOR SEGMENT INSTRUMENTATION
Chapter 6 Instruments for Anterior Segment Surgery   6.1
Michelle Glossip Lee T. Nordan, M.D.
Materials   6.2
Design   6.2
    Handle   6.2
    Working End   6.3
    Instruments   6.4
Conclusion   6.10

Chapter 7 Needles and Sutures   7.1
David W. Poley Peter A. Hatton
Needles   7.1
    Early Needles   7.1
    Anatomy   7.2
    Ethicon Needles   7.4
    Curvature, Radius, and Chord Length   7.5
    Lens Fixation and Iris Repair   7.8
    Alcon Needles   7.9
    Point Configurations   7.11
    Body Curvature   7.13
Ophthalmic Suture Materials   7.14
    Nonabsorbable Sutures   7.14
    Absorbable Sutures   7.16
Conclusion   7.17

SECTION III: SURGERY OF THE LENS
Chapter 8 Intraocular Lens Design   8.1
*Charles D. Fritch, M.D. Mathias Zirm, M.D.
David Dillman, M.D. Philippe Crozafon, M.D.
Lee T. Nordan, M.D.*
Posterior Chamber Intraocular Lenses   8.1
    Optic Size   8.1
    Haptic Material   8.3
    Haptic Design   8.5
Anterior Capsulotomy   8.7
Posterior Chamber Intraocular Lens
    Design Factors   8.7
Clinically Optimal Posterior Chamber
    Intraocular Lens Design   8.8
    Design Requirements   8.12
Trans-scleral Fixation of Posterior Chamber
    Intraocular Lenses   8.13
Anterior Chamber Intraocular Lenses   8.13
    Secondary Implantation of Anterior Chamber
    Intraocular Lenses   8.13
Multifocal Intraocular Lenses   8.13
    Mechanism of Action   8.14
Contrast   8.15
    Contrast Sensitivity   8.17
    Glare   8.17
    Modulation Transfer Function   8.18
    Profiling of Patients   8.20
Multifocal Intraocular Lens Styles   8.20
    Bulls-Eye   8.20
    Diffractive   8.20
    Aspheric   8.23
Conclusion   8.27

Chapter 9 Capsulorhexis, PC IOL Centration, and Trans-scleral PC IOL Fixation	**9.1**

David Apple, M.D. James A. Davison, M.D.
Lee T. Nordan, M.D.
W. Andrew Maxwell, M.D., Ph.D.

Capsulorhexis	9.1
Anatomy of the Lens and Zonules	9.2
Capsulotomy Methods	9.2
Can-Opener Capsulotomy	9.4
Continuous Circular Capsulorhexis	9.4
Anterior Capsular Radial Tears	9.5
Anterior Capsulotomy Considerations	9.6
PC IOL Centration	9.6
CCC Conclusion	9.7
Trans-scleral Fixation of Posterior Chamber Intraocular Lenses	9.8
Methods	9.8
Conclusion	9.11

Chapter 10 Extracapsular Cataract Extraction	**10.1**

Michael Blumenthal, M.D. Ehud I. Assia, M.D.

Surgical Anatomy	10.1
Anterior Chamber	10.1
Lens Capsule	10.2
Crystalline Lens Nucleus	10.4
Surgical Procedure	10.6
Maintaining the Anterior Chamber	10.6
Anterior Capsulectomy	10.7
Hydrodissection of the Nucleus	10.7
Hydroexpression of the Nucleus to the Anterior Chamber	10.7
Hydroexpression (Hydroextraction) of the Nucleus	10.8
Removal of the Epinucleus	10.9
Removal of Cortical Material and Implantation of Intraocular Lens	10.10
Conclusion	10.10

Chapter 11 The Mechanics of Phacoemulsification	**11.1**

R. Bruce Wallace, M.D. Lee T. Nordan, M.D.
Donald Fagen B.J. Barwick

Fluidics	11.2
Irrigation	11.2
Aspiration	11.4
Pumps	11.7
Peristaltic	11.7
Vacuum	11.9
Ultrasonic Handpiece	11.10
Phaco Power	11.11
Foot Pedal Function	11.11
Phacoemulsification Tip Design	11.12
Automated Anterior Vitrectomy	11.13
Desires and Reality: A Personal Perspective	11.13
Phacoemulsification Pumps	11.13
Power and Aspiration	11.14
The Future	11.16

Chapter 12 The Phacoemulsification Procedure	**12.1**

Lee T. Nordan, M.D.
W. Andrew Maxwell, M.D., Ph.D.

Outline of Phacoemulsification	12.2
Preoperative Preparation	12.2
Operating Room Setup	12.2
Patient Preparation	12.5
Surgical Procedure	12.6
Wound and Capsulotomy	12.6
Cataract Removal	12.6
Intraocular Lens Implantation	12.12
Wound Closure	12.12
Postoperative Regimen	12.13

Chapter 13 Cataract Removal by Phacoemulsification	**13.1**

James A. Davison, M.D.

In Situ Phacoemulsification	13.7
Capsular Bag Phacoemulsification	13.7
Intercapsular Phacoemulsification	13.8
Anatomic Considerations	13.8
Principles of Phacoemulsification	13.10
Phacoemulsification Surgical Procedure	13.11
Setup for Phacoemulsification	13.11
Wound Construction	13.15
Anterior Capsulotomy	13.18
Hydrodissection	13.24
Nucleus Strategy	13.24
Initial Phacoemulsification Steps	13.26
Capsular Bag Phacoemulsification: Strategy Selection	13.28
Selected Surgical Strategies	13.31
Aspiration of Cortex	13.40
Intraocular Lens Implantation	13.43
Wound Closure	13.44
Conclusion	13.46

Chapter 14 Small Pupil Phacoemulsification Techniques	**14.1**

I. Howard Fine, M.D. Samuel Masket, M.D.

Pupilloplasty Technique to Improve Cosmesis and Preserve Function After Cataract Surgery	14.1
Surgical Procedure	14.1
Clinical Results	14.3
Conclusion	14.4
Preplaced Iris Suture Technique for Small Pupil Management in Phaco and Fracture Endolenticular Phacoemulsification	14.4
Maintaining a Functional Pupil	14.4
Surgical Procedure	14.7
Conclusion	14.10

Chapter 15 Small Incision Intraocular Lens Implantation	**15.1**

Stephen F. Brint, M.D.

Surgical Procedure	15.3
Three-Piece Silicone Lens Implants	15.4
One-Piece Implants	15.10
Closure	15.12
Complications	15.14
Future Developments	15.14

Chapter 16 Comparison of Cataract
            Wound Sizes   16.1
Paul S. Koch, M.D.
The Scleral Flap Incision   16.1
   Depth   16.2
   Width   16.2
   Length   16.3
Vertical Corneal Instability   16.4
Conclusion   16.6

Chapter 17 Anterior Vitrectomy   17.1
Paul S. Koch, M.D.
Characteristics of the Vitreous   17.1
   The Vitreous in Phacoemulsification 17.2
Vitrectomy Principles   17.3
Bimanual Vitrectomy   17.4
   Cortical Aspiration   17.5
Results   17.6
Conclusion   17.6

SECTION IV: INNOVATIVE CATARACT SURGERY

Chapter 18 Chip-and-Flip Phacoemulsification   18.1
I. Howard Fine, M.D.
Surgical Procedure   18.1
Conclusion   18.8

Chapter 19 Radial-Transverse Cataract Incision 19.1
Steven B. Siepser, M.D.
The History of Cataract Surgery   19.1
Surgical Procedure   19.3
Clinical Considerations   19.4
Conclusion   19.5

Chapter 20 The Infinity Suture   20.1
I. Howard Fine, M.D.
Surgical Procedure   20.1
Conclusion   20.3

Chapter 21 Lensectomy with IOL Implantation
            and Phakic Hypernegative IOLs
            for the Correction of High Myopia   21.1
W. Andrew Maxwell, M.D., Ph.D.
Lensectomy and Intraocular Lens Implantation   21.2
   Preoperative Evaluation   21.2
   Surgical Procedure   21.2
   Results   21.3
Hypernegative Intraocular Lens Implants   21.4
   Lens Design   21.4
   Preoperative Evaluation   21.4
   Surgical Procedure   21.4
   Results   21.5
   Complications   21.5
   Conclusion   21.6
Summary   21.6

SECTION V: SURGERY OF THE CORNEA

Chapter 22 Radial Keratotomy   22.1
Fredric B. Kremer, M.D.
Mechanism of Action   22.1
   Optical Zone Size   22.3
   Incision Number   22.3
   Depth   22.4
   Bias   22.4
Preoperative Evaluation   22.4
Surgical Preparation   22.5
Anesthesia   22.7
Surgical Procedure   22.7
   Blade Preparation   22.9
   Incision Placement   22.9
Postoperative Management   22.10
Conclusion   22.11

Chapter 23 Astigmatism: Concepts
            and Surgical Approach   23.1
Lee T. Nordan, M.D. John D. Hofbauer, M.D.
Concepts and Principles   23.1
   Regular Astigmatism   23.1
   Irregular Astigmatism   23.7
Diagnosis   23.9
Correction   23.13
   Astigmatic Keratotomy   23.13
Surgical Strategy for Astigmatism Correction   23.18
   Congenital Astigmatism   23.18
Astigmatic Correction and Prevention During
   Cataract/IOL Surgery   23.23
   Against-the-Rule Astigmatism 23.24
Correction of Postcataract Extraction Astigmatism 23.27
   Aphakia   23.27
   Pseudophakia   23.29
Astigmatism Correction Following Penetrating
   or Lamellar Keratoplasty   23.29
   Penetrating Keratoplasty Astigmatism Strategy 23.30
Reoperation After Astigmatic Keratotomy   23.30
Conclusion   23.30

Chapter 24 Penetrating Keratoplasty   24.1
Roger F. Steinert, M.D.
Diagnosis and Evaluation   24.1
   Diagnostic Procedures   24.3
Preoperative Preparation   24.4
Surgical Procedure   24.4
   Trephining the Patient's Cornea 24.7
   Extracapsular Cataract Extraction and
      Intraocular Lens Implantation 24.9
   Intraocular Lens Removal   24.10
   Anterior Vitrectomy   24.10
   Anterior Segment Reconstruction 24.10
   Suturing the Transplant   24.10
Postoperative Regimen   24.13
Visual Rehabilitation   24.13
Complications   24.14
   Surface Disease   24.14
   Glaucoma   24.14
   Recurrent Disease   24.14
   Rejection   24.15
Conclusion   24.15

Chapter 25 Lamellar Keratoplasty	**25.1**
Roger F. Steinert, M.D. Lee T. Nordan, M.D.	
Overview	25.1
Indications for Lamellar Keratoplasty	25.2
Potential Problems	25.2
Surgical Procedure	25.2
Preparation	25.2
Recipient Lamellar Dissection	25.2
Lamellar Donor Preparation	25.6
Suturing	25.8
Postoperative Care	25.9
Tectonic Lamellar Keratoplasty	25.10
Surgical Procedure	25.10
The Donor Graft	25.10
Securing the Graft	25.10
Other Forms of Lamellar Keratoplasty	25.11
Intrastromal Alloplastic Implantation	25.11
Lamellar Keratoplasty for Hyperopia	25.13
Oblique Peripheral Keratotomy	25.14
Conclusion	25.14
Chapter 26 Laser Corneal Surgery	**26.1**
Roger F. Steinert, M.D.	
Laser Basics	26.1
Excimer Laser	26.2
Nd:YAG and Nd:YLF Laser	26.2
Excimer Laser Refractive Surgery	26.3
Delivery Systems	26.4
Procedure	26.4
Results	26.5
Complications	26.6
Directions for Future Development	26.6
The Picosecond Nd:YLF Laser	26.7
Conclusion	26.7
Chapter 27 Keratomileusis	**27.1**
Francis W. Price, M.D.	
Preoperative Considerations	27.1
Surgical Procedure	27.3
Non-Freeze Keratomileusis	27.8
New Developments	27.9
Complications	27.9
Conclusion	27.11
Chapter 28 Epikeratoplasty: Patient Selection and Surgical Technique	**28.1**
Daniel S. Durrie, M.D. Vance Thompson, M.D.	
Concepts	28.2
Aphakic Epikeratoplasty	28.5
Patient Selection	28.5
Surgical Procedure	28.5
Epikeratoplasty for Keratoconus	28.7
Patient Selection	28.7
Surgical Procedure	28.8
Visual Results	28.8
Potential Advances	28.10
Epikeratoplasty for High Myopia	28.10
Patient Selection	28.10
Surgical Procedures	28.10
Clinical Results	28.12
Present Status and Availability	28.14
Moderate Hyperopia Epikeratoplasty	28.14
Plano Epikeratoplasty	28.15
Conclusion	28.15

SECTION VI: SURGERY FOR GLAUCOMA

Chapter 29 Trabeculectomy	**29.1**
C. Eric Shrader, M.D.	
History of Filtering Surgery	29.2
Preoperative Considerations	29.2
Surgical Procedure	29.3
Preliminary Steps	29.3
Conjunctival Flap	29.3
Scleral Flap	29.5
Sclerectomy	29.5
Flap Closure	29.6
Postoperative Care	29.8
Laser Suture Lysis	29.8
Cataract and Glaucoma	29.9
Additional Treatment Possibilities	29.9
Argon Laser Trabeculoplasty	29.9
Laser Filtering Surgery	29.10
Wound Healing Inhibition	29.10
Shunts	29.11
Conclusion	29.12

SECTION VII: SURGERY FOR PTERYGIUM

Chapter 30 Pterygium Excision	**30.1**
Lee T. Nordan, M.D.	
Pathophysiology	30.1
Clinical Significance	30.2
Differential Diagnosis	30.2
Surgical Planning	30.2
Surgical Procedure	30.3
Excision of Primary Pterygium	30.3
Excision of Recurrent Pterygium	30.4
Conclusion	30.7

SECTION VIII: SURGERY OF THE LIDS

Chapter 31 Acquired Ptosis	**31.1**
Norman Shorr, M.D. Marc S. Cohen, M.D.	
Anatomy	31.1
Evaluation of the Acquired Ptosis Patient	31.2
Ptosis Following Cataract Extraction	31.2
Surgical Procedure	31.2
Müller's Muscle—Conjunctival Resection (Müllerectomy)	31.3
Fasanella-Servat Procedure (Tarsoconjunctival Müllerectomy)	31.6
Levator Resection (Anterior Approach)	31.9
Postoperative Care	31.12

CONTRIBUTORS

KEY

Training

P/U % = Private/university
R = Ophthalmology residency
F = Ophthalmology fellowship

Surgical Profile

RK = Radial/astigmatic keratotomy
LKP = Lamellar keratoplasty
K = Keratomileusis
Ex = Excimer laser photorefractive keratoplasty
LP = Lid plastic surgery

C = Cataract/IOL
PKP = Penetrating keratoplasty
T = Trabeculectomy
Epi = Epikeratophakia
P = Pterygium

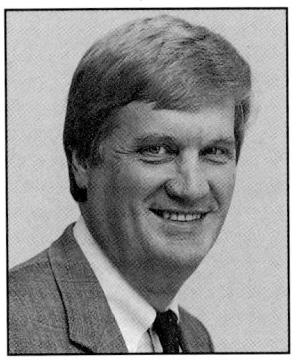

David J. Apple, M.D.
R = University of Iowa, Iowa City, 1977–80
F = Pathology, Armed Forces Institute of Pathology, Bethesda MD, 1969–70

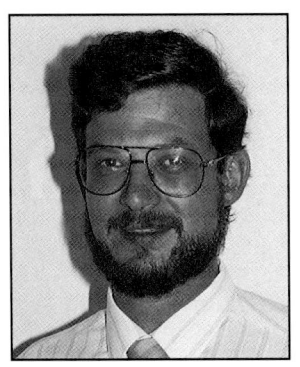

Ehud I. Assia, M.D.
R = Goldschleger Eye Institute, Sheba Medical Center, Tel-Hashomer Israel, 1988-90
F = Cataract/IOL, Center for Intraocular Lens Research, Storm Eye Institute, Medical University of South Carolina, Charleston, 1990-91
P/U = 0/100%
RK = 00%   C = 100%
LKP = 00%   PKP = 00%
K = 00%   T = 00%
Ex = 00%   Epi = 00%
LP = 00%   P = 00%

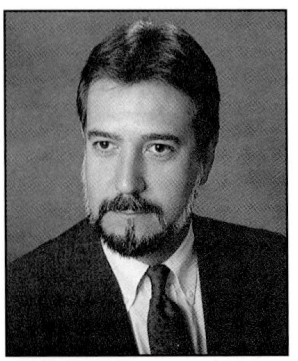

B.J. Barwick, Jr.
Optical Micro Systems Inc, President
Peabody MA

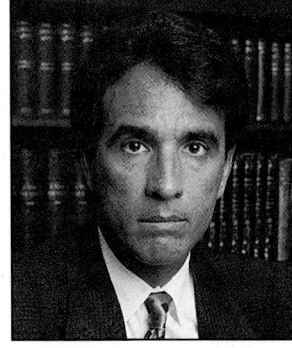

D.A. Benedetto, M.D.
R = Wills Eye Hospital, Philadelphia PA, 1978–1981
P/U = 85%/15%
RK = 00%   C = 98%
LKP = 00%   PKP = 01%
K = 00%   T = 01%
Ex = 00%   Epi = 00%
LP = 00%   P = 00%

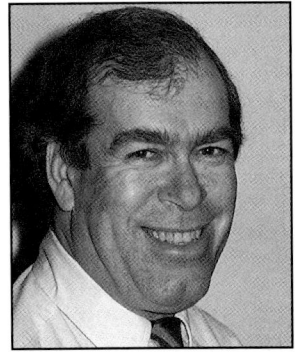

Michael Blumenthal, M.D.
R = Hadassah Hospital Medical School, Jerusalem Israel, 1962–64
F = Glaucoma, New York Medical College, New York NY, 1968–70
P/U = 100%/0%
RK = 05%   C = 85%
LKP = 00%   PKP = 05%
K = 00%   T = 05%
Ex = 00%   Epi = 00%
LP = 00%   P = 00%

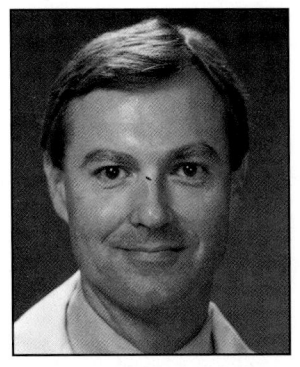

Stephen F. Brint, M.D.
R = Tulane University School of Medicine, New Orleans LA, 1974–1977
P/U = 95%/05%
RK = 20%   C = 75%
LKP = 00%   PKP = 02%
K = 00%   T = 02%
Ex = 01%   Epi = 00%
LP = 00%   P = 00%

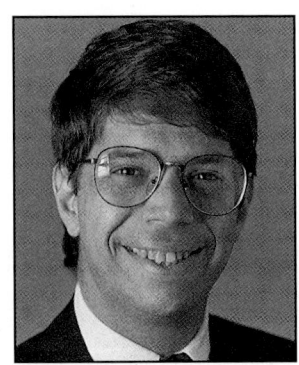

Marc S. Cohen, M.D.
R = Wills Eye Hospital, Philadelphia PA, 1985–88
F = Neuro-Ophthalmology, Wills Eye Hospital, 1988
F = Ophthalmic Plastics, Jules Stein Eye Institute, UCLA, Los Angeles CA, 1989–90
P/U = 50%/50%
RK = 00%   C = 00%
LKP = 00%   PKP = 00%
K = 00%   T = 00%
Ex = 00%   Epi = 00%
LP = 100%   P = 00%

Philippe Crozafon, M.D.
R = University of Grenoble, Grenoble France, 1976–77
P/U = 100%/0%
RK = 00%   C = 90%
LKP = 00%   PKP = 05%
K = 00%   T = 05%
Ex = 00%   Epi = 00%
LP = 00%   P = 00%

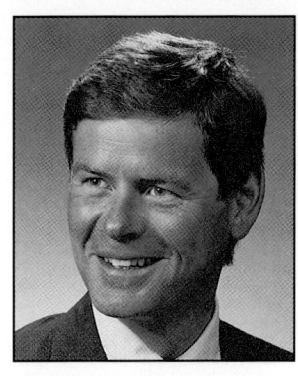

James A. Davison, M.D.
R = Mayo Graduate School of Medicine, Rochester MN, 1980
P/U = 100%/0%
RK = 05%   C = 60%
LKP = 00%   PKP = 00%
K = 00%   T = 05%
Ex = 00%   Epi = 00%
LP = 05%   P = 00%
Retina/Vitreous = 25%

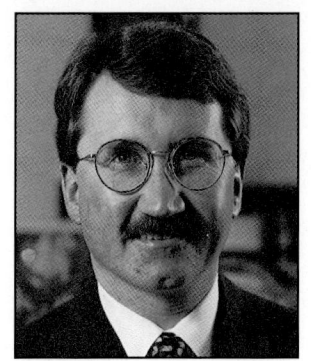

David M. Dillman, M.D.
R = Mayo Clinic, Rochester MN, 1980
P/U = 100%/0%
RK = 01%   C = 96%
LKP = 00%   PKP = 01%
K = 00%   T = 01%
Ex = 00%   Epi = 00%
LP = 00%   P = 01%

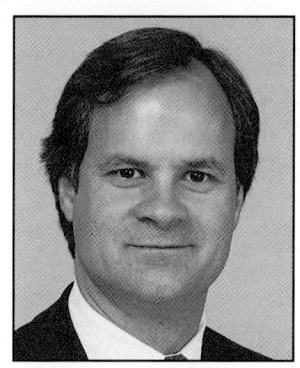

Daniel S. Durrie, M.D.
R = University of Nebraska Medical Center, Omaha, 1975–78
P/U = 90%/10%
RK = 60%   C = 00%
LKP = 00%   PKP = 30%
K = 00%   T = 00%
Ex = 02%   Epi = 05%
LP = 00%   P = 03%

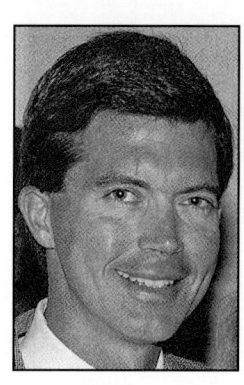

Donald Fagen
Southwest Texas State University, 1976
Alcon Surgical Inc
National Sales Director, Surgical Instruments

Kim Cooper MD
Stanford University
Dept. of Ophthalmology
Palo Alto, CA

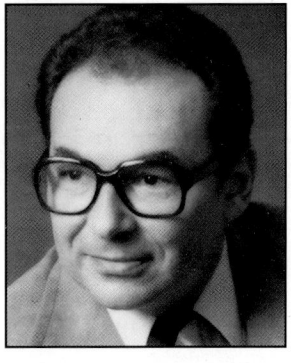

I. Howard Fine, M.D.
R = Boston University Medical Center, Boston MA, 1967–70
P/U = 100%/0%
RK = 01%   C = 95%
LKP = 00%   PKP = 03%
K = 00%   T = 01%
Ex = 00%   Epi = 00%
LP = 00%   P = 00%

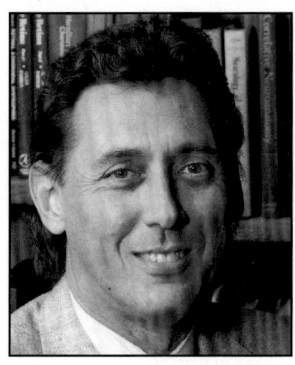

Charles D. Fritch, M.D.
R = UCLA, Los Angeles CA, 1974
P/U = 95%/5%
RK = 00%   C = 70%
LKP = 00%   PKP = 00%
K = 00%   T = 05%
Ex = 00%   Epi = 00%
LP = 00%   P = 00%
Retina/Vitreous = 20%

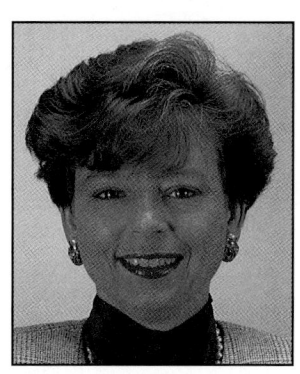

Michelle Glossip
Webster University, St. Louis MO, 1985
Storz Ophthalmics Inc
Senior Product Manager

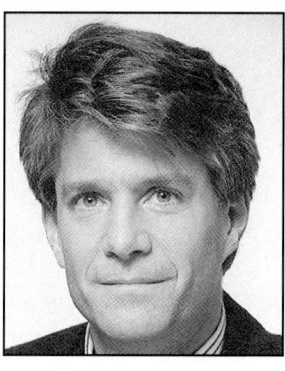

R. Bruce Grene, M.D.
R = University of Kansas, 1980–83
F = Cornea and External Disease, Massachusetts Eye and Ear Infirmary, Boston MA, 1983–84
P/U = 100%/0%
RK = 50%   C = 35%
LKP = 01%   PKP = 10%
K = 00%   T = 00%
Ex = 00%   Epi = 02%
LP = 00%   P = 02%

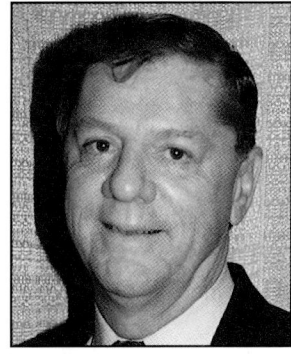

Peter Hatton
Northern Illinois University, Dekalb, 1971
Alcon Surgical Inc
Group Product Director

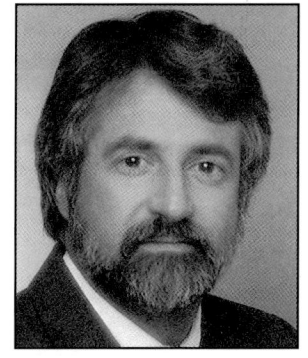

Jeffrey Hightower
University of Texas, Austin, 1969
Jeffrey Hightower Associates Inc
President

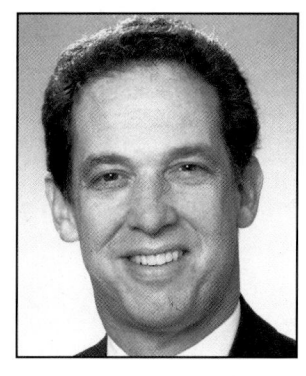

John D. Hofbauer, M.D.
R = Albert Einstein College of Medicine, New York NY, 1976–79
F = Cornea and External Diseases, Jules Stein Eye Institute, UCLA, Los Angeles CA, 1979–80
P/U = 95%/5%
RK = 05%   C = 60%
LKP = 02%   PKP = 20%
K = 00%   T = 00%
Ex = 00%   Epi = 00%
LP = 00%   P = 03%

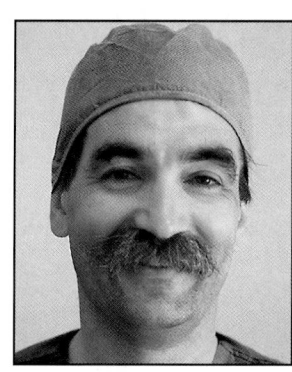

Edward Kane, M.D.
R = Anesthesiology, U.S. Naval Hospital, San Diego CA, 1970–73
P/U = 100%/0

XVII

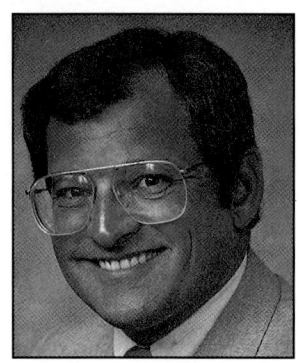

Paul S. Koch, M.D.
R = Manhattan Eye, Ear and Throat Hospital, New York NY, 1977–81
P/U = 100%/0
RK = 03%   C = 91%
LKP = 00%   PKP = 03%
K = 00%   T = 03%
Ex = 00%   Epi = 00%
LP = 00%   P = 00%

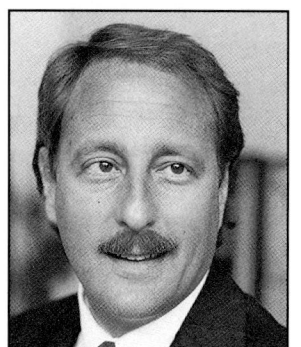

Fredric B. Kremer, M.D.
R = Wills Eye Hospital, Philadelphia PA, 1977–80
P/U = 95%/5%
RK = 40%   C = 40%
LKP = 02%   PKP = 03%
K = 05%   T = 03%
Ex = 00%   Epi = 01%
LP = 06%   P = 01%

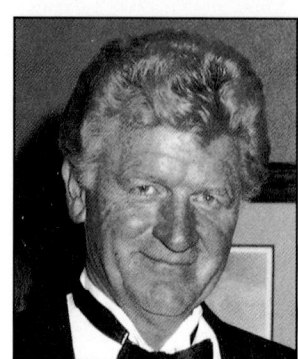

James H. Little, M.D.
R = Oklahoma University, 1963–66
P/U = 100%/0%
RK =00%   C = 95%
LKP = 00%   PKP = 00%
K = 00%   T = 05%
Ex = 00%   Epi = 00%
LP = 00%   P = 00%

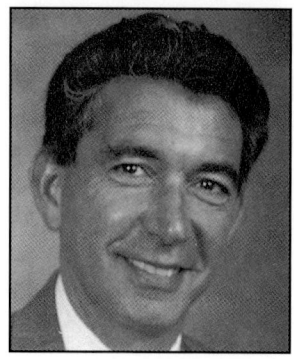

Samuel Masket, M.D.
R = New York Medical College, Valhalla NY, 1969–73
F = Strabismus, Harkness Eye Institute, Columbia University, New York NY, 1972–73
P/U = 90%10%
RK = 25%   C = 60%
LKP = 00%   PKP = 05%
K = 00%   T = 05%
Ex = 00%   Epi = 00%
LP = 00%   P = 05%

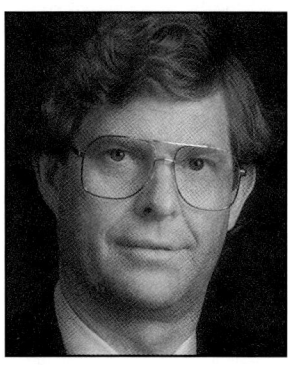

W. Andrew Maxwell, M.D., Ph.D.
R = Jules Stein Eye Institute, UCLA, Los Angeles CA, 1977–80
P/U = 100%/0
RK = 10%   C = 70%
LKP = 01%   PKP = 10%
K = 02%   T = 03%
Ex = 00%   Epi = 00%
LP = 03%   P = 01%

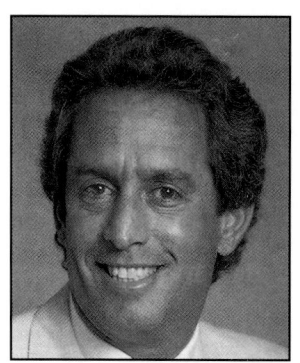

Lee T. Nordan, M.D.
R = West Virginia University Hospital, Morgantown, 1974–77
F = Cornea and External Disease, Jules Stein Eye Institute, UCLA, Los Angeles CA, 1977–78
P/U = 95%/5%
RK = 30%   C = 40%
LKP = 04%   PKP = 14%
K = 03%   T = 03%
Ex = 00%   Epi = 03%
LP = 00%   P = 03%

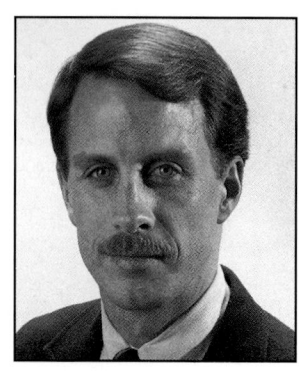

David Poley
Oregon State University, Corvallis, 1978
Ethicon Inc
Product Director, Ophthalmology

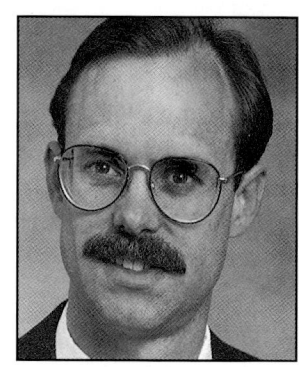

Francis W. Price, Jr., M.D.
R = Indiana University School of Medicine, Indianapolis, 1978–81
F = Cornea and External Disease, Tulane University, New Orleans LA, 1981–82
P/U = 100%/0%
RK = 05%   C = 04%
LKP = 02%   PKP = 50%
K = 01%   T = 15%
Ex = 00%   Epi = 01%
LP = 00%   P = 01%
IOL Exchange = 21%

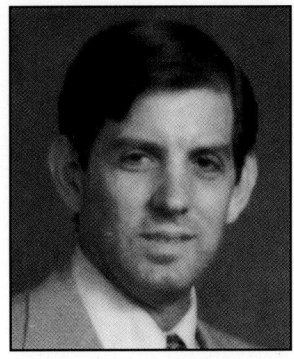

Norman Shorr, M.D.
R = Jules Stein Eye Institute, UCLA, Los Angeles CA, 1972–75
F = Ophthalmic Plastic and Reconstruction, Jules Stein Eye Institute, 1975–76
P/U = 90%/10%
RK = 00%   C = 00%
LKP = 00%   PKP = 00%
K = 00%   T = 00%
Ex = 00%   Epi = 00%
LP = 50%   P = 00%
Lacrimal = 25%   Orbit = 25%

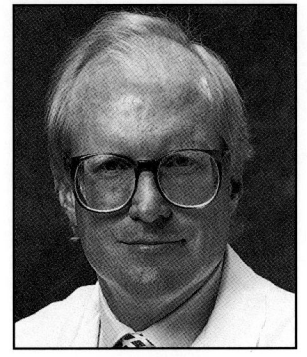

C. Eric Shrader, M.D.
R = University of Missouri, Kansas City, 1979–82
F = Glaucoma, Massachusetts Eye and Ear Infirmary, Boston MA, 1982–83
P/U = 100%/0%
RK = 00%   C = 66%
LKP = 00%   PKP = 00%
K = 00%   T = 34%
Ex = 00%   Epi = 00%
LP = 00%   P = 00%

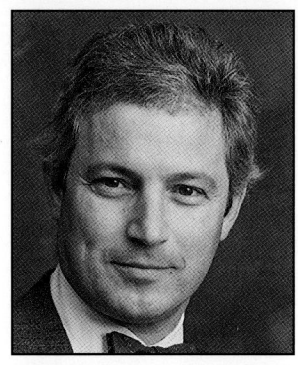

Steven B. Siepser, M.D.
R = Temple University, Philadelphia PA, 1976–79
P/U = 80/20%
RK = 01%   C = 80%
LKP = 00%   PKP = 02%
K = 00%   T = 10%
Ex = 00%   Epi = 00%
LP = 05%   P = 00%

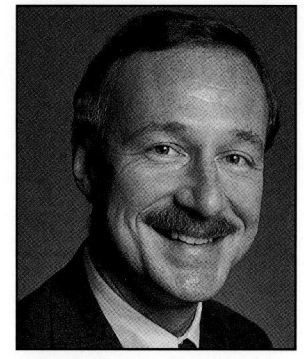

Roger F. Steinert, M.D.
R = Massachusetts Eye and Ear Infirmary, Boston MA, 1978–81
P/U = 0%/100%
RK = 01%   C = 50%
LKP = 05%   PKP = 40%
K = 00%   T = 00%
Ex = 02%   Epi = 01%
LP = 00%   P = 01%

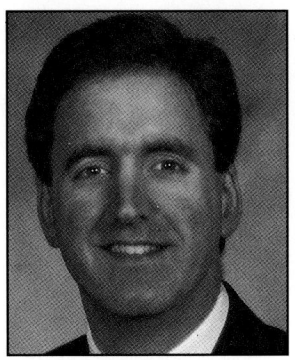

Vance Thompson, M.D.
R = University of Missouri, Columbia, 1987–90
P/U = 0%/100%
RK = 15%   C = 15%
LKP = 05%   PKP = 30%
K = 01%   T = 10%
Ex = 05%   Epi = 10%
LP = 09%   P = 00%

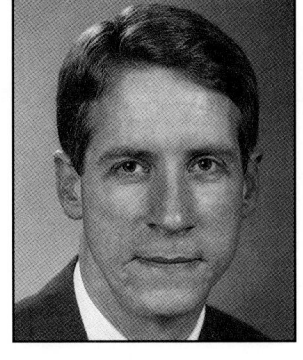

R. Bruce Wallace III, M.D.
R = Tulane Department of Ophthalmology, New Orleans LA, 1975–78
P/U = 95%/5%
RK = 03%   C = 95%
LKP = 00%   PKP = 01%
K = 00%   T = 00%
Ex = 00%   Epi = 00%
LP = 00%   P = 01%

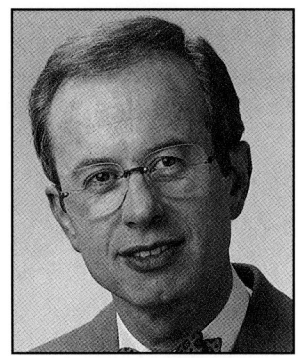

Mathias Zirm, M.D.
R = University Eye Clinic, Graz Austria, 1972–77
P/U = 50%/50%
RK = 00%   C = 90%
LKP = 00%   PKP = 03%
K = 00%   T = 03%
Ex = 00%   Epi = 01%
LP = 03%   P = 00%

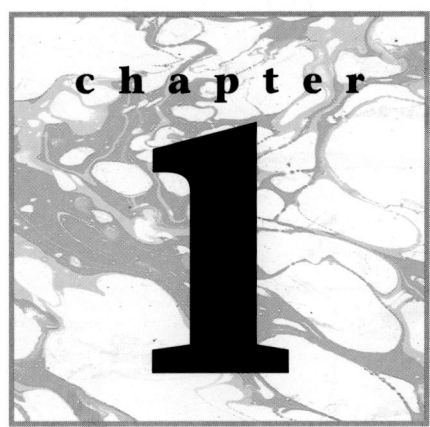

THE PHILOSOPHY OF EYE SURGERY

LEE T. NORDAN, M.D.   W. ANDREW MAXWELL, M.D., Ph.D.
JAMES A. DAVISON, M.D.

Creating a textbook such as *The Surgical Rehabilitation of Vision* demands that the editors and authors have a vision of the needs they hope it will fulfill. The goals of this project are:

• To provide the understanding and techniques necessary to perform state-of-the-art anterior segment surgery
• To present surgical techniques that allow the patient to achieve the *best possible appropriate uncorrected visual acuity*
• To integrate medical technology and surgical skills as they relate to anterior segment surgery into one reference work
• To instill the courage to strive for surgical excellence and to reinforce pride in surgical ability

The Art of Anterior Segment Surgery

In recent years, it has become apparent that a combination of disciplines is often mandatory when trying to achieve the best results in cataract/intraocular lens (IOL), corneal, and refractive surgery. For example: residual astigmatism is probably the most common limiting factor to good uncorrected vision after cataract surgery and IOL implantation. Can an ophthalmic surgeon be an excellent cataract surgeon without a working knowledge of astigmatic correction techniques, which have a foundation in refractive surgery? We think not. Astigmatic keratotomy should no longer be considered refractive surgery, rather part and parcel of sophisticated cataract/IOL surgery. The superb surgeon must master and be able to employ all techniques germane to the portion of the eye involved (Fig. 1.1 and Table 1.2). The classification of a surgical maneuver as specifically cataract or refractive is artificial and indicates separation rather than synergy.

We live during a time when information can be obtained from all corners of the world with incredible swiftness and precision. Photographic and videotape reproductions of ophthalmic microsurgery are exceptionally good at transmitting the techniques of a new procedure. The results of anterior segment surgery are readily quantifiable by refraction and keratometry. Often, computer analysis of this data can quickly provide trends to help the eye surgeon decide if a new idea is an improvement.

Spurred on by this worldwide instantaneous exchange of information, the last two decades have witnessed a significant change in the thinking of many ophthalmologists as they struggle to understand the legitimate goals of ocular surgery.

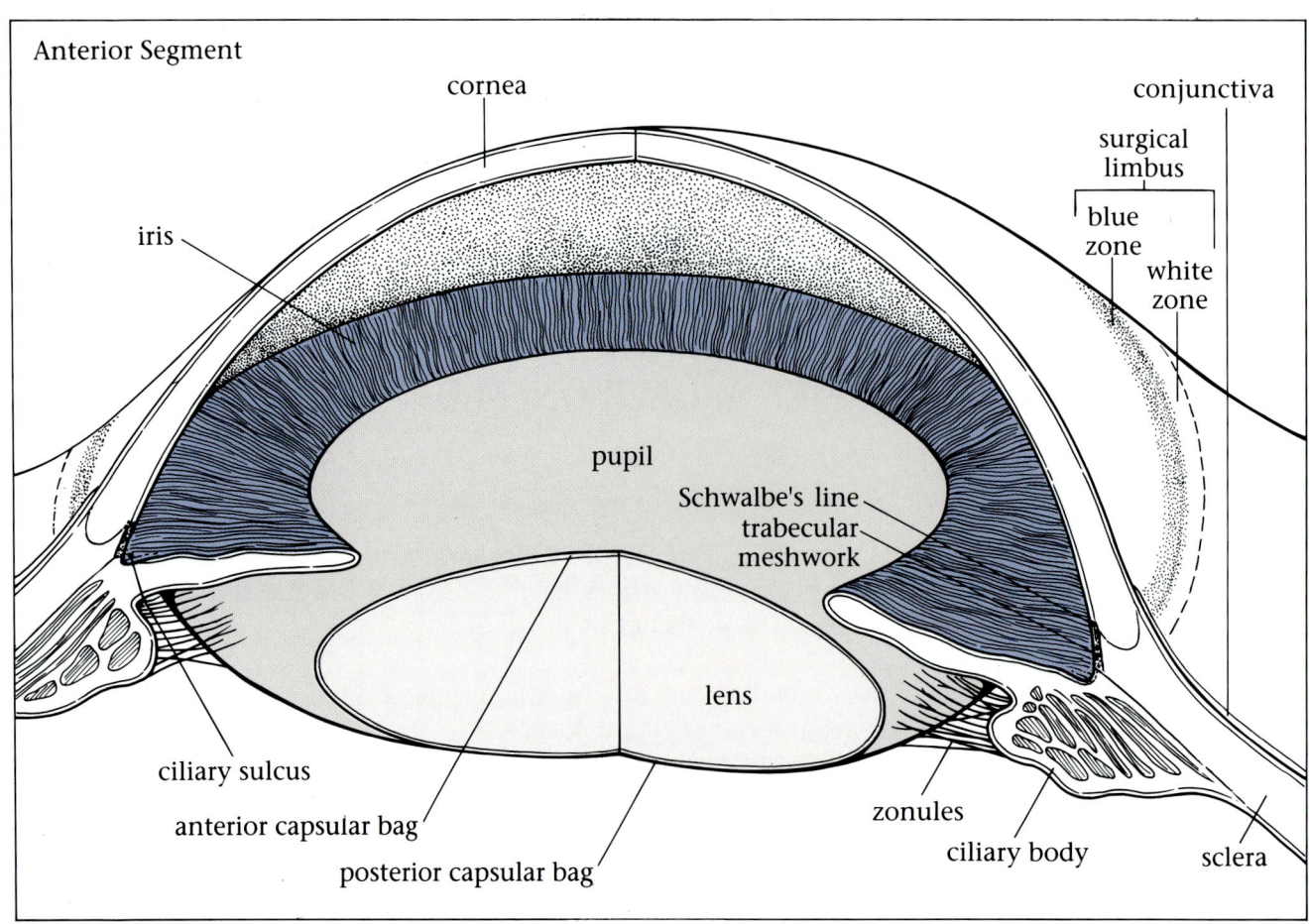

Figure 1.1 *The anterior segment of the eye.*

Table 1.2
Dimensions of the Anterior Segment (mm)

	Diameter	Thickness	Width	Height
Cornea	12.00			
Central		0.52		
Peripheral		0.70-0.85		
Limbus			1.00	
Lens	9.50	3.50		
Capsular Bag (after lens removal)	10.50			
Ciliary Sulcus	11.00			
Anterior Chamber	12.50			3.80

Up to now, eye surgeons have been trained to employ surgery as a means of curing obvious disease. Now, however, experience and technology may provide us with greater capabilities than before. The eye surgeon must confront the difficult issue of deciding whether reluctance to learn a new procedure that holds the promise of providing better visual function for the patient is based on a healthy skepticism after assessing the risk/benefit ratio of that procedure or a personal fear of not being able to perform the surgery.

The factors that make successful surgery possible are too often presented as a series of possibilities, thereby confusing the student with too many choices. When performing surgery, imitation of a known, successful technique is preferable to making decisions about which combination of factors to employ.

The student should be warned against attempting to "mix and match" the surgical techniques of various experts. The unique choice and order of steps of a surgical technique, created and modified according to the many complications encountered, comprise a master's procedure. Even imitation of an apparently simple surgical step can be very difficult. It soon becomes apparent that the art of anterior segment surgery is not immediately reproducible. After successful results with a given procedure can be produced reliably the learner can gradually progress to variations on that procedure. The original technique will then be a standard to which the surgeon can refer.

The Best Unaided Vision

Does 20/400 uncorrected visual acuity with 20/20 best corrected acuity represent a disease of the eye?

A cataract or bullous keratopathy certainly represents a disease state, but how should 4.00 mm of blepharoptosis, which does not significantly affect vision but is cosmetically undesireable, be classified?

How aggressively should a surgeon pursue the goal of providing the patient with best *uncorrected* visual acuity?

Is the choice of surgical procedure contemplated for a patient based on the most appropriate surgical techniques known to exist or on only those surgical procedures known to the surgeon?

These questions are intended to stimulate the reader, who then has to make fundamental decisions regarding personal philosophy and patient care. At the least, giving consideration to the definition of disease and the risk/benefit of certain surgical procedures teaches the surgeon about a propensity for accepting the norm or forging forward despite the increased risks associated with the greater benefits. Of course, change just for sake of change is of no value. It is far better for an eye surgeon to perform a time-tested surgical procedure well than a newer one poorly.

The words of Jose Barraquer, M.D., a great pioneer in refractive surgery, are interesting to consider:

The restoration of the physiological functions of the human being is the goal and raison d'etre of medicine and surgery. The achievement of superfunctions is still in the realm of utopia and probably in the clouds of DNA.

In accordance with this principle, the purpose of refractive surgery is restoring the visual function to ametropes, without the aid of prosthetic devices, since they—no matter how perfect or well tolerated they become, out of habit or resignation—continue to represent a handicap (when not a risk) in the performance of the functions proper to a normal life.

... Lister's maxim, 'Success depends upon attention to details' is particularly true because in them, the distance that separates success from unwanted complications or mediocre results is only a very small fraction of a millimeter.

The Goal: Excellence

Eye surgeons need be thinkers *and* doers. All ophthalmologists need the ability to periodically reassess their basic surgical techniques and to change them when warranted, based on objective data and personal observations. Either maintaining an outdated surgical technique or conversely, adhering to a technique that is imprudently aggressive and consistently causes needless injury is inappropriate. Because success and failure can easily trigger exhilaration or despair in the patient, the patient's family, and the eye surgeon, the ophthalmologist acquires a deep respect for those who achieve a measure of excellence in eye surgery and also for those who accept the challenge to achieve this goal.

SECTION ONE
RECENT DEVELOPMENTS

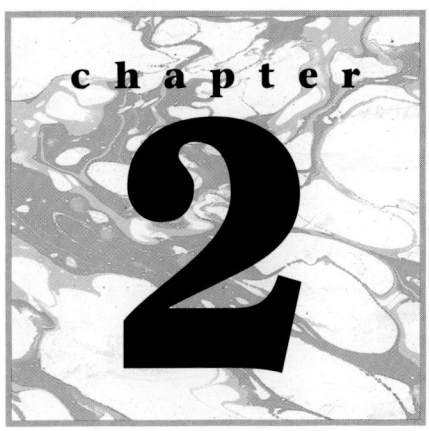

NEW OPTICS FOR THE EYE SURGEON

LEE T. NORDAN, M.D.

The introduction, maturation, and acceptance of several major developments in treating the anterior segment have occurred during the past decade. Radial keratotomy, epikeratoplasty, and multifocal intraocular lenses (IOLs) are examples of important innovations now used to obtain best uncorrected visual acuity in ametropes. *Aspheric optics* rather than the traditional system, *spherical optics*, is fundamental to these modalities. It has become apparent that some of the time-honored axioms and clinical implications that apply to spherical optics do not always apply to aspheric optics. This chapter discusses the significance of these new concepts in ophthalmic surgery using theory, clinical experience, and a discussion of corneal topography to illustrate various points.

Optical Mechanics

The normal cornea is essentially a central dome anchored to a circular base, the limbus. Although peripheral topography may vary, the central 5.00 mm to 6.00 mm of the cornea is generally spherical or mildly astigmatic.* Therefore, the amount of light focused on the macula is determined by the size of the pupillary aperture. Radial keratotomy, astigmatic keratotomy, myopic and hyperopic keratomileusis, myopic and hyperopic epikeratoplasty, alloplastic keratophakia, and laser corneal ablation all change the central or paracentral curve of the cornea to an aspheric curve (Fig. 2.1). This asphericity can have some very profound effects, both positive and negative, on visual function.

An aspheric curve's radius of curvature changes as may the location of the center of curvature, i.e., it is a spiral. A spherical curve,

---

*The term *spherical cornea* refers to the normal, unoperated cornea, which certainly possesses a small degree of clinically insignificant asphericity. The term *aspheric cornea* refers to a cornea with a marked degree of asphericity, which is clinically very significant but often unappreciated.

on the other hand, has a center of curvature and a radius of curvature that are constant (Fig. 2.2). When light strikes the surface of transparent material in an oblique fashion, the light's path is deflected due to the change in the velocity of light caused by this medium. The index of refraction (n) correlates to the density of a medium and the degree to which it reduces the velocity of light. The index of refraction for air is 1.00, which is the standard index of refraction. Refractive power in diopters (D) is defined as

$$\frac{n_1 - n}{r}$$

where n_1 and n are the indices of refraction of

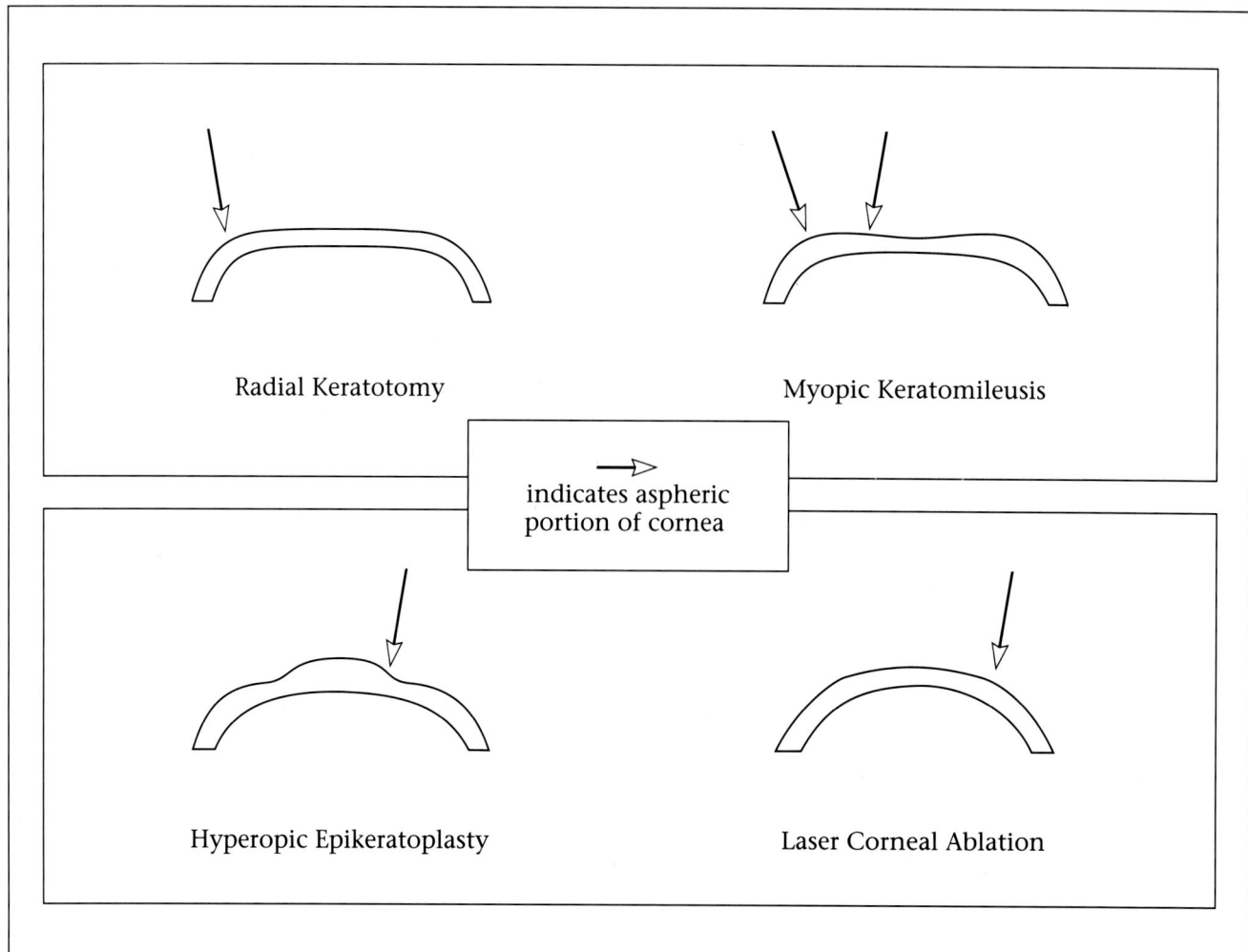

Figure 2.1 *The normal spherical curve of the cornea is converted to an aspheric curve by various types of corneal refractive surgery. The arrows indicate the portions of the cornea that are aspheric following radial keratotomy, myopic keratomileusis, hyperopic epikeratoplasty, and laser corneal ablation.*

the media at the refractive interface and r (in meters) is the radius of curvature at this interface.

A *diopter* is defined as the ability of a refractive surface to deviate the path of light one centimeter at one meter from a given surface and represents the amount light is bent by a lens. (When discussing optics relative to the eye, lens thickness is considered to be infinitely thin so no consideration is given to the small amount of refraction that occurs when light passes from the lens back to the original medium. This is known as

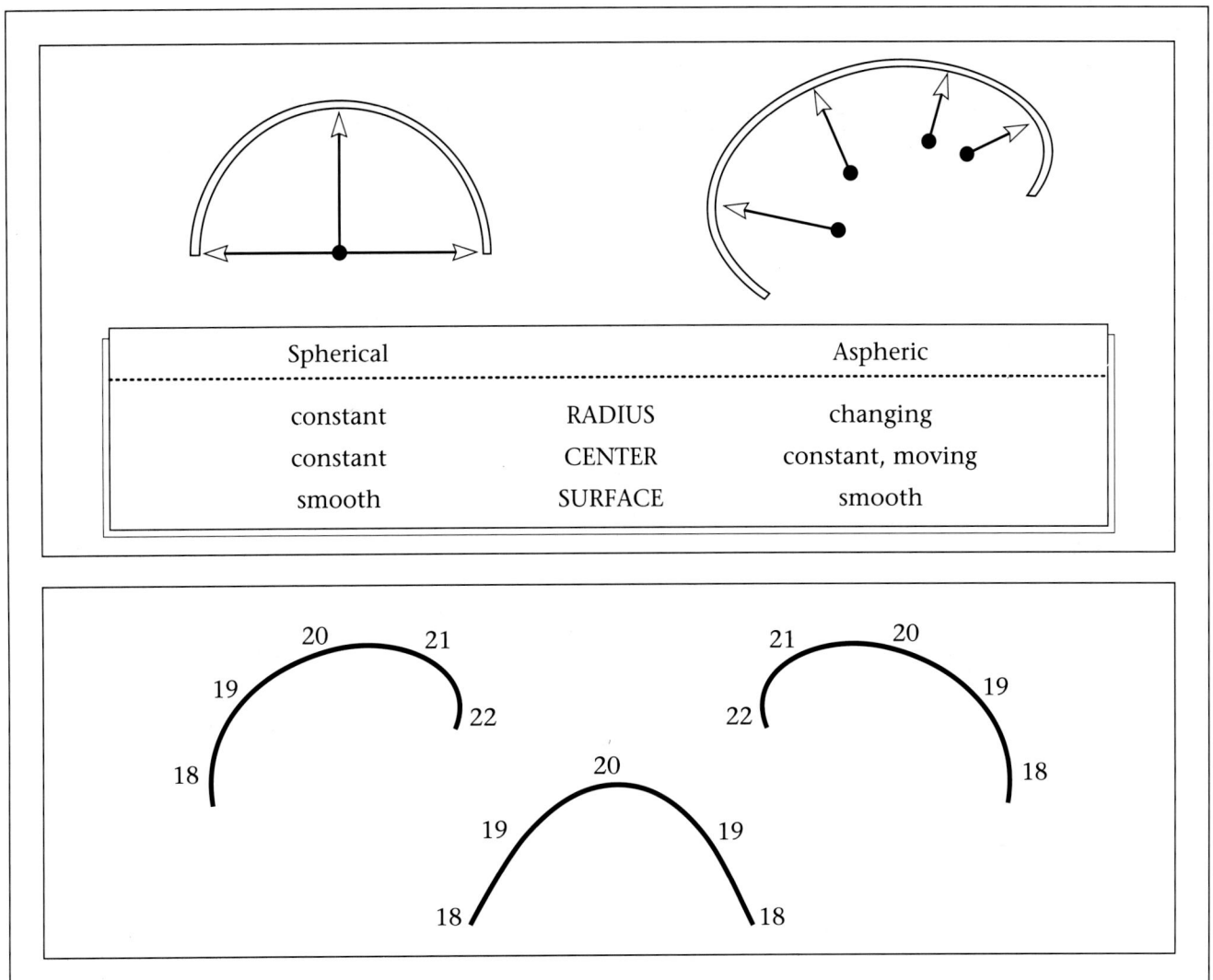

Figure 2.2 (Top) *In a spherical curve, the radius of curvature and the location of the center of rotation are constant.. In an aspheric curve, the radius of curvature is variable as may be the location of the center of curvature.* (Bottom) *An aspheric curve may present in various forms. The numbers represent the dioptric power at various points on the surface.*

first order optics.) The changing radius of curvature of an aspheric curve produces a different refractive power at every point on its surface (Fig. 2.3). A spherical curve produces a constant amount of refraction along its entire surface.

Several concepts become apparent when considering the aspheric cornea relative to visual function. These concepts are explicated below; several geometrical aspects of the aspheric cornea are described, each followed by an important clinical consideration based on that geometry.

Clinical Experience

1. Theoretical Concept. A spherical surface focuses all available light at one point. An aspher-

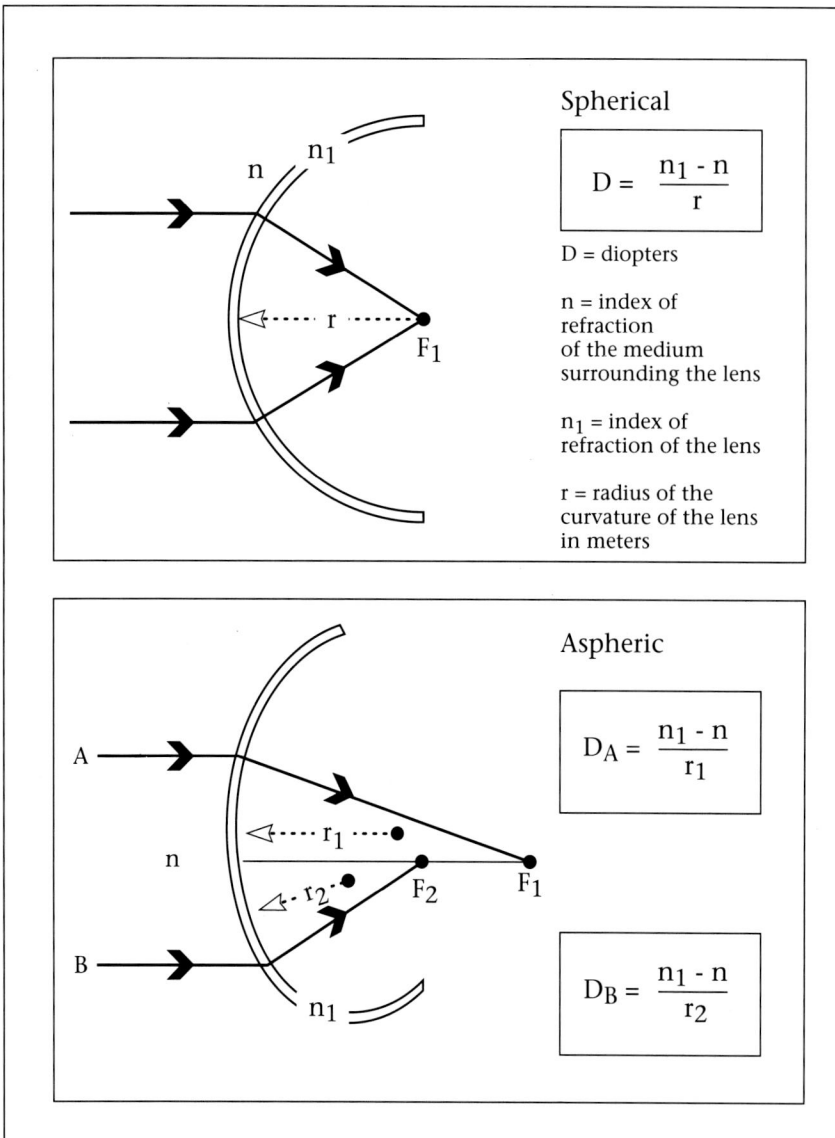

Figure 2.3 (Top) *A convex spherical lens refracts incoming parallel light rays to a point at the focal point (F_1) of the lens because the power of the lens is constant along its entire surface.* (Bottom) *An aspheric lens has a different refractive power for each location on its surface because the radius of curvature varies. Therefore, light refracted by an aspheric lens is focused at many points (F_1, F_2).*

ic surface uses only a portion of its surface to focus light at a given point. Therefore, only a portion of the aspheric cornea is used at a given time to provide 20/20 vision since only one dioptric value corresponds to the object under consideration (Fig. 2.4).

Clinical Consideration. After refractive surgery, patients commonly have excellent uncorrected distance acuity of 20/20 to 20/25, despite manifest refractions in the –0.75 D to –1.00 D range. These patients use a different portion of their aspheric cornea for unaided vision than they do for corrected vision.

Change in refraction may not correspond to change in keratometry following refractive surgery since the portion of the cornea used for refraction may not be in exactly the same location

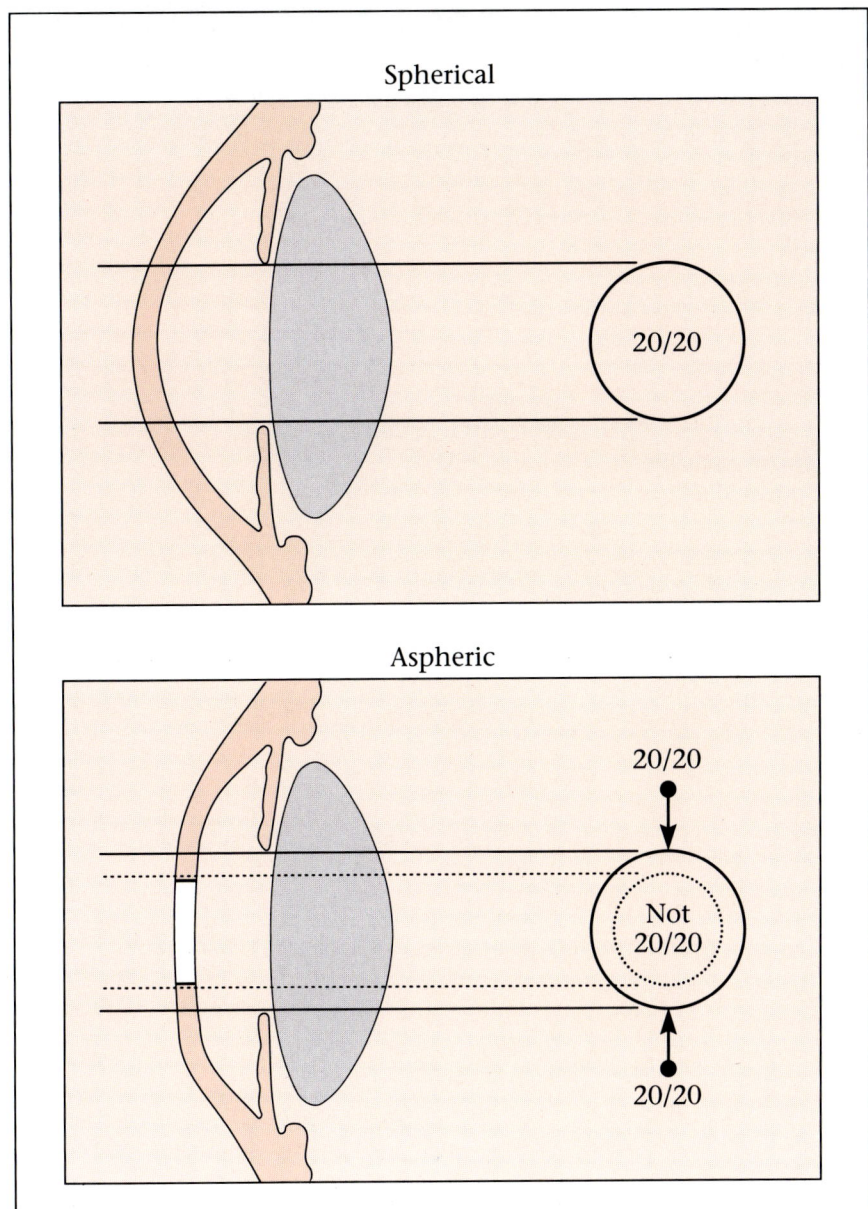

Figure 2.4 *The entire central portion of a spherical cornea focuses light on the macula. In contrast, only a certain portion of an aspheric cornea creates emmetropia.*

INTRAOCULAR LENS CALCULATION FOLLOWING KERATOREFRACTIVE SURGERY

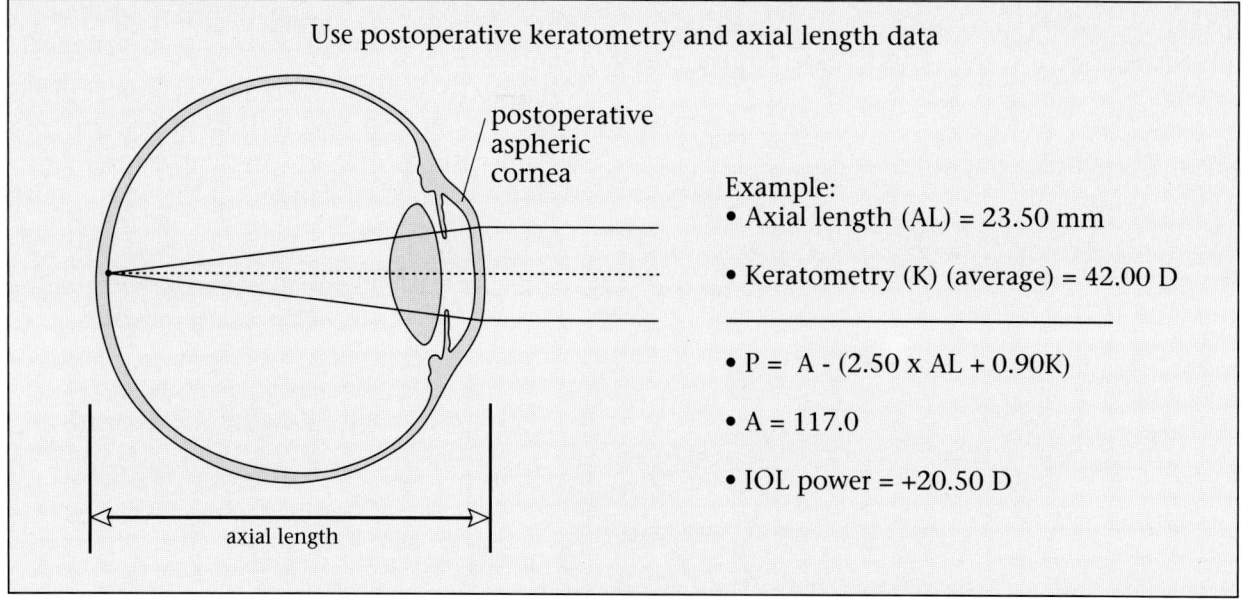

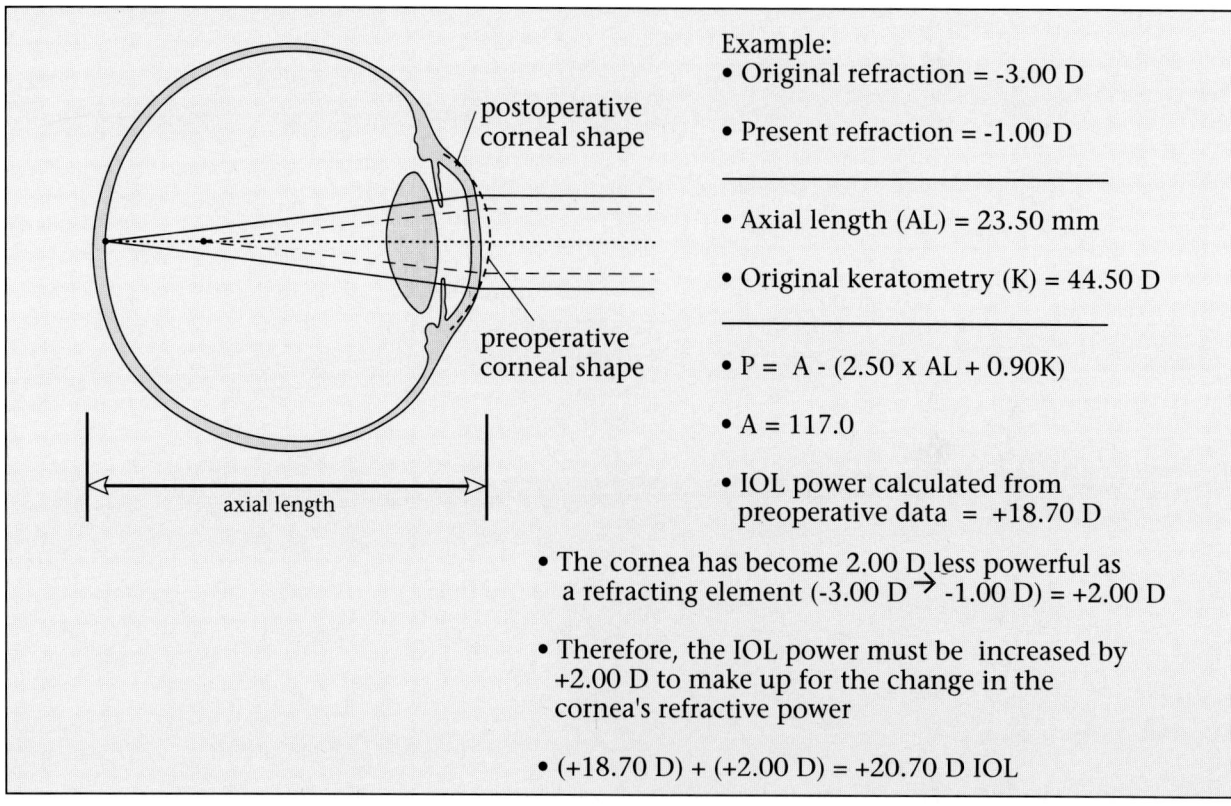

Figure 2.5 *Two methods for calculating IOL power following corneal refractive surgery. Comparing the results obtained from both methods may be useful. (Top) Postoperative keratometric and axial length data, which work rather well for mild to moderate myopia corrected by radial keratotomy. High refractive errors corrected by radial keratometry or other methods of refractive surgery may cause an error in IOL calculation by providing inaccurate keratometry data. (Bottom) If the preoperative refraction and keratometry are known, calculate the IOL power using the original data. Then determine the difference between the original refraction and the current refraction. Add this difference in refraction to the previously calculated IOL power (based on the preoperative data) if the patient was myopic; subtract this difference if the patient was hyperopic.*

as that measured by the keratometer. This disparity may be a very important issue when attempting to calculate an accurate IOL power for a patient who has previously undergone corneal refractive surgery (Fig. 2.5). Also, vision consists not only of focusing light on the macula but of integration and interpretation of the "image" by higher neurological elements. Thus, the slightly out of focus images created by an aspheric lens system may enhance or reduce contrast sensitivity and vernier discrimination.

2. Theoretical Concept. An aspheric cornea has its own built-in "add." If a particular portion of an aspheric cornea creates emmetropia, an adjacent area on this aspheric surface has a greater dioptric value (smaller radius of curvature) not creating emmetropia, even if the pupillary aperture allows light from this adjacent portion of the cornea to enter the fundus (Fig. 2.6).

Clinical Consideration. Presbyopic patients following refractive surgery become less presbyopic. This phenomenon, again, is due to the built-in "add" of the aspheric cornea.

3. Theoretical Concept. Monovision, defined as good distance visual acuity in one eye and good near visual acuity in the other, is often created using contact lenses so the presbyope will not need to wear spectacles. This is purposeful anisometropia. However, stereopsis is lost for both far and near since only one eye at a time functions effectively at each distance.

Clinical Consideration. Monovision following radial keratotomy in a 50-year-old, for example, can provide 20/20 acuity at distance and 20/30 at near in one eye and 20/30 at distance and 20/20 at near in the other with refractions of OD:plano and OS:−.75 D. This provides a truly

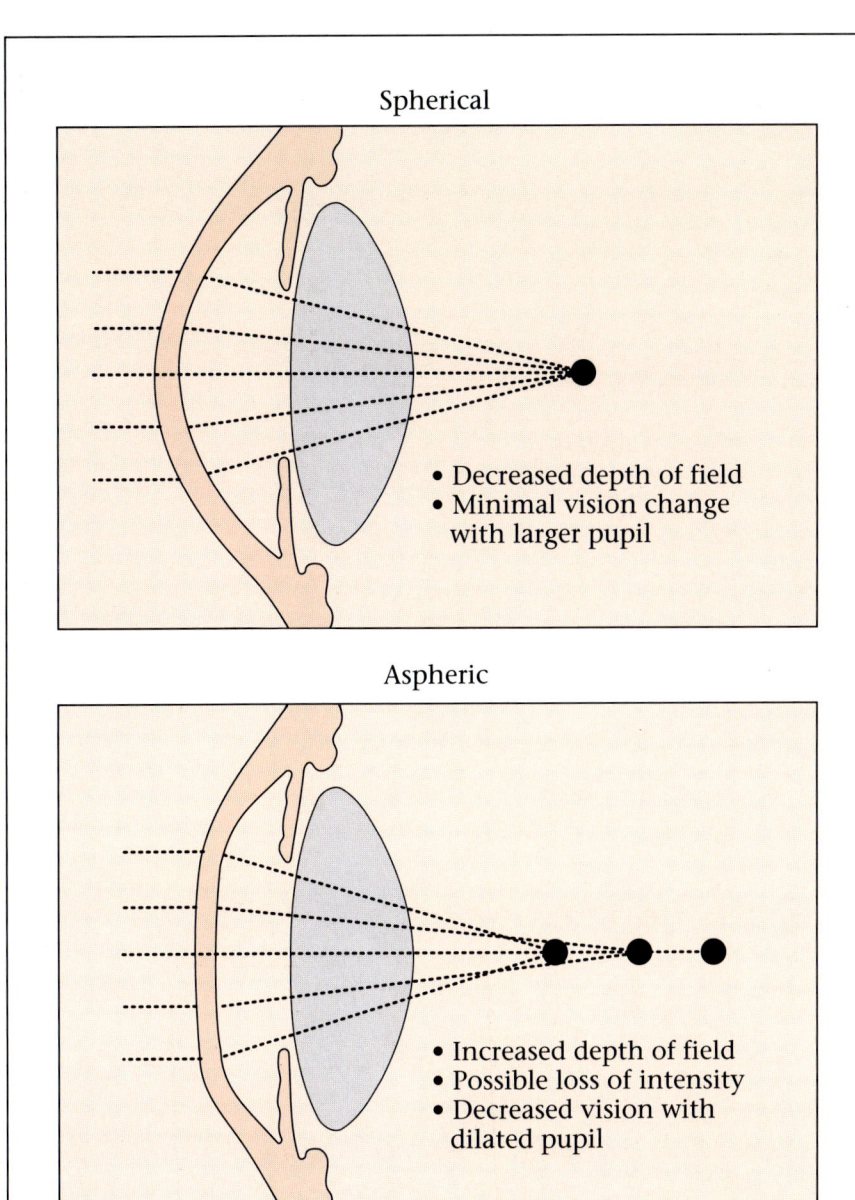

Figure 2.6 *An aspheric cornea minimizes presbyopia by creating a built-in optical "add." A portion of the corneal surface has a stronger refractive power than the portion used for emmetropia.*

functional result with stereopsis at near and far (Fig. 2.7).

4. Theoretical Concept. A dilated pupil often causes a greater decrease in the quality of visual acuity for an aspheric cornea than for a spherical cornea. The dilated pupil allows light from the paracentral knee to enter the fundus. This knee is a very strong, variable refractive surface that varies from emmetropia and may allow stray light and strongly defocused images to enter the eye and interfere with the quality of vision (Fig. 2.8).

Clinical Consideration. Mildly ametropic postoperative refractive surgery patients will often complain that their daylight vision is excellent but that they cannot drive at night or watch television easily. The change in vision from day to

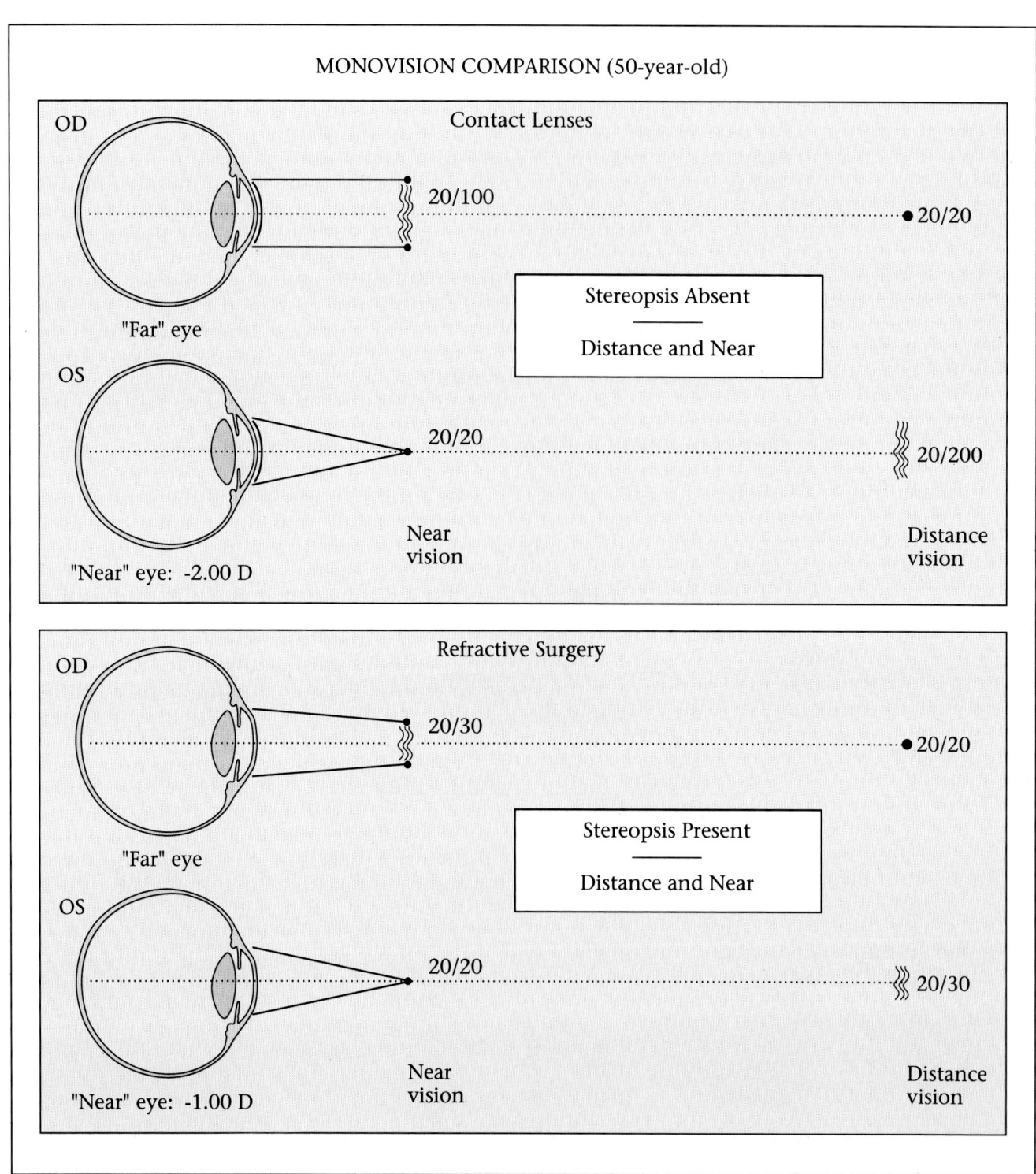

Figure 2.7 *A diagram depicting monovision created by disparate contact lens powers* (top) *and following radial keratotomy* (bottom). *Although monovision follows radial keratotomy, the patient is rewarded with stereopsis since the visual acuity for each eye is good at distance and near.*

night is much greater than experienced preoperatively when spectacle or contact lens correction had been slightly out of focus.

Topography

In recent years, there has been great interest in and effort expended to accurately portray the shape of the cornea. Documentation of the effect of anterior segment surgery on the refractive state of the cornea requires a quantifiable and reproducible corneal mapping system. The cornea can be mapped accurately only if the corneal topography instrumentation has a smooth corneal surface to measure (no irregular astigmatism). The keratometer (see Chapter 23), because of its high magnification and very precise mires, currently offers the most sensitive method for

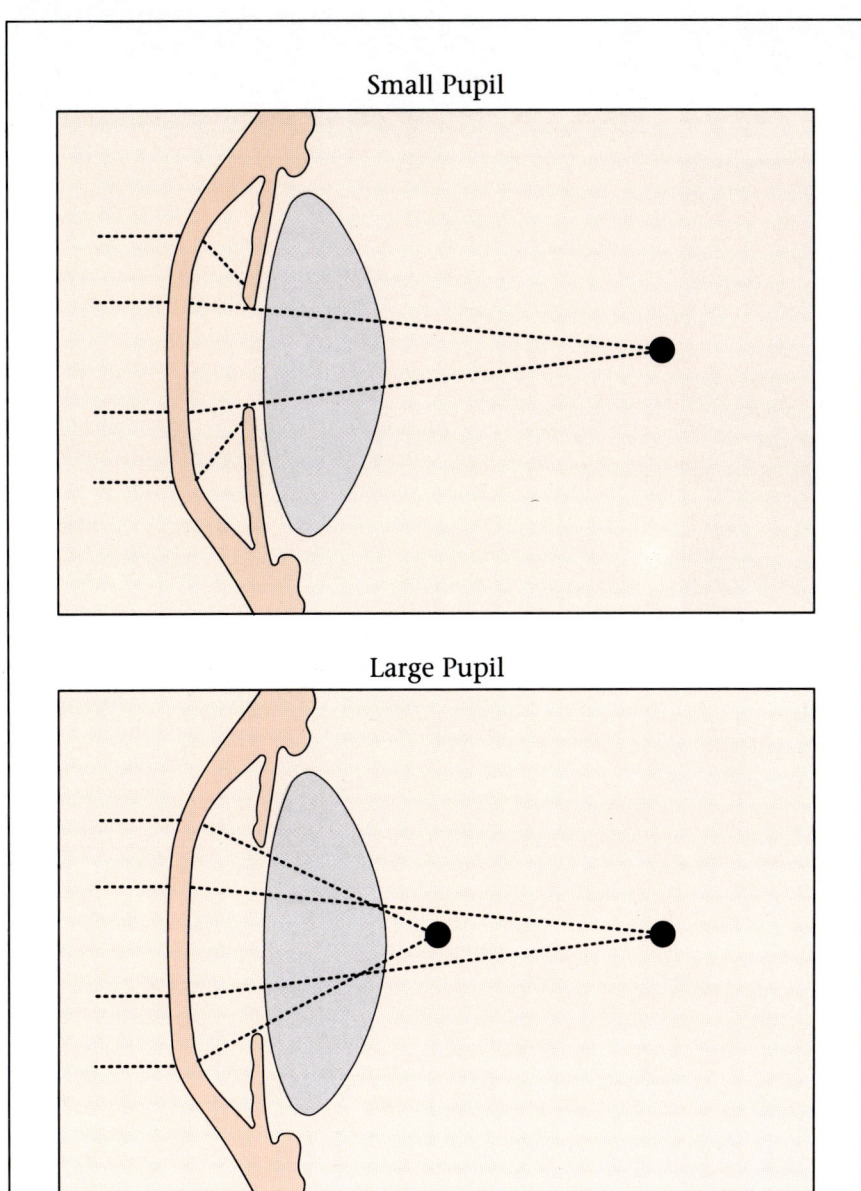

Figure 2.8 *The aspheric knee of the cornea, with its powerful refractive surface, may create unwanted optical effects when the pupil dilates.*

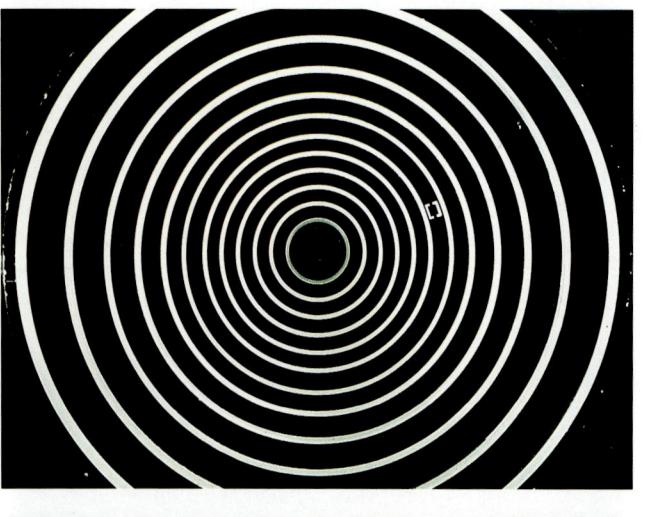
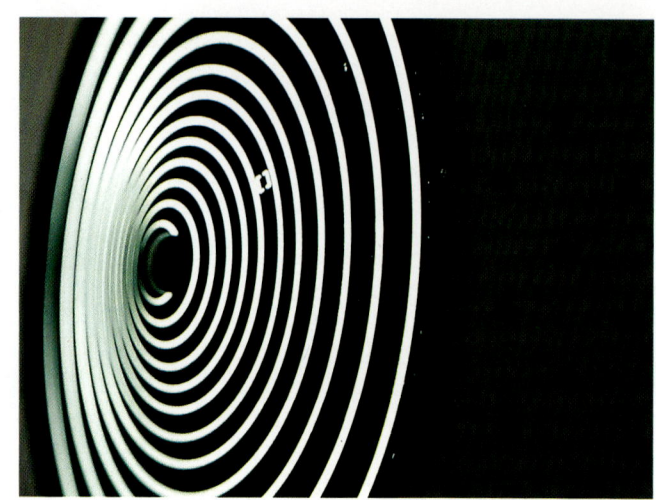
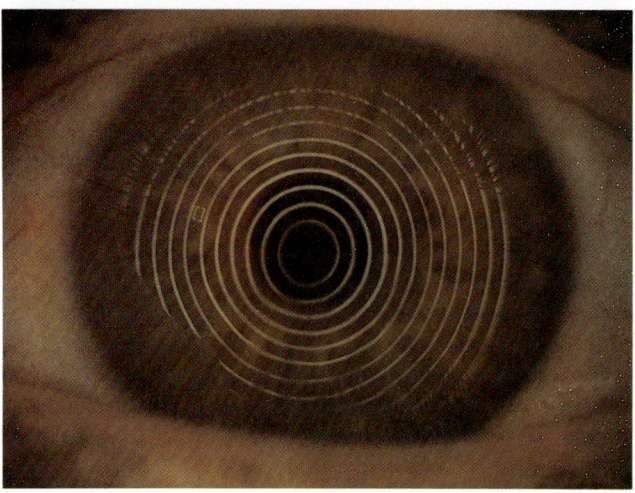

43.50 D x 80°

45.00 D x 170°

Figure 2.9 (Top left and right) *Corneoscope. Its circular object lights are arranged spherically and project a series of concentric circles on the cornea. A Polaroid camera is used to permanently record the reflected corneal mires.* **(Bottom left)** *A Corneoscope study of a patient with regular corneal astigmatism. Notice the slightly oval shape of the central mires.* **(Bottom right)** *A diagram showing the keratometry readings of the eye used for this Corneoscope study.*

documenting corneal irregular astigmatism in the visual axis.

A long-standing method of evaluating corneal topography is the Placido disc, which projects onto the cornea a series of concentric circles that are reflected back to the observer by the corneal surface. Photokeratoscopy, initially popularized by the Corneoscope, is a method of studying the corneal surface by using an instrument that, like the Placido disc, projects concentric circular objects onto the cornea but also preserves the reflections of these concentric light rings from the surface of the cornea using photography (Fig. 2.9). Unlike the Placido disc, which is flat, the Corneoscope's circular objects are dome-like—an attempt to maintain a constant distance between each object circle and the corneal surface. Actually, the least variation in the locations of the images that correspond to the object light rings is achieved when the object light rings are arranged in an elliptical manner.

By evaluating the relative widths of the reflected mires or the distance between mires, an observer can make a qualitative judgement as to the shape of the cornea. This process of evaluating corneal shape is similar to representing the earth's surface by a topographical map that uses lines to depict points of the same elevation. The steep surface of the mountain has rings close together (and narrow mires) and the flat plains have rings widely spaced (and broad mires) (Fig. 2.10). Corneal astigmatism is shown as oval rings, the shorter diameter depicting the meridian of greatest dioptric power (shorter radius of curvature) and the longer diameter representing the meridian of lesser dioptric power (longer radius of curvature).

Mathematical algorithms have been developed that attempt to quantify changes in the curvature of the cornea by assigning a dioptric value to the curved surface between adjacent rings. Recently, computer and printer technology has made it possible to represent these dioptric values by colors and then to print a colored topographical map of the cornea.

It is of concern, however, that although these colored topographical maps based on keratoscopy often provide a reasonable estimate of the general shape of the central cornea, they may not provide totally accurate and truly quantifiable information. The ability to digitalize a corneoscopy image accurately is difficult for several reasons:

1. Because the focal distance between the objects and the cornea varies (since the corneal shape does not exactly mimic the shape of the

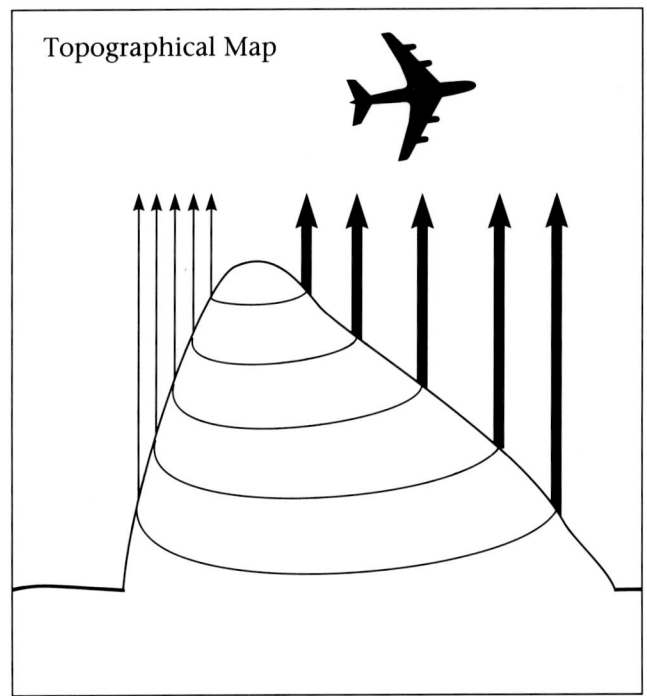

Figure 2.10 *A topographical map of the cornea resembles an aerial view of the earth's surface. Steep mountains (higher diopter values) have rings spaced closely together and narrow mires while the flat planes (low diopter values) have rings spaced widely apart and wide mires.*

keratoscope), the images of all the corneal mires cannot be in focus at the same time (Fig. 2.11). Therefore, the information provided by an analysis of some of the mires must be less accurate than others.

2. Assigning a specific dioptric value to mires that are either out of focus or reflected from an irregular corneal surface or tear film is difficult, since the instrument is designed to measure either mire width, mire/cornea contrast, or distance between mires (Fig. 2.12).

3. The accuracy of a color-coded topography display may be reduced up to half of its stated sensitivity since dioptric values represented by adjacent colors may be at the low end of the range for one color and at the high end of the range for another. When the desired level of sensitivity is about ±0.25 D, the "noise" inherent to the keratoscopy images may not allow for an interpretation that yields clinically useful information (Figs. 2.13 to 2.16).

Corneal topography is a developing technology that currently should be considered a qualitative, but not totally quantifiable, representation of the three-dimensional shape of the cornea. With the current level of photokeratoscopy, the central cornea can be more accurately mapped than the periphery. The presence of artifacts and inconsistent reproducibility because of tear film and corneal surface abnormalities should be considered. The data obtained from a patient's refraction, keratometry, and slit lamp examination provide the most useful information for the surgeon to make clinically relevant decisions. If corneal topography reinforces the clinical situation based on the previously mentioned data and helps further explain the clinical situation, then it is useful to the surgeon. However, if the topography study is at odds with

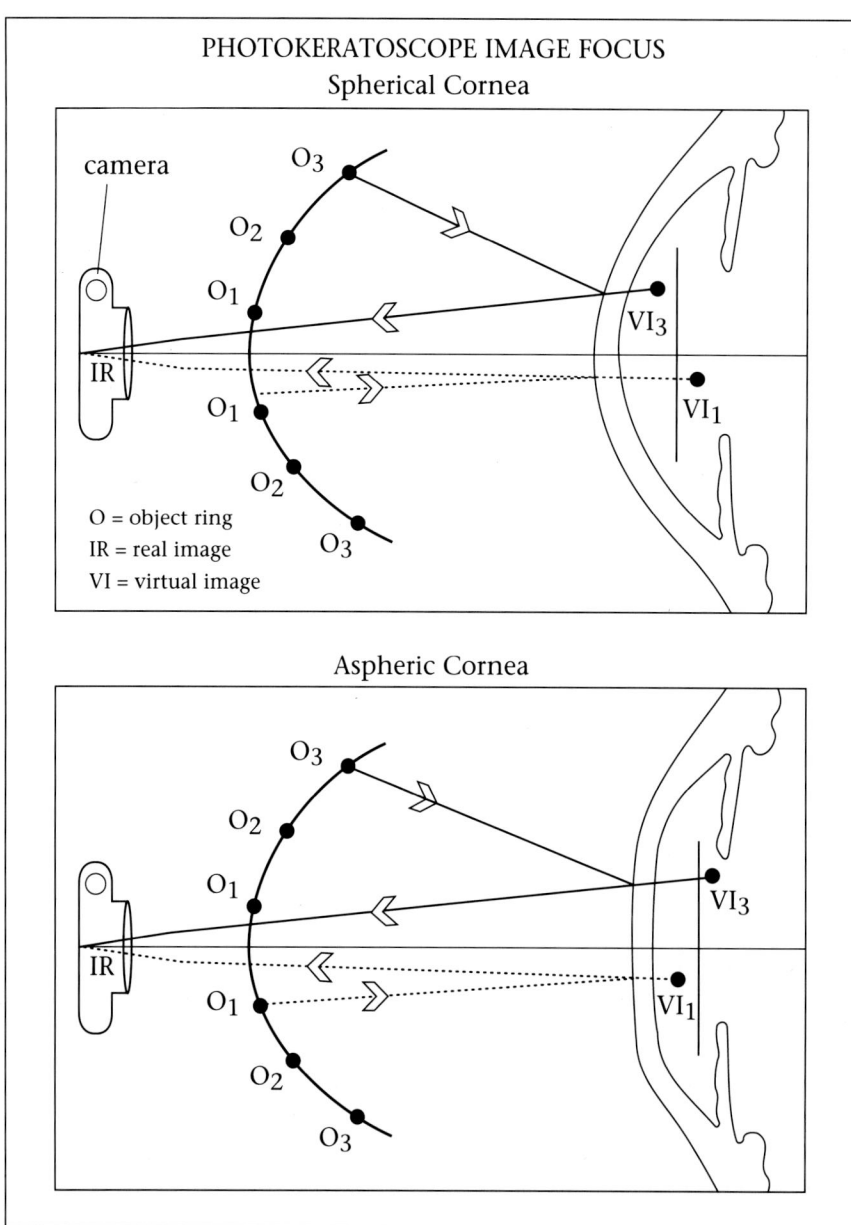

Figure 2.11 (Top) *The light circles of a photokeratoscope, the obects ($O_{1,2,3}$), are reflected by the corneal surface and create virtual images ($VI_{1,2,3}$). All of these images are not focused on the same plane. A corneal surface with a wide range of dioptric power, such as a cornea following RK* (bottom), *increases the magnitude of this problem. Arranging the object light rings in an elliptical pattern minimizes the image plane disparity when dealing with approximately spherical corneas.*

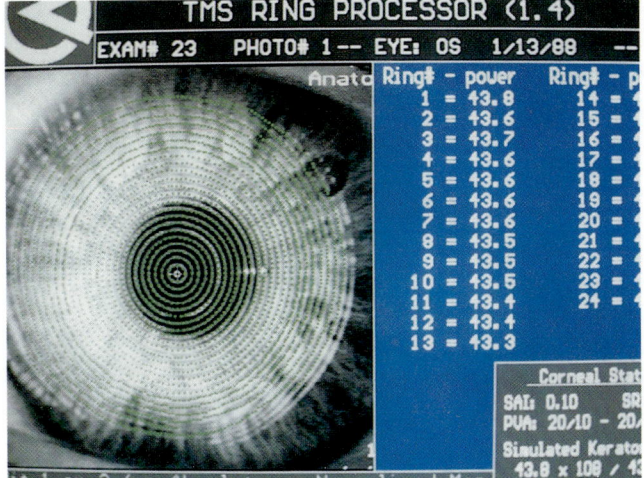 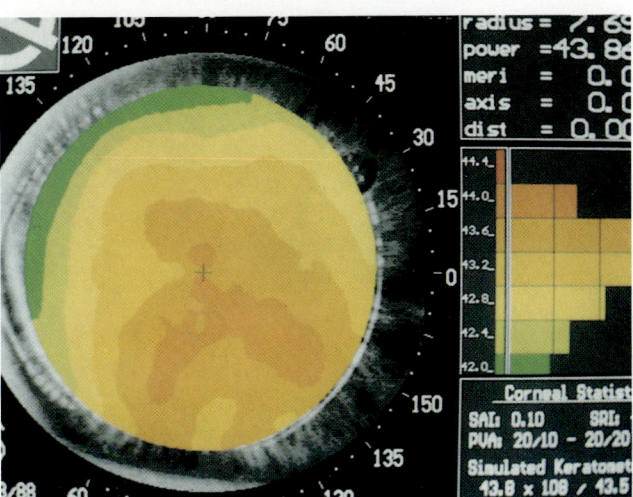

Figure 2.12 *Photokeratoscopic study* **(left)** *of a patient who underwent astigmatic keratotomy above and below the visual axis at 7.00 mm OZ was the basis for the color topography study* **(right)**. *Notice that the peripheral mires in the photograph, especially to the observer's left, are not of the same quality as the central mires. The centrifugal progression of orange to yellow to green in the topography study depicts a cornea that is becoming progressively flatter almost up to the limbus. This corneal configuration would necessitate that the cornea be extremely curved from 9 o'clock to 1 o'clock in order that it could reach the limbus, which is not confirmed clinically by slit lamp examination. Quantifying the dioptric power of the peripheral cornea is usually less accurate than it is for the central cornea.*

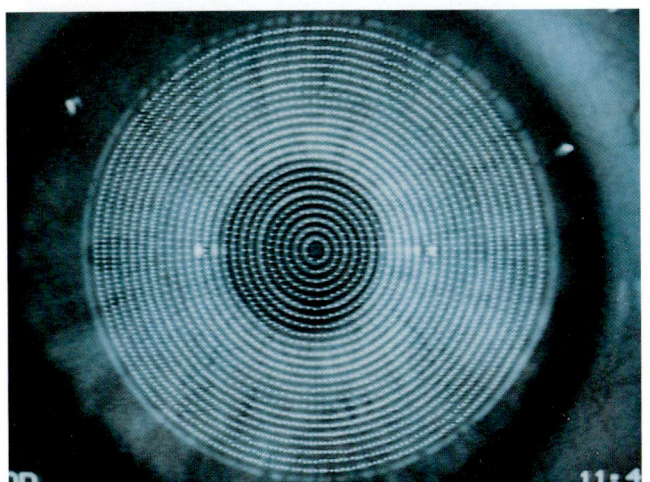 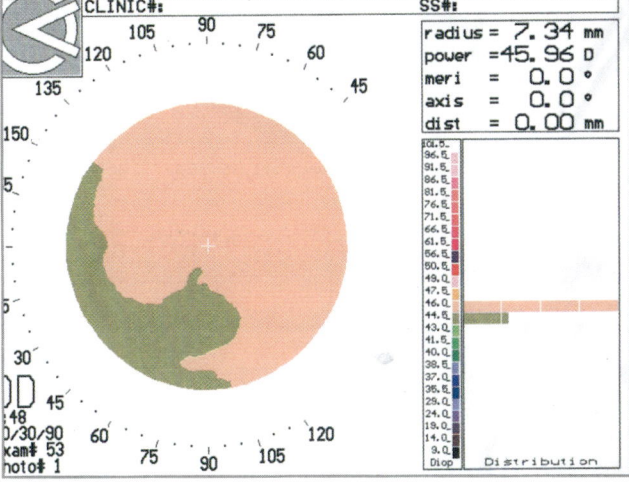

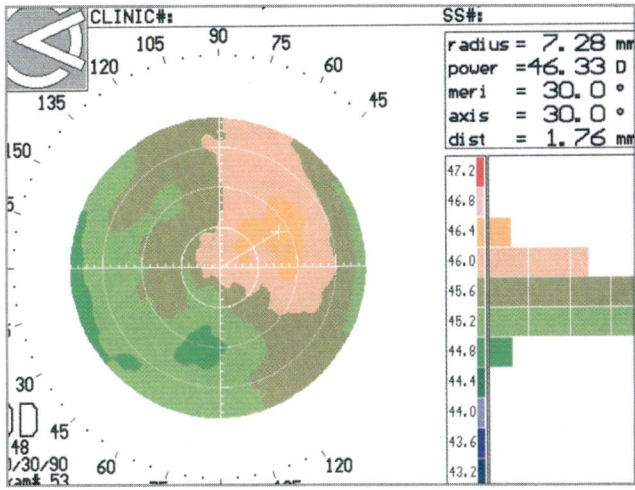

Figure 2.13 **(Left)** *Keratoscopy study used as a basis for topographical studies. The patient has a refraction of +0.50 −0.75 × 90 = 20/15 and the keratometry readings are 45.00 at 90 and 45.50 at 180. Topographical study of the patient generated with sensitivities of 1.50 D* **(top right)** *and 0.40 D* **(bottom right)**.

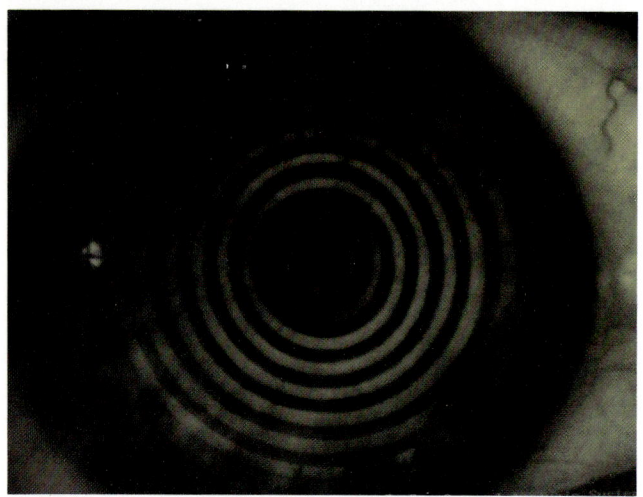

Figure 2.14 (top left) *A second photokeratoscopy study performed on the patient described in Figure 2.13, which served as a basis for topographical studies with a sensitivity of about 0.70 D* **(bottom left)** *and a sensitivity of about 0.40 D* **(right)**. *A comparison of the topographical studies in Figure 2.13 to Figure 2.14: Figure 2.14* **(bottom right)** *to Figure 2.13* **(bottom right)**; *Figure 2.13* **(top right)** *and Figure 2.14* **(bottom left)**, *all performed on the same cornea, reinforces the concept that these varied topographical representations may yield only limited clinically useful information unless correlated with refraction, keratometry, and slit lamp findings. The EyeSys topographical system uses corneal mire edge contrast as the basis for its calculations.*

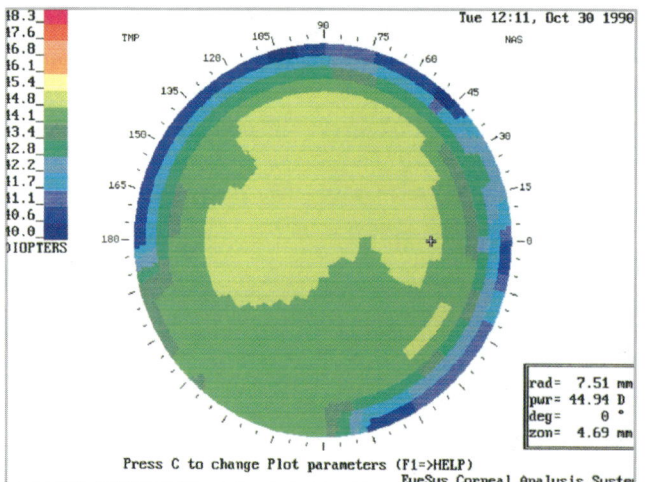

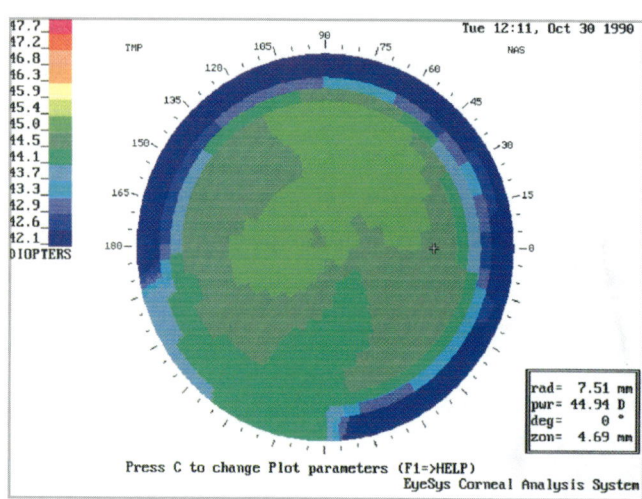

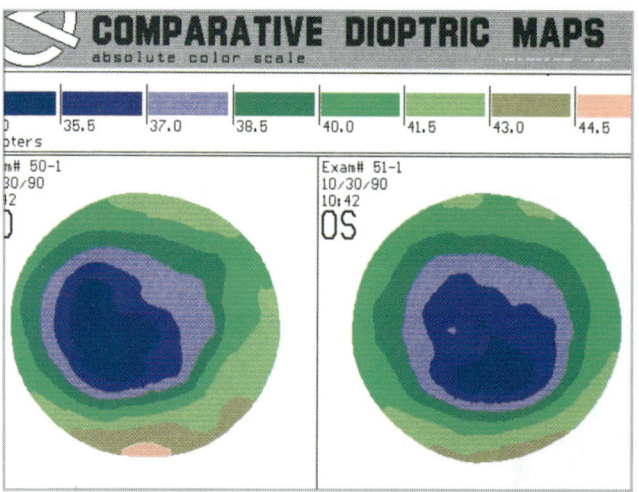

Figure 2.15 *Topographical study of a −5.00 D patient who underwent radial keratotomy bilaterally eight years earlier. This study demonstrates nicely the flattened central cornea, midperipheral steepening, and increased asphericity that occur after radial keratotomy. The clinician, however, does not know exactly which portion of this aspheric cornea in the visual axis is used by the patient for the best visual acuity.*

the above information, then the surgeon should rely on the refraction, keratometry, and slit lamp examination as a basis for clinical decisions. Keratometry remains the most accurate method of determining dioptric power, astigmatism, and quality of the corneal surface in the visual axis.

The limiting factor of current corneal topographical methods is the information provided by the reflected photokeratoscopy mires (explained above). Attempts at using hologram and other technology to represent the topography of the cornea are ongoing and have the promise of

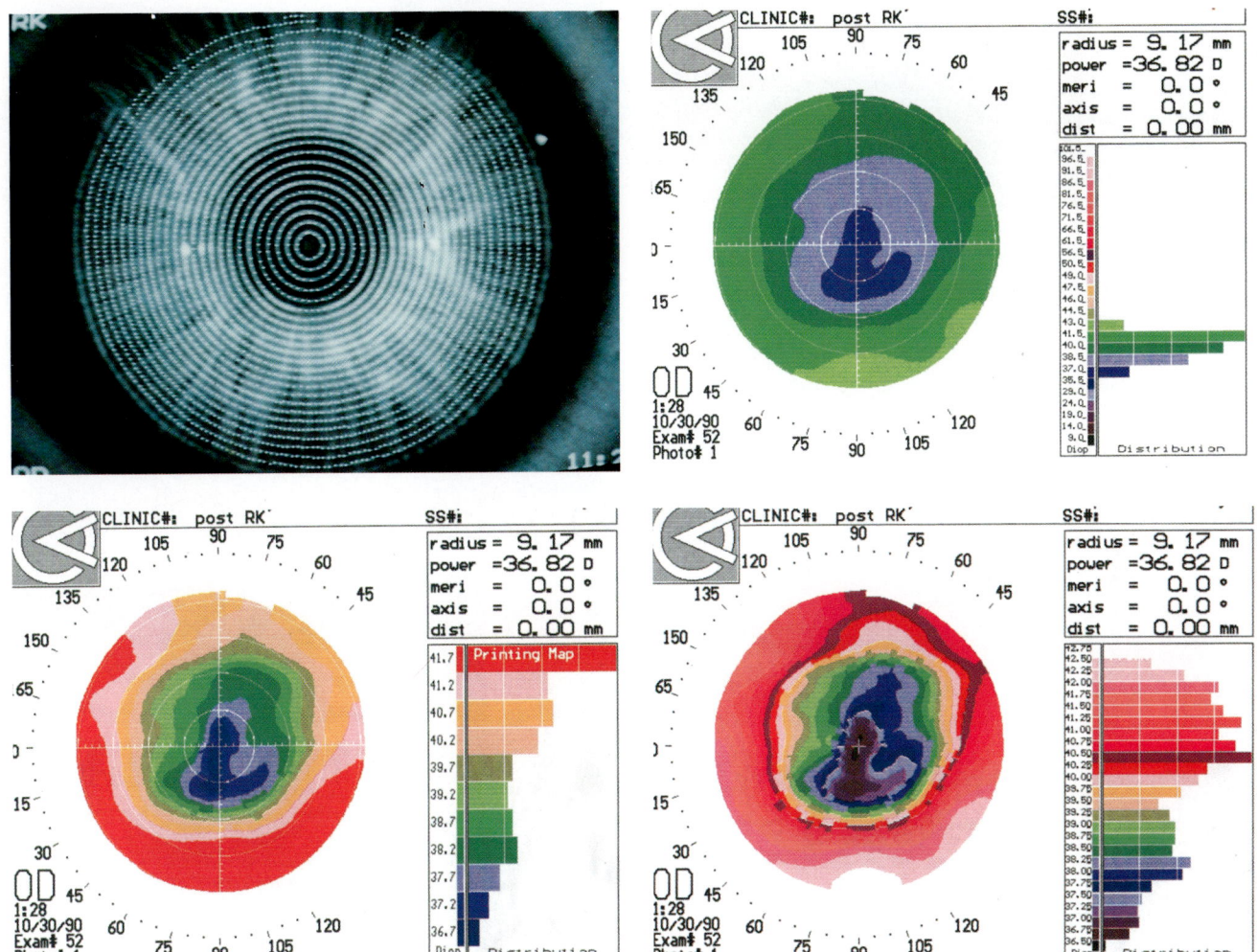

Figure 2.16 *(Top left) Corneoscope picture used to generate color topographical studies of a −5.00 D patient who underwent radial keratotomy one year previously with a sensitivity of 1.50 D* **(top right)**, *0.50 D* **(bottom left)**, *and 0.25 D* **(bottom right)**. *The general shape of the post radial keratotomy cornea is well demonstrated; however, at a sensitivity of 0.25 diopters, the "noise" of the mires limits the clinical usefulness of the topographical depiction since patients are refracted with lenses in 0.25 D increments.*

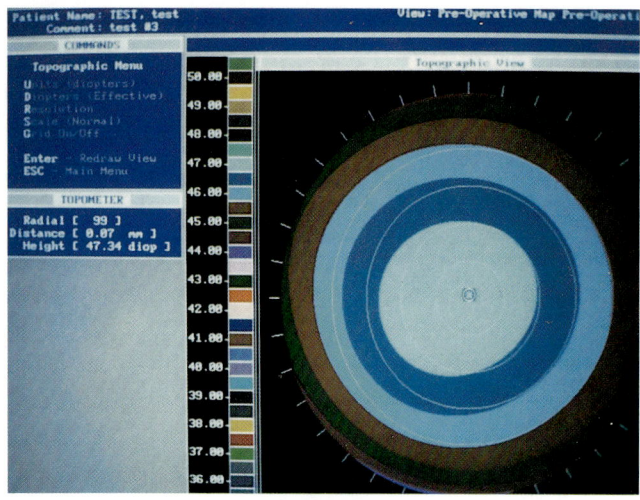
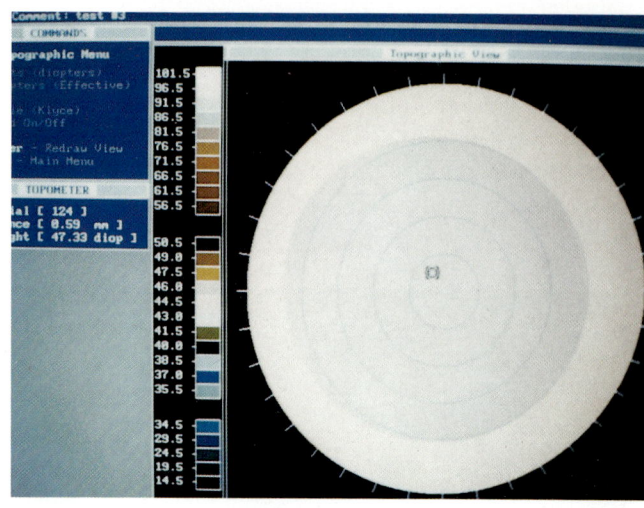

Figure 2.17 (**Left**) *Color-coded dioptric representation of a 47.00 D steel spherical test object with no irregular astigmatism generated by a holographic topography unit with a sensitivity of 0.50 D for each color. Notice that the accuracy of the measurements for the central portion of the test object is excellent, but the measurements of the peripheral aspects are significantly inaccurate, indicating a dioptric power of only 45.50 D. Also, a holographic pattern is so sensitive that it may be rendered inaccurate by minimal tear film irregularities.* (**Right**) *The same holographic topography data for the 47.00 D test object is presented with a sensitivity of 1.50 D for each color instead of 0.50 D. Notice that the spherical test object is depicted as spherical, but only because a range of up to 2.99 D of astigmatism may exist within the single color representation of the measured surface because of the system's low sensitivity.*

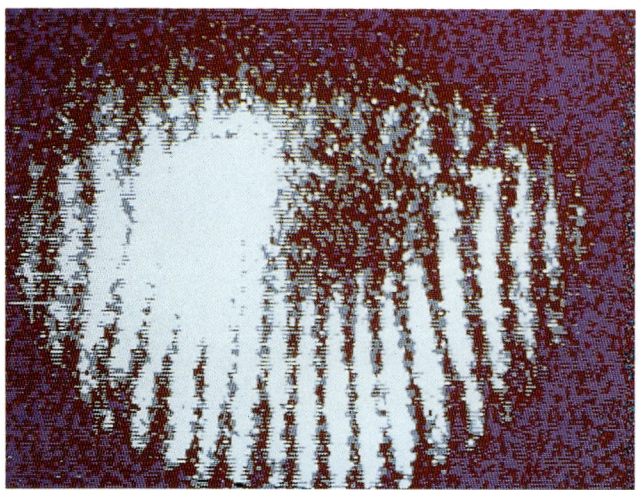
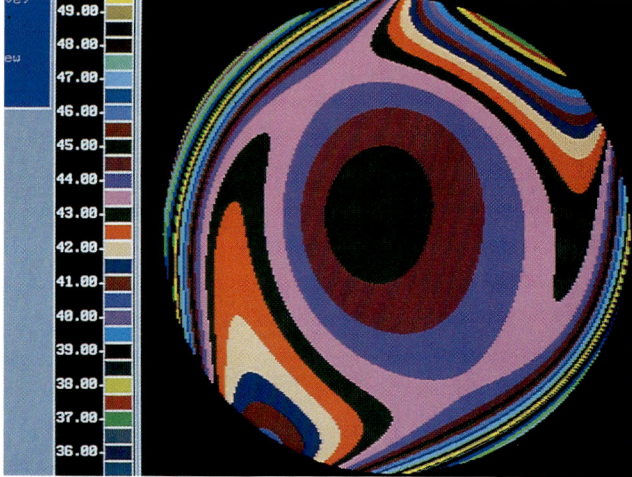
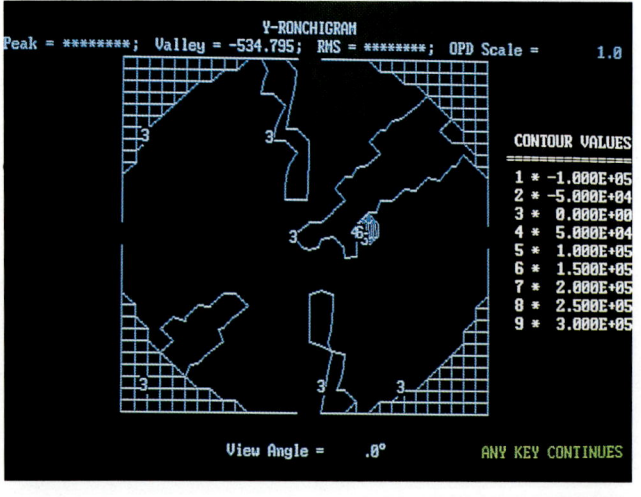

Figure 2.18 (**Top left**) *Interference pattern generated by a holographic topography unit while analyzing a post radial keratotomy cornea.* (**Right**) *Dioptric color representation of interference pattern.* (**Bottom left**) *Detailed analysis of the same interference pattern demonstrates local areas of corneal irregular astigmatism along four of the eight RK incisions.*

extreme precision but must be harnessed into a clinically useful format (Figs. 2.17 and 2.18). Subtraction topography, which depicts the amount of change induced at a corneal location, by mathematically and graphically subtracting the final corneal shape from the original, is coming of age. Subtraction topography correlated to the change in refraction should help determine which parts of the cornea are being used for best visual acuity after various surgical procedures. Of course, these studies can only be as accurate as the information provided by the photokeratoscopic method.

In the near future, the continued application of advanced technology to the present and proposed methods of photokeratoscopy should provide us with a corneal topographical system that can quantifiably represent at least the central 9.00 mm of the cornea and determine the quality of the corneal surface.

Additional Clinical Considerations

A time-honored dictum of refraction and spectacle lens dispensation is that despite clearer vision, a large change in axis or astigmatism can create asthenopia (which disappears after the patient has adjusted to new glasses.) However, I have never had a refractive surgery patient with a good result who complained about the loss of, say, 4.00 D of astigmatism, no matter what the original axis. This has led me to conclude that the changed refraction and reflection of light from the base curve of the periphery of the new lens, *not* the change in axis or power per se, may be the primary cause of asthenopia. In other words, when asthenopia occurs, the patient's previous visual acuity experience may be less of a factor than a different spectacle lens.

When the patient has a bilateral refractive problem, the surgeon must be aware of the disabling anisometropia that can result from uni-ocular surgery. Therefore, in high myopes or astigmats who are not contact lens wearers, bilateral radial keratotomy (assuming no entrance into the anterior chamber during the first surgical procedure) is desirable. The risk of infection after radial keratotomy is probably lower than the risk of infection from wearing a soft contact lens. If a noncontact lens wearer is a high myope and has surgery on only one eye, the patient will be incapacitated by a profound anisometropia that cannot be corrected by spectacles.

Asphericity plays an important part in multifocal IOLs as well. A description of this type of IOL is provided in Chapter 8.

Visual Function Index/Surgical Efficacy Index

As stated above, a patient with an aspheric cornea often has better uncorrected visual acuity than would usually be correlated with that refraction if it were based on a spherical cornea. The clinical matter of evaluating refractive surgery results is an important, yet difficult, task since the evaluator must decide which is more important—visual acuity or accuracy of refraction. Consider the example in Table 2.19: The 21-year-old is very happy with the result of the radial keratotomy and the 55-year-old is not. The 21-year-old's surgery has missed the goal of emmetropia by 50% (+1.00 D compared to an initial refraction of –2.00 D), but excellent uncorrected visual acuity predominates. This excellent result, however, will lose its effectiveness as the patient ages and the +1.00 D overcorrection will cause a decrease in visual acuity at distance and near.

The Visual Function Index (VFI) gives us another perspective.

VFI =
100 (Snellen acuity) – 10 [Spherical equivalent]

Table 2.19
Radial Keratotomy Goal: Emmetropia

	21-Year-Old	55-Year-Old
Preoperative	–2.00 sph = 20/20 V sc = 20/200	–2.00 sph = 20/20 V sc = 20/200
Postoperative	+1.00 sph = 20/20 V sc = 20/20	+1.00 sph = 20/20 V sc = 20/50

Postoperative VFI scores are assessed according to the following scale:

$$70 - \geq 100 = \text{excellent result}$$
$$40 - 69 = \text{good result}$$
$$20 - 39 = \text{fair result}$$
$$<20 = \text{poor result}$$

It is quickly ascertained that an emmetropic result (or result compared to the presurgical goal) with 20/20 visual acuity has a score of 100 (actually, 20/10 acuity would score 200). Since the VFI includes both the patient's visual acuity and current refraction, it is a dynamic measure of the visual status of a refractive surgery result. Also, the VFI allows the results from two patients to be compared objectively, represented by one number.

The VFI concept is also a good method of grading cataract/IOL surgery results. Consider our example again. The 21-year-old has a VFI = 90 and the 55-year-old has a VFI = 30 postoperatively, (Table 2.20). The difference between the postoperative and preoperative VFI defines the Surgical Efficacy Index (SEI):

SEI = VFI (postoperative) – VFI (preoperative)

SEI scores are assessed according to the following guidelines:

$$100 = \text{major change}$$
$$50 = \text{significant change}$$
$$0 = \text{no change}$$
$$<0 = \text{worsening}$$

Consider the SEI for the 21-year-old and the 55-year-old (Table 2.21). The SEI describes how effective the refractive surgical intervention has been, relative to the starting point. Consider the question: Which is "better" surgery, a radial keratotomy patient who started at –6.00 sph and ended up at –2.00 (V sc = 20/100) or a patient who started at –2.00 and ended up at –1.00 (V sc = 20/50)? Many surgeons instinctively consider the first case as "better" since the patient "improved" more. However, since the goal of 20/20 is a fixed standard, the second patient really has had more successful surgery because the final status is closer to 20/20.

An appropriate analogy would be two golfers, one facing a putt of 40 feet who leaves his ball six feet from the hole and the other facing a putt of nine feet who leaves her ball two feet from the hole. Who hit the better putt? The second player,

Table 2.20
Visual Function Index

21-year-old	55-year-old
$100 \left[\dfrac{20}{20}\right] - 10[+1.00] = 100 - 10 = 90$	$100 \left[\dfrac{20}{50}\right] - 10[+1.00] = 40 - 10 = 30$

Table 2.21
Surgical Efficacy Index

21-year-old	55-year-old
$100 \left[\dfrac{(20)}{200}\right] - 10[-2.00] = 10 - 20 = -10$	$100 \left[\dfrac{(20)}{200}\right] - 10[2.00] = 10 - 20 = -10$
Preoperative VFI = –10	Preoperative VFI = –10
Postoperative VFI = 90	Postoperative VFI = 30
Preoperative VFI = –10	Preoperative VFI = –10
SEI = 90 – (–10) = 100	SEI = 30 – (–10) = 40

because her ball is closer to the goal (the hole, 20/20), and her second putt will more likely be successful than the first player's second attempt. The fact that the first player's initial putt covered more ground is not the important issue since the goal is to stroke the ball into the hole at the end of two putts (Fig. 2.22).

So, a postoperative VFI defines the success of a surgical intervention and the SEI defines the difficulty of the attempt.

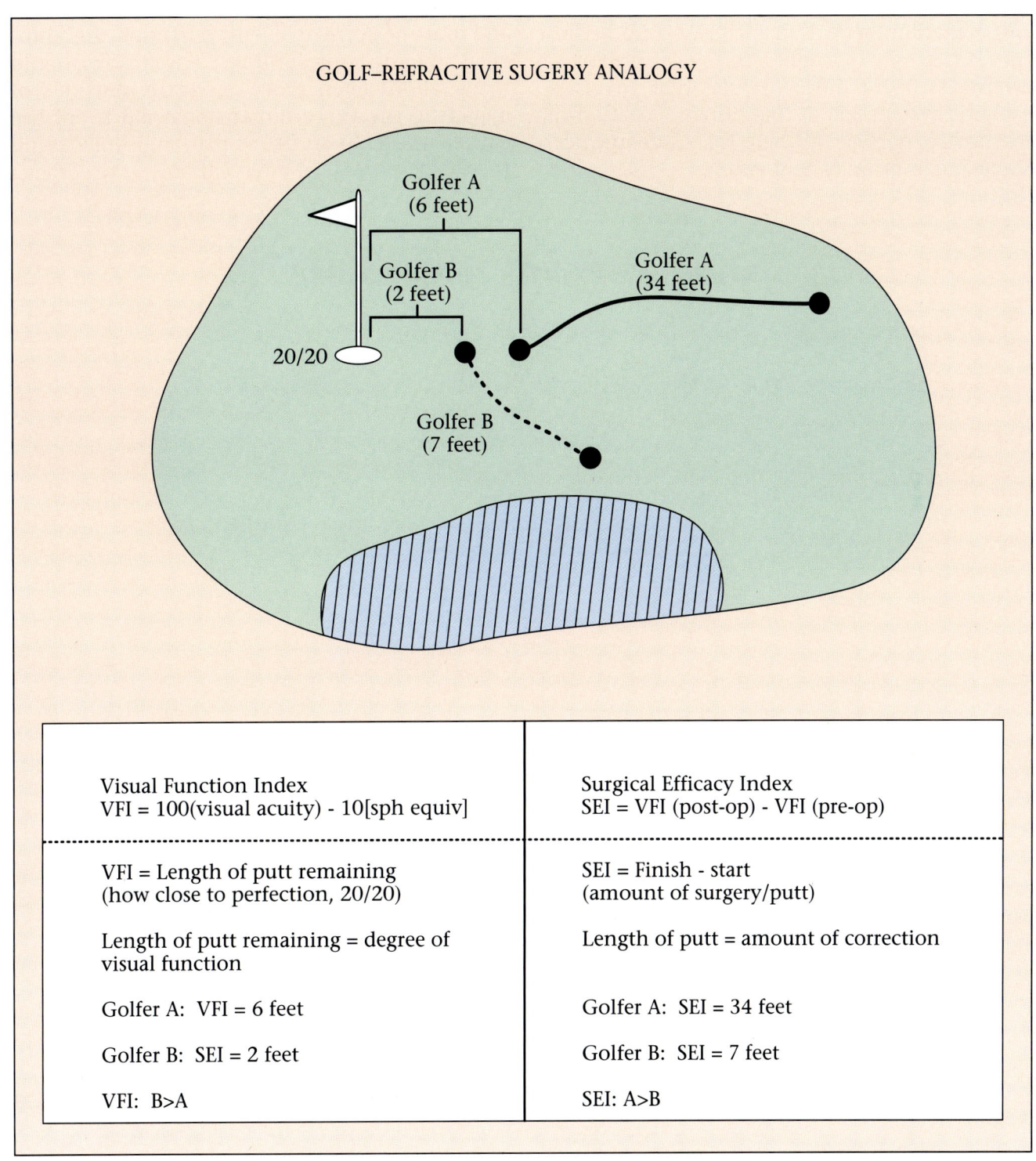

Figure 2.22 *This golf–refractive surgery analogy helps explain the Visual Function Index (VFI) and the Surgical Efficacy Index (SEI): Golfer A must attempt a longer putt (40 feet) than Golfer B (9 feet). (Patient A has a higher initial refractive error than Patient B.) Golfer A's putt travels almost five times as far as Golfer B's putt but ends up more distant from the hole; however golfer A has a much more difficult putt (6 feet) than Golfer B (2 feet) if he is to reach the hole with his next putt. (Patient A's refractive error has improved more than Patient B's, but Patient B has had more successful surgery since the end result is closer to the goal of 20/20.)*

Conclusion

Aspheric optics offer some important and interesting advantages and a few disadvantages for the patient. When dealing with an aspheric cornea, the surgeon must disregard several time-honored rules regarding refraction and presbyopia because they relate only to a spherical optical system. An awareness of the different rules that govern an aspheric system and of this system's relationship to clinical practice will help the surgeon understand and improve patient vision.

Great strides have been made in providing the clinician with an accurate topographical representation of the cornea. Present methods of topography are more qualitative than quantitative and must be correlated with refraction, keratometry, and slit lamp findings. The future should bring about even more accurate methods of depicting the three-dimensional nature of the cornea and help surgeons plan and understand the effects of surgical intervention on the cornea.

Clinical Points to Consider

☛ An aspheric corneal surface is created by all present methods of refractive surgery.

☛ An aspheric cornea can significantly affect visual function, both positively and negatively.

☛ Current corneal topography of the paracentral and peripheral portions of the cornea is more qualitative than quantifiable.

☛ The Visual Function Index (VFI) is a dynamic method of characterizing a patient's refractive error and best uncorrected visual acuity as a single number, which better represents visual function than a Snellen fraction alone.

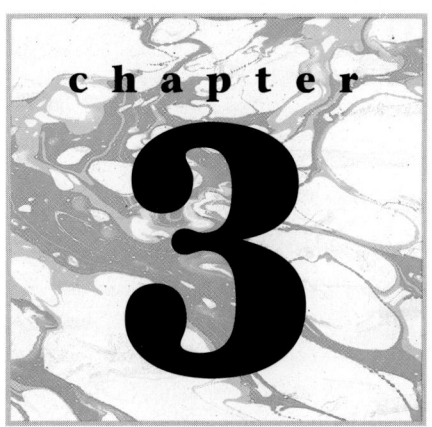

chapter 3

VISCOELASTICS

D. A. BENEDETTO, M.D.

In the 1950s viscoelastic solutions were introduced as vitreous substitutes and in the 1970s they were used for the first time in anterior segment surgery. The development of viscoelastic solutions for use in anterior segment procedures has been one of the most significant recent advances in ophthalmic surgery. Without viscoelastic solutions, it would be hard to imagine performing a 5.00-mm continuous circular capsulotomy or phacoemulsification or inserting a foldable intraocular lens (IOL) into the capsular bag. By reducing the morbidity associated with IOL implantation cataract surgery, viscoelastic solutions have directly influenced the replacement of aphakic spectacles and contact lenses with rigid and foldable posterior chamber IOLs.

The term *viscoelastic* refers to solutions that have dual properties — they act as viscous liquids as well as elastic solids or gels. The solutions predominantly used in ophthalmic surgery are clear aqueous solutions of the naturally occurring glucans, polymeric macromolecules composed of repeating units of disaccharides. The ideal viscoelastic solution should be viscous enough to resist collapse of the anterior chamber while at rest but liquid enough to be injected through small gauge cannulas. It should be elastic and shock absorbing, possess mild surface activity, enhance coating properties, and not affect intraocular pressure. Finally, the ideal solution should be cohesive enough so that it can be easily aspirated from the anterior chamber at the flow rates and vacuum pressures of routine irrigation and aspiration. If a viscoelastic is too cohesive, however, it may be completely aspirated and not provide optimal protection to the endothelial cells during surgery.

Principles and Concepts

Hyaluronic acid (HA) is the ideal biological shock absorber. In mammals HA is the major component of synovial fluid. A basic understanding of the chemistry and rheology of this major tissue polysaccharide and related structures, e.g., chondroitin sulfate (CS), can serve as a basis for a discussion of viscoelastic agents in general and as an introduction to the principles and concepts involved in the clinical use of viscoelastic solutions.

HA is a naturally occurring polysaccharide with an extremely long chain length that exists in animals as a folded, fluid, ribbon-like structure. It is found mainly in soft or loose connective tissue (e.g., vitreous and synovial fluid) in a completely free state unassociated with protein. CS, on the other hand, is a component of harder connective tissue like cartilage and the cornea. It is almost always associated with protein in the form of a proteoglycan. It is more rigid and rod-like and has a short chain length. In the extracellular matrix of tissues, these gel-like polysaccharides have a water-bed effect—they surround cells and fibers, dispersing shock and protecting delicate tissues and cells from permanent deformation and harm.

In solution, HA and CS form different geometric structures, the result of their different primary chemical structures. In most physiologic solutions, depending on chain length and concentration, these polysaccharides form secondary helical structures of variable dimensions. Compared to CS, the HA found in nature has a long chain length and fewer negative charges, giving HA greater conformational freedom to develop a highly folded but flexible tertiary structure while in solution. Individual HA molecules sweep through very large domains while in solution, occupying a space one thousand times the volume of the anhydrous molecule—this expanded molecular structure gives HA its shock-absorbing capacity. On the other hand, the greater negative charge and shorter chain length of CS cause its molecules to be more separated and rigid in solution. Related polymers with bulky side chains (for example, some cellulose derivatives such as hydroxypropyl methylcellulose) have less freedom to rotate about their central axis. These polymers are also rigid in solution and have less elastic or shock-absorbing capacity. Being more rigid and rod-like, CS and cellulose molecules are more likely to align themselves in parallel configurations. In nature this is an ideal conformation for making fibers since parallel molecules can readily be linked by hydrogen bonds.

The structure that polymers assume in solution affects their rheological, or flow, properties. Viscoelastic solutions resist flow (are viscous) and recover their original shape after being stretched (are elastic). When stress is applied to a solution of high molecular weight HA, it resists flow because energy is necessary to deform the highly folded, spheroid, tertiary structure of the molecule (Fig. 3.1). As stress increases, the spheroid molecule deforms and begins to unfold, making the solution less gel-like and more liquid. Increasing stress causes the molecule to completely unfold so a liquid state is achieved. When stress on the solution is released, the molecules recover their original shape, thus exhibiting their elastic behavior. This transformation from a solid or gel to a liquid, with accompanying change in molecular structure, is termed *pseudoplastic behavior*. Pseudoplastic behavior indicates the ability of a solution to reduce its viscosity with applied stress. For HA, pseudoplasticity decreases with decreasing chain length. Solutions of HA with a molecular weight of less than 100,000 exhibit little pseudoplastic behavior.

Elastic and pseudoplastic behavior, or the lack of it, directly affect the important clinical properties of viscoelastic solutions, such as space maintenance, tissue manipulation, shock absorption, and ease of injection. These properties as well as tissue coating, solution aspiration characteristics, and the effects on intraocular pressure will be discussed in light of the physical characteristics of each of the commercially available viscoelastic solutions.

By knowing the chemical composition, molecular chain length, degree of pseudoplasticity, and surface activity of a viscoelastic solution, the general behavior of that solution can be predicted. Table 3.2 lists currently available and investigational viscoelastic agents and some of their chemical and physical properties. All information contained in this table was obtained from package inserts or directly from the manufacturer. The pH and osmolality of all solutions listed, while not included, are compatible with ocular tissue.

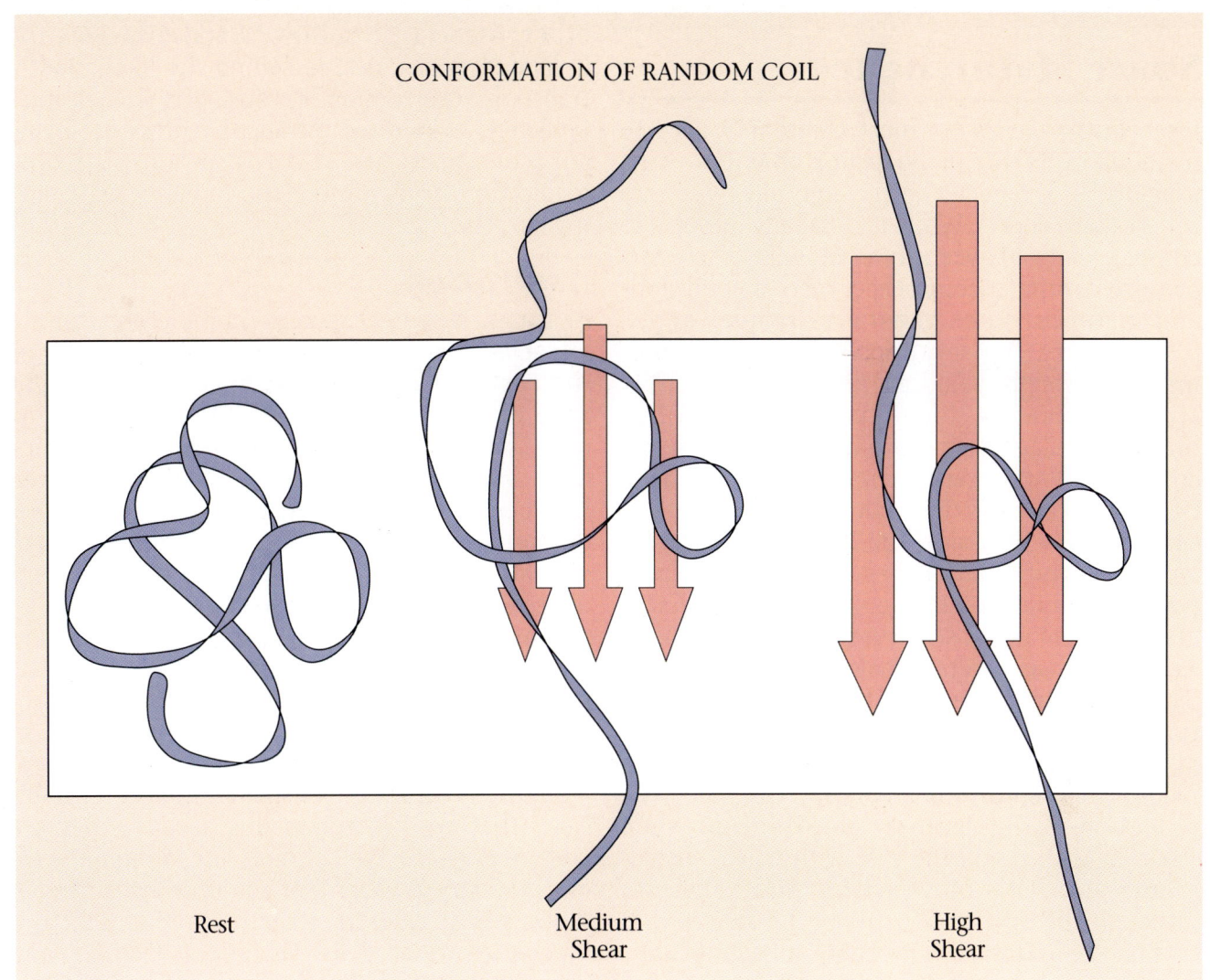

Figure 3.1 *Conformation of a flexible random coil molecule at rest* (left) *and at medium* (center) *and high* (right) *shear rate.*

Table 3.2
Currently Available and Investigational Viscoelastic Agents

Solution	Manufacturer	Chemical Compound	Molecular Weight (average)	Concentration mg/mL (percent)	Viscosity (cp) (shear rate) 0	Viscosity (cp) (shear rate) 2 sec^{-1}	Surface Tension (dynes/cm)	Contact Angle on PMMA (degrees)
Healon	Pharmacia	HA	4,000,000	1.40	200,000	26,250	70	70
Healon GV	Pharmacia	HA	5,600,000	1.40	2,000,000	80,500	55-70	60-70
AmVisc Plus	Iolab	HA	2,000,000	1.60		40,125	70	70
Viscoat	Alcon	HA	500,000	3.00		51,000	55	60
		CS	25,000	4.00				
Occucoat	StorzCoburn	HPMC	86,000	2.00		4,000	40	60
Vitrax	Weck	HA	500,000	3.00	40,000			
Ocugel	Surgidev	HPMC	100,000	2.75		12,500		
		CS	25,000	0.50				
Orcolon	Optical Radiation	Polyacrylamide	950,000	0.50		30,400		

Space Maintenance

Viscoelastic agents are most commonly used to form the anterior or posterior chamber. This property is dependent on the solution's viscosity at rest (zero shear). While it is usually difficult to compare data between different manufacturers because of differences in experimental conditions and methods, some general principles apply. When comparing solutions of HA, the higher molecular weight solutions have higher viscosity at rest. Laboratory studies have determined that high molecular weight HA (4,000,000) has a viscosity of 200,000 centipoise (cp) at zero shear. Lower molecular weight HA (50,000) has a viscosity of only 500 cp, a 400-fold difference. This becomes significant during surgery when there is positive orbital or intraocular pressure. Viscoelastic substances with very high molecular weight, such as Healon, Healon GV, AmVisc Plus, and Viscoat are more likely to maintain the anterior chamber under such circumstances.

For most of the solutions listed, viscosity is reported at a shear of 2 seconds^{-1}. This value is a reflection of the viscosity of a solution when stress is applied and the ease with which instruments and IOLs move within the solution. Although the difference between the solutions is as much as fivefold, it is probably not significant.

Intraocular Pressure

When viscoelastic solutions are placed in the eye, they are cleared in an unmetabolized state by filtration through the trabecular meshwork. Although not completely understood, the elevated intraocular pressure that occurs in the presence of viscoelastic solutions is thought to be due to the solution's molecular configuration as well as its viscosity. Large globular molecules that do not deform easily and are larger than the pore size of the trabecular meshwork could theoretically block the exit of aqueous and cause elevated intraocular pressure. In contrast, a molecule that deforms easily might be able to exit the eye even though its size is larger than that of the trabecular pores. Solutions made of rigid, rod-like molecules that are smaller than the trabecular pore size could also cause significant outflow obstruction similar to a log jam in a flowing river.

To avoid intraocular pressure elevations, it is advisable to aspirate viscoelastic solutions from the anterior chamber as completely as possible. This can be accomplished by using a solution that is highly cohesive (i.e., has a high molecular weight HA). Furthermore, injecting a balanced salt solution into the anterior chamber dilutes other viscoelastic solutions and disperses the individual molecules, lessening the likelihood of trabecular obstruction. Because of a viscoelastic's tendency to increase intraocular pressure, many surgeons prescribe short-term antiglaucoma medication following the use of viscoelastic during surgery.

Aspiration

At times, it is necessary to completely aspirate viscoelastic material from either the anterior or the posterior chamber. Such conditions might arise when a patient is known to have glaucoma or a traumatic injury to the anterior segment that might produce trabecular clogging from intraocular debris. In such instances, solutions of polymers of extremely long chain length should be considered because the entanglement of individual molecules makes them more cohesive and easier to aspirate. Aspiration forces are transmitted throughout the solution as if the individual polymer molecules were attached to one another, allowing for complete aspiration of the viscoelastic.

Solutions consisting of smaller molecules; solutions that are heterogeneous because they are composed of one type of molecule, although each one may vary in weight; or solutions consisting of molecules of different structure and length (i.e., Viscoat, AmVisc Plus, Occucoat, Ocugel, and Vitrax) are less likely to be aspirated completely during surgery because they are less cohesive. When suction is applied, fracturing of these solutions takes place because of the decreased interaction of individual molecules, leaving part of the gel behind.

When such a viscoelastic solution coats the endothelium, problems may occur with visualization. An irregular interface forms at the viscoelastic–aqueous juncture, which may cause unwanted glare from light scatter. This phenomenon is occasionally seen with Viscoat and Occucoat.

Ease of Injection and Tissue Manipulation

The ability of a solution to become less viscous when stress is placed on it (pseudoplastic behavior) is a desirable property as it pertains to the injection of viscoelastic material through small gauge cannulas and tissue manipulation. Solutions of high molecular weight HA exhibit the most pseudoplastic behavior. Solutions of low molecular weight HA (less than 50,000) are similar to pure solutions of CS in that they have no pseudoplastic character. Solutions of short chain molecules, such as Vitrax, Occucoat, and Ocugel, similarly exhibit less pseudoplastic behavior. Solutions that are not pseudoplastic require significant force on the syringe plunger to express the solution from the tip of the cannula. This can decrease control of precision movements during microscopic surgery. A combination solution such as Viscoat, while exhibiting some of the properties of a pure hyaluronic acid solution, is less pseudoplastic than a pure solution of HA because of the presence of CS.

The ability of a viscoelastic solution to manipulate tissue, i.e., maintain space, is directly related to its viscosity when at rest. The higher its viscosity at rest—Healon GV has the highest—the greater the tissue manipulation capability. Thus, as viscoelastic passes through a small gauge cannula, it is liquid-like because it is being subjected to high shear. As it exits the cannula, shear immediately drops to zero and the solution becomes very viscous, more solid and gel-like, resists flow, occupies space, and exerts a force on or displaces tissue.

Shock Absorption

The ability of a solution to absorb shock and protect intraocular tissues from instruments or IOLs is a function of the solution's elasticity, that is, its ability to recover its original shape after being deformed by stress. This ability, in general, is related to the structure and concentration of molecules in solution (as is pseudoplastic behavior). Molecules of long chain length (like those found in Healon, Healon GV, AmVisc Plus, Viscoat, and Vitrax) are highly folded, have elasticity, and are shock absorbing in solution. (Healon and Healon GV have the most elasticity and shock-absorbing capability.)

Surface Coating

Surface coating in anterior segment surgery should prevent damage from irrigation or endothelial touch. Ideally, a viscoelastic agent would form a thin coating on the IOL, the instruments, and the endothelium. A solution's ability to coat a surface is often confused with its viscosity. Viscous solutions often appear to adhere to surfaces. While it is generally true that viscous solutions are unlikely to flow from a surface when applied, this does not necessarily mean that there is an interaction between the viscous material and the surface. Whether or not a given solution coats a surface depends on the solution's surface tension and its interaction with the surface tension of the solid surface it is intended to coat. Viscosity is not a property that applies to surface spreading or coating. When the surface tension of an aqueous solution of viscoelastic polymers interacts with a hydrophobic surface such as a PMMA IOL, the lower the solution's surface tension the greater the spreading of the solution on the IOL surface. Thus, solutions with low surface tension (e.g., Viscoat and Occucoat) are able to coat IOLs and instruments to a greater degree than solutions with high surface tension (e.g., Healon or AmVisc Plus).

It is not understood how the surface tension of a solution affects endothelial coating because the surface properties of the corneal endothelium have yet to be well characterized. Clinically, solutions such as Viscoat, Occucoat, and Vitrax form an endothelial coating visible under the operating microscope. Whether this coating is present as a result of surface spreading of viscoelastic molecules on the endothelium or weak molecular interactions, such as hydrogen bonding, is not known. It is known that the corneal endothelium possesses a 1200 Å glycocalyx that extends from its surface. It is possible that viscoelastic molecules bind to this structure, and in fact this may be the binding site on the endothelium reported for Healon. Yet, clinically Healon does not appear to coat the corneal endothelium. In addition to chemical binding, a solution's cohesive properties also play a role in the ability of a solution to form a grossly visible endothelial coating. Protection of the endothelium from irrigation damage by a viscoelastic coating has recently been demonstrated.

One undesirable property of solutions with low surface tension is its tendency to form bubbles. Bubbles are air that has been encapsulated by a thin film of surface active molecules. The numerous interfaces produced by bubbles cause unwanted reflection and poor visualization of intraocular structures and instruments; thus, such a solution is not desirable where repeated instillation of viscoelastic and air is necessary or in traumatic cases involving blood and tissue debris in the anterior chamber, which further impair visibility.

While first-generation viscoelastics have pushed anterior segment and IOL surgery into another era, no single solution presently available can satisfy all of a surgeon's requirements. It is likely that viscoelastic solutions of the future will be made for more specific uses. Viscoelastic solutions with different physical properties are likely to be used during different stages of anterior segment surgery to optimize surgical performance and decrease ocular morbidity.

Clinical Points to Consider

☛ The space-occupying qualities of a viscoelastic can improve the ease and reduce the trauma of many surgical procedures in the anterior chamber.

☛ Because the clinical properties and optimal uses of viscoelastics differ, the surgeon should be familiar with various types.

☛ Viscoelastic that remains in the anterior chamber can augment postoperative pressure rises, thus oral or topical short-term antiglaucoma medications are indicated at the time of surgery.

Computers and Ophthalmic Surgery

JEFFREY HIGHTOWER

Most of us, at one time or another, have been awestruck by the growing presence of computer technology in our daily lives. The ability of computers to simplify and automate complex tasks and to vastly shorten the time required to electronically process and accurately analyze information is amazing. Microprocessors, computers the size of a tiny electronic chip, are capable of controlling the operation of mechanical implements, ranging from rocket control guidance systems to children's toys. In past years, this computing power was used only by governments, universities, and giant corporations; however, it has rapidly found its way into homes and offices.

All of this computer power, speed, and accuracy is made possible by a simple binary technology—put simply, a computer works by detecting either the presence or absence of an electrical charge at a particular electronic location, or address. Every computer's electronic components include millions of these addresses. The presence or absence of electrical charges at these addresses combine to create letters, numbers, and commands that in turn combine to become stored information, or instructions, for the computer. They can be processed by the computer millions of times per second. *Software* is the set of customized instructions that harness the computer's power into specific applications.

Today's ophthalmic practice can benefit from advanced computer technology in almost all administrative, diagnostic, clinical, and surgical activities. One of the most useful computer capabilites is the *database*, a computerized electronic filing system in which patient records can be stored electronically. Any and all information can be searched, recalled, analyzed, and printed in whole, in part, or in any desired combination. A computer is capable of analyzing a database in seconds while a manual analysis and summary of the same information might take months.

Computer-Designed Cataract and Refractive Surgery

Spherix is one example of state-of-the-art personal computer technology for the ophthalmic surgeon that combines processing power and database capabilities.

The expressed goal of Spherix is the promotion of surgical consistency and improved surgical results through methodical presurgical planning and analysis of postoperative results. Even minimal preoperative patient data allows Spherix to offer possible surgical options for cataract/intraocular lens (IOL) surgery, astigmatic surgery, and radial keratotomy (Fig. 4.1). Surgical options for a specific patient are processed using a database of assumptions constructed by a consensus of the Spherix Advisory Board, which is made up of ophthalmic surgeons. Spherix automatically creates an easily maintained database of pre- and postoperative patient information. This database not only becomes a useful and reliable set of patient records, it also becomes the material for evaluating surgical results and consistency.

The spherix software is found in three fully integrated modules:
Cataract/IOL Surgery Module
Refractive Surgery Module
Evaluation Module

Cataract/IOL Module

The cataract/IOL surgery section of Spherix provides a consistent approach to IOL power and astigmatism control. IOL power is automatically computed on the basis of the SRK II, the Binkhorst, and the Collenbrander-Hoffer formulas.

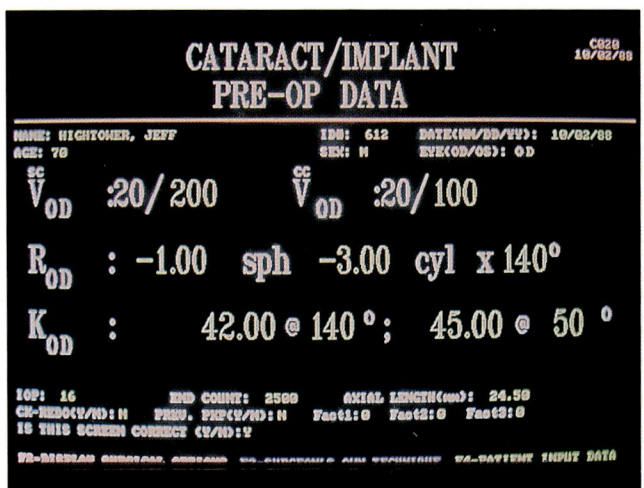

Figure 4.1 Cataract/implant *computer screen containing preoperative information necessary for cataract/IOL surgery.*

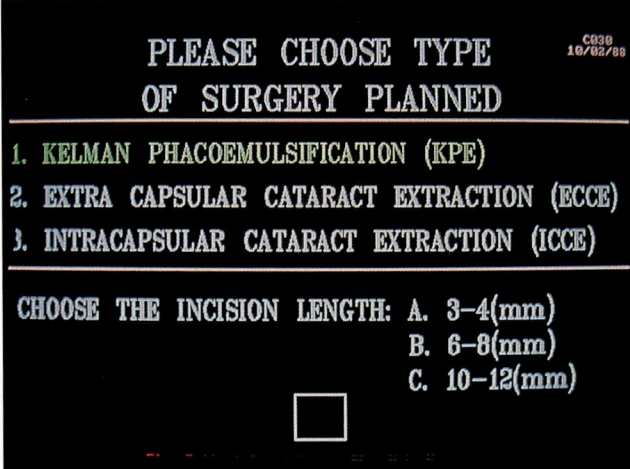
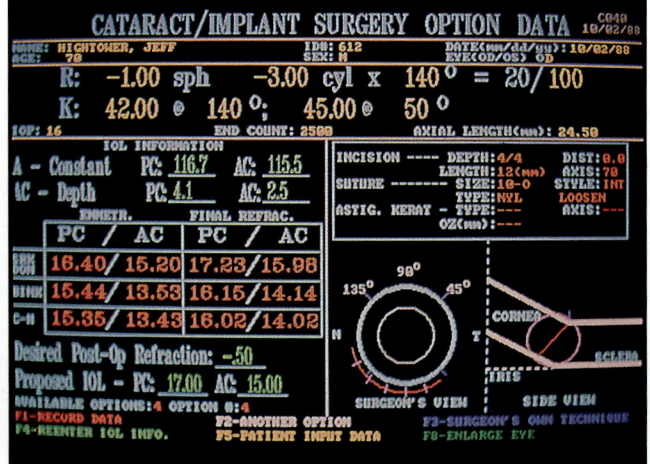

Figure 4.2 (Left) *Computer screen showing cataract procedure and wound length options.* **(Right)** *An overview of the* Surgical Planning *screen. Note that the preoperative keratometry and refraction, intraocular pressure selection data, and surgical option diagram are all presented on one screen. Each segment of this screen may be enlarged and isolated as desired. The surgical option offered on this screen is for an ECCE with a 10.00-mm to 12.00-mm wound.*

The IOL power necessary to achieve emmetropia, or any other desired final refraction, are displayed in a table that presents the differences between the three formulas as the eyes become increasingly hyperopic or myopic (Fig. 4.2).

Astigmatism control, which consists of either preservation of low presurgical astigmatism or correction of high presurgical astigmatism, is achieved by wound and suture combinations and/or astigmatic keratotomy. Wound variables are length, location, and suturing style (Fig. 4.3); astigmatic keratotomy variables include achieved corneal depth, length, optical zone, and axis of incision. In generating surgical options, the Spherix protocol assumes that long-term correction of significant against-the-rule astigmatism cannot be achieved by using tight sutures with a wound located in the flatter meridian. Surgical options are offered that require recession of an incision along the steeper meridian, allowing the steeper meridian to flatten and provide long-term astigmatic correction. Spherix is programmed to assume that the maximum astigmatic correction from the recession of various wounds is as appears in Table 4.4.

When appropriate for against-the-rule astigmitism, the surgical options provided by Spherix include a temporal incision to allow wound recession of the steeper meridian and an option that combines a superior wound with a horizontal astigmatic keratotomy (Fig. 4.5). Astigmatic keratotomy options employ transverse incisions (T-cuts) or modifications of the Ruiz procedure, depending on the severity of the preoperative astigmatism.

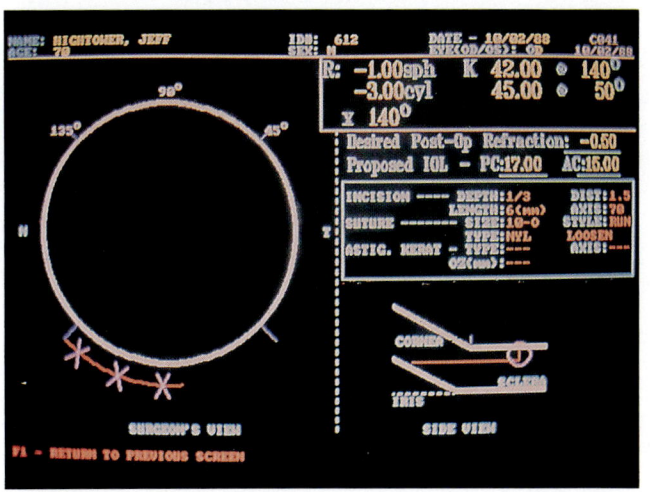

Figure 4.3 *Another surgical option for the patient in Fig. 4.2: phacoemulsification and a 6.00-mm wound. Notice that the wound is centered on the steeper meridian of the cornea.*

Table 4.4
Maximum Astigmatic Correction

Length of wound by wound recession (mm)	Dioptric correction obtained by wound recession
3.00	0
4.00	1.50
6.00	3.00
10.00–12.00	6.00

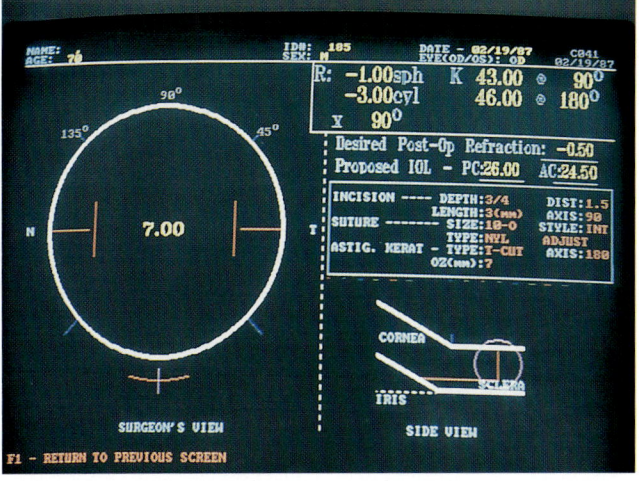

Figure 4.5 *A surgical option using a 3.50-mm wound and an astigmatic keratotomy.*

Refractive Surgery Module

The refractive surgery section of Spherix provides surgical options for the performance of radial keratotomy combined with astigmatic keratotomy, as desired (Fig. 4.6). Spherix bases its surgical options on an analysis of patient variables, which include the following preoperative factors:

Refractive surgical equivalent
Desired refractive result
Gender
Intraocular pressure
Corneal thickness
Preoperative keratometry

Evaluation Module

For a single patient or a composite group of patients, the evaluation section creates an overlaid graph of postoperative results (sphere, cylinder, and spherical equivalent over time) (Fig. 4.7). The cylinder regression profile, which can help predict the results of wound healing and suturing techniques done by any given surgeon, is especially useful. Cataract/IOL or radial keratotomy patients can be easily identified using various criteria. The surgeon can visualize how changes in preoperative, intraoperative, and postoperative techniques will affect the composite cylinder regression profile, final spherical equivalent, or IOL selection accuracy. Changes that improve results and consistency and lessen the frequency of complications can be readily identified.

Conclusion

Computers offer many advantages for the ophthalmic surgeon and office staff, with computer technology easily integrated into record keeping, surgery, and postoperative evaluation. All efforts are aimed at achieving improved patient care and surgical results. Perhaps the computer's most important function is its ability to evaluate, enabling the surgeon to accurately learn from previous experience and compare results with colleagues.

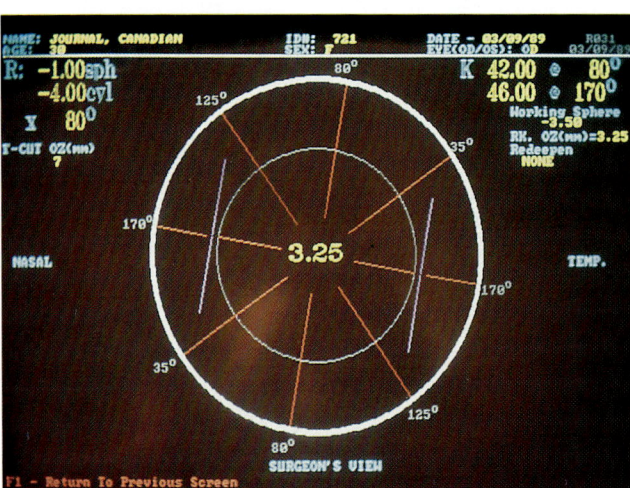

Figure 4.6 *A surgical option for a refractive patient–radial keratotomy combined with astigmatic keratotomy.*

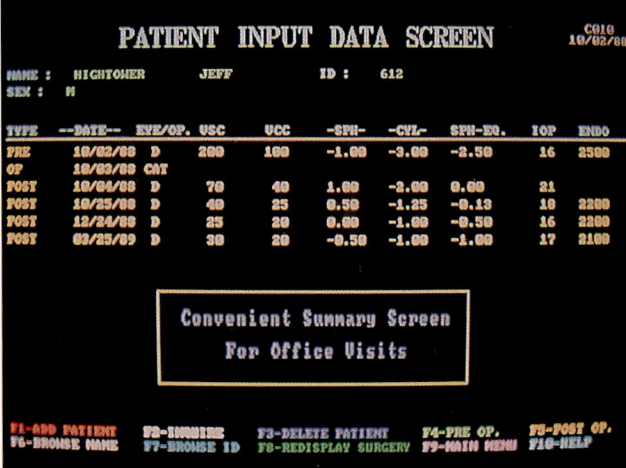
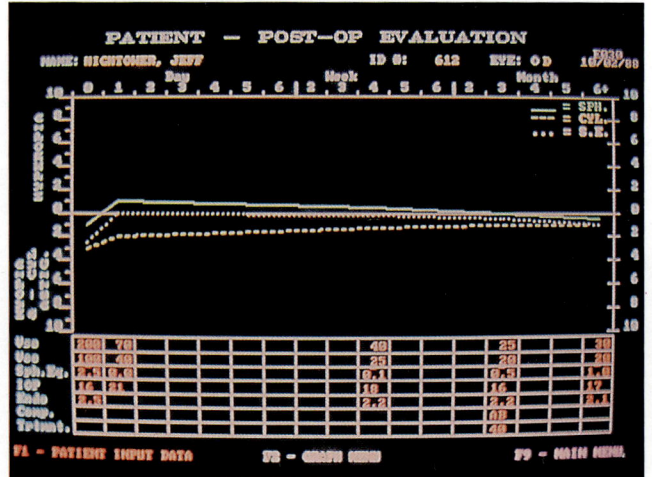

Figure 4.7 (Left) *A written evaluation screen showing the clinical course of a cataract patient.* **(Right)** *A graphic evaluation screen showing the clinical course of a cataract patient for six months. This graph allows easy evaluation of astigmatism and IOL power for an individual patient or a group of patients.*

Clinical Points to Consider

☛ Long-term astigmatism or IOL power is generally the factor that precludes excellent uncorrected visual acuity for postoperative cataract/IOL patients.

☛ Access to cataract/IOL surgical results enables the surgeon to adjust the IOL power calculation nomogram and surgical technique.

☛ Refractive surgery planned by a computer increases the consistency of radial and astigmatic keratotomy plans.

chapter 5

OCULAR SURGERY ANESTHESIOLOGY

EDWARD KANE, M.D.

Although the ophthalmologist is responsible for the outcome of ocular surgery, a well-coordinated operating room team (anesthesiologist or anesthetist, scrub nurse, and circulating nurse) helps insure a safe and successful surgical experience. With the available surgical techniques, facilities, and medications, the patient having anterior segment surgery under local anesthesia should be able to leave for home shortly after surgery. This chapter will describe how the anesthesiologist can contribute to the desired safety and success of the surgery.

Preoperative Considerations

NPO Policy

Many hospitals require that patients having surgery, under either general or local anesthesia, refrain from eating or drinking for at least eight hours prior to surgery. The difficulty with this rule is that the elderly cataract patient scheduled for surgery at 11:00 AM will not have eaten from bedtime the previous night (about 13 hours). Because the risks of aspiration during local anesthesia are not the same during general anesthesia, a more lenient policy of allowing a glass or two of juice or clear liquid up to within four hours of surgery seems appropriate. In fact, recent studies suggest that patients have emptier stomachs if they drink water two hours before surgery rather than six to eight hours before surgery.

Topical Medications

Immediately prior to anterior segment surgery, an antibiotic as well as medication to control pupil size is usually given. Mydriasis is necessary for cataract extraction, and Cyclogyl (cyclopentalate) 2% and Neo-Synephrine (phenylephrine) 2.5% or 10% provide the strongest, yet easiest to reverse, dilating combination. Pilocarpine 2% or 4% may be used if miosis is desired for phakic penetrating keratoplasty, trabeculectomy, or other procedures such as epikeratoplasty and lamellar corneal transplant, in which centration of the corneal graft on the visual axis is important. For secondary implantation of an anterior chamber intraocular lens (IOL), at which time an anterior vitrectomy may be necessary, the surgeon may wish to use the moderate mydriasis caused by the retrobulbar block and then create miosis with Miochol (acetylcholine) or Miostat (carbachol). Many surgeons prefer to include a form of corticosteroid and/or a nonsteroidal anti-inflammatory agent, such as Ocufen (flurbiprofen), in their topical medication regimen.

The preferred preoperative topical anesthetic is proparacaine (Ophthaine, Alcaine, AK-taine) because it does not sting after each application, and it does not cause the epithelium to become irregular. Anesthetic drops should be administered to both eyes. This serves a dual purpose. First, the patient will not feel successive medications applied to the operative eye. Second, administering the anesthetic to both eyes insures an absent blink reflex, which increases patient compliance during the retrobulbar or peribulbar injection. Topical medications should never be left with their tops off because this increases the chance of bacterial contamination.

The patient scheduled for the first surgery in the morning must be adequately dilated. To accomplish this, a mixture of antibiotic and dilating agents may be provided to be instilled at home by the patient on the day of surgery.

Intravenous Line

Several studies have concluded that the least enjoyable and, unfortunately, most memorable aspect of cataract surgery under local anesthesia is the pain associated with starting the intravenous (IV) line. The anesthesiologist or designee must develop a technique that allows for the most painless insertion of the IV catheter, since the patient can not yet be more fully sedated. A local skin wheal created by 0.5% Xylocaine (lidocaine) without epinephrine, administered through a 30-gauge needle, may help keep the pain at a minimum. Of course, a friendly, confident manner on the part of the anesthesiologist is an important factor while starting the IV line.

The patient should urinate before surgery. The IV line should be at a "keep open" rate when not needed for administering medication so that excessive amounts of fluid do not enter the patient's circulation. Alternatively, a heparin lock ("heplock") IV may be used to minimize both the amount of fluid administered and the cost of IV solution.

IV mannitol is usually employed for penetrating keratoplasty, secondary anterior chamber IOL implantation, and glaucoma filtering procedures because it shrinks the vitreous by pulling fluid into the hypertonic bloodstream by osmosis. It takes at least 20 minutes for IV mannitol to affect the vitreous. Rather than administer 500 cc of a 20% mannitol/normal saline combination over one-half to one hour, two 50 cc ampules of 25% mannitol administered via the IV line over two to three minutes will achieve the same effect without making the patient need to urinate or significantly changing blood pressure. Mannitol is a sugar that is not metabolized and is safe for use in diabetics.

Analgesia/Sedation/Amnesia

Once the IV line has been established, analgesia, sedation, and short-term amnesia may be accomplished using the appropriate agents. A combination of Sublimaze (fentanyl) or one of its congeners with similar action (Sufenta, Alfenta) and Versed (midazolam) causes the patient to be slightly detached, cooperative, and mildly amnestic during both the block and surgical procedure (Fig. 5.1). Some anesthesiologists feel that narcotics such as fentanyl should not be given to elderly patients; however, in small, judicious doses (i.e., fentayl 10 µg to 50 µg) respiratory depression and other undesirable side effects of narcotics are rarely encountered.

Midazolam has caused many instances of excessive sedation and respiratory depression in elderly patients, but almost always with high doses. For ocular anesthesia, 0.50 mg to 1.50 mg of Versed is generally all that is required. In small amounts, midazolam has great amnestic properties, which are apparent long before signs of clinical obtundation are present, i.e., slurred speech, disorientation, and the inability to cooperate or follow commands. Unwanted side effects occur at doses frequently given to patients undergoing endoscopy (i.e., almost 10.00 mg). Obviously, each patient requires gentle titration of these medications to achieve the desired effect.

Brevital (methohexital) is often used by anesthesiologists to sedate the patient before the anesthetic block; however, it makes patient cooperation impossible and does not cause sedation for the duration of the procedure. Similarly, Diprivan (propofol), a frequently used new agent, causes hypnosis and makes it impossible for patients to follow commands. Propofol can also cause significant hypo-tension in elderly patients.

Each anesthesiologist should develop a routine for providing local anesthesia that allows the patient undergoing ocular surgery to leave the facility shortly after the procedure without feeling drowsy or nauseated.

RETROBULBAR/PERIBULBAR

The debate between the pros and cons of retrobulbar and peribulbar anesthesia rages on in ophthalmic circles, and no attempt will be made to decide the issue in this chapter. Although peribulbar anesthesia is safer than retrobulbar anesthesia, I prefer retrobulbar because it is my perception that more complete anesthesia, lack of motility, and less ptosis is achieved more consistently than with peribulbar infiltration.

The pain associated with retrobulbar anesthesia usually occurs when penetrating the skin, which is rich in nerve fibers. The potential spaces be-tween the wall of the orbit, Tenon's capsule, and the globe allow fluid to be injected slowly and virtually without sensation. Therefore, the use of a 1¼ inch 27-gauge needle to administer the retro-bulbar anesthetic is advantageous, since quick penetration through the skin causes minimal sensation. The surgeon should be sure to palpate the inferior orbital rim and displace the globe slightly upward with the index finger of the free hand to create a safe space for the needle as it passes the equator of the globe (Fig. 5.2). A blunt 23-gauge needle (Atkinson) hurts as it passes through the skin and is more likely to tear an orbital blood vessel than a 27-gauge needle is liable to puncture one because orbital blood vessels are loose and tend to roll away from contact.

The patient should be asked to look with the nonoperative eye at a target held by an assistant.

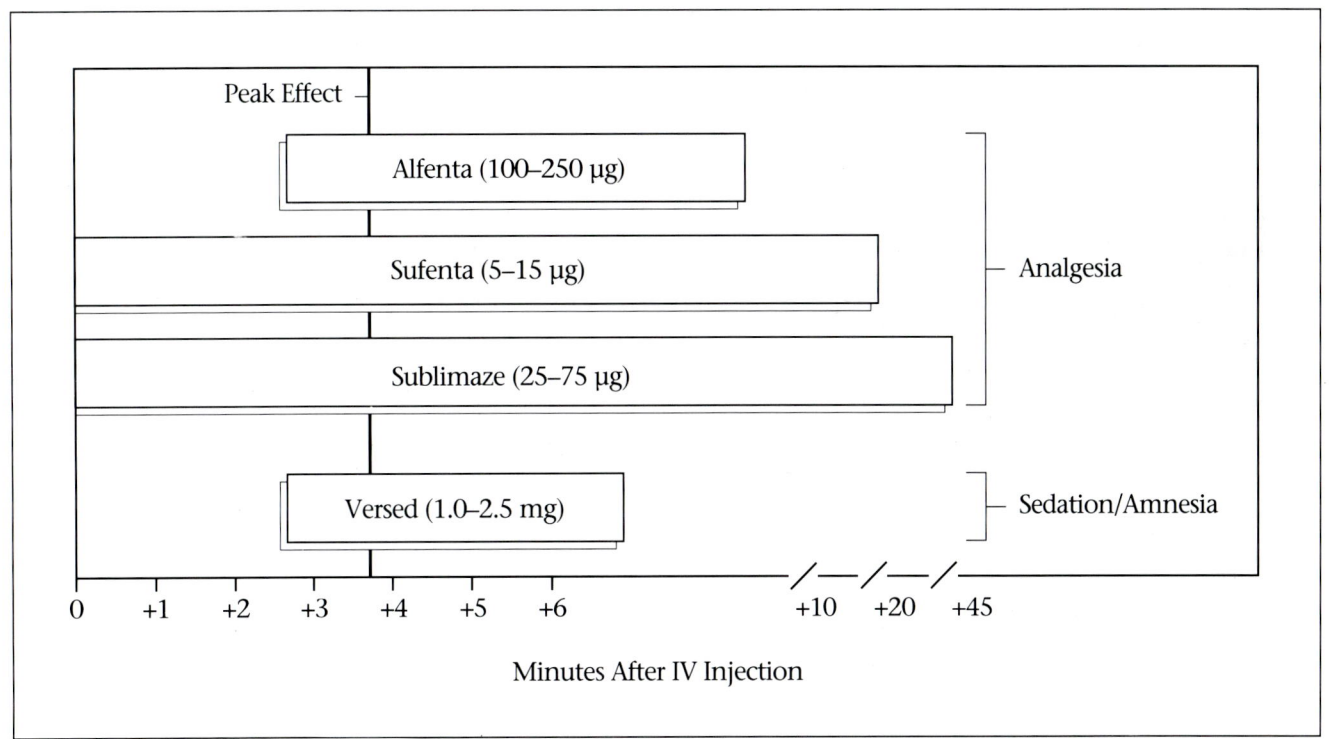

Figure 5.1 *Well-timed administration of sedatives and narcotics will enable simultaneous peak effects.*

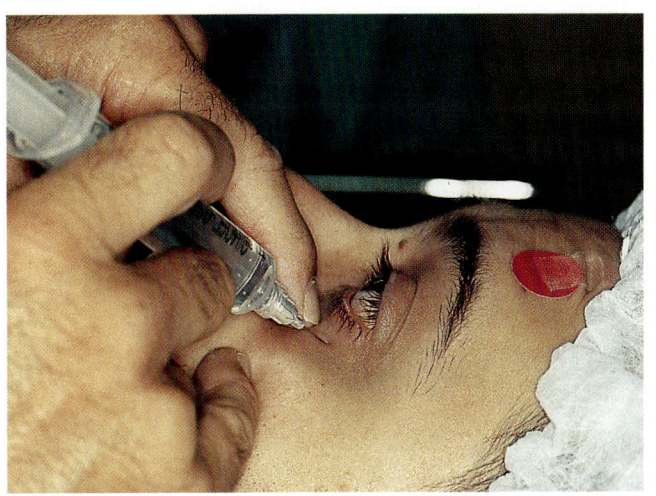

Figure 5.2 *A retrobulbar block being initiated with a 27-gauge needle. Notice that the index finger of the left hand displacing the globe superiorly to define a space between the inferior aspect of the globe and the inferior orbital rim.*

This will put the operative eye in the proper position for the retrobulbar block. In the past, the favored position was "up and in," but many surgeons now feel that a straight-ahead position minimizes the chance of the needle engaging the optic nerve. Only the person performing the block should give instructions so that the patient is not confused by multiple voices and commands.

A lid block, which affects the superior portion of the seventh nerve, may be achieved by injection of an anesthetic agent near the lateral canthus (O'Brien, van Lint, Iliff) or behind the ear between the stylomastoid process and the mandible (Nadbath), where the combined branches of the seventh nerve exit the skull (Fig. 5.3). The Nadbath is favored because it does not cause lid or facial edema; however, it may not be effective if the patient has had a face lift, since the scar behind the ear may prevent the anesthetic agent from affecting the seventh nerve as it courses upward around the front of the ear. In that case, the Iliff block—three injections of the anesthetic agent, 1.00 cc to 2.00 cc, subdermally through a skin wheal at the lateral canthus—may be used. One injection should be directed posteriorly toward the upper portion of the earlobe, one angled downward, and one angled upward. The anesthetic is injected as the long 27-gauge needle is withdrawn. About 3.00 cc to 5.00 cc of anesthetic is used for the combined injections.

For the Nadbath block, 5.00 cc of a 50/50 mixture of 0.5% Marcaine (bupivicaine) and 2% Xylocaine is injected behind the ear using a 25-gauge short (5/8-inch) needle aimed at the lateral canthus of the ipsilateral eye but directed across the skull (Fig. 5.4). A swelling in front of the ear indicates an accumulation of the anesthetic agent that will affect the seventh nerve as it courses up and around the ear. The Nadbath block should be performed very slowly to minimize pain.

At most operating facilities, surgeons perform their own blocks, but at others the anesthesiologists or anesthetists are responsible for administering them. Blocking two patients before the

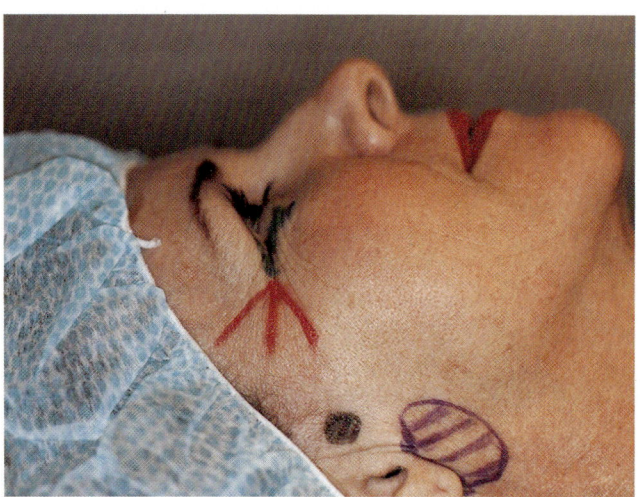

Figure 5.3 *A representation of various lid blocks: green, van Lint; black, O'Brien; red, Iliff; purple, accumulation of anesthetic agent from Nadbath block.*

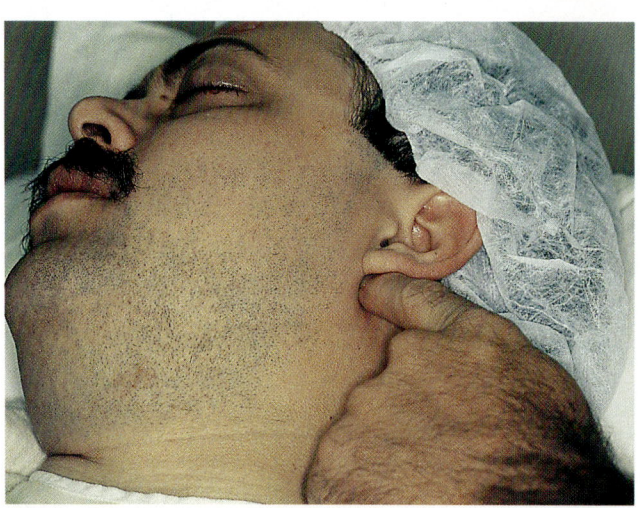
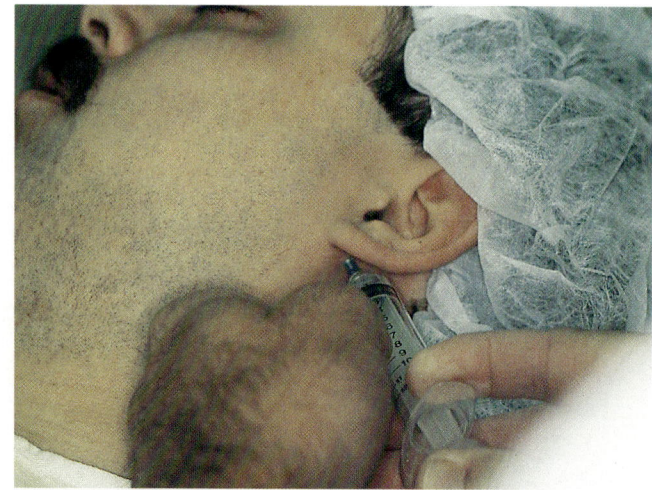

Figure 5.4 (Left) *Identify the space between the stylomastoid process and the mandible for the Nadbath injection.* (Right) *The Nadbath block is performed with a short 25-gauge needle.*

first surgery will allow the second patient to be ready immediately and the staff to stay one patient ahead. Each patient will be able to receive medication, the block, and the pressure balloon in a controlled and relaxed fashion.

The anesthesiologist must be prepared for a vagal response or activation of the oculocardiac reflex during the retrobulbar block, characterized by a sharp drop in the patient's pulse rate and blood pressure, nausea, and faintness. Treatment consists of increasing the IV flow rate, lowering the head of the bed and elevating the foot to restore blood flow to the brain, and administering IV atropine (0.50 mg to 1.00 mg) to increase the heart rate. Supplemental oxygen is useful. A complete retrobulbar or peribulbar block supposedly protects a patient from a vagal response initiated by anterior segment surgery.

Ocular Pressure Device

A pressure device that administers about 30 mm Hg of external pressure to the globe insures a soft eye during surgery. Six to eight minutes allows for adequate aqueous to be expelled from the anterior segment. In cases of severe glaucoma, a pressure device should not be used, since even a slight increase in the intraocular pressure might cause a venous or arterial occlusion. Of course, an ocular pressure device is not indicated in cases of traumatic ocular perforation or suspected perforation.

A pressure device should be placed on the eye after the anesthetic block. It is fruitless, and also painful, to soften the eye by means of a pressure device and then inject anesthetic fluid behind the eye for the block, again raising the intraocular pressure.

Blood Pressure

Once the patient is in the operating room in the proper surgical position, the patient's blood pressure should be noted. The ophthalmologist should know what systolic limit is acceptable, since high systolic blood pressure may cause unexpulsive hemorrhage. The limit is usually from 160 mm Hg to 170 mm Hg.

A new agent that reduces blood pressure is labetalol (Normodyne, Trandate). It is a nonselective beta blocker and selective alpha blocker. The systolic pressure is reduced more than the diastolic pressure and the heart rate is also lowered. The onset of action is about two minutes with a peak affect of five minutes and a half life of about six hours.

Apresoline hydralazine is more potent agent for lowering blood pressure, but it can cause a sudden reduction in systolic and diastolic blood pressure levels as well as orthostatic hypotension after the procedure. Apresoline can also cause a reflex tachycardia, which is undesirable in patients who often have clinical or subclinical cardiac disease.

A new agent, Brevibloc (esmolol), can be used in patients with tachycardia and high blood pressure. Brevibloc is a beta-selective adrenergic blocking agent with a very short duration of action–the half life is only nine minutes.

Intraoperative Considerations

Patient Position and Draping

The patient is placed on the operative bed or reclining chair. The top of the head should be aligned with the top edge of the bed. A bend in the bed at the knees or a pillow placed under the knees will prevent discomfort in the lumbar area of the back and make the patient generally more comfortable. A device (neck support) that provides support *under the neck* so that the head tilts backward and the airway stays open is preferable to a headrest (Fig. 5.5). Headrests that limit

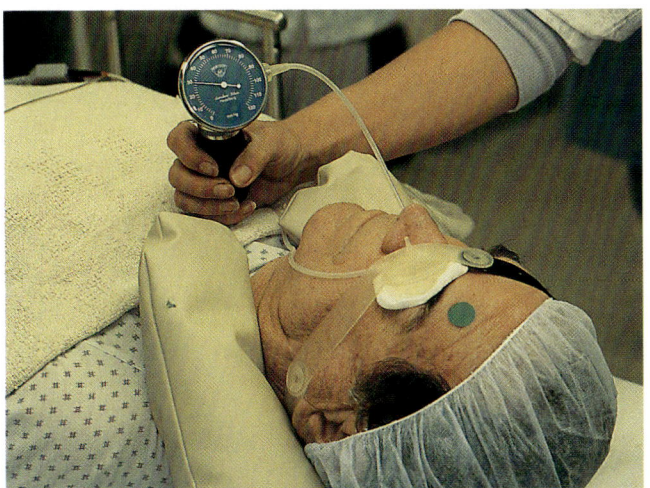

Figure 5.5 *The patient's ocular pressure device is about to be removed and the left eye prepared for surgery. A neck support makes the patient comfortable, opens the airway, and elevates the chin, which increases accessibility for the surgeon. When air is aspirated from the neck rest, it is firm yet comfortable and stabilizes the patient's head.*

the lateral motion of the head and even provide music or messages to the patient via earphones are available.

At this time it is useful for the anesthesiologist to provide the patient with a nonverbal method of communication (for example, raising a finger or squeezing a hand). This will allow the patient to be attended to by the anesthesiologist, who will be asking most of the questions, and the patient will be less likely to move his or her head, which happens instinctively while talking. Also, the patient can be instructed that the surgeon will use the patient's name when addressing the patient to avoid confusion as to whether the discussion is among the operating team only or includes the patient.

The surgeon's draping style should allow an open airway and easy access to to the patient's mouth (Fig. 5.6). Covering the patient's mouth with a sheet and then forcing air/oxygen under this claustrophobic tent is pointless and limits the anesthesiologist's view and access to the mouth. (In fact, the surgeon and anesthesiologist should lie on the operating table with the ocular drapes placed in various ways so they can experience firsthand the advantages and disadvantages of the proposed methods.)

The operating room should be arranged to provide the best service possible. If the microscope stand is nearby, which is common, the anesthesiologist must take care not to use it as a footrest. Even the slightest movement of the base will disrupt the surgeon's field of view.

Blood Pressure Cuff

The major goal of preparing an eye for anterior segment surgery is to achieve and maintain low intraocular pressure. When the stomach muscles tense, the intraocular pressure rises by the Valsalva mechanism.

Patient movement or talking can cause changes in the eye that are noticeable under the microscope. Using an automatic blood pressure cuff during a critical time when the eye is open (a corneal transplant, for example) is extremely undesirable—the surprise and discomfort caused by the constricting cuff may result in a significant Valsalva mechanism. If the patient has stable vital signs, the anesthesiologist should monitor the patient using nonverbal clues during the vulnerable portions of the procedure and avoid methods (blood pressure cuff) that create excessive external physical stimuli.

Sedation/Coughing

The anesthesiologist is often in the best position to judge the patient's level of discomfort. The surgeon and anesthesiologist should prearrange the method by which the anesthesiologist will administer medication. If a surgeon notices a gradual increase in patient anxiety and movement, an attentive anesthesiologist will have noticed it as well and asked the surgeon if action is warranted. Judicious doses of Versed, with its short duration of onset and action, is usually the first drug of choice for intraoperative anxiety. Many times, all that's needed to solve the problem is a reassuring

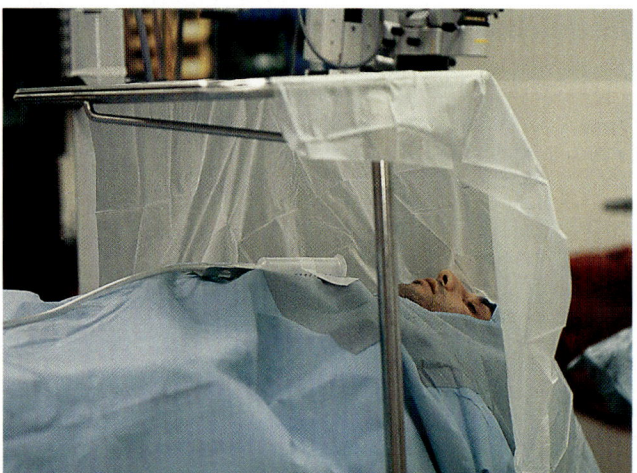

Figure 5.6 *This draping method allows the patient ample space and the anesthesiologist easy access to the patient's airway.*

word from the surgeon or anesthesiologist. Telling a patient to lie still in an increasingly loud voice will not help.

If the patient has a propensity to cough, the safest approach is to keep the patient as awake as possible so that clear communication between the patient and surgeon can be maintained. Small IV doses of narcotic may help if coughing develops intraoperatively. Preoperatively, if the patient cannot abstain from coughing, deep IV sedation and/or general anesthesia can be used. Deep IV sedation can be quite risky, resulting in respiratory arrest, prolonged sedation, and disorientation. In addition, the patient may wake suddenly during the procedure and move or cough violently because of a collection of secretions, saliva, or postnasal drip. Deep IV sedation should be administered by anesthesiologists who are experienced with the technique and have the appropriate monitors available. A pulse oximeter should be used on *all* ocular anesthetic cases.

Postoperative Considerations

Postoperative treatment should facilitate the transition from the operating center to home. After the eye has been patched, the patient's vital signs should be checked and the IV line removed. The patient should then get dressed or take off the jump suit provided at the surgical facility.

The surgeon may give cataract patients Neptazane (methazolamide) or Diamox (acetazolamide) in order to control postoperative intraocular pressure. If Marcaine is used in the block, the patients will probably not experience pain for about eight hours after the block. Pain medication may be dispensed after this time if necessary.

The staff should review the postoperative instructions with the patient (i.e., activity limitations, sleeping position) and what to do for pain or other problems. The patient should be given an appointment for the following day. Since patients will be hungry, juice and a light snack should be offered by the staff. Hot beverages, such as tea and coffee, should not be served immediately because lip sensation and movement may be dulled by the anesthesia.

Conclusion

The performance of virtually all anterior segment surgery on an outpatient basis has been made possible by improved surgical and anesthetic techniques. Anesthesia via a local block and IV sedation has made surgery safer and less unpleasant for the patient. A safe and successful surgical experience depends not only on new technology and the opthalmologist but also on the abilities and attitudes of the anesthesiology and nursing staffs.

Clinical Points to Consider

☛ Preoperative medications that induce short-term analgesia, sedation, and amnesia are desirable.

☛ Often the most painful steps of an ocular operation performed under local anesthesia are starting the IV line and performing the lid block.

☛ A neck support, rather than a head rest, and an appropriate draping method greatly facilitate ocular surgery as well as insure patient comfort and safety.

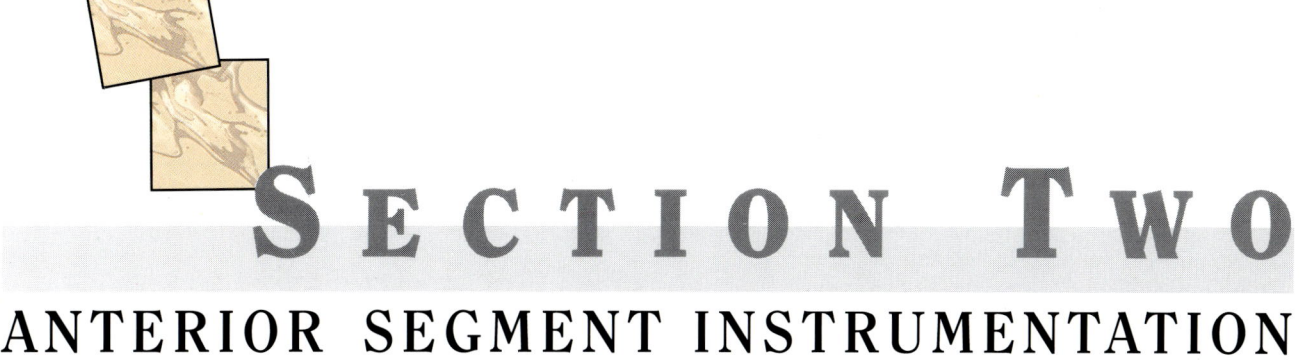

SECTION TWO
ANTERIOR SEGMENT INSTRUMENTATION

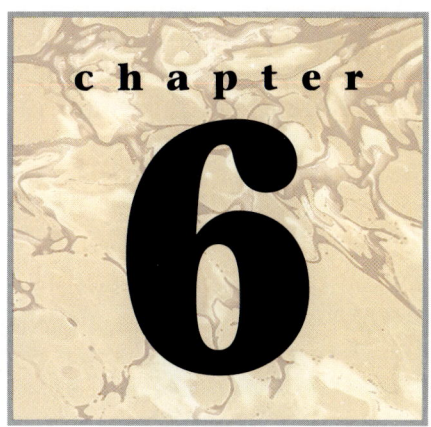

INSTRUMENTS FOR ANTERIOR SEGMENT SURGERY

MICHELLE GLOSSIP   LEE T. NORDAN, M.D.

Ophthalmic surgery is continually being revolutionized by surgeons who develop and perfect surgical techniques, which often require new or modified instruments. The surgeon and the instrument manufacturer's skilled craftspeople work together to create instruments that will facilitate these special surgical techniques and procedures. A new instrument may represent a complete change from the previous model or only a minor change in detail. The changed characteristics may involve material, overall dimension, handle design, tip design, or port location.

Over the past two decades there have been notable changes as basic instrument designs have developed into the elegant microsurgical micro-instrumentation needed to perform the most delicate of anterior segment procedures. Currently, the ophthalmic surgeon may select from over 2000 surgical instruments, depending on the procedure being performed and individual preference.

Each instrument is designed for a specific function, its special features usually determining its use; however, many instruments have multiple uses, and a surgeon may opt to use one instrument for several functions. A surgical instrument is often named for the surgeon who designed it, or the hospital or university where it originated. As an instrument is modified, a second or third name may be added.

Instruments are manufactured by various methods, ranging from mass production to handcrafting. Old-world craftsmanship of instruments was brought to the United States over 200 years ago. The instrument maker, a master craftsperson who understands metal working, handcrafting, and a variety of manufacturing machinery, devotes five years to an apprenticeship in order to qualify as a surgical instrument maker. There are no schools in the United States that teach this fine art.

Surgical instruments vary in quality, material, and workmanship. Instruments that are made of inferior materials or are the product of poor workmanship will not withstand normal use and will affect the surgeon's ability to perform surgery. Currently, there are no agencies in the United States that set or review standards of quality for materials, accuracy, or the copying or reproduction of instruments from the original designer and manufacturer. The formation of a standards committee, which would represent a concerted effort by physicians and the ophthalmic industry to standardize ophthalmic instrumentation, would be an important milestone in the advancement of ophthalmic instrumentation.

The surgical instrument is the means by which the skills of the surgeon are optimized for the patient's benefit; thus, a thorough knowledge of anterior segment surgical instrument concepts and designs is most important for the anterior segment surgeon. This chapter brings the design and function of anterior segment surgical instrumentation to the surgeon's attention and describes major anterior segment instrument categories, including nomenclature, working end, handle, function, materials, and manufacturer. Also, a few suggestions covering basic instrument selection and use will be made.

Materials

In the manufacture of surgical instruments, a variety of materials are necessary (e.g., stainless steel, titanium, plastics) to produce the many types and designs required. Stainless steel is the most commonly used material, although carbon steel and titanium, which are processed and heat-treated to insure quality and durability, are also used often. Instruments are generally finished in either a bright, smooth, polished chrome or a sandblasted satin. In addition, some instruments feature carbide tips, jaws, or blades that provide extra strength, gripping ability, or long-lasting edges.

Titanium is lightweight, noncorrosive, reduces glare under the microscope, and retains alignment. However, stainless steel retains a "feel" that is most comfortable for the majority of surgeons and provides a finer cutting edge for quality surgical scissors. Plastics may provide new capabilities for instrument manufacture.

Design

A hand-held ophthalmic surgical instrument used for anterior segment surgery has three important parts: the handle, the shaft, and the working end (Fig. 6.1). This section will describe the attributes of various handle and working-end designs of some basic instruments.

Handle

Length. A microsurgical anterior segment instrument must be short enough to clear the end of the microscope, which is usually about eight inches from the eye, and long enough to provide the surgeon with a stable grasp. Most instruments are between 8.00 cm and 13.00 cm in length. A stable grasp is best achieved with the rear end of the handle resting in the anatomical snuffbox between the base of the thumb and the tissue proximal to the base of the second digit (Fig. 6.2). Virtually all anterior segment surgery instruments should be held like a pencil to allow for ease of manipulation with maximal support. Short instruments do not allow for maximal stability (Fig. 6.3).

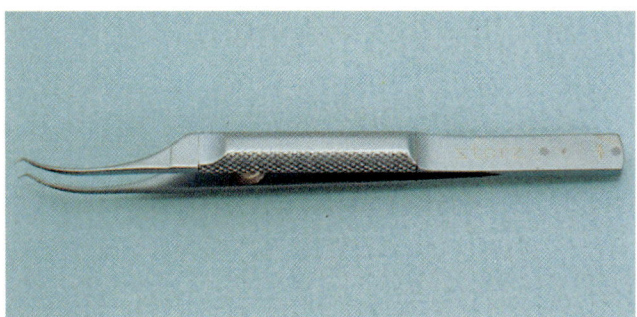

Figure 6.1 *Working end* (left), *connected to the shaft, which is connected to the handle* (right).

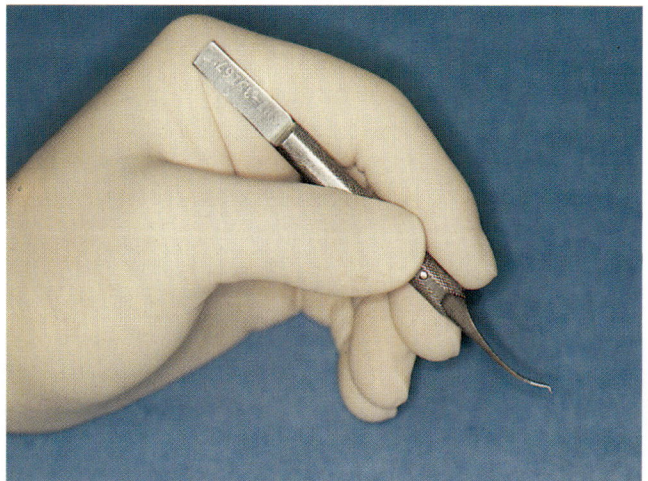

Figure 6.2 *A stable platform, which provides excellent instrument control, can be created by three-point fixation, involving the fingers and the anatomical snuffbox of the hand.*

Shape. A round handle allows for ease of rotation with the fingers only, while a flat handle needs pronation of the entire wrist. However, the flat handle provides a convenient reference point by feel since the surgeon knows the alignment of the working end of the instrument relative to the flat aspect of the handle. A handle that combines a flat and round shape offers the advantages of both configurations.

Squeeze Action. The most delicate control for a forceps or needle holder is obtained by a direct squeeze action that causes closure when pressure is exerted. The instrument should have enough closure resistance to allow for optimal control but obviously not too much resistance, which might cause fatigue.

Scissors have two opposing blades that are open while at rest and closed when the handle is squeezed together. Certain forceps, such as those designed for foreign body extraction or intraocular lens (IOL) implantation, use a cross-action squeeze handle that is in the closed position when at rest. This design allows for manipulation of the forceps without the need to exert additional finger pressure.

Working End
TOOTHED FORCEPS

Teeth. The grasping end of a toothed forceps uses either interdigitating teeth (Fig. 6.4) or opposing single teeth (Pierse) that are designed to minimize tissue damage but may provide slightly less fixation of the tissue (Fig. 6.5). The teeth of an anterior segment microsurgical instrument are usually 0.12 mm in length and may protrude from the shaft of the instrument at either a right angle or an obtuse angle (Fig. 6.6). Under the microscope, it is evident that 0.30-mm and 0.50-mm teeth may create unnecessary tissue damage, except for tasks such as grasping a rectus muscle for placement of a fixation suture.

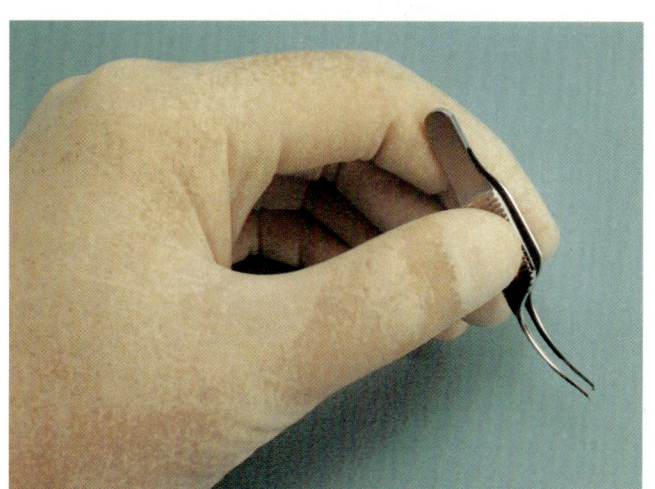

Figure 6.3 *Two-point fixation of an instrument may not provide for optimal control.*

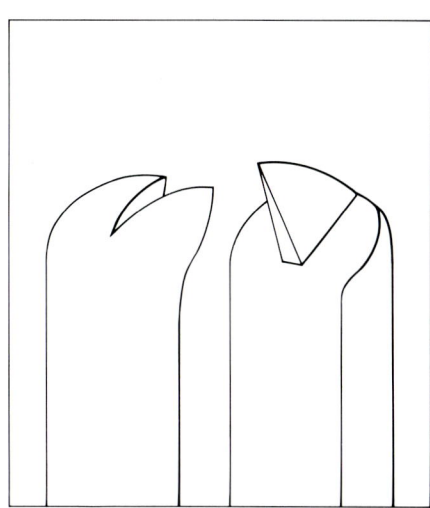

Figure 6.4 *The one-into-two pattern of interdigitating teeth is the standard of toothed anterior segment ophthalmic instruments.*

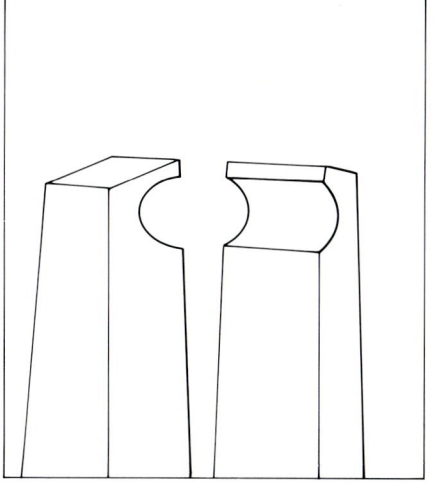

Figure 6.5 *Pierse forceps use opposing flat surfaces for fixation and a hollowed out area near the point of fixation to accommodate tissue.*

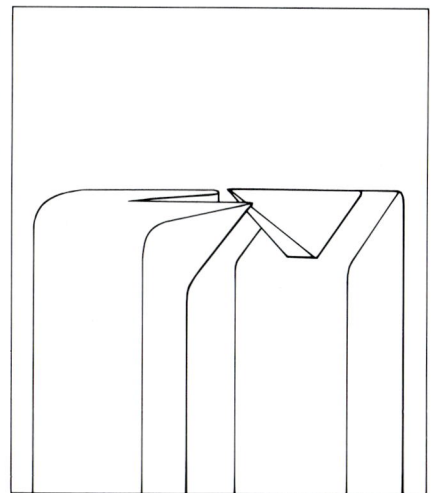

Figure 6.6 *Teeth protruding at a right angle from the shaft. (In Fig. 6.4 the teeth protrude at an obtuse angle.)*

Angle. An angle at the end of the instrument shaft just preceding the teeth can allow for easier manipulation and more effective function when working at various angles in the anterior segment. A straight shaft may be appropriate for anterior chamber work as well as wound manipulation when the area of concern is directly in front of the surgeon.

The most common form of toothed forceps used in anterior segment surgery is the Colibri forceps, which combines 0.12-mm teeth with a tying platform (Fig. 6.7). (Colibri means little bird in Italian and refers to the winged shape of the original handle.) A Colibri forceps can be used to grasp and control corneal and scleral tissue, and it is used during the suturing process. Also, the small 0.12-mm teeth are useful for grasping the iris during peripheral iridectomy and positioning the conjunctiva. Some surgeons, however, believe that only smooth forceps should be used for manipulation of the conjunctiva during filtering procedures so that no unnecessary holes are placed in the conjunctiva. In addition, the Colibri forceps may be rotated 180 degrees and used to grasp a needle after suture placement when controlling the needle with the needle holder is awkward (Fig. 6.8).

Instruments

SMOOTH FORCEPS

One of the major uses of smooth forceps in anterior segment surgery is to tie sutures. Tying for-

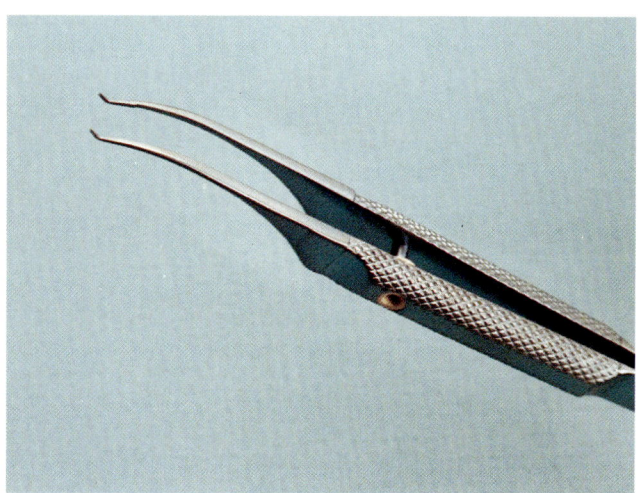

Figure 6.7 *A Colibri forceps, which combines 0.12-mm teeth with a tying forceps. The angled working end enables the surgeon to grasp tissue from a wide range of angles.*

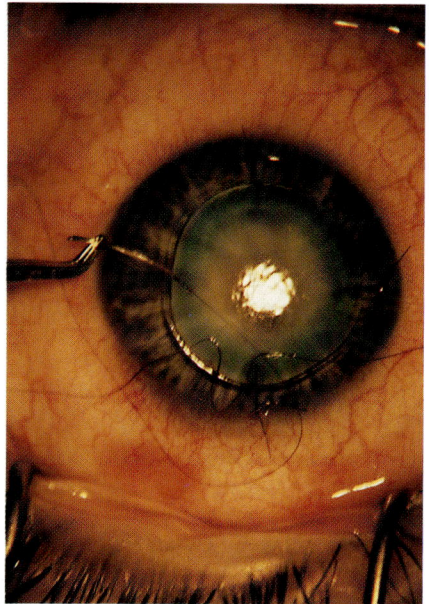

Figure 6.8 *A Colibri forceps pulling a suture needle through its track during a myopic keratomileusis procedure. A right handed surgeon might find it awkward to use a needle holder to perform this task without damaging the point of the needle.*

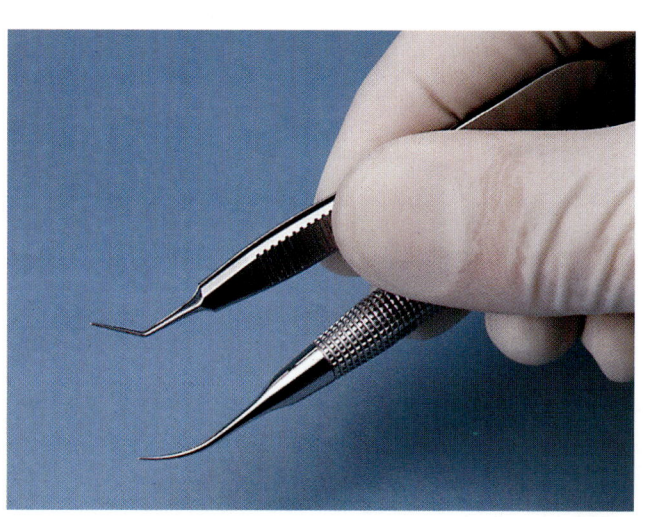

Figure 6.9 *Straight, angled, or curved forceps may be used for tying fine suture. Usually, a set of tying forceps has one straight and one curved forceps. Curved tying forceps (bottom) allow for better visibility of the tips of the forceps than do the angled McPherson forceps (top) since the straight end of an angled forceps may block visibility of the tip when positioned between the tip of the instrument and the microscope ocular. Angled forceps, such as long and short McPherson forceps, are very useful for manipulating tissue and other objects within the anterior chamber.*

ceps are often used in pairs—a straight forceps and a curved or angled forceps. A gentle curve at the working end provides greater visibility than an angled end. The curved or angled tying forceps is usually held in the dominant hand during knot tying, and the curve or angle allows for easier capture of the suture as it is looped around the instrument (Fig. 6.9).

The width of the tying forceps must be small enough to allow for easy capture of fine 10-0 and 11-0 nylon suture but not so narrow or pointed that it can cause kinking and potential break points in vulnerable sutures (Fig. 6.10), especially when a running suture is being tightened and multiple regrasping of the suture may take place.

Angled McPherson forceps (long and short) are fine, smooth forceps with a bend in the shaft 6.00 mm to 10.00 mm from the end. These forceps are excellent for anterior chamber work since they can fit through a small wound and still be opened and closed (Fig. 6.11).

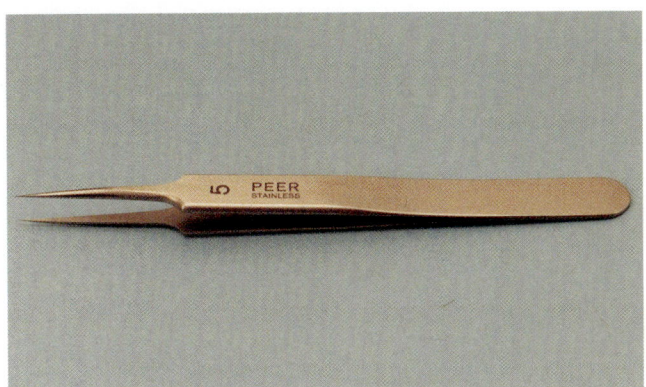

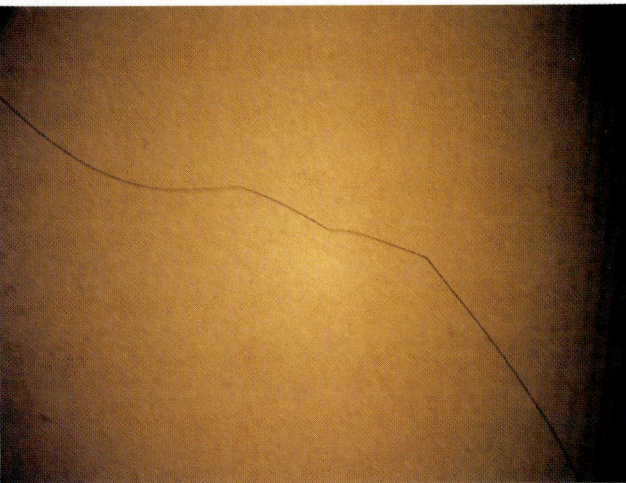

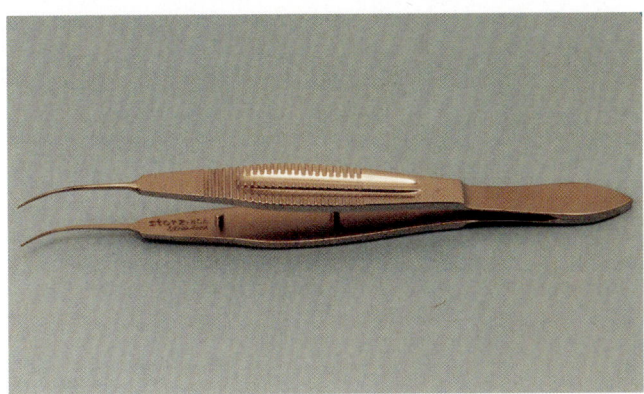

Figure 6.10 *Excessive pressure transmitted through the very narrow tips of a smooth forceps, such as jeweler's forceps* **(upper left)**, *may create a kink in thin, nylon suture. The kinks made in 10-0 nylon suture* **(right)** *by improper manipulation with pointed tying forceps are weak spots that may break unexpectedly. The tips of the tying forceps* **(lower left)** *are slightly blunted and broader than those of the jeweler's forceps. Suture should always be grasped with the inner edges of the tying forceps parallel to the suture.*

Figure 6.11 *McPherson forceps have a long, narrow working end and are useful for manipulating tissue inside the anterior chamber.*

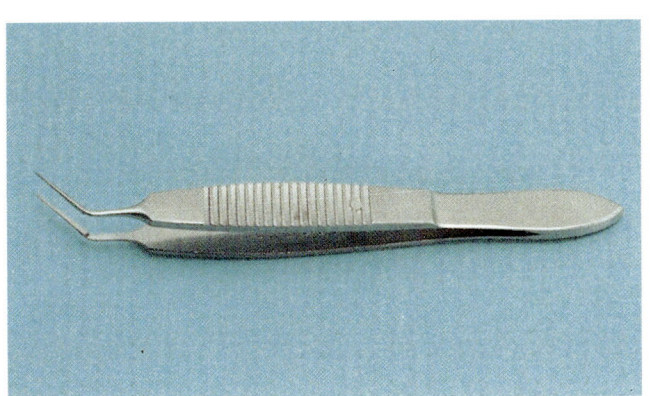

NEEDLE HOLDER

The jaws of the microscopic needle holder must be fine enough not to distort the small curved needles they grasp but wide enough to provide adequate fixation of the needle so that it does not wobble during suture placement. The straight outer jaw of a needle holder must make contact with a curved needle at only one point, if the needle is not to be distorted (Fig. 6.12). Ideally, the jaws of the needle holder should conform to the shape of the tying forceps as much as possible so that the needle holder can be used for tying fine sutures as well (Fig. 6.13).

The jaws of a microscopic needle holder may be straight or curved. The curved needle holder is useful when the surgeon is working at locations other than directly ahead. On the other hand, when a straight needle holder grasps a needle, the

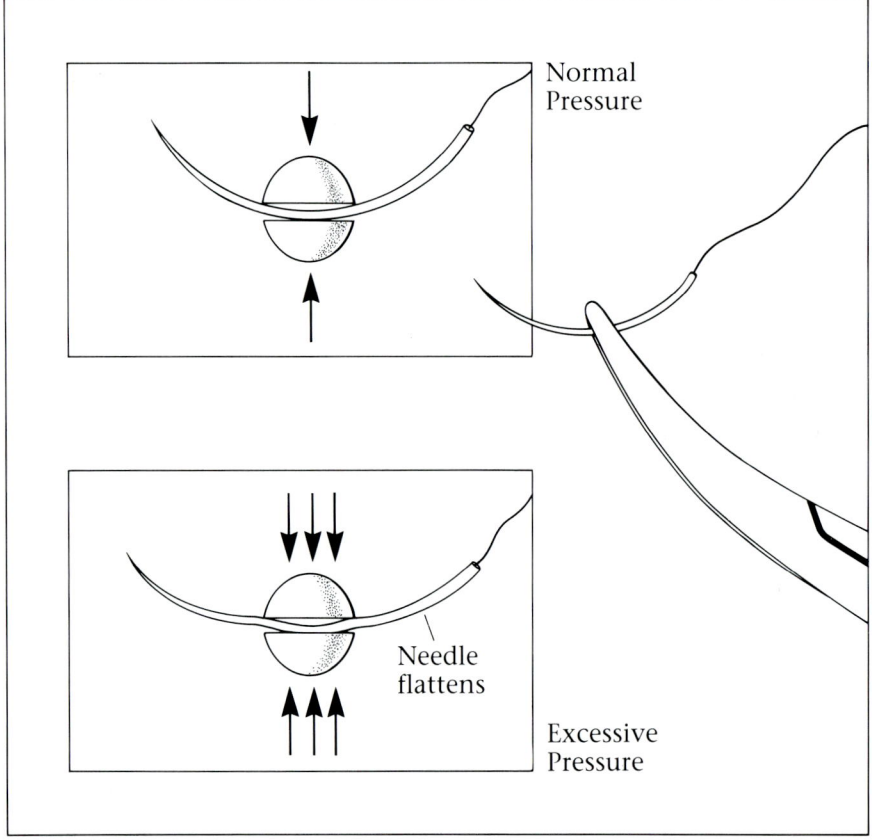

Figure 6.12 *A diagram showing how the flat edges of a needle holder fixate a curved needle at three points. Excessive pressure will bend the needle.*

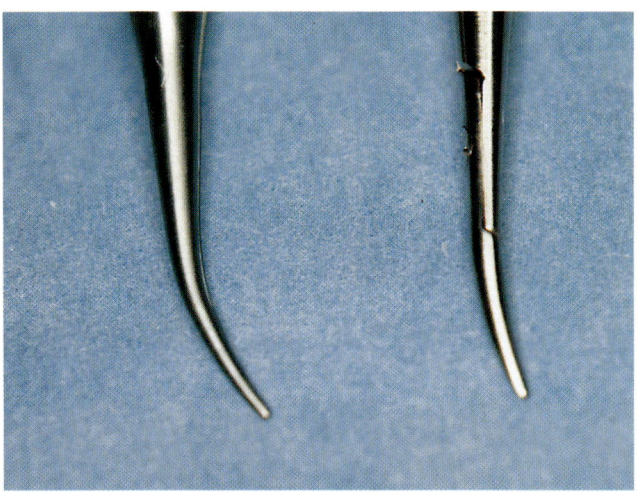

Figure 6.13 *The shape of the jaws of a tying forceps* (left) *and a needle holder* (right) *may be similar. The needle holder and the Colibri forceps may be used together for both placing and tying suture, which is more efficient than using different sets of instruments for these two tasks.*

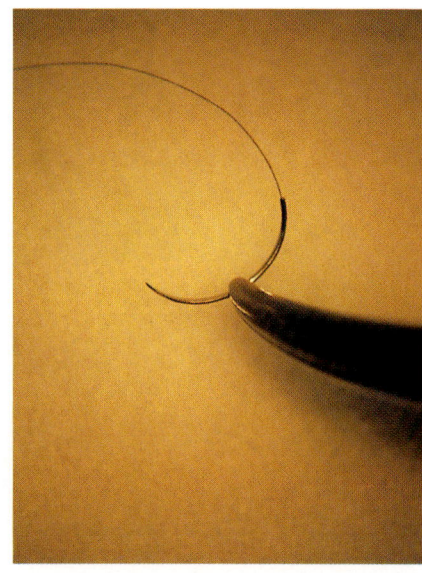

Figure 6.14 *A curved needle should be grasped at its center by the needleholder.*

needle holder is always properly positioned for the next suture, but a curved needle holder must be reoriented. Also, good microscopic surgical technique demands the use of a nonlocking needle holder to avoid the tissue distortion caused by needle movement as the surgeon attempts to unlock the needle holder after placing each suture. The needle should be grasped at its center by the needle holder for maximum control during the initial pass of the needle (Fig. 6.14).

SCISSORS

Conjunctival scissors should have slightly blunted points and some curve so that there is no danger of injuring the globe during dissection. Conjunctival scissors may also have millimeter markings that can aid the surgeon in judging conjunctival and scleral incisions (Fig. 6.15). It has become a trend to use scissors smaller than the traditional Westcott scissors for conjunctival work because they are easier to view under the microscope and are better for the small peritomies necessary for small cataract wounds.

Corneoscleral scissors have a lower blade outside the upper blade, which creates a beveled incision, while corneal scissors have the lower blade inside the upper blade, which creates a vertical wound during corneal transplantation (Fig. 6.16).

Vannas scissors are extremely fine scissors with narrow blades that can be placed into the anterior chamber and operated through a very small incision. Vannas scissors may be curved or straight (Fig. 6.17).

DIAMOND BLADES

During the last several years, the trifaceted diamond blade has emerged as a very popular and useful instrument for creating a corneoscleral groove and dissecting a scleral flap for a trabeculectomy or a phacoemulsification wound. The

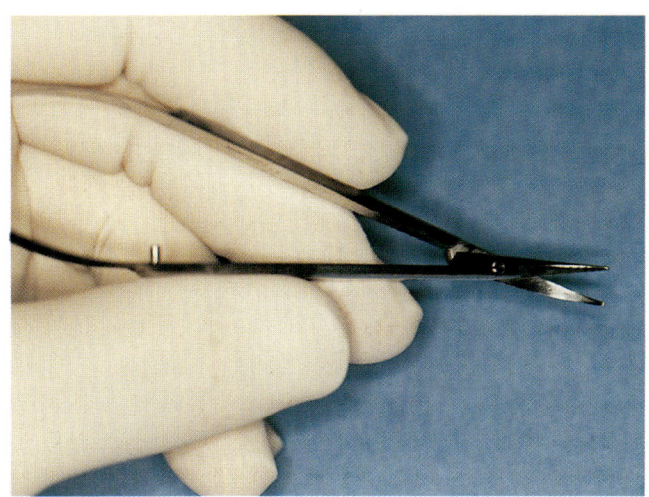

Figure 6.15 *A Shepard scissors has lines along the blade that mark off six millimeters in one-millimeter increments.*

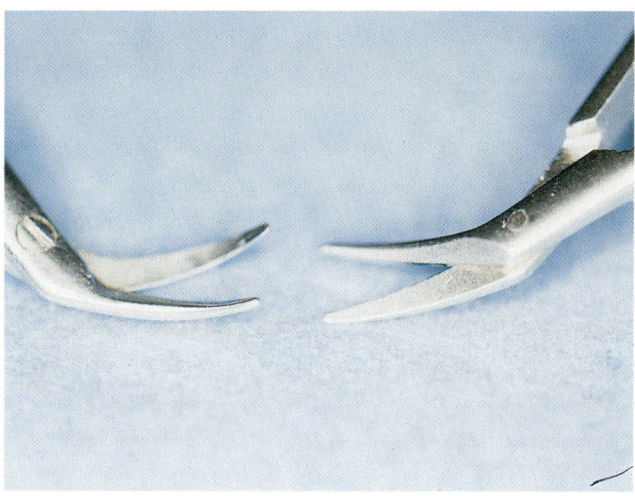

Figure 6.16 (Right) *Corneoscleral scissors are constructed with the lower blade outside the upper blade in order to create the beveled incision desired for cataract surgery.* (Left) *Corneal scissors have the lower blade inside the upper blade to create the perpendicular incision desired for penetrating keratoplasty.*

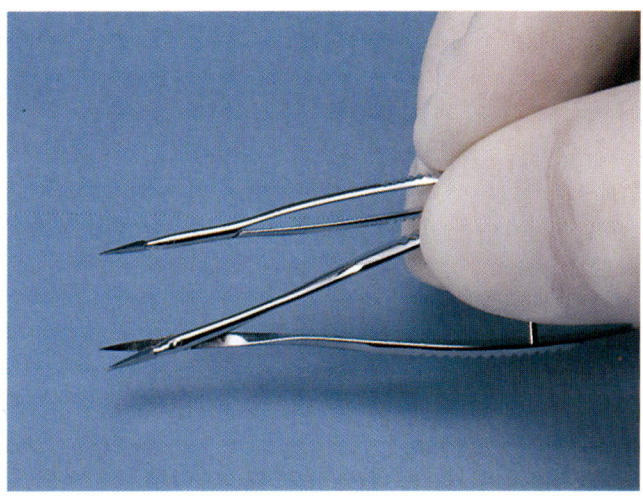

Figure 6.17 *Vannas scissors are very delicate scissors used inside the anterior chamber. The shaft narrows at the pivot of the blades to minimize fluid loss from the anterior chamber while the blades are activated.*

blade has three unequal edges, which enable the surgeon to create grooves with the angle between the edges and to dissect with either lateral edge (Fig. 6.18).

Most surgeons control metal blades by tactile and visual feedback. A high-quality diamond blade is so sharp that there is virtually no tactile feedback, and the surgeon must learn to control the trifaceted blade through visual clues only. It is not uncommon for a diamond blade to last through 600 to 800 operations, thereby making these exquisite instruments very cost effective.

CAPSULORHEXIS INSTRUMENTATION

Capsulorhexis has become the preferred method of anterior capsulostomy for phacoemulsification. Virtually all surgeons use either a cystotome or forceps or both to control the anterior capsule while performing capsulorhexis.

Capsulorhexis forceps, commonly referred to as Utrata forceps, have a long, thin working end that terminates with a small right-angled portion for grasping the capsule.

The original Kelman cystotome designed for anterior capsulotomy is a 23-guage shaft with a curved tip. The sharp edge facing the surgeon can be used to cut the capsule, and the two flat lateral sides create enough resistance to tear and manipulate the capsule. Cystotomes created by bending the tip of a needle have sharp lateral edges and flat surfaces facing toward and away from the surgeon.

A cystotome designed by Michael Blumenthal, M.D., has a distal end that is bent backward 90 degrees and then rotated 90 degrees to produce a configuration that allows for increased control of the anterior capsule during capsulorhexis (Fig. 6.19).

SPECULUM

The Kratz-Barraquer wire lid speculum provides blepharostasis for cataract/IOL implantation,

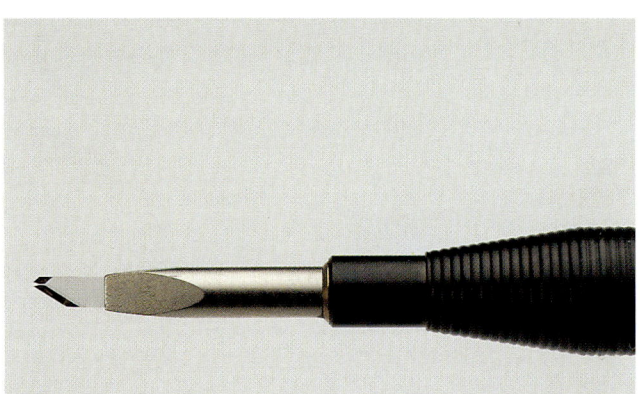

Figure 6.18 (Left) *A trifacet diamond blade can be used for making a corneoscleral groove or creating a scleral flap.* **(Right)** *The ASICO trifacet diamond blade allows*

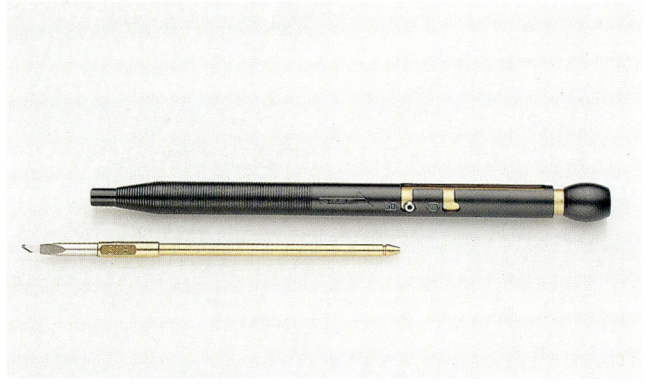

the stylus and blade to be removed from the handle so that replacement blades can be changed easily and independently from the handle.

Figure 6.19 *The tip of the Visitec cystotome has a backward bend and a 90-degree twist to allow for better control of the anterior capsule during capsulorhexis.*

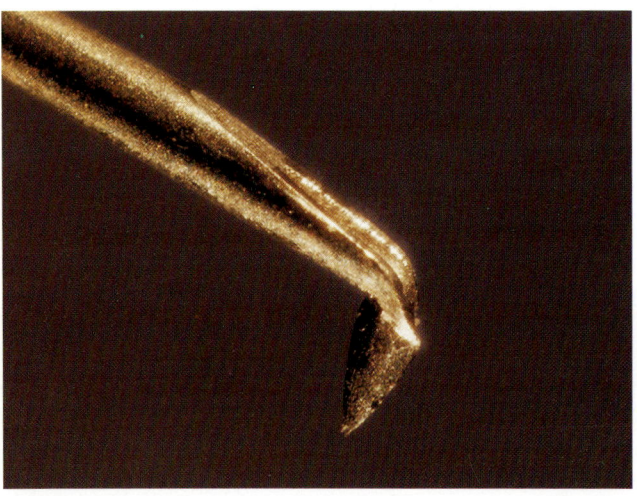

lamellar corneal transplantation, pterygium removal, conjunctival procedures, and other anterior chamber endeavors. This speculum is especially useful during phacoemulsification because there is no bar that can make contact with the phacoemulsification handpiece and transmit undesired pressure to the globe (Fig. 6.20). This speculum obviates the need for a lid speculum that has separate blades for each lid and unwieldy elastic extensions that attach above and below each lid.

The solid-bladed Guyton-Park lid speculum is useful during penetrating corneal transplantation because the blades can be supported independently in order to transmit the absolute smallest amount of pressure possible to the globe (Fig. 6.21). This lack of pressure is extremely important because the globe is open and much more vulnerable than during other anterior segment procedures. It is important that the blades of the Guyton-Park lid speculum be maintained in a horizontal position by supporting its lateral end with a folded gauze pad so that minimal pressure is transmitted to the globe. This speculum is not indicated during most forms of cataract extraction since it is too bulky and may interfere with automated nucleus and cortical removal.

The Lancaster speculum is very valuable during radial keratotomy procedures. This procedure is performed under topical anesthesia, and the Lancaster speculum prevents voluntary or involuntary lid closure (Fig. 6.22).

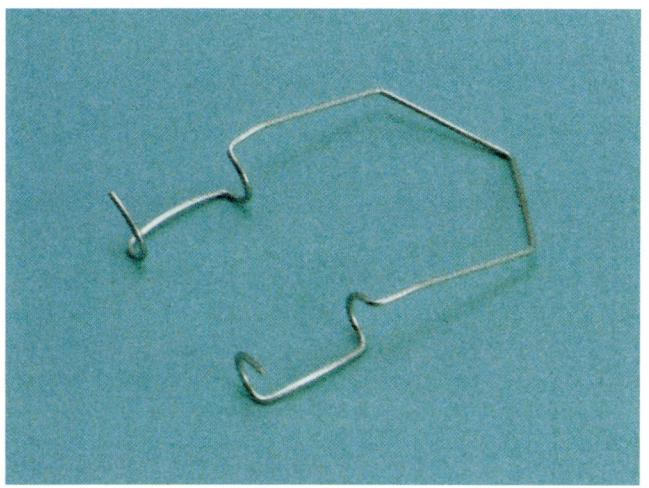

Figure 6.20 *The Kratz-Barraquer lid speculum has no bar above the lids and is an efficient, simple means of obtaining blepharostasis. This speculum is useful during many types of anterior segment procedures and is especially well-suited for phacoemulsification since it does not transmit pressure to the globe by contact between the phacoemulsification handpiece and the speculum.*

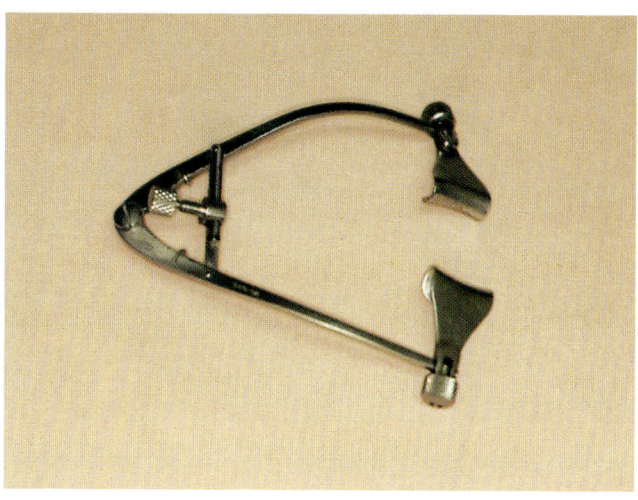

Figure 6.21 *The Guyton-Park lid speculum is valuable during penetrating keratoplasty since the adjustable blades can be elevated to keep pressure off the globe. A solid blade keeps the lashes and surgical drape well away from the operative field.*

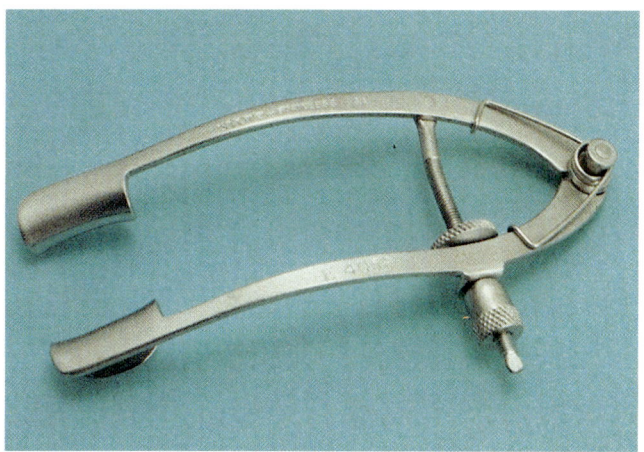

Figure 6.22 *The Lancaster lid speculum provides excellent blepharostasis during radial keratotomy and other procedures requiring only topical corneal anesthesia and those in which a strong blink reflex must be controlled.*

Conclusion

For a basic set of microscopic anterior segment surgical instruments, the surgeon might consider including an angled Colibri forceps with a wide tying platform, a gently curved fine needle holder, and a matching pair of curved and straight tying forceps (Fig. 6.23).

The Colibri forceps and needle holder allow the surgeon to suture and to tie knots without changing forceps after each needle placement. The tying forceps are useful when manipulating a running suture during cataract or corneal transplant surgery, cutting suture, or for tasks requiring smooth forceps. These instruments as well as various styles of scissors, a few blades, irrigation cannulas, and manipulators can be used to efficiently perform almost all anterior segment surgery.

In the future, the anterior segment surgeon will have more options in instrument selection. Disposable instruments, plastic instruments, and color-coded instruments should be available in the very near future. The anterior segment surgeon is urged to assemble a personalized set of instruments and to keep them in good repair. These instruments will allow the surgeon to produce the best results possible.

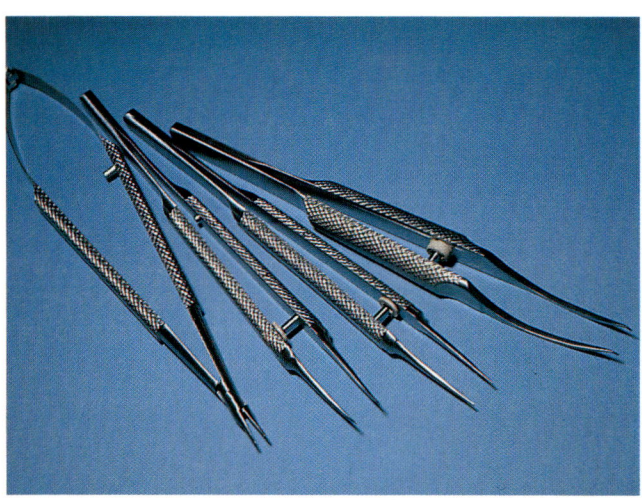

Figure 6.23 *A basic set of instruments for surgery on the anterior segment might contain an angled Colibri forceps with 0.12-mm teeth, a needle holder with a shape similar to a curved tying forceps, and a straight and curved pair of tying forceps. The surgeon should also consider the material and length of the instruments.*

Clinical Points to Consider

☛ Stainless steel and titanium both have advantages and disadvantages as a material used to construct anterior segment surgical instruments.

☛ It is useful for the surgeon to be able to tie 10-0 nylon suture with a needleholder and fixation forceps, instead of always changing to tying forceps.

☛ Various lid specula are well suited for diverse anterior segment surgical procedures.

NEEDLES AND SUTURES

DAVID W. POLEY   PETER A. HATTON

Needles and suture materials used in ophthalmic surgery have undergone an extraordinary evolution since the early 1950s, when there were no ophthalmic needle/suture combinations. The development of fine wires, needles, and microsutures for ophthalmologic use can be attributed to Wendell L. Hughes, M.D. and Ramon Castroviejo, M.D., physicians who pushed United States manufacturers to produce miniature needles sharpened to a fineness not available previously.

For wound closure in anterior segment surgery prior to the 1960s, ophthalmic surgeons were, for the most part, using eyed Grieshaber needles and threading the eye in the operating room, often with 6-0 silk suture (Fig. 7.1). The large eye and double suture created problems, and the development of a manufacturing process to produce a swaged-on suture was a quantum leap in the development of ophthalmic products. In the past ten years, major changes have been made in wire materials, wire size, point configurations, suture materials, and just about every other aspect of ophthalmic needles and sutures. These advances and developments have enabled surgeons to use needles and sutures in a greater variety of ophthalmic procedures than was possible previously. Fine surgeons have become even better, and advancements in ophthalmic surgery exceed by far those in all other microsurgical specialties.

The following overview traces the development of ophthalmic needles and suture materials, focusing on anterior segment surgery, from the threading of needles in the 1950s to the wide variety of precision wound-closure products available today.

Needles

Early Needles

The most apparent disadvantage of the early needles was that the suture had to be threaded through the eyes. The resultant double strand of suture and the comparatively large needle and suture gauges traumatized delicate eye tissue. In 1954, in response to this situation, Ethicon created a Surgical Advisory Panel, which helped develop the kinds of needle/suture combinations needed by ophthalmic surgeons. The first significant advancement was the introduction in 1955 of the Micro-Point surgical needle (G [Grieshaber] series), a reverse-cutting ophthalmic needle that was preswaged to the suture (Fig. 7.2) and a major improvement in strength and sharpness. These needles are now used primarily for traction and oculoplastic procedures.

The next major advancement in ophthalmic needles, the Micro-Point spatula needle (GS [Grieshaber spatula] series), occurred in the early 1960s. The primary difference between the spatulated and reverse needles was that the third cutting edge on the bottom or outer curve of the needle was eliminated (Fig. 7.3). Spatulated needles offer three advantages for anterior segment, retinal detachment, and strabismus surgery:

1. The flattened cutting surfaces permit the needle to split the layers of tissue rather than cut through them
2. The removal of the outer cutting edge makes it less likely that the needle will accidentally penetrate too deeply
3. The point configuration of the spatula needle is smaller and less traumatic

Anatomy

Ophthalmic needles, like all other surgical needles, have three parts—the swage (connection point for the suture), the body, and the point—and are made of stainless steel. The stainless steel most commonly used, designated 420 by the steel industry ratings, has been chosen because of its superior ability to be shaped, sharpened, and hardened.

The needle has five geometric aspects (Fig. 7.4):

Length. The distance along the circumference from the tip of the needle to the swage of the needle.

Chord Length. The distance of the straight line from the tip of the curved needle to the swage of the curved needle. This measurement determines the width of the suture bite.

Radius. The length of the line from the center of the circle (that would be formed if the curved needle continued 360 degrees) to the periphery.

Wire Diameter. The thickness of the wire provided by the steel manufacturer prior to needle construction.

The diameter of an ophthalmic needle is measured in mils ($\frac{1}{1000}$ of an inch). In the metric conversion, one mil equals roughly 25 μ. To close corneal-scleral tissue in anterior segment surgery, 8-mil, 6-mil, and 4-mil needles are now used. As needle technology and microsurgical technique have advanced, surgeons have started using finer wire diameters. The difficulty that surgeons encounter when using the larger wire diameter needles is the additional tissue trauma, as well as the additional force required for penetration. Figure 7.5 shows a 10-0 nylon suture swaged to an 8-mil, 6-mil, and 4-mil needle. The

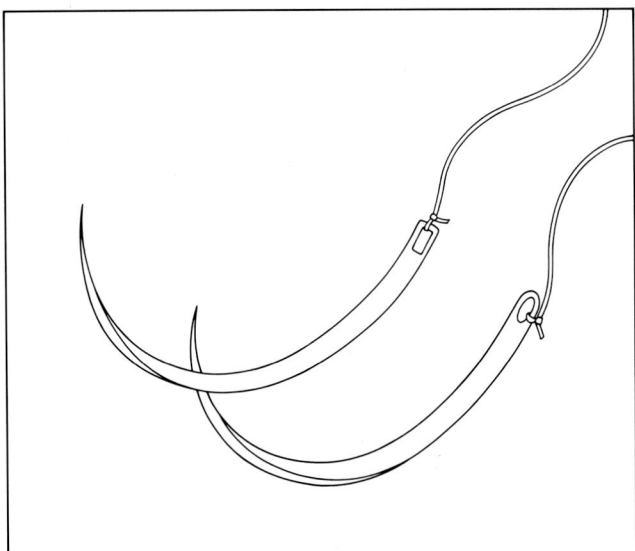

Figure 7.1 *The original ophthalmic sutures used eyed needles.*

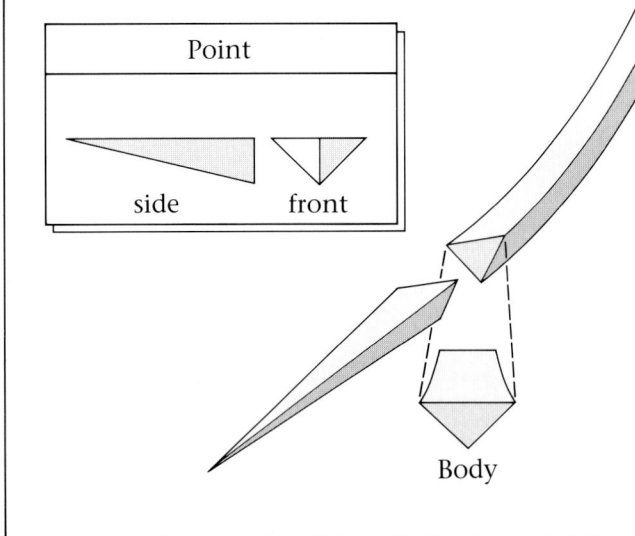

Figure 7.2 *Swaging the suture to the needle has vastly improved the quality of ophthalmic sutures.*

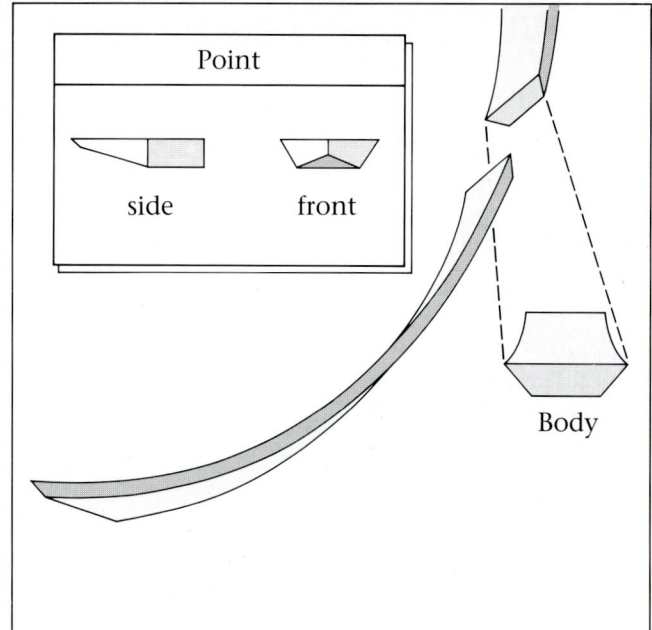

Figure 7.3 *The spatula needle, which provides cutting surfaces on the edges rather than the bottom of the needle, has further improved the quality of ophthalmic needles. (Compare the spatula needle configuration to the cutting needle configuration in Figure 7.2.)*

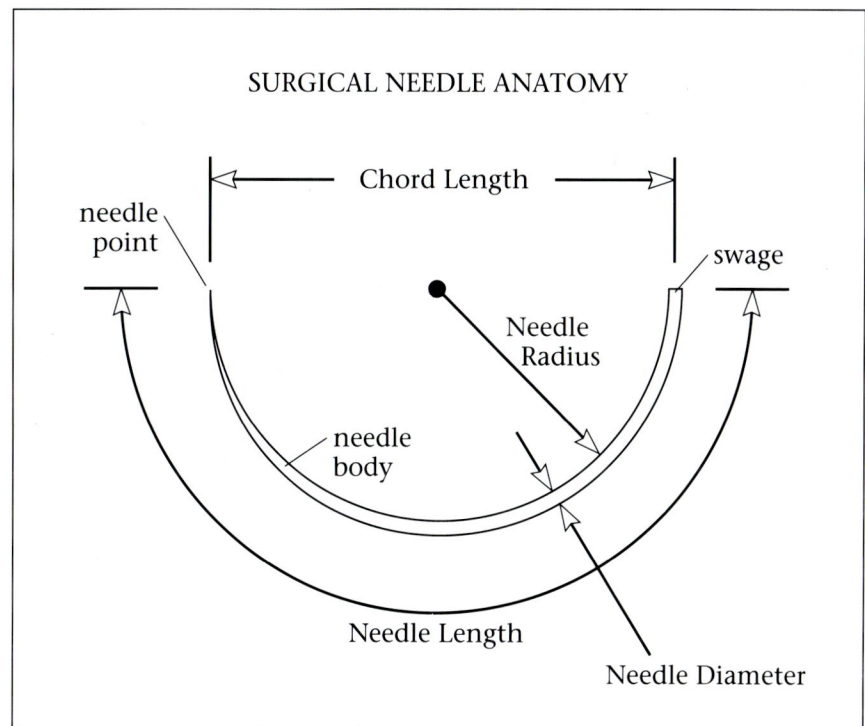

Figure 7.4 *Surgical needle anatomy.*

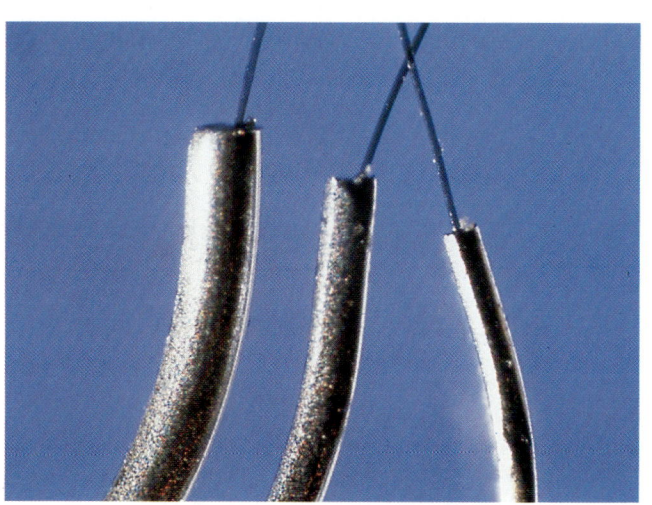

Figure 7.5 *A 10-0 nylon suture swaged to an 8-mil, 6-mil, and 4-mil needle. The difference in tissue penetration is dramatic.*

6-mil needle and, even more dramatically, the 4-mil needle provide a smaller needle track, a better needle/suture ratio, and easier penetration since less needle mass must be driven through the tissue.

Bicurve. Two radii on a single piece of wire, where the radius near the point is shorter than the radius of the body closer to the swage.

Ophthalmic needles undergo a process of forging, bending, and annealing prior to having the suture attached to the swage. Each needle is inspected many times during the manufacturing process. The end result is a fine wire needle that is sharpened at the widest point to withstand multiple suturing passes by the ophthalmic surgeon.

After a section of wire, taken from a coil, is straightened and cut into short pieces, the wire is cold forged and the desired tip configuration, body shape, and swage area are incorporated into the needle blank. The desired curve is added to the wire. Cleaning, electropolishing, and heat-treating follow. Throughout the manufacturing process, the needles are inspected and reinspected. They are protected from the environment through the use of special forceps and ultraclean manufacturing areas.

Fine nylon, silk, polyester, or polypropylene sutures are attached by hand with the wire crimped around the suture. The completed double- or single-armed suture is wrapped around a foam pack and packaged in a plastic Tyvek pouch. This Assist-OR package, developed by Alcon, was the first lint-free ophthalmic suture package. Its design has since become the industry standard and is now provided in one form or another by all suppliers.

Ethicon Needles

While the reduced mass of finer wire needle provides easier penetration, there is a reduction in strength; consequently, the needles are more likely to bend, particularly on repeated passes through tough corneal-scleral tissue. To overcome this difficulty, Ethicon developed a new series of anterior segment surgery needles in the early 1980s, the TG (transverse grind) Plus series. To strengthen this new generation of needles and thereby minimize difficulties with bending, an exclusive 455 stainless steel alloy was used rather than the standard 420 stainless steel alloy. Additionally, the body of the needle was side flattened, displacing more mass in the direction of the curve and increasing its rigidity.

Perhaps the most critical characteristic of corneal-scleral needles is ease of penetration, particularly after repeated passes. A new transverse grind honing process, developed with the TG Plus series of needles, produced more defined cutting edges that could slice through tissue with the cutting effect of a serrated steak knife. In effect, greater edge definition was achieved with the newer TG honing process than with the former smooth GS honing process.

Ophthalmic wire diameter needles have become smaller in order to minimize trauma and provide easier penetration. Also important when selecting a corneal-scleral needle is the surgeon's suturing technique. While finer wire needles provide easier penetration, they make a smaller hole, which makes it more difficult to rotate or bury the suture knot in the needle track. This is especially important with an interrupted suturing technique, which is made up of multiple knots, rather than with a continuous or shoelace suturing technique, where generally only one knot is rotated.

While knot burial is relatively easy with the larger 8-mil wire needle, it was recognized that knot burial could be made easier yet by modifying the spatula tip geometry of a 6-mil wire needle. The result was the TGW (transverse grind wide) series: 6-mil wire needles with wider spatula tips. The wider needle track created by this needle makes it easier to rotate or bury the suture knots. It is important to note that the TGW geometry makes a wider needle track, as opposed to a larger needle track (Figs. 7.6 and 7.7). While both needles have a 6-mil wire diameter, the spatula tip of the TGW needle has more mass displaced in the horizontal plane than in the vertical plane. In effect, the TGW needle slices a wider, thinner hole whereas the TG Plus needle punctures a hole with a more even diameter. The elastic nature of the corneal-scleral tissue permits rotation of suture knots more readily into the sliced TGW hole.

The most recent corneal-scleral needles produced by Ethicon (CS Ultima) incorporate a geometric shape that improves tissue penetration. These ophthalmic spatula needles have improved and modified forms of the original trapezoid spatula geometry (Fig. 7.8). The CS Ultima needle incorporates concave spatula geometry (i.e., significantly reduced angles on the needle edges). The reduced edge angles enable the needle to glide through corneal-scleral tissue with minimal resistance; in fact, 50% less force than was necessary previously for a similar needle. This needle is the same width as the TGW needle and produces a needle track that facilitates knot rotation or burial as well as ease of penetration.

Curvature, Radius, and Chord Length

The curvature, radius, and chord length of anterior segment surgery needles affect the ease with

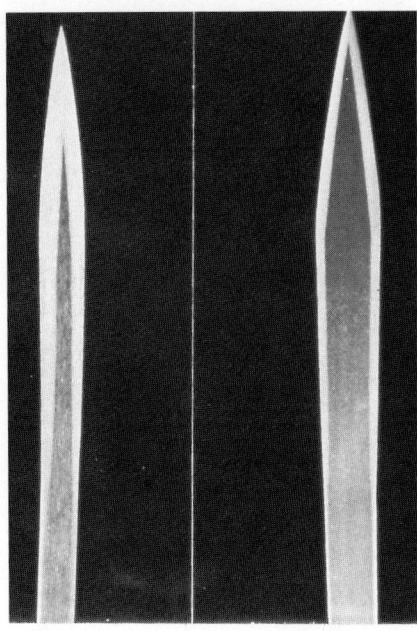

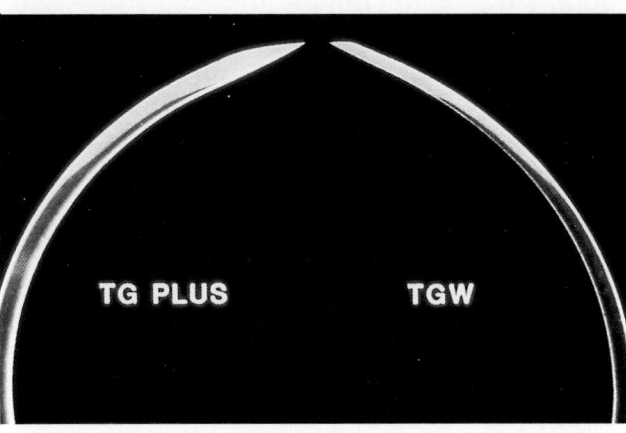

Figure 7.6 *A 6-mil, TG Plus needle compared to a 6-mil TGW needle. The TGW needle was designed to create a wider, flatter wound that allows for knot rotation into the wound.*

Figure 7.7 *Notice that the TGW needle is flatter than the TG Plus needle, even though they are both 6 mil.*

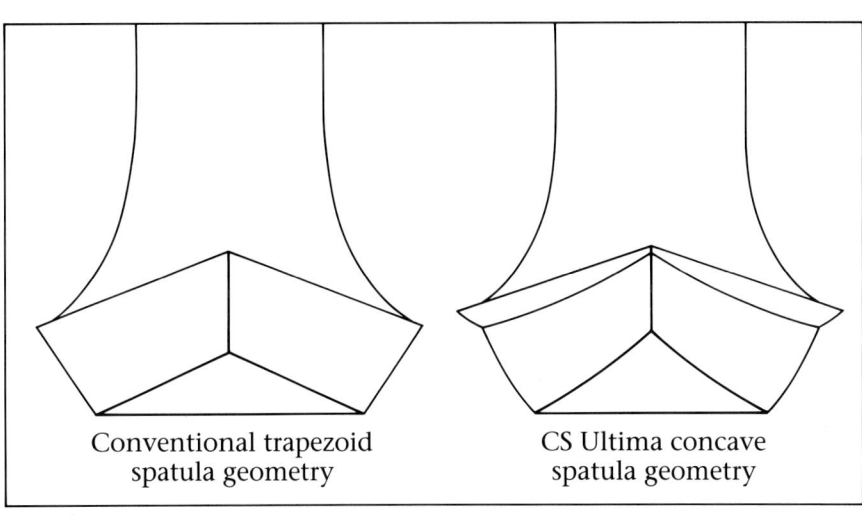

Figure 7.8 *Standard trapezoidal spatula needle and CS Ultima needle.*

which the surgeon achieves the desired length and depth of bite into corneal-scleral tissue (Fig. 7.9). A summary of the needles we have discussed is provided in Table 7.10.

LONG/SHALLOW BITES

Surgeons often use the larger radius 140-degree-curve needle for the long/shallow bites that are preferred when closing scleral pocket-type incisions in cataract surgery, particularly with a horizontal suturing technique or in corneal transplant surgery. An example of this needle in a 6-mil wire diameter is the CS-140-6. This corneal-scleral, 140-degree curve, 6-mil wire needle has a radius of 2.50 mm and a chord length of 4.75 mm.

SHORT/DEEP BITES

To assure posterior wound apposition, anterior segment surgeons often desire essentially full depth closure. Full depth closure with a needle that has a radius larger than 2.50 mm requires a tissue bite that is longer than 2.50 mm. If the sutures are tied too tightly, tissue compression is affected and the resultant corneal distortion is amplified.

On the other hand, a needle with a shorter radius (e.g., the 160-degree curve, 2.00-mm radius needle) facilitates full depth closure without requiring a long pass. If the sutures are inadvertently overtightened, a shorter bite will result in less corneal distortion and less with-the-rule astigmatism than would result with an overtightened long bite suture. For this reason, the most commonly used corneal-scleral needle is the short/deep bite, 160-degree needle, an example of which, in 6-mil wire, is the CS-160-6 needle, which has a 2.00-mm radius and a 4.00-mm chord length.

As a compromise between the 140-degree and 160-degree curve needles, the 175-degree curve needle was developed. While this needle has a longer curve length than the other curve needles, its radius of 2.30 mm and chord length of 4.60 mm reflect its appropriateness for bites of medium depth and length. Figure 7.11 illustrates actual needles representing three traditional curves just discussed and summarizes the tech-

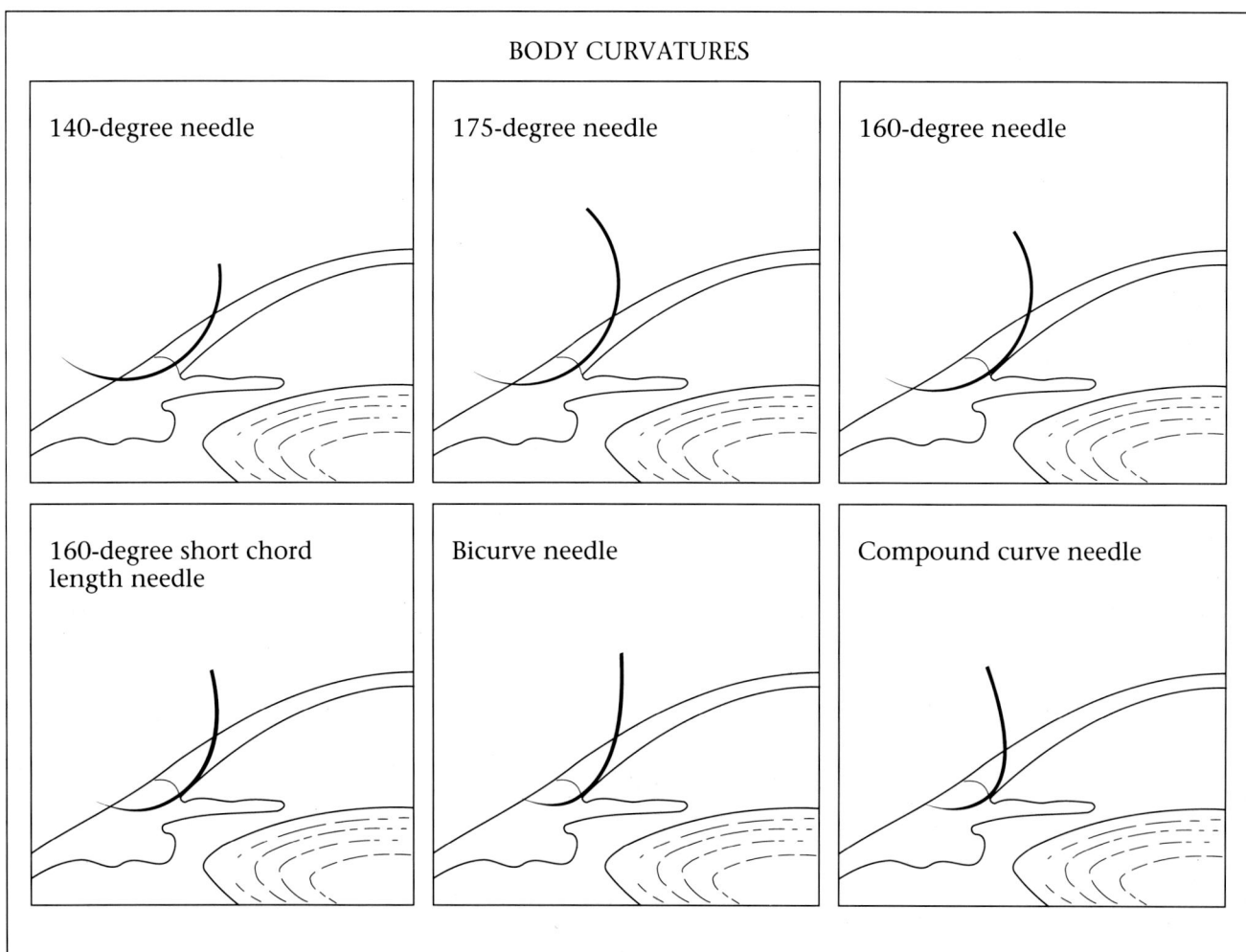

Figure 7.9 *The relationship between needle curvature and suture bite.*

Table 7.10
Ethicon Corneal-Scleral Needles

TRADITIONAL CURVATURES			MODIFIED SHORT/DEEP CURVATURES		
140-Degree	175-Degree	160-Degree	Minicurve	Bicurve	Compound Curve
		8-mil			
TG-140-8	TG-175-8	TG-160-8	—	—	—
CS-140-8	CS-175-8	CS-160-8	—	—	—
		6-mil			
TG-140-6	TG-175-6	TG-160-6	TG-160-6-3M	TG-6-S	TG-6-C
TGW-140-6	TGW-175-6	TGW-160-6	TGW-160-6-3M	TGW-6-S	TGW-6-C
CS-140-6	CS-175-6	CS-160-6	CS-M-6	CS-B-6	CS-C-6
		4-mil			
TG-140-4	—	TG-160-4	TG-160-4-3M	TG-4-S	TG-4-C
CS-140-4	—	CS-160-4	CS-M-4	CS-B-4	CS-C-4

Length/Depth of Bite	Curvature	Radius (mm)	Chord Length (mm)	Needle
long/shallow	140°	2.54	4.75	TGI-140-6
				CS-140-6
medium/medium	175°	2.28	4.57	TG-175-6
				CS-175-6
short/deep	160°	2.00	4.00	TG-160-6
				CS-160-6
very short/deep	minicurve	1.50	3.00	TG-160-6-3M
				CS-M-6
very short/deep	bicurve	1.39/2.54	—	TG-6-S
				CS-B-6
very short/deep	compound	1.39/2.54	—	TG-6-C
				CS-C-6

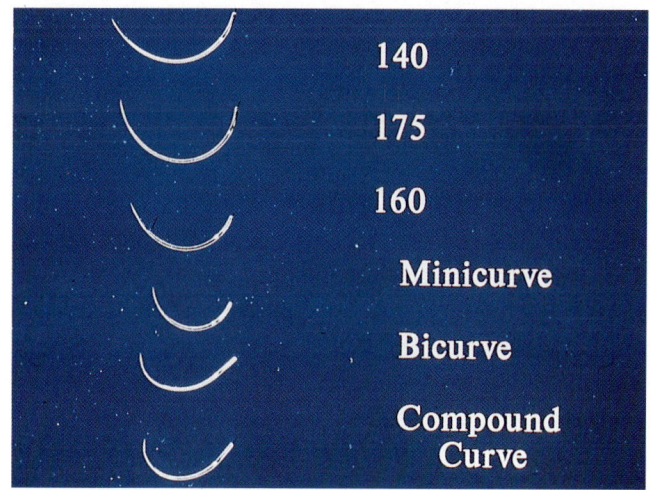

Figure 7.11 *Comparison of 140-, 160-, and 175-degree curve needles with other forms of corneal-scleral needles.*

niques and specifications associated with these traditional curvatures. Note the decreasing radius from 140 degrees to 175 degrees to 160 degrees.

VERY SHORT/DEEP BITES

To control astigmatism, surgeons make very short, deep bites of tissue. The bites should be equidistant from the incision. Various needle curvatures help the surgeon achieve this aim.

Minicurve. The 160-degree minicurve or short chord length needle is similar to the more traditional needles mentioned above. It has a continuous, nonchanging radius throughout the curve. To facilitate shorter bites, this needle has a tight 1.50-mm radius compared to the 2.00-mm radius of the traditional CS-160-6 needle.

Bicurve. The bicurve needle (e.g., CS-B-6), unlike the needles mentioned above, does not have a continuous single radius throughout the entire length of the needle body. Instead, the body of the bicurve needle incorporates an initial 2.54-mm radius from the swage to the middle portion, followed by a much tighter 1.39-mm radius toward the point of the needle. The tighter radius of the bicurve needle allows quick turnout and a deep bite. The more gradual curve toward the swage permits easier handling and exit from the tissue.

Compound Curve. The compound curve needle (e.g., CS-C-6) is very similar to the bicurve needle in curvature and radius. The compound curve needle differs, however, in that the reduced 1.39-mm radius at the tip becomes angled inward even further by a sharp, straight point. This straight point facilitates the initial entrance and depth of penetration, while the tight curvature behind the tip permits rapid, accurate needle rotation at the selected depth. The compound curve needle is an excellent tool for achieving very short, deep bites of tissue equidistant from the incision. In order to achieve this a straight-jawed, round-bodied needle holder is recommended. The needle tip should penetrate vertically to the desired depth before any rotation of the needle is made. The round-bodied needle holder is rotated before exiting.

Lens Fixation and Iris Repair

Needles used for transscleral or transchamber suturing are frequently used for intraocular lens

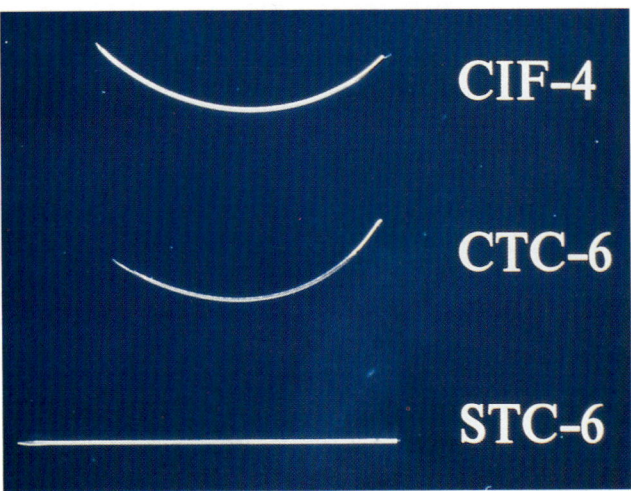

Figure 7.12 *The CIF-4, CTC-6, and STC-6 needles are designed for transscleral and anterior chamber fixation of IOLs.*

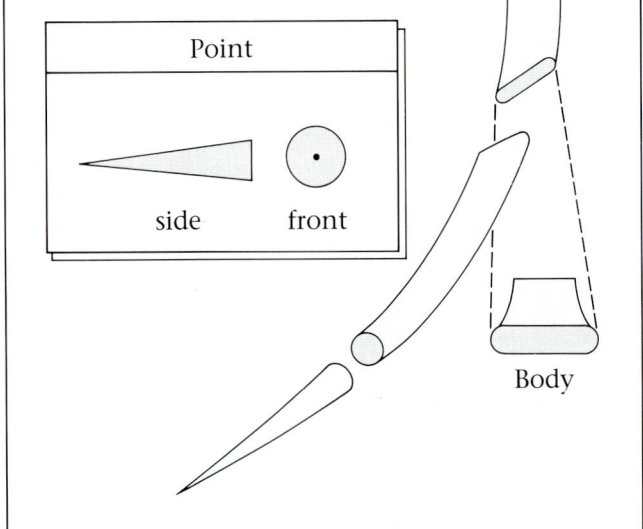

Figure 7.13 *Taperpoint needles minimize soft tissue trauma and are commonly used for placing iris sutures.*

(IOL) fixation and for closed-chamber iris suturing. These needles (Fig. 7.12) include:

1. CIF-4: 88-degree curve, 13.00 mm long, 8-mil wire diameter, taper cutting point
2. The newly developed curved TransChamber CTC-6: 88-degree curve, 12.00 mm long, 6-mil wire diameter, spatula cutting point
3. Straight TransChamber STC-6: 16.00 mm long, 6-mil wire diameter, spatula cutting point

When suturing iris tissue in an open chamber, such as during cataract or keratoplasty procedures, or when performing iris fixation techniques for lens fixation, many surgeons recommend the use of noncutting taper point microsurgery needles, often referred to as BV needles since they were originally developed for microsurgery of blood vessels. These atraumatic taper point needles (Fig. 7.13) help minimize trauma and tearing of the delicate iris tissue. An example of this needle is the taperpoint BV-100-4.

Alcon Needles

Because of the unique nature of ophthalmic surgery, needles with special point configurations have been designed and developed specifically for ophthalmic surgery (Table 7.14). Following are

Table 7.14
Alcon Corneal-Scleral Needle Code Descriptions

	Designation	Description
Series	A	Advanced corneal closure needle: side cutting, spatula trapezoid body
	C	Corneal closure needle: side cutting, spatulated flat bottom
	S	Superior corneal closure needle: side cutting, spatulated flat body
	B	Reverse cutting needle
	R	Retina/posterior segment needle: diamond point, side cutting
	T	Scleral side cutting spatulated needle
	P	Bridle suture needle: taper point, round tip, flat body
	PC	Bridle suture needle: taper point cutting, round tip, flat body
Wire Diameter	U	Ultra-thin (4-mil or 6-mil)
	1	4-mil
Radius of Curvature	1–5	(1 = longest radius and 5 = shortest radius)
Example		Each needle designation includes one or two capital letters separated by a hyphen from a one- or two-digit number, e.g., CU-15:
		C = Side cutting, spatulated, flat bottom
		U = 4- or 6-mil
		1 = 4-mil
		5 = shortest radius curvature

Table 7.15
Alcon Corneal-Scleral Needles

Needle	Wire Diameter (inch)	(mm)	Included Angle† (circle)	Length (inch)	(mm)	Radius (inch)	(mm)	Chord (inch)	(mm)
Side Cutting									
AU-1/CU-1/SU-1	.006	0.15	140	.244	6.19	.100	2.54	.187	4.75
AU-2/CU-2/SU-2	.006	0.15	175	.275	6.98	.090	2.28	.180	4.57
AU-5/CU-5/SU-5 (CU-5C)	.006	0.15	160	.217	5.51	.078	1.98	.158	4.01
			105			.034	.86		
AU-6/CU-6/SU-6	.006	0.15	85	.243	6.17	.122	3.10	—	—
			90			.060	1.52		
AU-8/CU-8/SU-8	.006	0.15	50	.190	4.83	.110	2.79	.146	3.71
AUM-5/CUM-5/SUM-5	.006	0.15	160	.166	4.22	.060	1.52	.118	3.00
AU-11/CU-11	.004	0.10	140	.244	6.19	.100	2.54	.187	4.75
AU-15/CU-15	.004	0.10	160	.217	5.51	.078	1.98	.158	4.01
AUM-15/CUM-15/SUM-15	.004	0.10	160	.166	4.22	.060	1.52	.118	3.00
A-3/C-3/S-3	.008	0.20	137	.258	6.55	.109	2.77	.204	5.18
A-4/C-4/S-4	.008	0.20	175	.281	7.13	.094	2.39	.187	4.75
A-5/C-5/S-5	.008	0.20	160	.217	5.51	.078	1.98	.158	4.01
A-7/C-7/S-7	.008	0.20	—	.280	7.11	.055*	.14*	—	—
			90			.060	1.52		
C-8	.008	0.20	50	.190	4.83	.110	2.79	.146	3.71
Reverse Cutting									
B-1	.008	0.20	110	.312	7.92	.157	3.98	.256	6.50
B-2	.008	0.20	165	.312	7.92	.109	2.77	.218	5.54
BO-1	.013	0.33	135	.435	11.04	.187	4.75	.346	8.79
BO-2	.017	0.43	155	.515	13.07	.187	4.75	.366	9.30
Center Point Side Cutting									
R-1	.014	0.35	90	.312	7.92	.200	5.08	.283	7.19
R-2	.018	0.45	90	.312	7.92	.200	5.08	.283	7.19
R-3	.014	0.35	180	.312	7.92	.100	2.54	.200	5.08
R-5	.011	0.28	90	.240	6.10	.153	3.88	.216	5.49
R-7	.015	0.38	90	.258	6.55	.164	4.16	.232	5.89
Side Cutting Scleral									
T-1	.013	0.33	90	.312	7.92	.200	5.08	.283	7.19
T-2	.017	0.43	90	.312	7.92	.200	5.08	.283	7.19
T-3	.013	0.33	180	.312	7.92	.100	2.54	.200	5.08
T-5	.011	0.28	90	.240	6.10	.153	3.88	.216	5.49
T-6	.015	0.38	90	.312	7.92	.200	5.08	.283	7.19
T-7	.015	0.38	90	.258	6.55	.164	4.16	.232	5.89
Taper Point									
P-1	.011	0.28	137	.485	12.32	.203	5.16	.377	9.59
P-5	.015	0.38	137	.485	12.32	.203	5.16	.377	9.59
Cutting Taper Point									
PC-1	.014	0.35	135	.555	13.99	.234	5.90	.437	11.0
PC-5	.015	0.38	135	.555	13.99	.234	5.90	.437	11.0

†Angles are in degrees
*Dimension of needle beyond 90° bend

the major point styles produced by Alcon for use in ophthalmology (Tables 7.15 and 7.16).

Point Configurations

CUTTING TAPER POINT

Three microfacets forged into a point facilitate this needle's passage through Tenon's capsule. The absence of cutting surfaces on the remainder of the point and the body make the needle ideal for passing the bridle suture underneath the superior and/or inferior rectus muscle. The needle is referred to as the PC (point cutting) needle (Fig. 7.17).

SPATULA SIDE CUTTING

Developed for ophthalmic surgery, this needle is designed to be used for corneal and scleral wound closure. The needle is sharpened on the side with a small cutting facet at the front and, generally, is flat on the top and bottom with a trapezoidal body

**Table 7.16
Most Recent Alcon Needles: The Excalibur Series**

Needle	Curve (degrees)	Chord length (mm)	Suture	Product No.
SU3-Solitaire	44°	6.00	10-0, BMN 3″, SA	8065-2184-01
SU-5	160°	4.01	10-0, BMN 6″, DA	8065-2180-01
SU-2	175°	4.57	10-0, BMN 12″, DA	8065-2182-01
SU-5	160°	4.01	9-0, BMN 12″, DA	8065-2185-01
SU-5	160°	4.01	10-0, PP 12″, DA	8065-2187-01
SU-8	90°–50°	3.71	10-0, BMN 8″, DA	8065-2190-01
SU-6	105°–85°	—	10-0, BMN 12″, DA	8065-2193-01
SUM-5	160°	3.00	10-0, BMN 8″, DA	8065-2194-01
SU-18	90°–50°	3.71	10-0, BMN 8″, DA	8065-2198-01
SU-5*	160°	4.01	10-0, BMN 12″	8065-2140-01
PC-5*	135°	11.00	4-0, BBS 18″	

BMN = black monofilament nylon
PP = polypropylene
BBS = braided black silk
DA = double armed
SA = single armed
*Pair-Pak II

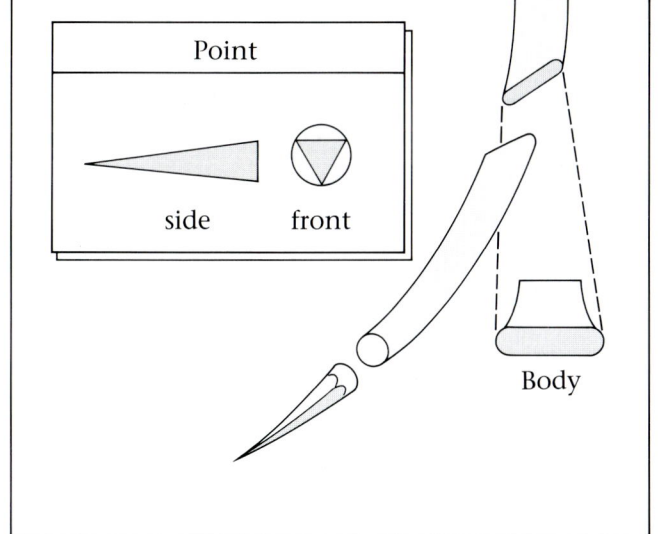

Figure 7.17 Cutting taper point needle. This needle is commonly used to pass a silk fixation suture under a rectus muscle.

(A series) or rectangular body (C series). Wire diameters are 8-mil, 6-mil, and 4-mil (Fig. 7.18).

REVERSE CUTTING NEEDLE

This needle is used most often in oculoplastic procedures. It is characterized by a triangular point with the cutting surface on the edges and the lower front. This design makes it useful in penetrating the epidermis. It is sometimes used for the rectus scleral fixation suture, but the cutting taper-point or spatula side cutting needle are preferred for this because their cutting surfaces tend not to penetrate the sclera (Fig. 7.19).

CENTER POINT SIDE CUTTING

Characterized by a center point and side cutting surfaces along the horizontal median plane, this R series needle is designed for use in the posterior segment. It is sharp along the edges and flat on the top and bottom so that it cuts between layers of scleral lamellae. Its design allows for good control with a shallow bite (Fig. 7.20).

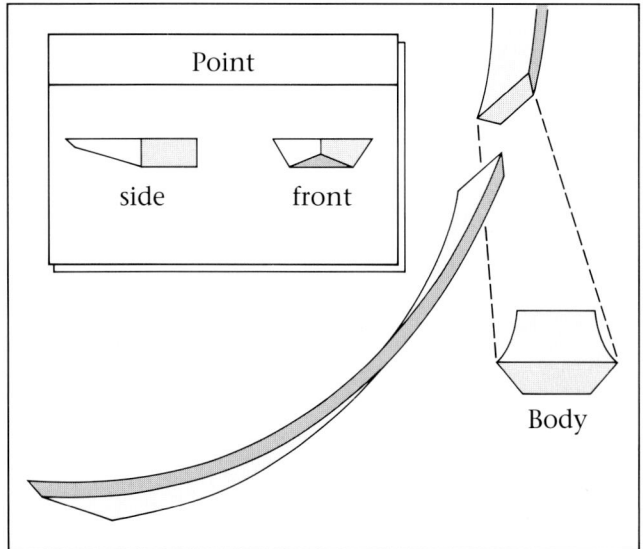

Figure 7.18 *Spatula side cutting needle. This is the preferred needle for corneal and scleral wound closure in the anterior segment since it can penetrate deeply yet maintain a constant depth between corneal lamellae. This needle may also be useful for placement of an episcleral fixation suture.*

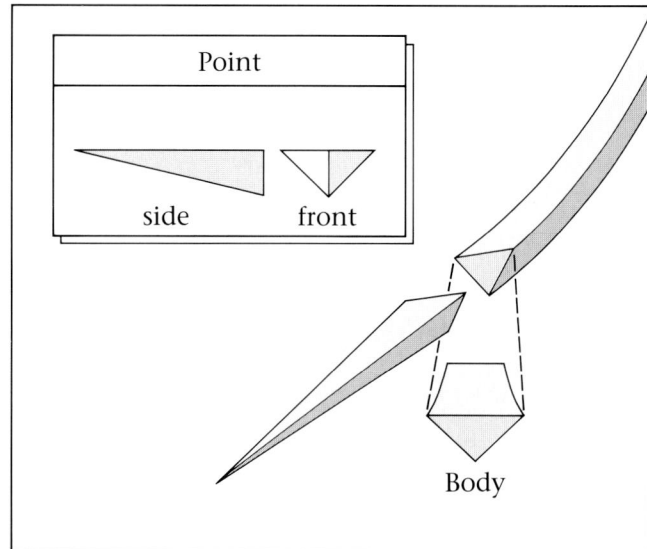

Figure 7.19 *Reverse cutting needle. This needle is most often used in oculoplastic surgery, although it is not the needle of choice when placing a fixation suture since the inferior cutting edge tends to penetrate more deeply into the sclera.*

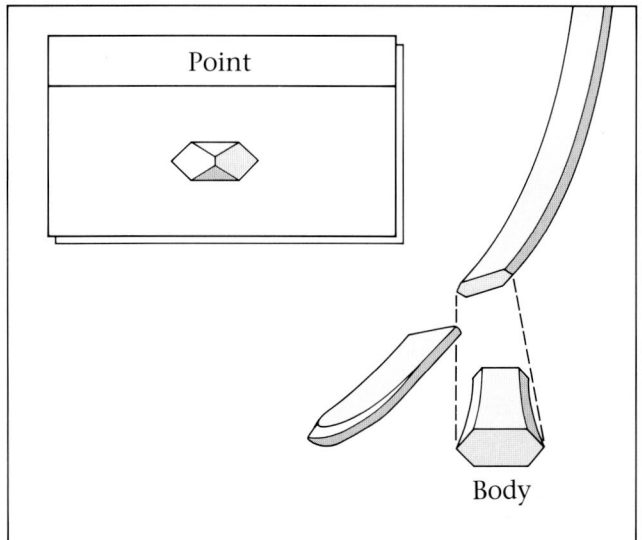

Figure 7.20 *Center point cutting needle. This needle is used for posterior segment surgery when a shallow scleral bite is desired, such as strabismus surgery or placement of a scleral encircling band or buckle.*

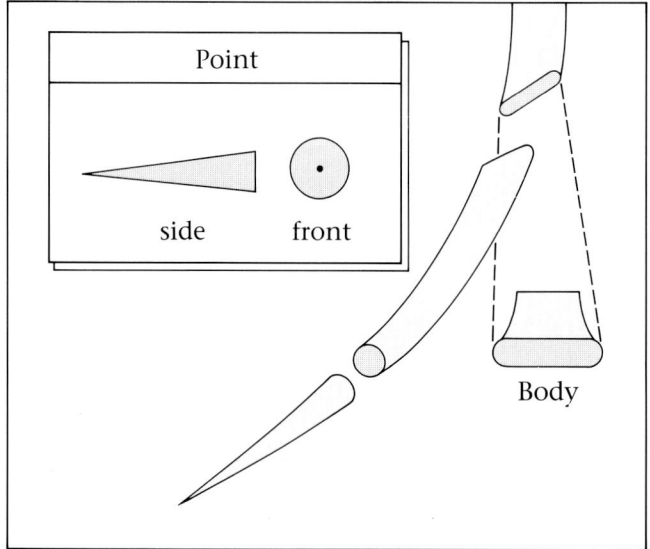

Figure 7.21 *Taper point needle. This needle is used for iris repair or placement of a rectus fixation suture.*

TAPER POINT

This P series needle has a point similar to a sharp pencil and has no cutting surfaces. The body is flat for easy grasping and it is generally used for iris repair or under the superior rectus muscle (Fig. 7.21).

Body Curvature

The depth of the bite in corneal-scleral tissue is determined by the curve of the needle (Table 7.22). The more curved the needle, the deeper the bite. The bicurved needle produces both the deepest and the shortest bite with the least amount of tissue distortion. This is accomplished by the distal curve of the needle, which penetrates deeply and surfaces quickly. David McIntyre, M.D., developed both the needle and the suturing technique for Alcon in 1985. Theoretically, the deeper and shorter the suture bite, the less astigmatism produced during cataract/IOL surgery.

Corneal surgery, however, (e.g., lamellar and penetrating keratoplasty) requires intrastromal bites longer than required for cataract surgery to minimize wound leaks and the pulling out of sutures from unhealthy recipient tissue. Also, the bicurve shape is not applicable to situations in which sutures must be placed in a 360-degree manner, because the mechanism of action is the rotation of the needle toward the surgeon. A needle such as the Alcon CU-1 is excellent for longer corneal suture bites and has the strength to withstand 16 to 20 passes of a running suture. When a shallow, long bite is needed, as in posterior segment surgery, a 90-degree needle is generally used.

The Solitaire needle (SU-3) is designed for closing a 3.00-mm to 5.00-mm small incision cataract wound with a mattress or horizontal suture (Fig. 7.23). Since the arc of this needle is only 44 degrees, it will routinely penetrate less than

Table 7.22
Corneal-Scleral Needle Shapes and Function

Type	Degrees	Narrow Bite	Wide Bite	Deep Bite	Shallow Bite
Bicurve "fishhook"	105/85	X		X	
Open bicurve	90/50	X		X	
One-half circle	160/175	X		X	
Three-eighths circle	130/140		X		X
One-quarter circle	85/110		X		X

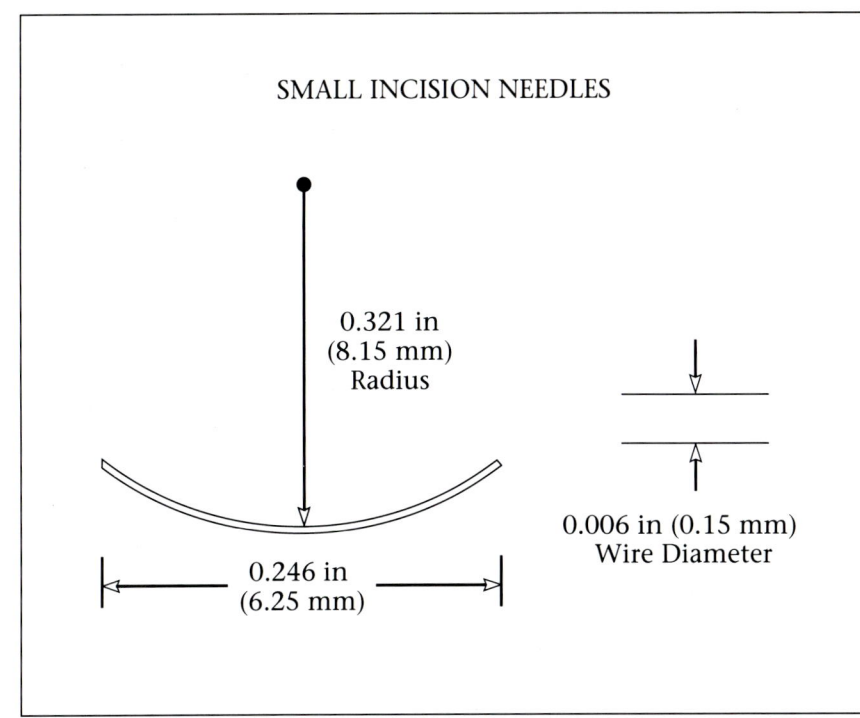

Figure 7.23 *Alcon Solitaire needle (SU-3). This needle is designed to close the 3.00-mm to 5.00-mm wound used in small incision cataract surgery.*

0.025 mm into the sclera and will produce a bite 3.00 mm to 5.00 mm in length. The dimensions of the SU-3 are as follows:

Wire size	0.006 (0.15 mm)
Arc length	6.00 mm
Chord length	6.25 mm
Degree of circle	44

Ophthalmic Suture Materials

Advancements in polymer and suture technology have resulted in a number of innovations in the fine size suture materials used in ophthalmic surgery (Table 7.24). The fine size sutures used in corneoscleral closure include 9-0, 10-0, and 11-0 diameter sizes. These sizes are United States Pharmacopeia (USP)* ranges, specifying 30 μ to 39 μ for 9-0, 20 μ to 29 μ for 10-0, and 10 μ to 19 μ for 11-0 (Fig. 7.25).

Nonabsorbable Sutures

Nonabsorbable suture materials are not degraded into their simple elements and absorbed into the body as are absorbable materials. If tolerated, they are encapsulated within the tissue. If the sutures are not tolerated, the body will reject them. Rejection is often manifested by the suture migrating to the surface. The diameter and knot pull limitations of ophthalmic sutures are dictated by the USP (Table 7.26). All nonabsorbable sutures, regardless of the material, must conform to these standards.

*The USP is a United States government publication that sets official standards for quality of medications and various surgical items.

Table 7.24 Closure Materials

Suture Material	Mono-filament	Braided	Twisted	Virgin	Coated	Absorbable Yes	Absorbable No	Use
Nylon	X						X	AS/PS
Silk		X	X	X	X		X	AS
Polyester	X	X			X		X	AS/PS
Polypropylene	X						X	AS
PD6		X				X		AS
PGA		X			X	X		AS
Gut	X				X	X		AS

AS = Anterior Segment   PS = Posterior Segment

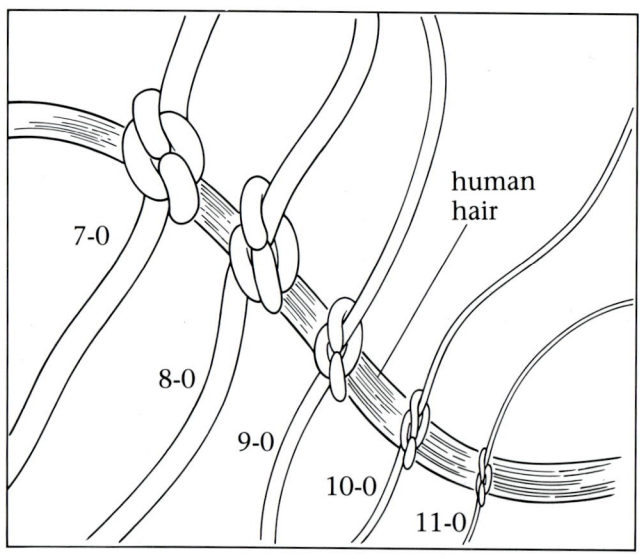

Figure 7.25 *Comparison between the thickness and knot size of human hair and various sutures used in corneoscleral closure. Notice that the volume of the knot formed by 9-0 nylon is about three times that of a knot formed by 10-0 nylon. The degree of neovascularization caused by a nylon suture is determined almost entirely by the volume of the knot.*

SILK

Through the 1960s and into the early 1970s, the standard choice for primary closure in anterior segment surgery was silk suture, primarily 7-0, 8-0, and 9-0. Additionally, 7-0 and 8-0 silk sutures have been widely used as preplacement or safety sutures in cataract surgery and as cardinal sutures in corneal transplant surgery. Although silk suture handles and ties easily, by one year after surgery it has lost its tensile strength.

Fine size silk suture is available in two forms: virgin and braided. Virgin silk retains the silk's natural serecin coating to enable smooth passage through tissue. It is available in 8-0 and 9-0 only and is used primarily for corneal-scleral closure in cataract surgery. To help reduce reactivity to the natural serecin "gum" and to increase the strength of the suture, braided silk sutures are also available. The silk is degummed before braiding to more effectively remove the serecin gum and to allow for a tighter braid of the fibers. In cataract surgery, 7-0 and 8-0 braided silk are used as preplacement or safety sutures, while 4-0 through 6-0 are widely used for traction and for closure in oculoplastic and retinal detachment procedures.

NYLON

Nylon is the suture material of choice for closing corneoscleral wounds. It is classified as nonabsorbable suture by the USP. In 1968 the first needle/suture combinations, incorporating fine size nylon suture, were introduced. During the 1970s nylon gradually replaced silk as the standard primary closure material in anterior segment surgery. Unlike the twisted or braided fibers of silk suture, the monofilament construction of nylon enables smoother passage through the delicate corneal-scleral tissue. The 10-0 monofilament nylon suture has helped ophthalmologists overcome intraoperative breakage while tying. No other suture material offers the combination of thinness, mild elasticity, ease of passage, and secure knot tying found in nylon.

POLYPROPYLENE (PROLENE)

Although all nylon suture is classified as nonabsorbable, suture undergoes a gradual process of hydrolysis, resulting in postoperative relaxation, and, often, suture fragmentation. Where permanent or long-term wound support is needed, nylon may not be the material of choice for many surgeons. (The fact that cardiovascular surgeons use Prolene rather than nonabsorbable nylon to perform vascular anastomoses illustrates this.) In cataract surgery, iris repair, and IOL fixation, 9-0 and 10-0 Prolene have become popular for anterior segment procedures where permanent or long-term support is needed.

Table 7.26
USP Specifications For Suture Sizes
(Nonabsorbable Suture)

USP Size	Metric Size (Gauge No.)	Limits on Diameter (mm) Min	Max	Limits on Knot Pull*
11-0	0.1	0.010	0.019	0.005
10-0	0.2	0.020	0.029	0.016
9-0	0.3	0.030	0.039	0.036
8-0	0.4	0.040	0.049	0.06
7-0	0.5	0.050	0.069	0.11
6-0	0.7	0.070	0.099	0.20
5-0	1.0	0.10	0.149	0.40
4-0	1.5	0.15	0.199	0.60
3-0	2.0	0.20	0.249	0.96
2-0	3.0	0.30	0.339	1.44
1-0	3.5	0.35	0.399	2.16

*Class I - silk or synthetic fibers of monofilament, twisted, or braided construction. Tensile strength (kg).

POLYESTER (MERSILENE)

As mentioned above, some of the concerns expressed by anterior segment surgeons in using nylon suture include tensile strength/intraoperative breakage, hydrolysis/postoperative fragmentation, and hydrolysis/short-term wound support. While nylon sutures solve these problems, the elastic or stretchy nature of both nylon and polypropylene make it difficult for the surgeon to achieve precise and consistent tension along the wound. When closing with 10-0 nylon, surgeons tend to tie the sutures tightly, inducing some with-the-rule astigmatism. This seems preferable, if not necessary, because the nylon sutures loosen or stretch, and if the suture is not initially tight, stretching may result in some against-the-rule astigmatism. Occasionally, however, sufficient loosening does not occur and the tight sutures must be cut in order to reduce the with-the-rule astigmatism.

Mersilene 10-0 and 11-0 polyester fiber sutures have helped anterior segment surgeons who have problems with intraoperative breakage, postoperative fragmentation, tensile strength degradation, and elasticity—all of which are associated with nylon and/or polypropylene. Mersilene suture does not biodegrade or hydrolyze postoperatively, virtually eliminating the inconvenience of having to remove irritating suture fragments from the eye several months after the procedure. Mersilene suture is also the strongest monofilament suture available; thus, suture breakage while tying or handling is minimal. Mersilene suture is also less elastic than nylon suture, i.e., stretches minimally. Additionally, because Mersilene suture does not hydrolyze or biodegrade, it provides reliable long-term wound support.

Absorbable Sutures

Absorbable suture materials are classified as either natural or synthetic. Natural absorbable sutures include gut and collagen. Synthetic absorbable sutures include coated Vicryl (polyglactin 910) and PDS II (polydioxanone). The mechanism for absorption of absorbable sutures depends on their source of origin. Natural absorbable sutures are digested by cellular and tissue enzymes, while synthetic absorbable sutures are hydrolyzed by tissue fluids.

GUT

Surgical gut suture, produced from the serosa and/or submucosa layer of beef or sheep intestine, provides in vivo wound support for approximately ten to 21 days. These sutures are used in oculoplastic and strabismus surgery. Today, there is limited use of this suture material in anterior segment surgery.

COLLAGEN

Collagen suture is produced from the flexor tendon of sheep and is a purer proteinaceous suture material. Because this suture elicits less tissue reaction than surgical gut suture, 7-0 or 8-0 is good for closing conjunctiva. Collagen suture will also provide tensile support to the wound for approximately ten to 21 days.

POLYGLACTIN 910 (COATED VICRYL)

Coated Vicryl suture, primarily 5-0 and 6-0, is very popular for suturing muscles in strabismus surgery, and 7-0 and 8-0 coated Vicryl are popular as a preplacement or safety suture in cataract surgery. This braided synthetic absorbable suture material retains its in vivo tensile strength up to 28 days, contrasting with gut and collagen sutures, which hold up to 21 days. Many ophthalmologists prefer to use a synthetic absorbable suture because its hydrolysis generally elicits less reaction than a suture absorbable by enzymatic action. Having supported the wound for 35 days, coated Vicryl suture will be absorbed in 56 to 72 days. Additionally, coated Vicryl suture provides significant benefits over other braided synthetic absorbable suture materials: smoother passage through tissue, knots that snug down and hold, and superior handling. Vicryl suture is also available in a monofilament construction, in sizes 9-0 and 10-0, and is used primarily for conjunctival/scleral closure.

POLYDIOXONONE (PDS)

Another major advancement in wound closure is the result of the 9-0 PDS suture. Prior to the development of PDS suture, 28 days was the longest in vivo tensile strength provided by an absorbable suture. Many ophthalmologists did not feel that 28 days was long enough to cover the critical wound-healing period for cornealscleral tissue following cataract surgery. The development of PDS suture provided in vivo tensile strength support for twice as long as any other absorbable suture material used in ophthalmic surgery (Fig. 7.27). At 42 days, generally considered the critical wound-healing period for ocular tissue, PDS suture still has roughly 25% of its original tensile strength remaining. Having supported the wound through the critical healing period, PDS suture is absorbed via hydrolysis, eliminating the need to cut and remove sutures postoperatively. As mentioned earlier, one of the difficulties surgeons experience with nylon suture is the postoperative fragmentation that results from hydrolysis. Clinical studies indicate that PDS suture in corneal-scleral tissue is essentially absorbed within 180 days postoperatively, and therefore can help minimize this difficulty.

Conclusion

Needles and sutures used in ophthalmology have come a long way in the past twenty years, with accelerated growth occuring in the past decade. Advancements in ophthalmic surgical technique have in turn demanded parallel advancements in ophthalmic needle and suture technology. Suturing is still the closure method of choice for anterior segment surgery; however, other forms of closure are currently being investigated (e.g., cyanoacrylate glues, biological glues, and staples). Whether any of these materials will be used routinely in ophthalmic surgery is now only speculation. Any method or material that will prove advantageous to the patient and the surgeon will certainly be accepted as long as it is safe and efficacious.

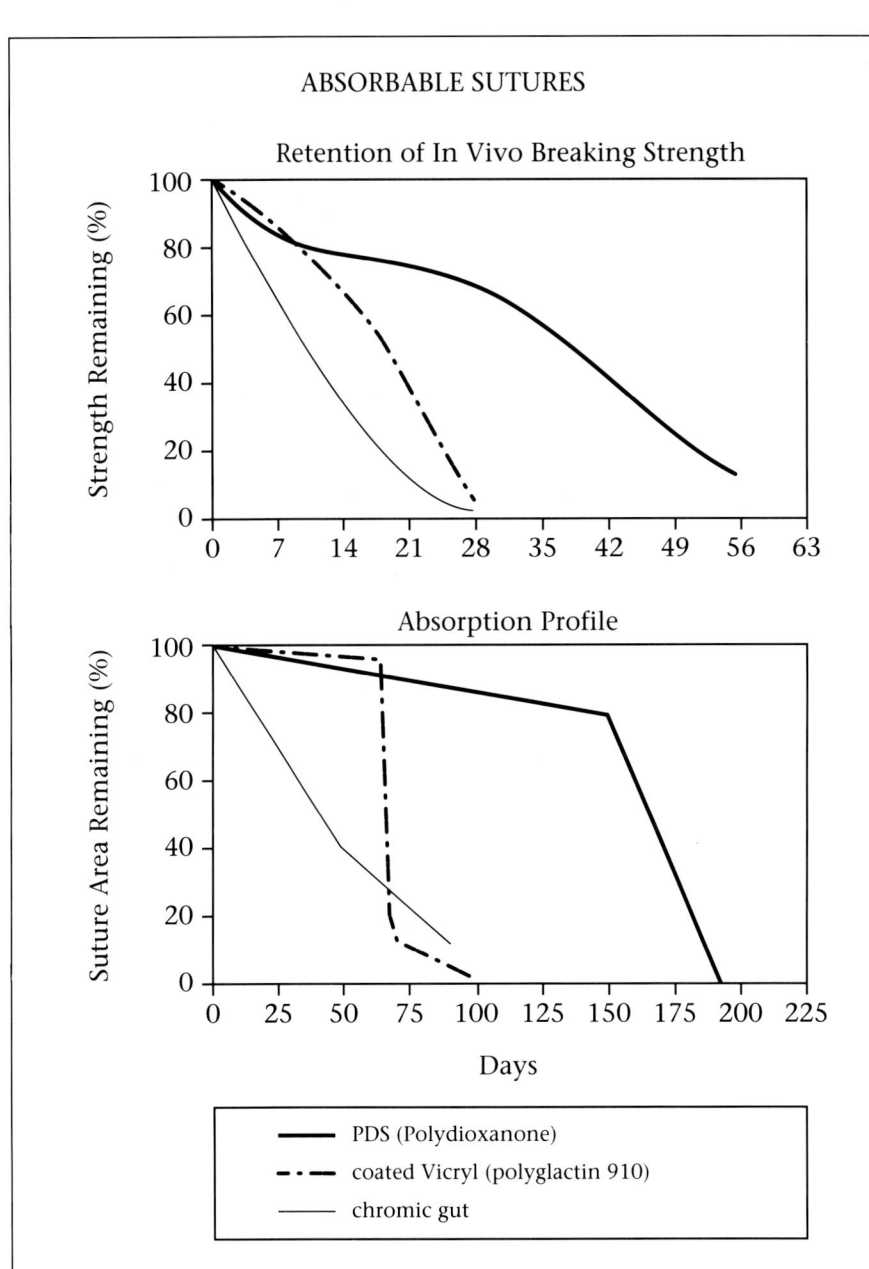

Figure 7.27 *Comparison between in vivo breaking strength of PDS and other absorbable sutures.*

Clinical Points to Consider

☞ Spatula needles are routinely used for corneal and corneoscleral wound closure due to excellent penetration and minimal damage.

☞ The anterior segment surgeon should be familiar with the various needle configurations used for corneoscleral closure and their intended uses.

☞ Nylon has become the most widely used suture in anterior segment surgery because it is strong, slightly elastic, easily tied, and minimally biodegradable.

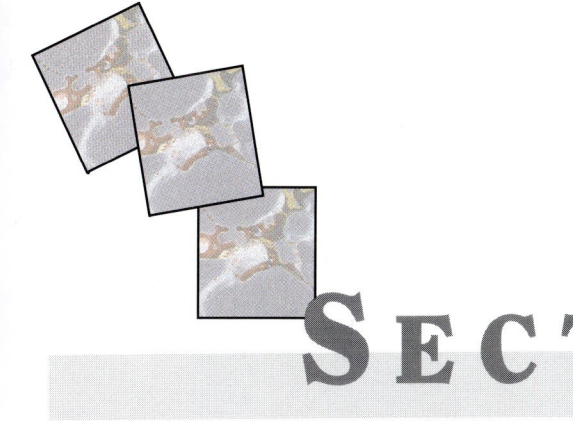

SECTION THREE
SURGERY OF THE LENS

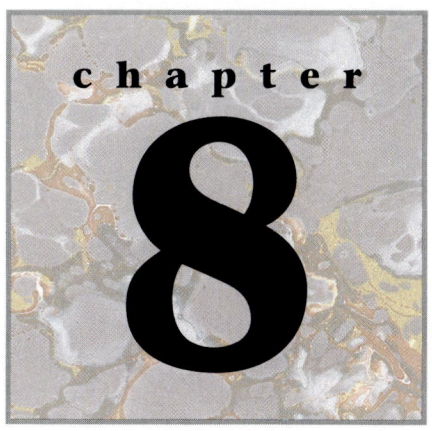

Intraocular Lens Design

CHARLES D. FRITCH, M.D.   MATHIAS ZIRM, M.D.
DAVID DILLMAN, M.D.   PHILIPPE CROZAFON, M.D.   LEE NORDAN, M.D.

Ocular function after cataract extraction has been revolutionized by intraocular lens (IOL) implantation. Virtually all cataract surgery currently performed in a sophisticated medical setting incorporates IOL implantation. Except in rare circumstances, aphakic spectacles and contact lenses and their associated problems have vanished. The advantages provided by current IOLs, however, have not been gained without great struggle. Many eyes were damaged by complications created by the early IOLs. Most chronic complications were related to IOL design and occurred despite appropriate surgical technique. This chapter presents IOL design considerations and attempts to correlate these designs with clinical IOL successes and limitations. Also, possibilities for future IOL designs, such as a posterior chamber (PC) IOL with a haptic diameter more suited for in-the-bag implantation and multifocal IOLs, will be discussed.

Posterior Chamber Intraocular Lenses

The PC IOL has become the standard IOL for use after uncomplicated forms of extracapsular cataract extraction (ECCE), which preserves the posterior capsule that supports the PC IOL. Not all PC IOL designs and materials can be included in this chapter, but concepts and specifics that pertain to most PC IOL designs will be considered.

Optic Size

The 6.00-mm optic with no positioning holes is the best choice when trying to limit edge glare caused by decentration and postoperative astigmatism caused by a longer incision length. Positioning holes can be a source of glare and the site of posterior synechiae. IOLs with 7.00-mm optics do well with planned ECCE, but the idea that high myopes require an optic of this diameter because it supports the vitreous face to a significantly greater degree than a 6.00-mm optic has been based on intuition rather than statistical evidence (Fig. 8.1).

Several factors must be considered when positioning an ovoid IOL (usually 5.00 mm × 6.00 mm) during implantation. Rotation of the optic horizontally may be advantageous since the pupil and, therefore, the center of the visual axis are usually positioned about 0.60 mm nasal to the geometric center of the cornea. Since the capsular bag is concentric with the cornea, an IOL implanted properly within the capsular bag will be slightly "decentered" with respect to the visual axis (Fig. 8.2), although the horizontal positioning assumes the capsulorhexis to be well-centered. If the capsulorhexis is decentered superiorly, which is most often the case, the surgeon must consider that late contracture of the capsulorhexis opening may cause vertical decentration of the optic (see Chapter 9, Fig. 9.11), a scenario that dictates vertical placement of the haptics.

Ovoid IOLs minimize postoperative astigmatism because they require an incision of only 5.00 mm for insertion. A 4.00-mm incision can be used when implanting a foldable IOL, but the surgical technique may require maneuvers considerably more difficult. It makes sense to use ovoid IOLs, if the surgeon is able to consistently implant an IOL with both haptics inside the capsular bag, even with a small pupil, and perform a well-centered capsulotomy. However, the edge of a vertically implanted ovoid IOL will be at the pupillary border when the pupil is 3.80 mm in diameter, assuming the 0.60 mm decentration mentioned above. A horizontally implanted ovoid IOL can accommodate a 4.80-mm pupil. This is a very significant difference because the pupils of elderly patients rarely have a physiologic mydriasis of 4.50 mm or greater; however, the surgeon

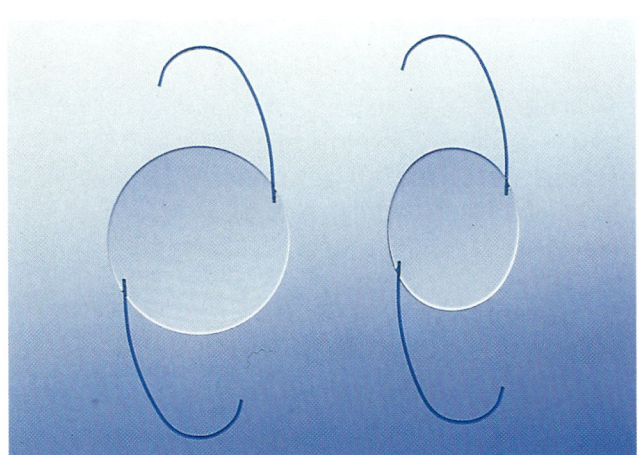

Figure 8.1 *Two IOLs, one with a 7.00-mm circular optic* (**left**) *and one with a 5.00 × 6.00 mm oval optic* (**right**).

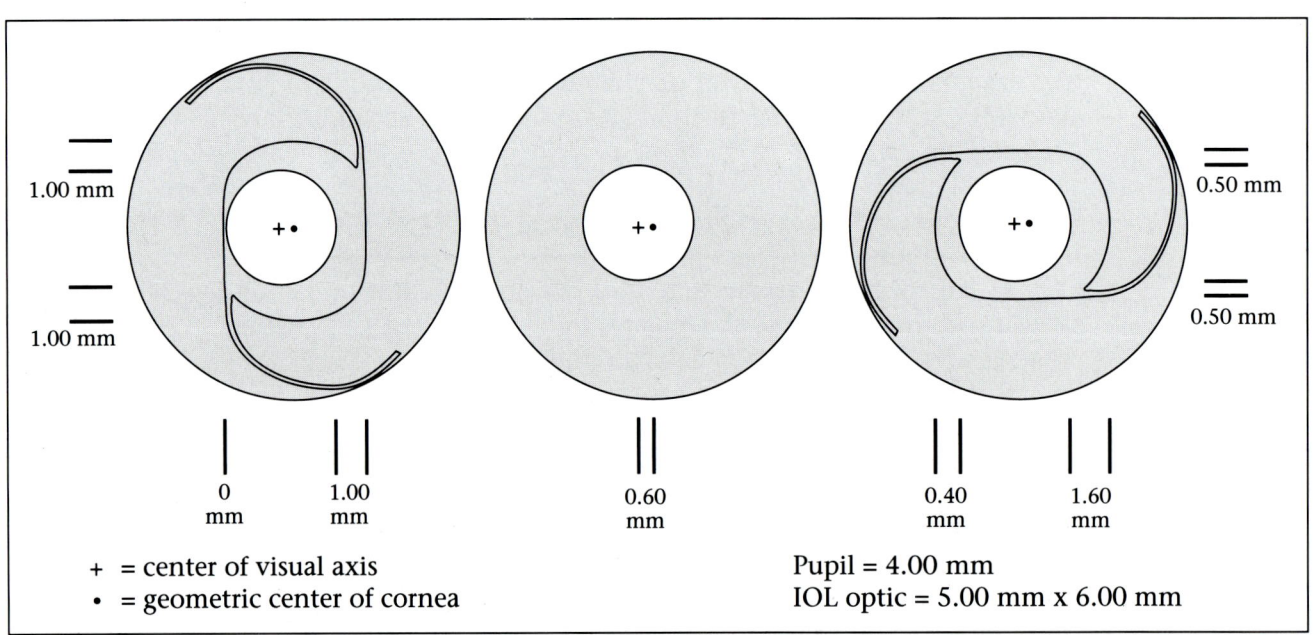

Figure 8.2 *The visual axis is usually nasal to the geometric center of the cornea. Therefore, if the IOL remains centered, an ovoid IOL, which is placed horizontally, runs less risk of producing edge glare with a pupil size greater than 4.00 mm than an IOL placed vertically.*

should consider whether the forces causing late vertical IOL decentration will outweigh the advantage of placing the IOL horizontally.

DECENTRATION

The centration of a PC IOL optic is determined by the haptic configuration, assuming an adequate anterior capsulotomy. The most important haptic factors that prevent significant decentration, even if one haptic is positioned inadvertently in the ciliary sulcus and the other in the capsular bag, are the acute angle between a haptic and the optic as well as a flexible haptic. The acute angle makes it more likely that the optic will *rotate* rather than be *displaced* as the flexible haptics conform to asymmetrical haptic implantation (Fig. 8.3). The limit of this acute angle is determined by structural considerations that must be taken into account when staking the haptic into the optic and by how much room is needed for the positioning hook (Sinskey, Graether, etc.) so it does not get stuck when manipulating the IOL during implantation.

Haptic Material

Traditionally, IOLs with 4-0 or 5-0 polypropylene (Prolene) haptics have been the most commonly used, but during the late 1980s there was a significant trend toward one-piece as well as three-piece PMMA IOLs (Figs. 8.4 and 8.5). Three-piece PMMA IOLs incorporate a PMMA optic into which are staked separate PMMA optic haptics. These three-piece and thinner one-piece PMMA IOLs are replacing the older one-piece PMMA IOLs,

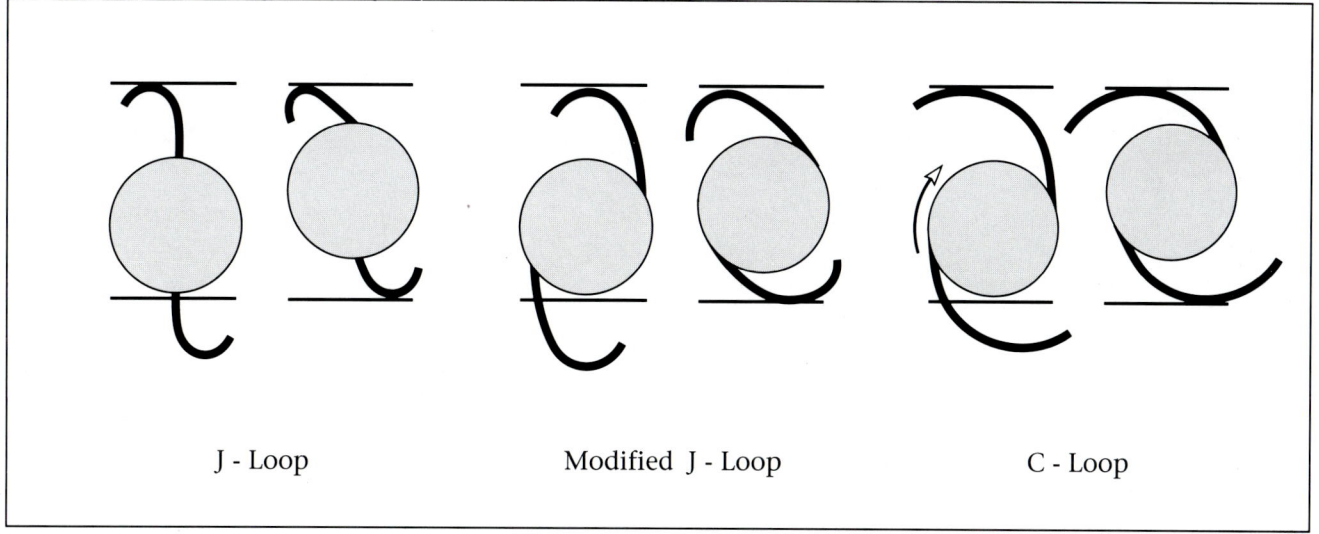

Figure 8.3 *For PC IOLs of similar construction, the more acute the angle between the haptic and the optic, the less pressure necessary to compress the haptics and the greater the tendency for the optic to rotate rather than decenter. A PC IOL with an overall haptic diameter of 12.00 mm requires less haptic compression than a PC IOL with an overall haptic diameter of 13.00 mm to 14.00 mm.* **(Left)** *Original J-loop (Shearing),* **(center)** *modified J-loop (Sinskey), and* **(right)** *C-loop (Simcoe) PC IOLs.*

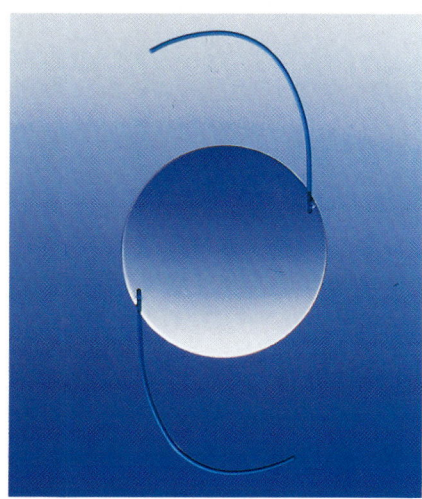

Figure 8.4 *Three-piece PC IOL with PMMA haptics.*

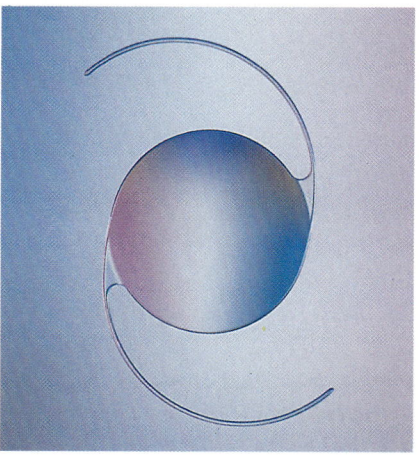

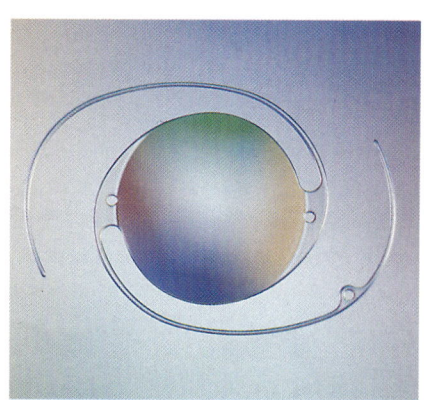

Figure 8.5 (Left and right) *One-piece PMMA PC IOLs.*

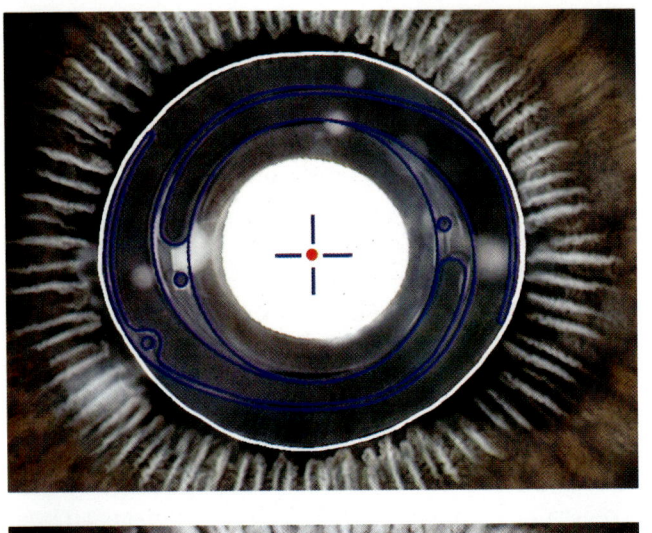
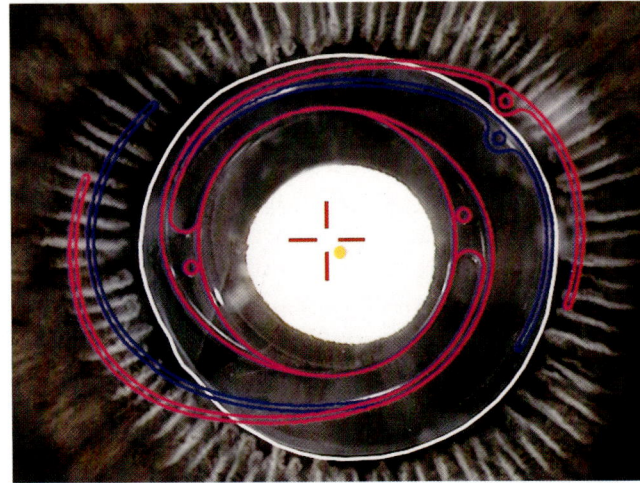
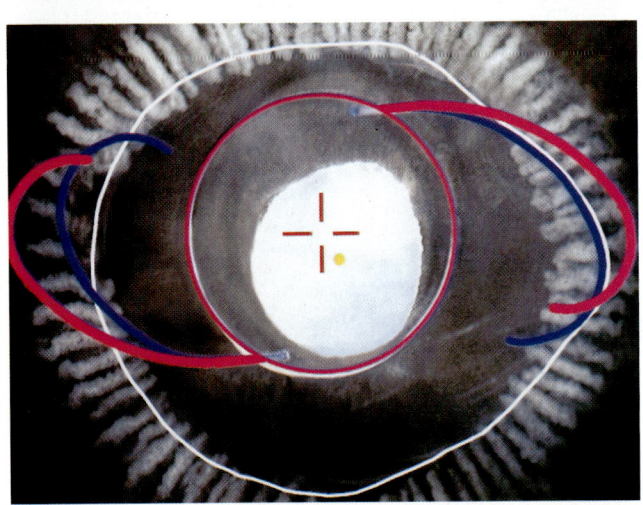
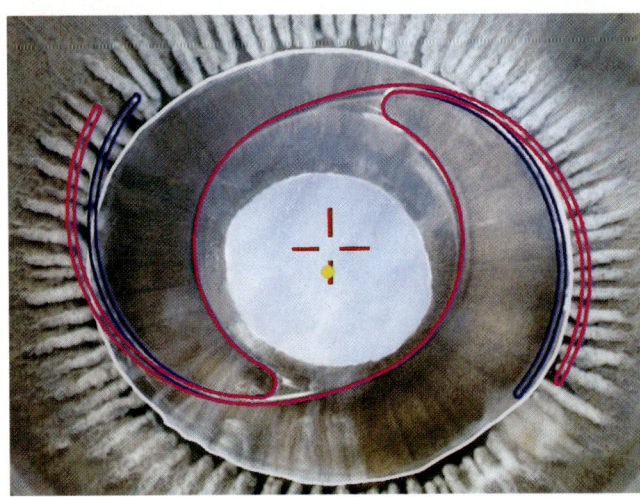
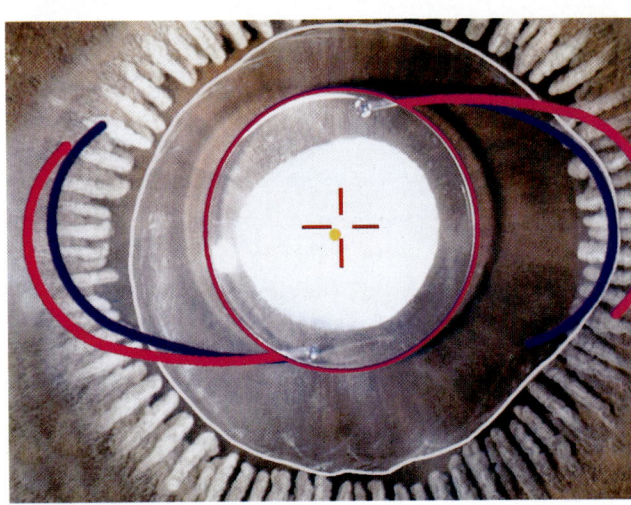
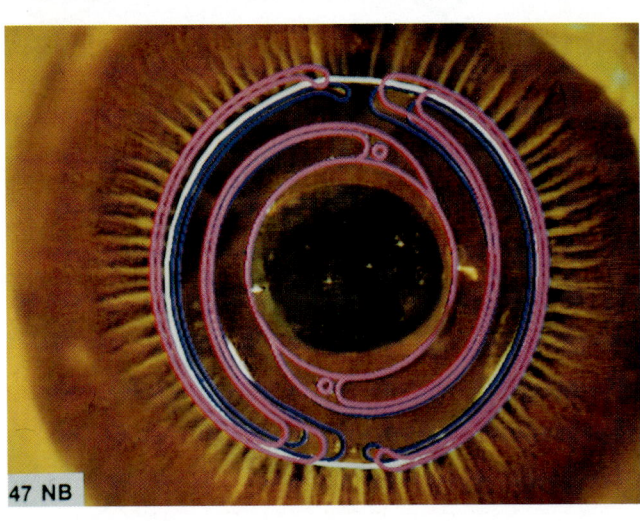

Figure 8.6 *A one-piece PMMA IOL implanted within the capsular bag shows excellent centration despite ovalization of the capsular bag* **(top left)**. *The center of the IOL optic (cross) is perfectly aligned with the optical axis of the eye (dot). This IOL and globe are used to analyze the asymmetric implantation of the IOL, caused by a tear in the anterior capsular bag. An SFVT (Synchronous Film Video Technique) and Visualeyes (Visitec) study shows that the center of the IOL optic (cross) is now displaced only about 0.50 mm from the optical axis (dot) because of the relatively flexible haptics* **(top right)**. *There is less compression of the haptic in the ciliary sulcus than the one in the capsular bag. The pink lines indicate the shape of the IOL haptics before implantation and the blue lines indicate the shape of the haptic after implantation. Various shaped haptics cause an IOL optic to shift location differently under the conditions of assymetrical implantation. Modified J-loop Prolene haptics—vertical/horizontal shift* **(middle left)**. *C-loop haptic one piece PMMA IOL—vertical shift only* **(middle right)**; *short-C Prolene haptic—almost no shift* **(bottom left)**. *An IOL with a multicurved haptic creates a beautifully spherical capsular bag after implantation with minimal compression of the haptics* **(bottom right)**. *However, consistent implantation of this style IOL into the capsular bag (with or without a tear) through a contracting pupil, small capsulorhexis, or 6.00 mm wound might tend to be difficult.*

which have thicker, stiffer haptics near the optic. Some older one-piece PMMA IOLs center very well because they exert a large degree of force on the scleral wall of the eye, but it is also possible that this large degree of force exerted on the capsule, choroid, and sclera can cause increased zonular stress or erosion into the ciliary body and sclera.

A desirable property of Prolene is that it loses its compressibility several months after implantation and will not create stress on the zonules or capsular bag. However, Prolene haptics are not able to resist the forces of late optic decentration, which may be generated by contracture of an asymmetrical capsulorhexis.

Thin PMMA haptics are almost as flexible as Prolene haptics but do not lose their compressibility completely. PMMA is thought to be more biologically inert, possibly causing less inflammation. Prolene has never been proved to cause acute or chronic iritis following PC IOL implantation, although there has been speculation that it may cause inflammation in the anterior chamber as a result of exposure to limited amounts of ultraviolet (UV) radiation. Also, electron microscopy has detected significant pitting and erosion of the Prolene loops of PC IOLs that have been implanted for several years.

Haptic Design
SHAPE

The distal shape of the haptic is important, as is the angle between the haptic and the optic (Fig. 8.6). A C-loop (Simcoe) configuration may provide more contact area and fill out the capsular bag more completely than a modified J-loop style (Fig. 8.7). However, a stiff C-loop, with its long radius of curvature, may be more difficult to

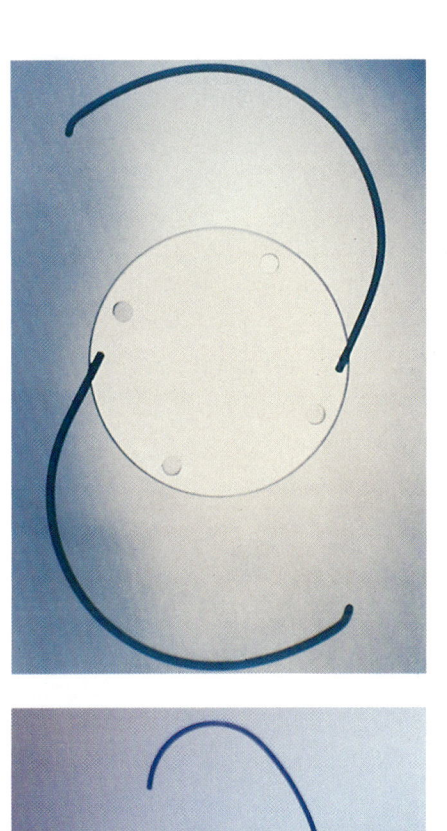
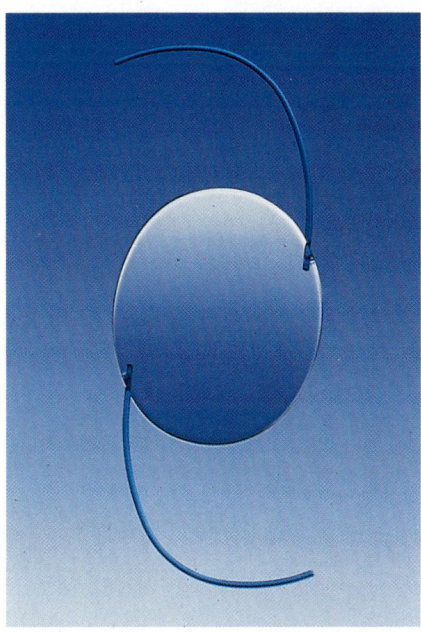

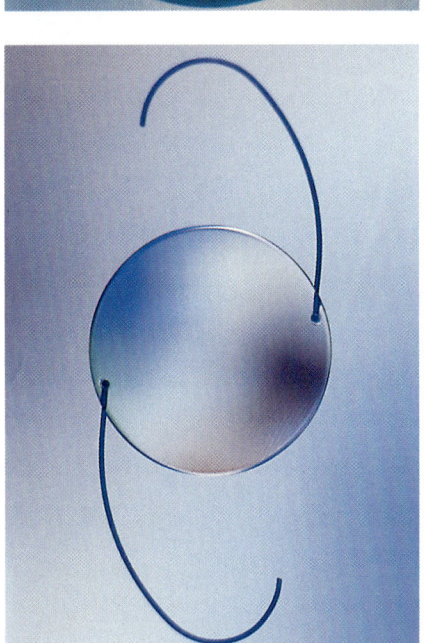

Figure 8.7 *Comparison of PC IOLs with C-loop and J-loop haptics. A C-loop (Simcoe) haptic* **(top left and right)** *may provide more support yet be more difficult to insert into the capsular bag through a small capsulotomy than a modified J-loop haptic, with its more curved distal portion* **(bottom left and right).**

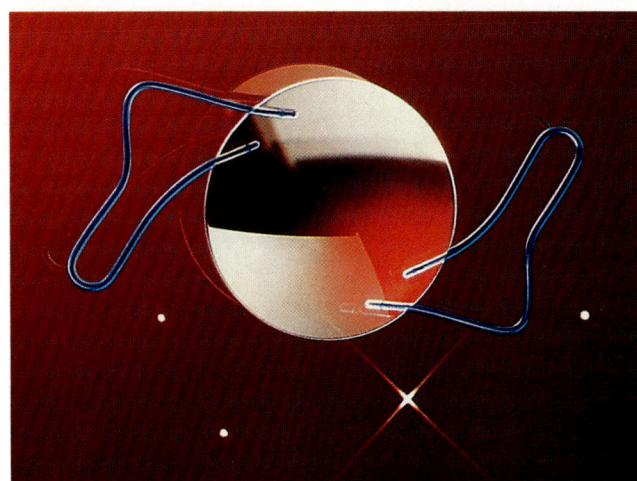

Figure 8.8 *PC IOL with closed loop haptics (3M–Style 30).*

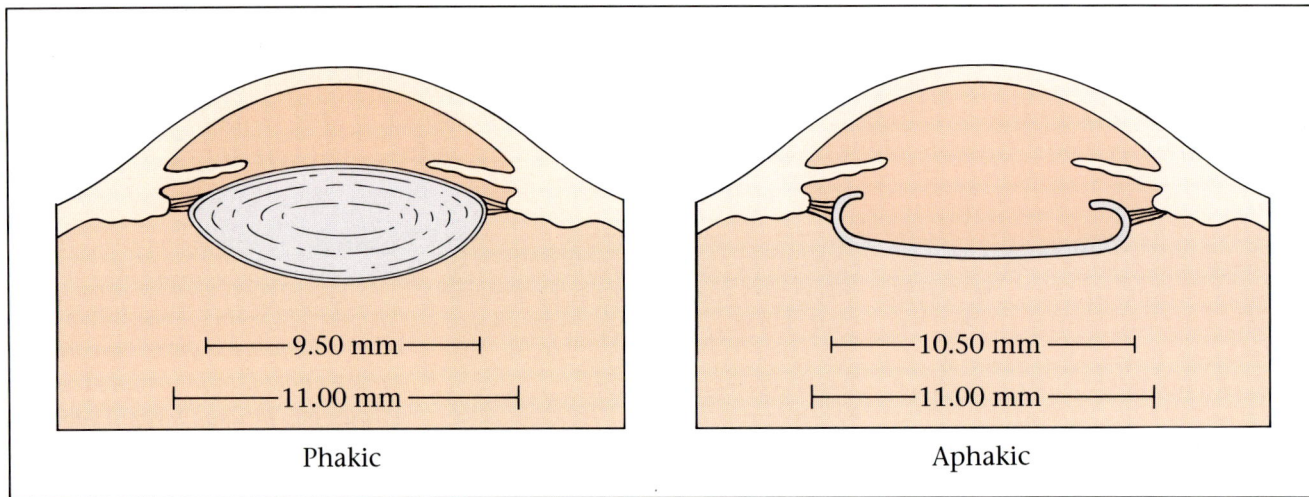

Figure 8.9 *The dimensions of the capsular bag and its relationship to surrounding structures, before and after cataract removal. A PC IOL with a 12.00 mm to 12.25 mm overall haptic diameter can be well stabilized even with asymmetrical implantation.*

Figure 8.10 *PC IOL haptic angulation ranges from 0 (planar) to 10 degrees.*

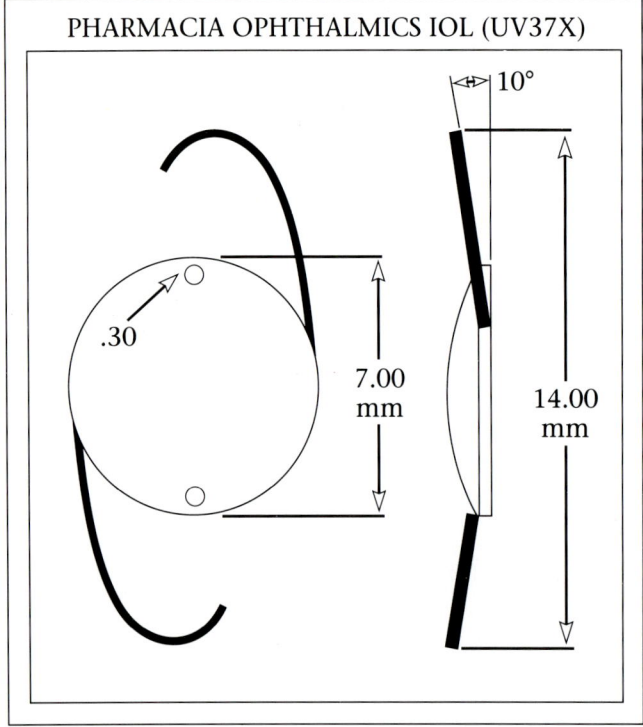

insert into a small capsulorhexis, especially if the pupil constricts during surgery and no positioning holes are present to allow for a "dialing" insertion technique.

Closed loop haptics for PC IOLs create more contact pressure than an open loop, and since they are often more difficult to insert into the capsular bag probably offer no special clinical advantage (Fig. 8.8). IOLs without haptics (disc optics) or IOLs with a continuous ("steering wheel") haptic might offer excellent centration within the capsular bag. However, excellent centration requires that the diameter of all capsular bags be equal and the absence of anterior capsular radial tears, which might extend during the insertion. Despite the theoretical advantages, implantation of this style IOL is so difficult that it probably will not be acceptable for routine use.

OVERALL DIAMETER

The human lens is about 9.50 mm in diameter and about 4.00 mm thick. The lens is suspended from the zonules directly opposite the pars plicata of the ciliary body. After a cataract has been removed, the diameter of the empty capsular bag enlarges to approximately 10.50 mm and the diameter of the ciliary sulcus remains 11.00 mm (Fig 8.9). A PC IOL with a haptic diameter of 12.00 mm to 12.50 mm allows for implantation in-the-bag and adequate centration even if one haptic is inadvertently positioned in the ciliary sulcus. In-the-bag implantation does not require the 13.50 mm to 14.00 mm haptic diameters that were created as sulcus fixation IOLs.

ANGULATION

A mild haptic angulation of about five or six degrees allows for easy implantation of the PC IOL into the capsular bag. The final position of the IOL should be posterior enough to prevent the iris from rubbing on the anterior surface of the optic (Fig. 8.10). Marked haptic angulation may necessitate excessive optic manipulation and create posterior capsular tension while jockeying the haptics into the capsular bag.

Anterior Capsulotomy

Ciliary sulcus positioning of the haptics has served many patients well for years. However, sequestering the haptic in the capsular bag provides potential long-term advantages because the interaction between the choroid and haptic is minimized. Since cataract patients may commonly live 15 to 20 years after surgery, in-the-bag implantation seems advantageous as long as the surgical technique has been mastered. A can-opener anterior capsulotomy is adequate for in-the-bag implantation, but it should be recognized that radial tears often extend peripherally from the edge of the capsulotomy (usually superiorly) and are a key factor in late PC IOL decentration (see Chapter 9).

A smooth, complete capsulorhexis is an important factor in providing long-term IOL centration (see Chapter 9). However, a capsulorhexis is more difficult to learn than a can-opener capsulotomy, and it tends to have a smaller diameter, which makes phacoemulsification and ECCE more difficult. Often, the neophyte phaco surgeon must choose between a 6.00-mm capsulorhexis, with a superior tear necessary for prolapse of the nucleus, or a larger can-opener capsulotomy without the tear. Similarly, in-the-bag phaco is desirable but may lead to a higher rate of complications than iris plane phaco, especially with a harder nucleus.

Posterior Chamber Intraocular Lens Design Factors

No PC IOL design is ideal, but consider the following factors, which pertain to IOL function:

Optic diameter:
- 5.00 mm diameter—small wound (less induced astigmatism); greatest chance of producing edge glare.
- 6.00 mm diameter—middle-sized wound; minimal chance of edge glare.
- 7.00 mm diameter—largest wound; least chance of edge glare.

Optic shape:
Plano-convex; convex-concave (meniscus); biconvex—probably no clinically significant difference. Some surgeons believe that a biconvex shape reduces the incidence of secondary posterior capsule opacification.

Haptic material:
- Prolene—no long-term outward pressure; possible long-term biodegradation; easily decentered.
- PMMA—slight long-term outward pressure; minimal biodegradation; resists decentration.

Haptic configuration:
- Modified J-loop—haptic more easily implanted through a small capsulorhexis or pupil; capsular bag not evenly distended.
- C-loop—haptic may be more difficult to implant through a small capsulorhexis or pupil with dialing technique; distends capsular bag more evenly.

Haptic diameter:

11.00 mm—demands in-the-bag implantation.

12.00 mm to 12.50 mm—less capsular and zonular stress for in-the-bag implantation. Adequate centration with asymmetrical implantation.

13.00 mm to 14.00 mm—designed for ciliary sulcus fixation. More difficult to implant in the presence of a small capsulorhexis.

Clinically Optimal Posterior Chamber Intraocular Lens Design

A foldable IOL with a 6.00-mm, no hole, silicone or acrylic optic implanted through a 4.00-mm incision that can be closed by a single horizontal suture is the state of the art design for minimizing induced surgical astigmatism and maximizing the use of the small incision PC IOL (see Chapter 15) (Fig. 8.11) However, many questions remain as to the optimal haptic design for a PC IOL.

In 1984, James A. Davison, M.D., set out to determine and document the optimal PC IOL haptic configuration for in-the-bag implantation. Previous clinical and postmortem observations revealed the advantages of reducing haptic contact with choroidal tissue by placing the PC IOL inside the capsular bag (Fig. 8.12). The goal of secure fixation within the capsular bag associated with the least degree of capsular and zonular stress favored an overall haptic diameter in the 12.00 mm range (Figs. 8.13 to 8.15)

Next, the shape of the haptic had to be determined. PC IOL prototypes were produced and implanted in cadaver eyes at the Center for Intraocular Lens Research (Charleston, South Carolina; David Apple, M.D., Director). The Miyake camera technique with still photography and videotape was used, and the implantation of various IOLs was observed by IOL designers and engineers. A PC IOL with a 14.00-mm overall haptic diameter and 7.00-mm haptic (Pharmacia UB-89; Obstbaum), despite being oversized, demonstrated a good relationship between the distal haptic and the capsular bag; i.e., the distal haptic did not stick out or curl up within the capsular bag (Figs. 8.16 and 8.17). A steering wheel PC IOL, with its continuous haptic, also demonstrated a good haptic/capsular bag configuration (Fig. 8.18).

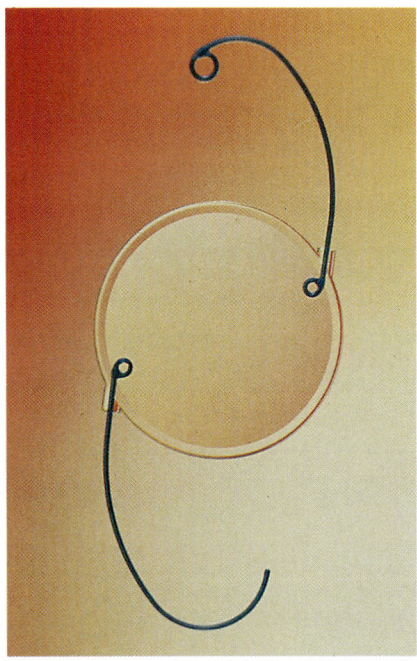 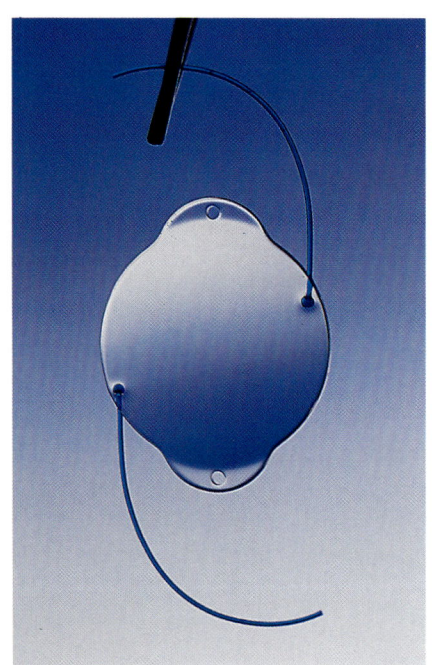 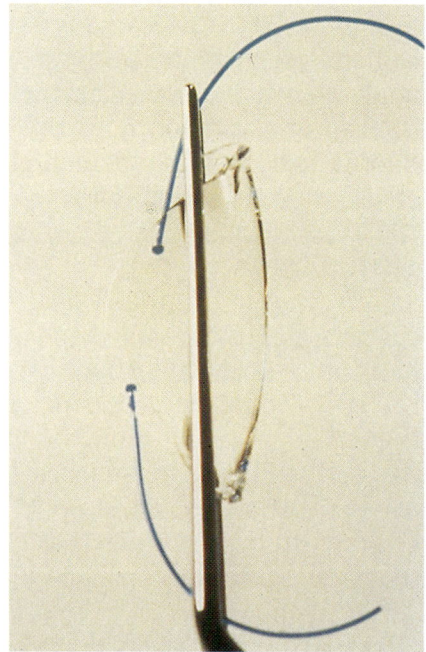

Figure 8.11 *A PC IOL with a foldable, silicone optic (AMO SI-18NB) in the unfolded position* **(left)** *has the same appearance as its PMMA counterpart. The Ioptex Research acrylic optic PC IOL (ACR-365) in the unfolded position* **(middle)** *and the folded position* **(right)**.

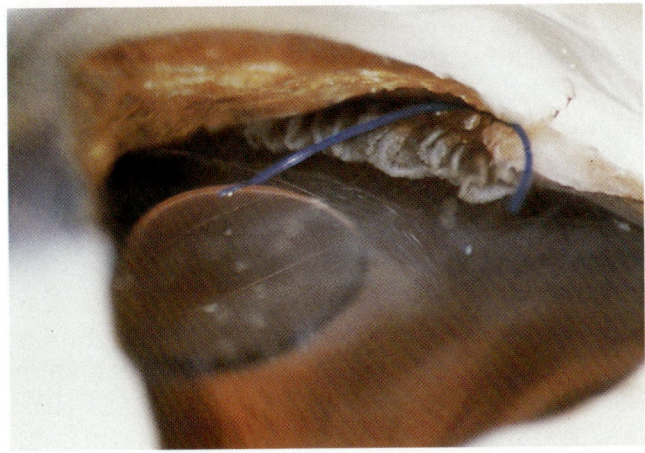

Figure 8.12 *Three-piece PC IOL with the haptic in the ciliary sulcus. Problems related to uveal tissue irritation are well known.*

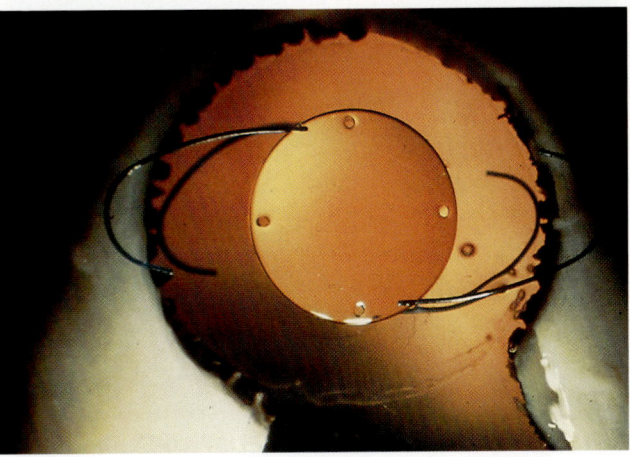

Figure 8.13 *Two PC IOLS, each with a 6.00 mm optic but one with an overall haptic diameter of 12.00 mm. One is positioned nicely in the capsular bag and the other with a 14.00 mm overall haptic diameter placed on the preparation for comparison.*

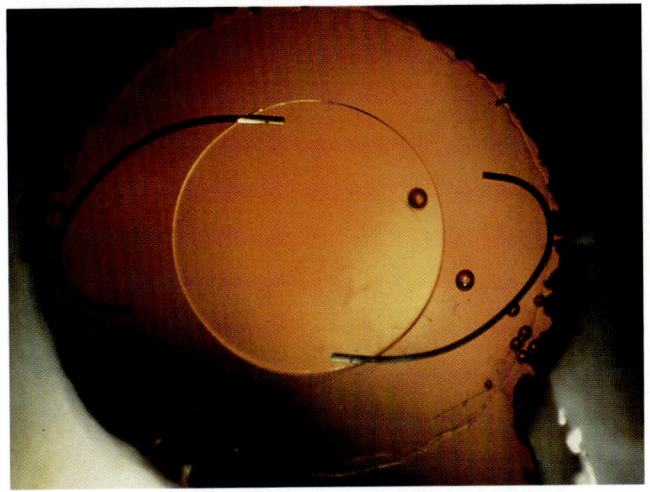

Figure 8.14 *A three-piece PC IOL with overall diameter of 12.00 mm has sufficient length to center well within the capsular bag.*

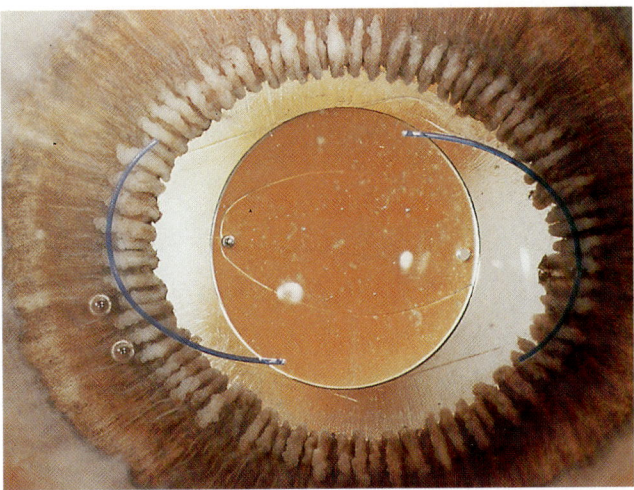

Figure 8.15 *Asymmetric stretching of the capsular bag with a 14.00-mm, Prolene haptic PC IOL in position.*

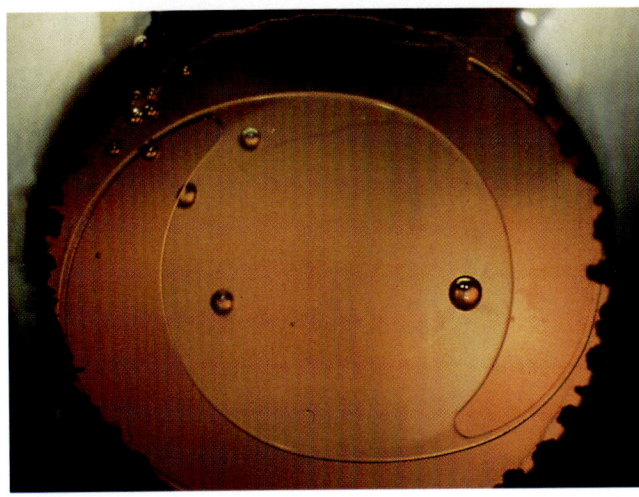

Figure 8.16 *This PC IOL (Pharmacia UB 89) with a 7.00-mm optic and 14.00-mm overall haptic diameter is slightly oversized, yet positions well within the capsular bag.*

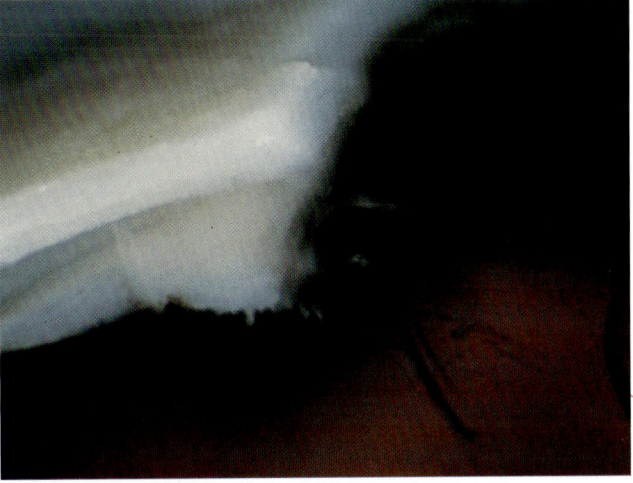

Figure 8.17 *This view of the Pharmacia UB-89 PC IOL haptics demonstrates that the distal haptic is in broad contact with the capsular bag, and the haptic does not create a focal stress point.*

A new Pharmacia PC IOL (UB 120; Davison) was developed with the following design characteristics (Figs. 8.19 and 8.20):

Overall haptic diameter: 12.00 mm
Composition: One piece PMMA
Optic diameter: 6.00 mm
Optic shape: biconvex
Haptic design: soft C-loop
Haptic angulation: 6 degrees

Implantation of the UB-120 centered well within the capsular bag, even when one or two radial tears were created in the anterior capsular leaf in an attempt to purposely compromise the integrity of the capsulorhexis. Further examination, however, revealed that striae were produced in the posterior capsule, the result of focal stresses produced in the equatorial portion of the capsular bag by the haptic of this IOL. The portion of the haptic nearest the optic, "the shoulder," was too stiff. Broad support from the entire length of the haptic was not achieved.

The engineers then designed a second curve into the shoulder of the haptic, similar in appearance to a haptic modification being evaluated by Philippe Crozafon, M.D., of Nice, France (Fig. 8.21). Implantation of this new IOL design revealed that the distal portion of the haptic was too stiff (Figs. 8.22 and 8.23). Another change in the secondary curve of the haptic, with computer design assistance, yielded an IOL (Pharmacia 811; Davison) that supported itself with broad, even haptic contact within the capsular bag. This IOL was even easier to insert through a 5.50 mm diameter capsulorhexis than other haptic designs (Figs. 8.24 and 8.25).

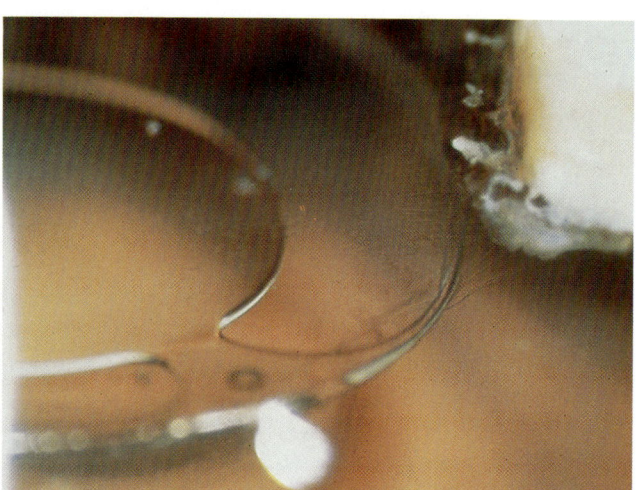

Figure 8.18 *A "steering wheel" PC IOL has a circular haptic. This haptic fits nicely within the capsular bag and does not create areas of focal stress.*

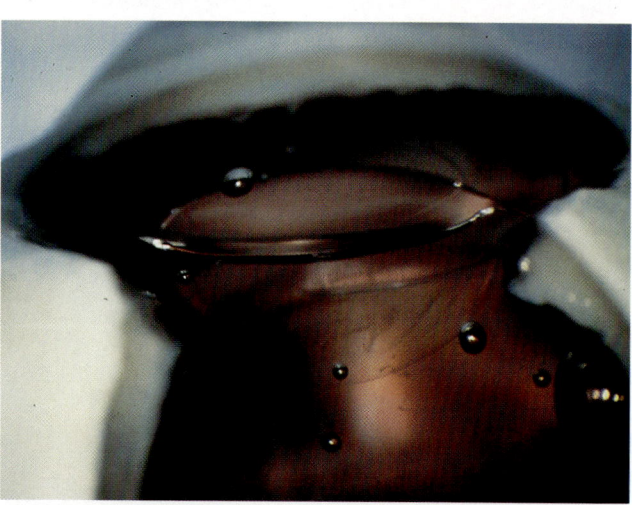

Figure 8.19 *This prototype PC IOL (Pharmacia UB 120) centers well within the capsular bag, but the distal portion of the haptics has not been recruited to resist the compressive force of capsular bag fibrosis. Positioning of this IOL within the capsular bag approaches "two-point fixation" —the distal haptic is not being used.*

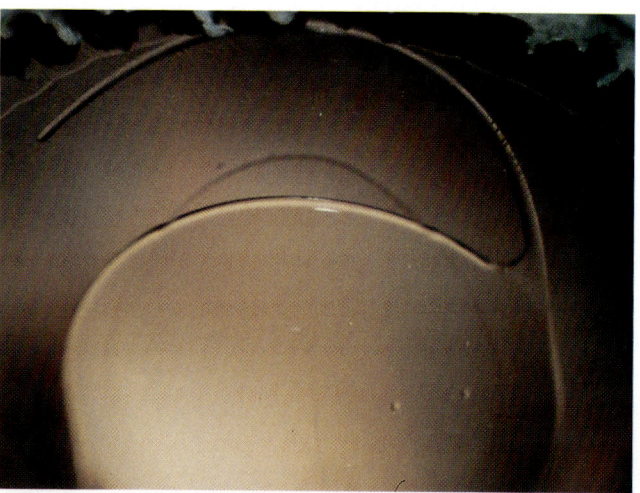

Figure 8.20 *A close up of the distal haptic of the UB 120 IOL shows that it is not contributing to the fixation of the PC IOL.*

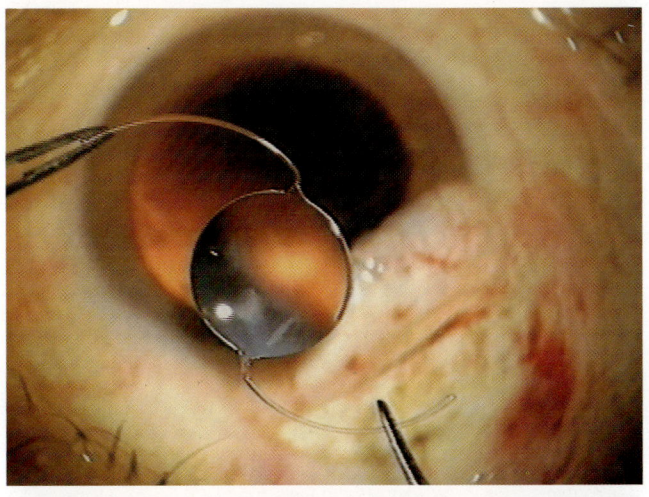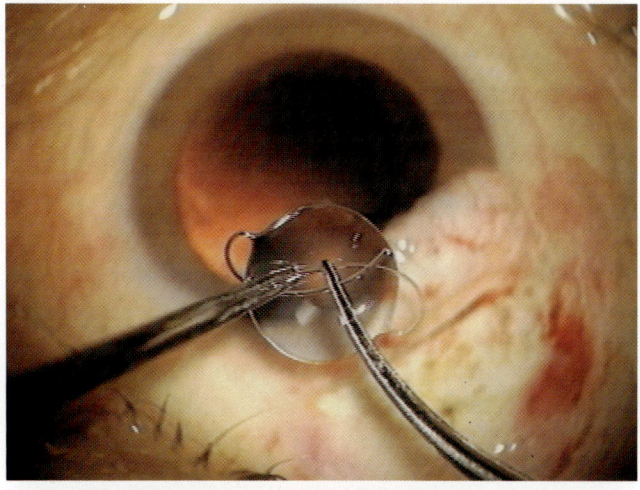

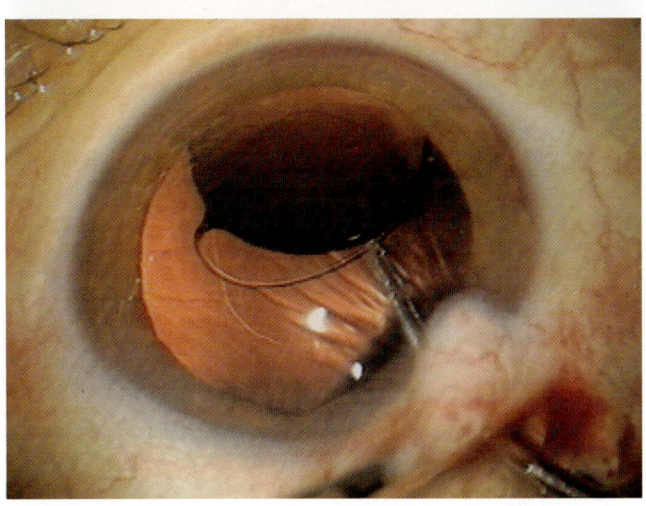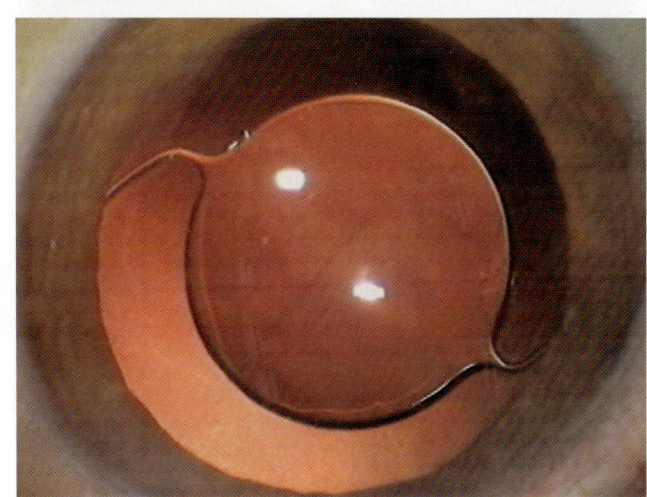

Figure 8.21 *The Pharmacia 740-P is a one-piece, PMMA PC IOL with a 5.00-mm diameter optic, primary and secondary haptic curves* **(top left)**, *and broad, very flexible haptics* **(top right)**. *The haptics require extreme displacement of the optic and creation of considerable* zonular stress for the IOLs implantation into the capsular bag through a 4.50 mm capsulorhexis. The Pharmacia 740-P centers itself well within the capsular bag as the anterior chamber is formed **(bottom left and right)**.

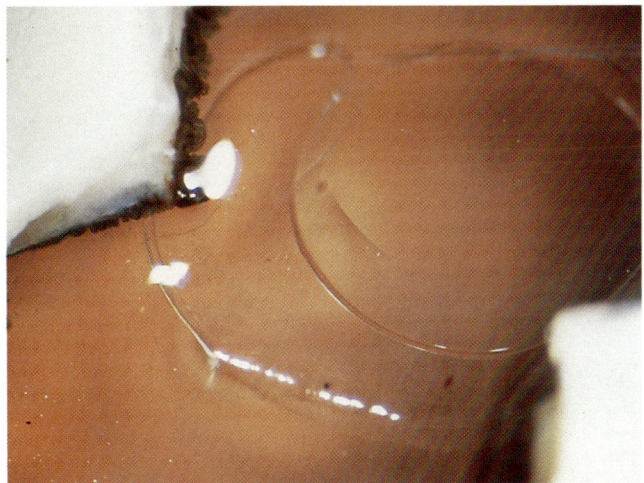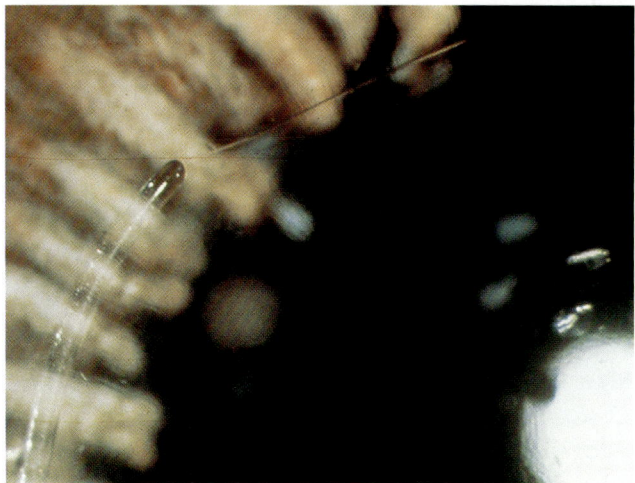

Figure 8.22 *Further modification of the haptic "shoulder" produced a prototype PC IOL (Pharmacia 811). Too much pressure is exerted on the capsular bag by the distal haptic, causing distention of the capsular bag toward the ciliary body.*

Figure 8.23 *Further modification of the haptic "shoulder" yielded the final form of the Pharmacia 811 PC IOL. The haptic fits the capsule in a broad arc, without distention or bowing in of the capsular bag or haptic.*

Design Requirements

PC IOLs must fulfill three essential requirements. First, the IOL must provide superior optical performance. Second, the IOL's residence within the capsular bag must not generate complications. Third, the IOL must be implanted easily, successfully, and consistently. Experience has shown that a 6.00-mm optic affords the patient a reasonable compromise between long-term IOL optic performance and induced astigmatism caused by the surgical wound. Of course, a foldable 6.00-mm optic inserted through a 3.50-mm to 4.00-mm wound provides even more advantages for many patients.

Further research by Davison and colleagues, as well as Apple, Blumenthal, and others showed that haptic diameters of 13.50 mm to 14.00 mm, which were designed originally for ciliary sulcus implantation of PC IOLs, could cause decentration when implanted within the capsular bag. The decentration is caused by the excessive pressure exerted by the IOL, which causes the capsular flap defects to unfold, resulting in undesired protrusion of the haptic outside the capsular bag (see

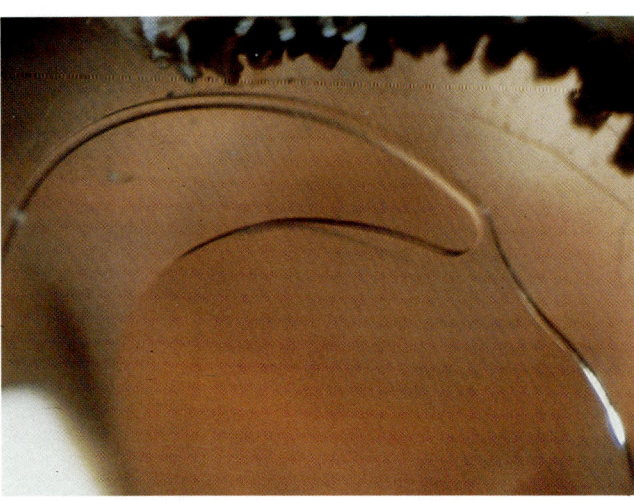

Figure 8.24 *Pharmacia 811 PC IOL within the capsular bag.*

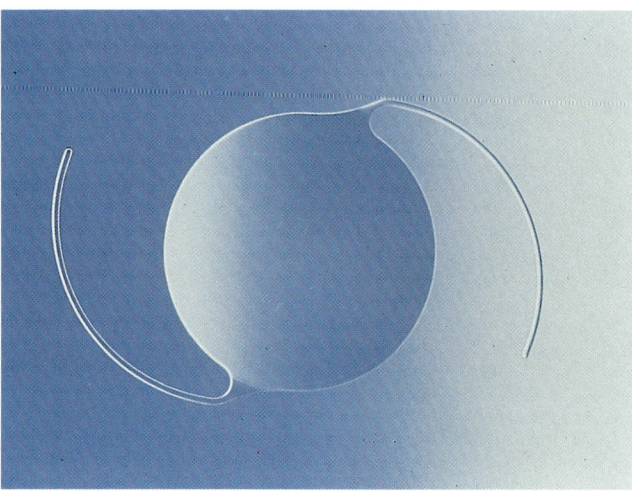

Figure 8.25 *Pharmacia 811 PC IOL.*

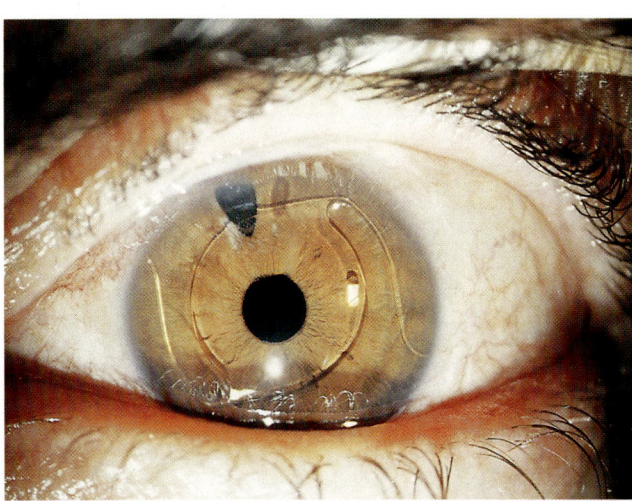

Figure 8.26 *An AC IOL was placed in the eye of a 50-year-old male following cataract extraction by phacoemulsification. The posterior capsule had been ruptured six months preoperatively during attempts to eradicate vitreous floaters with a YAG laser. Traumatic retinal detachment and repair by encircling element followed the phacoemulsification/AC IOL surgery. The original AC IOL was replaced to correct the resulting myopia. Four years after the last surgery, visual acuity is 20/25 without correction and 20/15 with correction. Sporadic episodes of low grade iritis are of concern.*

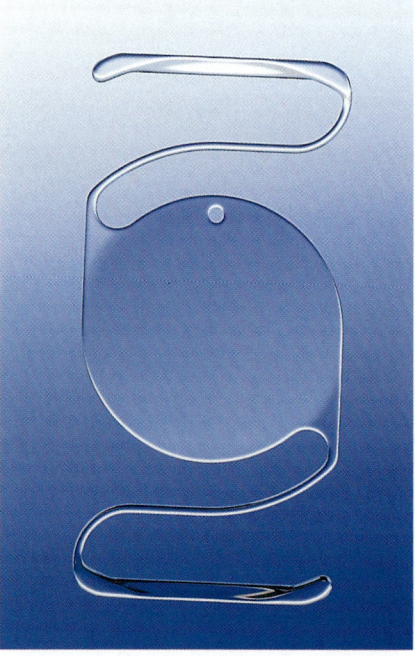

Figure 8.27 *The Ioptex Research version of the Kelman Multiflex AC IOL.*

Chapter 9). The ciliary sulcus is about 11.00 mm in diameter, and a 12.00 mm overall haptic length has been shown to sufficiently insure adequate centration in the event of asymmetrical implantation (one haptic in the capsular bag and one in the ciliary sulcus). In the presence of multiple anterior capsular radial tears a flexible, 12.00-mm, C-loop haptic offers a better chance of in-the-bag implantation than a stiff, 14.00-mm, one piece PMMA IOL. This longer haptic is more likely to stress the capsular bag and cause an anterior capsular flap to unfold, which allows one haptic to reside in the zonules, ciliary body, or vitreous.

A PC IOL with a 6.00-mm optic (foldable or not), 12.00-mm overall haptic diameter, very flexible PMMA haptics, soft C-loop design with appropriate secondary curve, and 6-degree haptic angulation should be considered seriously as the design of choice for IOL implantation within the capsular bag. This PC IOL style affords the patient and surgeon an excellent compromise between reasonable ease of insertion combined with excellent centration and full, almost symmetrical distension of the capsular bag with just enough haptic force to counteract the forces of capsular bag contraction.

Trans-scleral Fixation of Posterior Chamber Intraocular Lenses

When necessary, PC IOLs may be implanted despite the absence of a capsular bag by anchoring the haptic of the PC IOL in the ciliary sulcus with Prolene suture. Routinely, an anterior chamber (AC) IOL is preferred, but aniridia or extensive synechiae may leave a trans-sclerally fixated PC IOL as the best hope of rehabilitating an eye. The techniques for sewing in a PC IOL are similar to the suturing techniques used to correct PC IOL decentration (see Chapter 9).

Anterior Chamber Intraocular Lenses

AC IOLs are not preferred for primary cataract extraction since they cause a higher incidence of iritis, glaucoma, pupillary distortion, anterior synechiae, and cystoid macular edema than PC IOLs. Nevertheless, AC IOLs are very useful in complicated primary cataract extractions and other cases in which PC IOL implantation is not possible, such as penetrating keratoplasty and secondary IOL implantation (Fig. 8.26).

The parameters that should be followed when designing an AC IOL have been presented by Charles Kelman, M.D., and are time-tested. Indeed, Kelman's Multiflex design has proven to be the best AC IOL and is manufactured by virtually every major IOL company (Fig. 8.27). An effective AC IOL must possess the following characteristics:

1. Haptics with no closed loops
2. Slightly bowed haptics, to avoid optic contact with the iris
3. Peripherally flat, wide haptics to avoid synechiae and encapsulation of haptic by surrounding iris
4. Flexible haptics that can adjust to the micromovements of the eye

Secondary Implantation of Anterior Chamber Intraocular Lenses

Secondary implantation of an AC IOL following an intracapsular cataract extraction is becoming less common as more ECCEs are performed. Whenever a secondary AC IOL is necessary, the surgeon should be aware of the astigmatism, which is usually against-the-rule. The wound should be oriented on the flatter meridian and the limbus reconstructed to its original anatomic structure. Sutures should be placed under keratometric control to create a slight with-the-rule astigmatism.

Multifocal Intraocular Lenses

Several companies have produced multifocal IOLs that are at various levels of clinical investigation. A brief description of the major multifocal IOLs is provided along with an explanation of the optical testing parameters that may be used to test a multifocal IOL in vitro. Of course, in vivo clinical trials still provide the most important data, since actual function is of prime importance. *To be a valuable asset, multifocal IOLs must not significantly compromise distance vision and must provide comfortable 20/40 or better near vision, without near correction.*

The 20/40 or better uncorrected near vision provided by a multifocal IOL allows a patient to perform without spectacles many up-close tasks that cannot be performed well with a monofocal IOL, which is emmetropic for distance and allows for 20/80 uncorrected near vision. When using monofocal IOLs, most surgeons aim for a residual refraction of about −0.50 D to −1.00 D, which allows for a reasonable compromise between uncorrected distance and near vision. A mild degree of astigmatism may provide "pseudo-accommodation," but postoperative astigmatism greater than about 1.75 D significantly reduces the quality of vision.

The fact that an individual may still wear glasses to obtain 20/20 at near does not negate the usefulness of a multifocal IOL. A patient with one monofocal IOL and one multifocal IOL does well with a bilateral "add" based on the monofocal IOL refraction. Success does not demand perfection, only a significant improvement over existing treatment. Some European studies demonstrate that patients who have undergone bilateral implantation with multifocal IOLs of a diffractive design may have better uncorrected vision at near and distance than patients with only one multifocal IOL of this design. This phenomenon is commonly found also with refractive surgery. Yet, initial trials with aspheric multifocal IOLs have shown great patient satisfaction with a monofocal-multifocal IOL combination.

The surgeon must be wary when evaluating results of multifocal IOL studies because it is difficult to know the quality of near vision. A patient can be coaxed to 20/30 vision at near with a multifocal IOL even though comfortable visual acuity at near is really 20/50 and the patient wears reading glasses most of the time.

Mechanism of Action

Some portion of a multifocal IOL that does not change shape must be capable of focusing a distant object on the macula and another portion must be capable of focusing a near object on the macula. Macular confusion, a state of having two *discrete* images focused on the macula simultaneously, does not occur for two reasons. First, reading material or other near objects are opaque, and no image from a distant object can be focused through the multifocal IOL to fall on the macula. (If reading material were written on transparent paper, everyone would have macular confusion because they would also be viewing somewhat distant objects through the reading material.) Second, when viewing a distant object, the multifocal IOL patient, or even a person *without a pseudophakos*, will not allow an image to encroach on the macula-object line, since this would block the view of the distant object.

In distance vision, the near focusing portion of the multifocal IOL causes the object to be focused as a large, blurry image that cannot compete with the sharp image on the macula (Fig. 8.28). The same phenomenon occurs in reverse with near vision. All near objects not on the macula-object line are focused as blurry images on the periperipheral retina. Visual and neural perception pathways allow those with normal vision to routinely disregard peripheral blurry images in favor of the sharp image focused on the macula.

The phenomenon of so-called selective vision *does not exist.* A multifocal IOL patient is *never* forced to choose between two sharp images focused on the macula simultaneously. In addition, invoking a theory of selective vision to

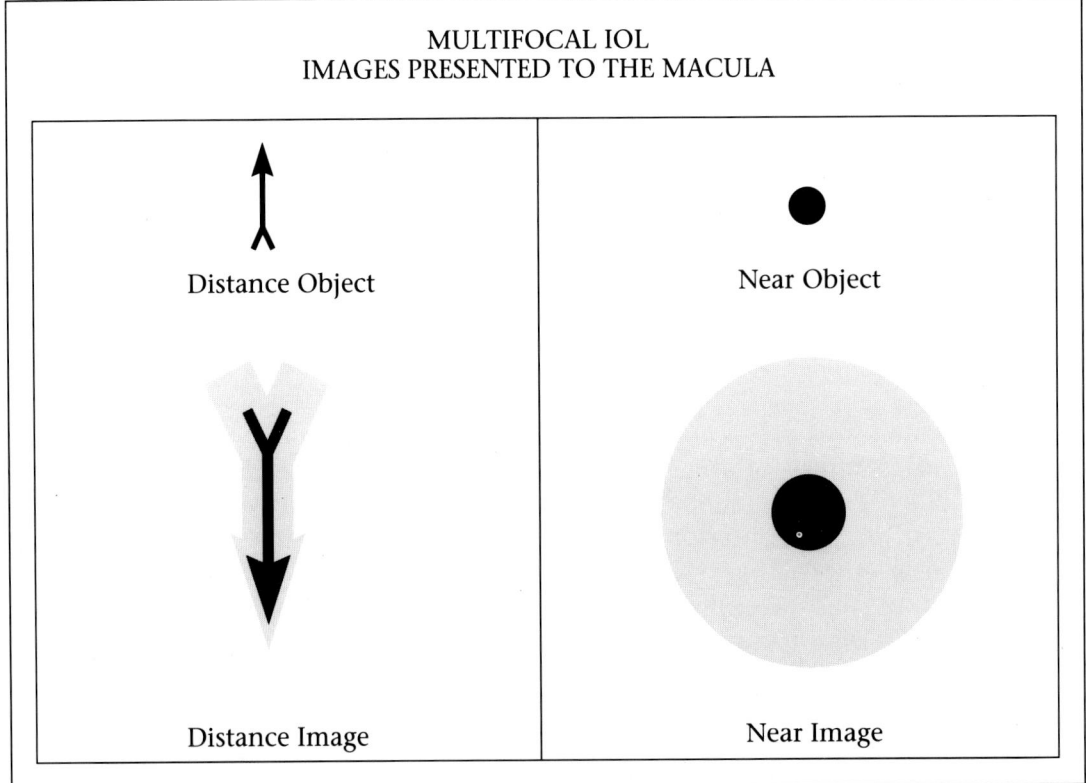

Figure 8.28
Visual confusion does not occur with a multifocal IOL since two equally clear images are not presented to the macula simultaneously. The blurry image projected onto the macula and surrounding retina, however, causes a decrease in contrast sensitivity.

explain multifocal IOL function implies that the brain could relearn its mechanisms of vision. This runs counter to all clinical experience.

Contrast

Evaluating multifocal IOLs requires an understanding of contrast and contrast sensitivity. The following discussion is designed to correlate some of the theoretical concepts of contrast and light transmission through a lens system to the efficacy of the visual system in general and the clinical performance and testing of multifocal IOLs in particular.

Light passing through a lens may be either transmitted or absorbed. Transmitted light may be refracted cleanly and pass through the lens unaltered to a focal point, or it may be altered and pass through the lens as diffuse (nonfocused) light or as glare (random scattered light) (Fig. 8.29). An increase in diffuse light increases the translucency (the transmission of nonfocused light) of a lens. As the human lens ages and cataract formation occurs, the lens's transmission capability decreases as absorption and translucency increase. As will be explained below, it is perhaps surprising to discover that translucency of the lens is usually more important than absorption in affecting visual acuity.

Contrast, as a factor in determining visual function, is defined as the variation in luminance (brightness; the amount of light reflected by a surface) between a darker target of lower luminance (L_{min}) and a lighter background with higher luminance (L_{max}), according to the relationship

$$\frac{100\ (L_{max} - L_{min})}{(L_{max} + L_{min})}\ \%.$$

To analyze contrast in an idealized setting, a background is assigned a value of 100% luminance (all incident light is reflected). The targets (letters) on the background may range from very dark (luminance = 0%; all incident light is absorbed) to barely discernible (luminance = 99%; almost all incident light is reflected). Of course, if the target reflects as much light as the background, the target is invisible because it is identical to the background.

A standard Snellen chart has a contrast of about 92%. Therefore, using the formula for contrast stated above, the luminance of the dark letters must be about 4% since

$$\frac{100 - 4}{100 + 4} = \frac{96}{104} = 92\%.$$

An increase in absorption of light by the lens decreases the amount of light striking the macula. Assume that absorption increases to 80% but there is no increase in translucency, as with a pinhole. When viewing a Snellen chart under these conditions contrast would be defined as

$$\frac{20 - 4}{20 + 4} = \frac{16}{24} = 67\%.$$

Thus, a large decrease in the amount of light reaching the macula reduces contrast a relatively small amount. However, when the translucency

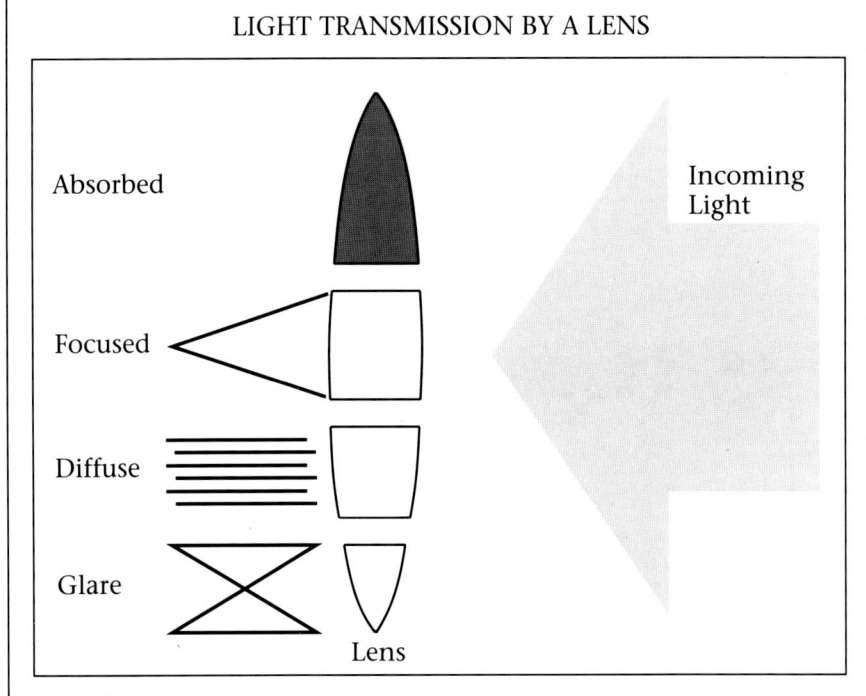

Figure 8.29 *Light striking the lens may be either absorbed or transmitted. The transmitted light may be focused clearly by the lens, made diffuse, or be scattered as glare.*

of the lens is increased to 20% and there is no change in absorption, contrast is also defined as

$$\frac{100-20}{100+20} = \frac{80}{120} = 67\%.$$

Notice that a relatively small increase in translucency has drastically decreased contrast. This decrease in contrast occurs because the diffuse light of translucency blankets the retinal images of both the target and background and has the effect of making the target appear lighter compared to the background, which is already reflecting as much light as possible (Fig. 8.30).

Consider a multifocal IOL and its effect on contrast. Even though the transmission of light through the optic is essentially 100%, only about 40% to 50% of the optic is dedicated to focusing light for near or distance vision. The other portion of the multifocal IOL creates a nonfocused image blur on the entire posterior retina. This is the equivalent of increasing translucency, the effect of which is to decrease contrast.

Even though the entire visual axis of a multifocal IOL is not dedicated to distance or near vision, designs that allow clinically good vision are likely to emerge. The quality of vision with a multifocal IOL is similar to that of a 60-year-old with minimal nuclear sclerosis of the lens and

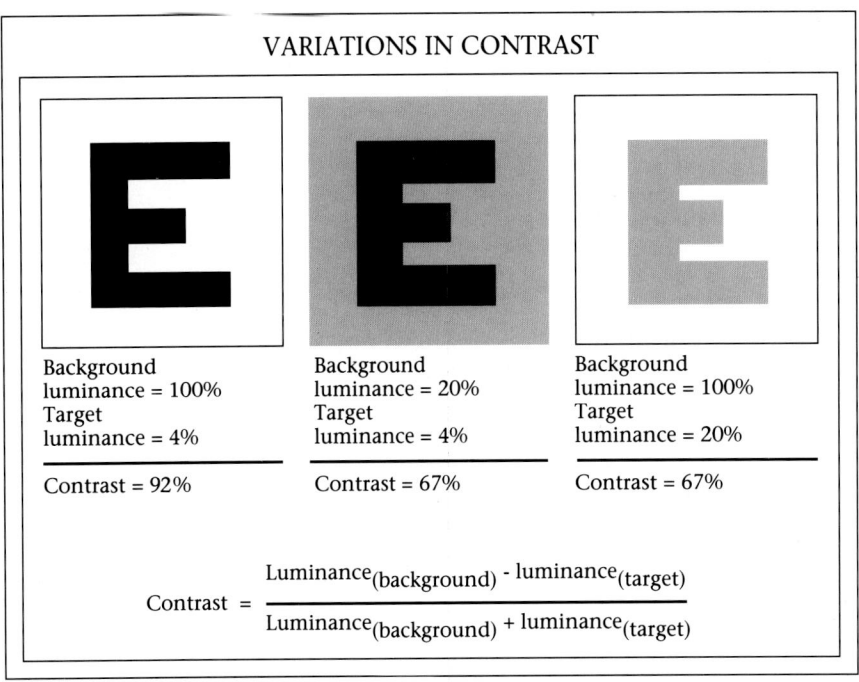

Figure 8.30 *Notice that an equal reduction in contrast from the 92% contrast* (left) *may be caused by either an 80% decrease in background luminance* (center) *or a 16% increase in target luminance* (right).

Table 8.31
Functional Comparison: Clear Lens, Mild Cataract, and Multifocal IOL

	Age 10	Age 60	Multifocal IOL
Visual acuity	20/20	20/20	20/20
Lens–clarity	Clear	1 + nuclear sclerosis	Clear
Lens–transmission of light	100%	60%	100%
Lens–absorption of light	0%	↑	0%
Lens-translucency	Low	Increased	Increased
Contrast sensitivity	High	Slightly reduced	Mildly reduced
% of incoming light available for distance or near vision	100%	60%	40–50%

The minimally nuclear sclerotic lens of a 60-year-old with 20/20 visual acuity affords the macula only about 60% of the light available through the clear lens at age ten because of increased translucency and absorption of light by the sclerotic lens. The degree of contrast between the image and the background as presented to the macula is of paramount importance.

20/20 acuity who may have lost the capacity to effectively focus on the macula 40% of the light presented to the lens (compared to the lens at age ten) because of an increase in absorption and the translucency of the lens. This increased absorption and translucency reduce contrast sensitivity significantly, yet the patient is capable of clinically acceptable 20/20 acuity (Table 8.31).

The Regan Low Contrast Acuity Charts are an example of a low contrast acuity test. Four charts, one each for high contrast (96%), intermediate contrast (25%), low contrast (11%), and very low contrast (4%), may be presented to the patient under constant illumination (Fig. 8.32). Typically, the normal eye will lose about four lines of Snellen acuity from the high contrast (96%) to the low contrast (11%) chart and seven lines from the high contrast (96%) to the very low contrast (4%) chart. A patient's loss of acuity between the higher and lower contrast charts is then compared to the norm (Fig. 8.33).

Contrast Sensitivity

The best visual acuity possible for a given contrast is known as contrast sensitivity. Contrast sensitivity is defined as the reciprocal of the contrast that barely allows a certain acuity. For example, if contrast is 100% (100/1), then contrast sensitivity is 1/100 = 0.01; if contrast is 4% (1/25), then contrast sensitivity is 25/1 = 25. If a graphic plot of the lowest contrast values for a range of threshold visual acuities is made, the resultant curve is known as a contrast sensitivity curve. A contrast sensitivity curve describes a patient's visual function just as an audiogram describes a patient's hearing function. In an audiogram, the loudness (contrast) is increased for a certain frequency of sound (visual acuity) until the threshold is reached and the tone becomes audible to the patient. Reduced contrast sensitivity may indicate certain diseases (e.g., multiple sclerosis, glaucoma, and various maculopathies).

Glare

Glare may be defined as that randomly scattered light striking the retina perceived by the viewer. When conditions increase the contrast of the glare (e.g., nighttime), vision is usually adversely affected. Glare may be caused by an external source such as a car headlight or by an intraocular source such as a cataract or the optical discontinuity of an IOL edge or multifocal IOL. Glare can be tested by plotting a contrast sensitivity curve while increasing a known amount of glare directly into the eye by an external source of light, such as the BAT (Brightness Acuity Tester), or glare onto the target, as with the Miller-Nadler Glare Test, and comparing the results to previously determined norms.

Although glare is an extremely important factor in reducing visual acuity, it is often rather difficult clinically to quantify the exact effect of glare on a patient's visual ability for at least two rea-

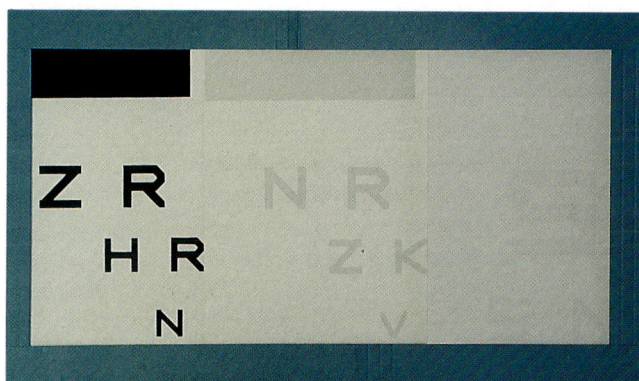

Figure 8.32 *The Regan Low Contrast Acuity Charts. These charts, from left to right, present letter/background contrasts of 96%, 11%, and 4%.*

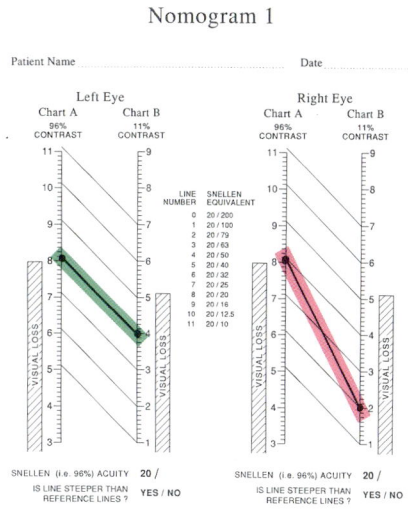

Figure 8.33 *The patient's performance when viewing the Regan charts compared to a standardized nomogram. The normal eye, without loss of contrast sensitivity, loses four lines of visual acuity when comparing the 96% to the 11% contrast sensitivity chart. A line (red) steeper than than the norm (green) indicates a loss of contrast sensitivity.*

sons. First, glare testing depends on a patient's willingness and ability to guess at the target under glare conditions with the same degree of confidence as under the baseline high contrast conditions. Second, pupil size, which may be dictated during the glare testing, may not correlate to the patient's clinical situation. Nevertheless, an awareness of glare's detrimental effect on visual acuity emphasizes that visual function is not well described by a high contrast Snellen test alone. Contrast sensitivity testing in moderate and low contrast conditions and glare testing more accurately assess a patient's visual profile.

Modulation Transfer Function

Optimal multifocal IOL design should minimize the loss of contrast caused by the diffuse, out-of-focus images created by the various optical elements of a multifocal IOL. The multifocal IOL Investigational Device Exemption (IDE) protocols of the Food and Drug Administration (USA) require that visual function be evaluated under high, intermediate, and low contrast conditions. The modulation transfer function (MTF) is a valuable way to describe the function of a lens system under varying contrast conditions.

A mathematical function, the MTF is used by engineers to describe the efficiency of a lens system. The MTF is related to a contrast sensitivity curve, except that it plots the ratio of image contrast to object contrast (modulation) instead of contrast sensitivity against visual acuity threshold (spatial frequency) (Fig. 8.34) As the modulation decreases, the image contrast decreases. The MTF describes how a patient with better visual acuity can function with a lower object contrast than a patient with a poorer visual acuity threshold. 1.5 cycles (1 cycle equals a dark/light line combination) per degree represents about 20/400 visual acuity and 24 cycles per degree represents about 20/25 visual acuity.

The human eye may require a modulation of only about 10% to 15% to perform detailed tasks and to achieve excellent vision at a given spatial frequency under certain conditions. A monofocal IOL can provide a modulation of about 50% to 80% at a given spatial frequency. Pupil size, illumination, and spatial frequency can all influence the image contrast obtained through an IOL.

The MTFs and the image quality of the color spectrum for a monofocal PC IOL and various PC multifocal IOLs as measured in water by Jack Holladay, M.D., et al., are presented in Figures 8.35 and 8.36. As might be predicted from MTFs, a monofocal IOL produces better quality vision than a multifocal under the same conditions. At issue is whether patients will trade a slight drop in intensity of vision for the ability to function well without spectacles at distance and near.

It must be remembered that an MTF describes the efficiency of a lens system and does not correlate exactly with a patient's visual satisfaction. This situation exists because functional vision consists not only of focusing a clear image on the macula but also involves phenomena such as suppression, summation, and enhancement of contrasting edges by higher elements of the visual system, starting with the ganglion layer of the retina. Therefore, although optical bench testing of an IOL is valuable, one should not presuppose that it exactly predicts clinical function and patient satisfaction.

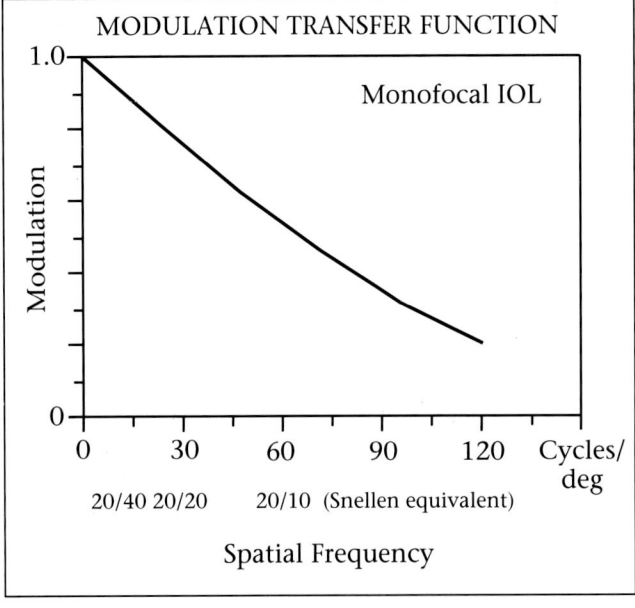

Figure 8.34 *Modulation transfer function of a typical monofocal IOL.*

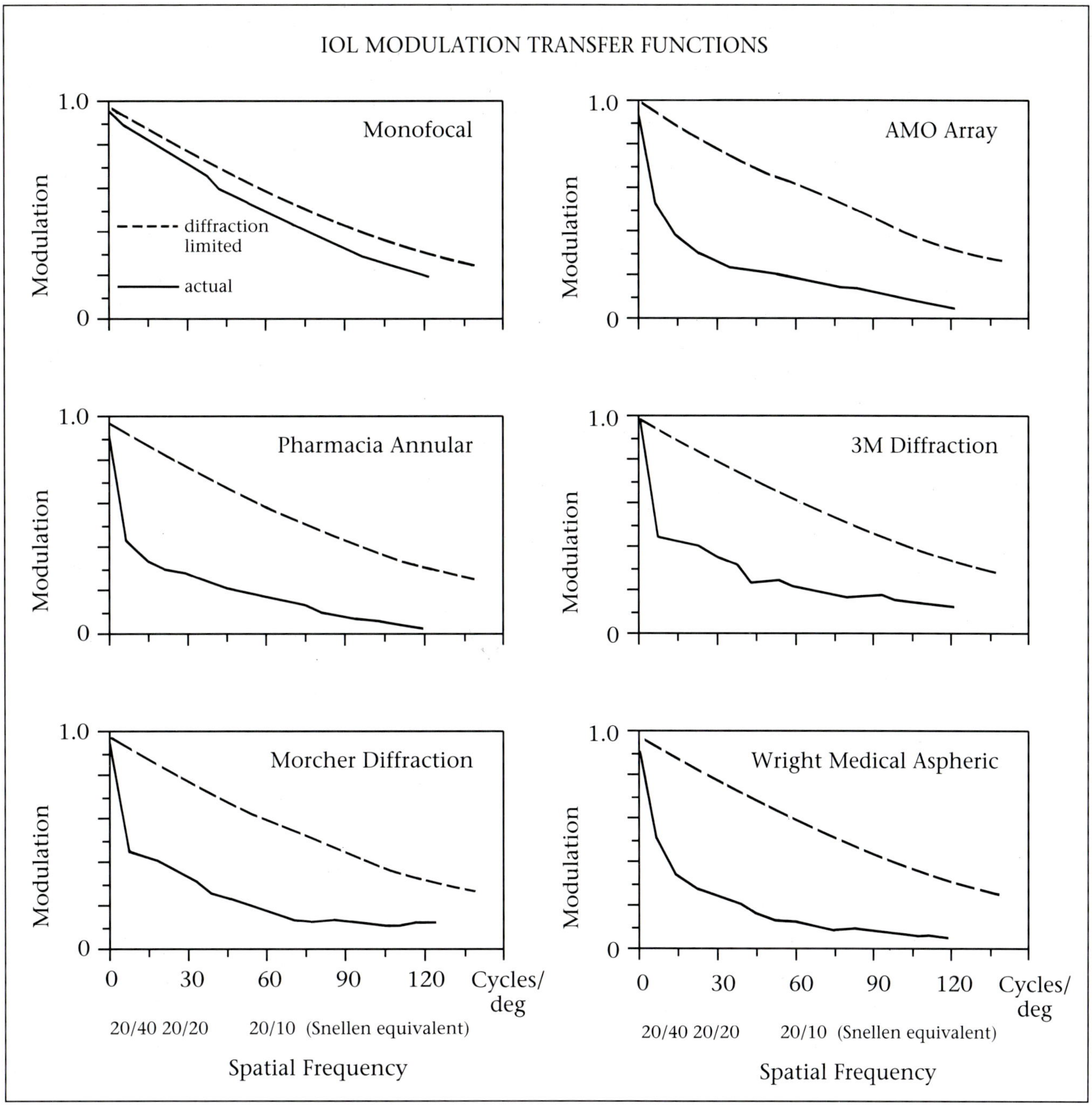

Figure 8.35 *Modulation transfer functions of several multifocal IOLs.*

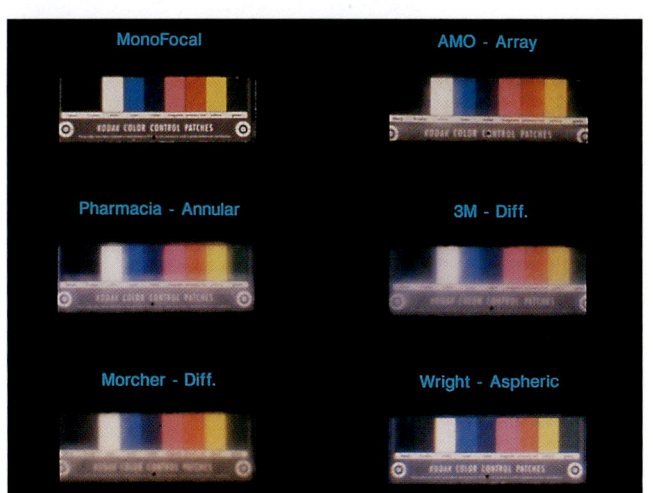

Figure 8.36 *The color spectrum viewed by a camera through a monofocal IOL and various multifocals.*

Profiling of Patients

Multifocal IOLs must accomplish their mission of satisfactory visual acuity near and far, corrected and uncorrected, compared to monofocal IOLs or they will fall into disuse. It is not practical or feasible to profile patients based on macular function or job description and predict the future. A 65-year-old with a normal macula may develop senile macular degeneration three years after IOL implantation. Multifocal IOLs will not be widely accepted and become the standard of care if they function well only under a narrow set of conditions because these conditions may change. Otherwise, they will be considered no more than an interesting attempt at improved IOL technology.

Multifocal Intraocular Lens Styles

Bulls-Eye

IOLAB NUVUE BIFOCAL IOL

This bulls-eye IOL, originally designed by Precision Cosmet, in conjunction with J. McHenry Nielson, M.D., and Richard Keates, M.D., was the first multifocal IOL produced. It was first implanted by Mr. John Pearce in England in 1986 and then by Keates in the United States in 1987. The lens consists of a 2.00-mm diameter central spherical add portion and a peripheral spherical portion for distance (Fig. 8.37). This design is sensitive to pupil size since the distance vision may be compromised when the pupil becomes miotic. Therefore, this IOL functions better when the lens is decentered relative to the visual axis. The transition zone between the central and peripheral segments may be responsible for glare and, also, for an improved depth of field due to its variable refractive surface.

This IOL is historic, but is probably not viable in its present form due to the above mentioned limitations. A second variation has been offered that has a distance segment in the center of the add portion. However, the problems associated with the optical discontinuity created by the junction of two spherical curves still remain.

PHARMACIA MULTIFOCAL IOL

This concentric design is the reverse of the Iolab lens; it has a central distance portion surrounded by an annular near portion that is again surrounded by a distance zone (Fig 8.38). There is concern that the optical discontinuities created by the intersection of the spherical curves may cause glare. Also, near vision may vary according to pupil size.

Diffractive

3M MULTIFOCAL IOL

This diffractive IOL has been in use since 1988. By 1990, about 10,000 lenses were implanted in

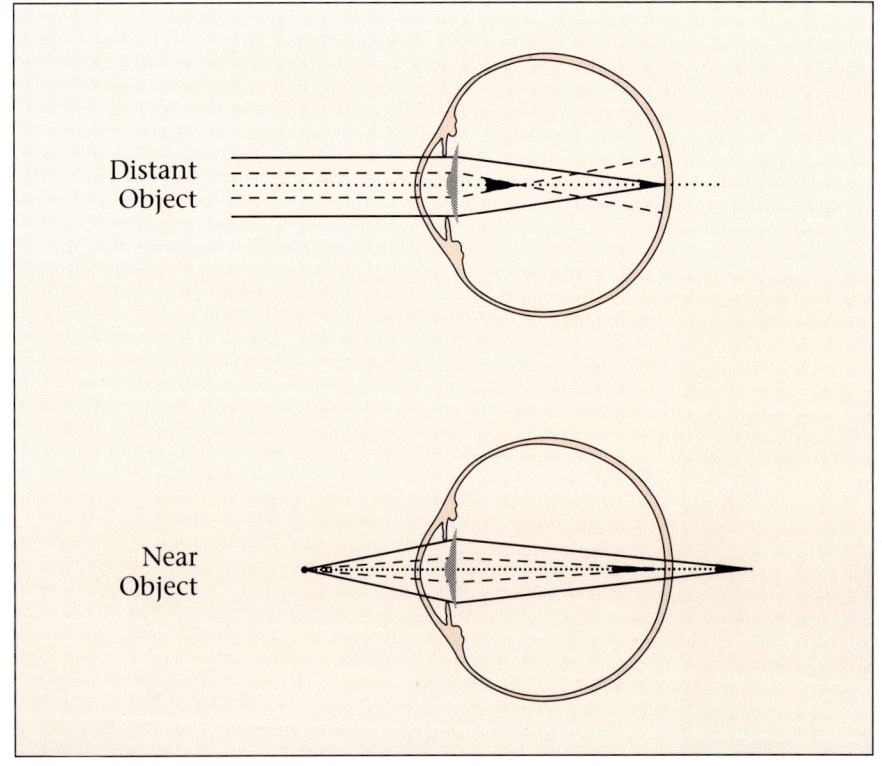
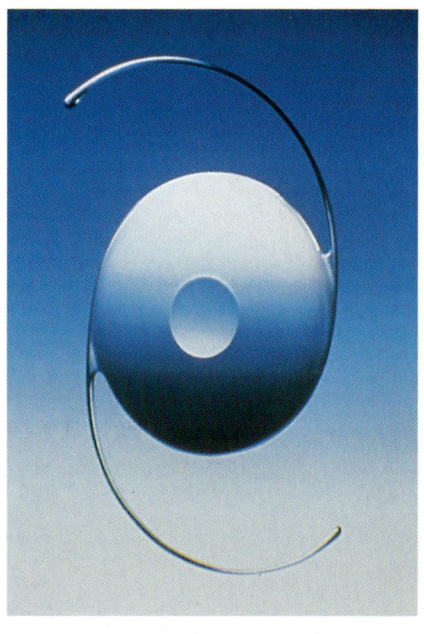

Figure 8.37 *The Iolab Nuvue multifocal PC IOL design* **(left)** *and IOL* **(right)**.

Europe and several hundred in the United States. This IOL functions for near by focusing light on the macula by diffraction rather than refraction.

Diffraction is the phenomenon of light bending as it passes near an edge. The shape of the edge can determine the amount of bending. The waves of light can be made to augment or suppress each other by constructive or destructive interference, respectively (Fig. 8.39). With this IOL, diffraction is caused by circular microridges on its posterior

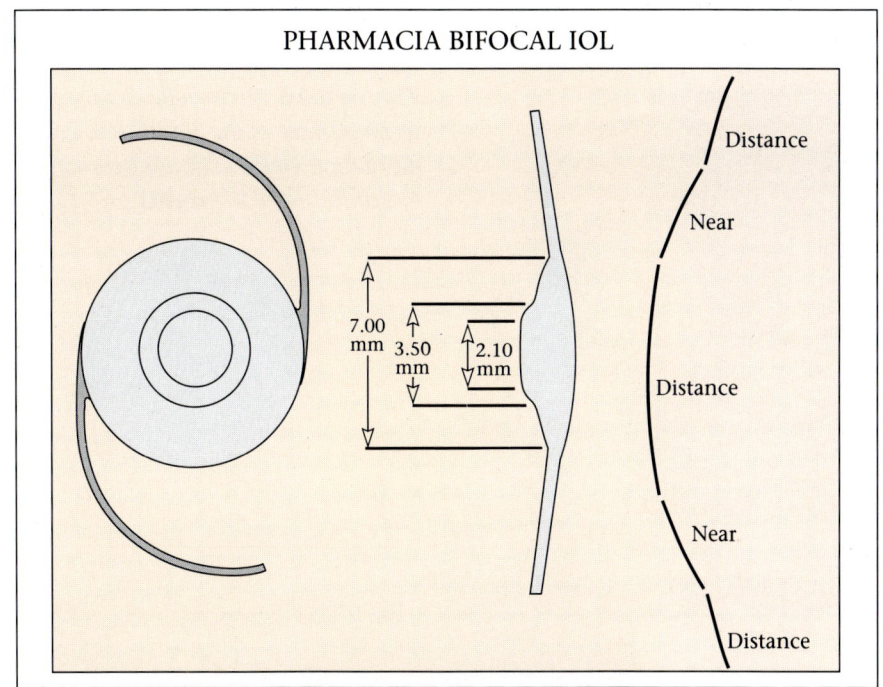

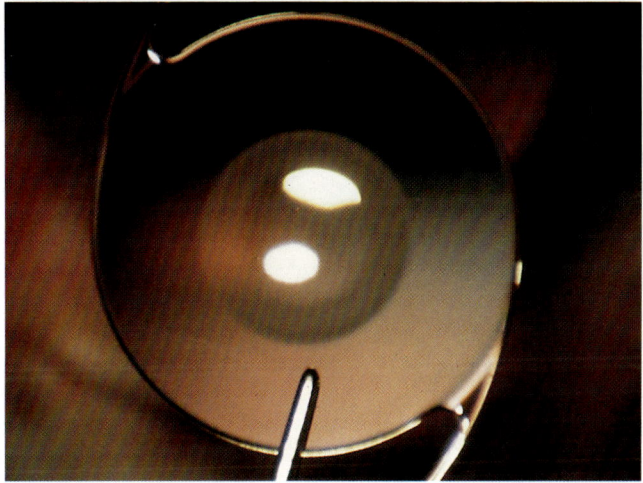

Figure 8.38 *The Pharmacia Multifocal PC IOL design* **(top)** *and IOL* **(bottom)**.

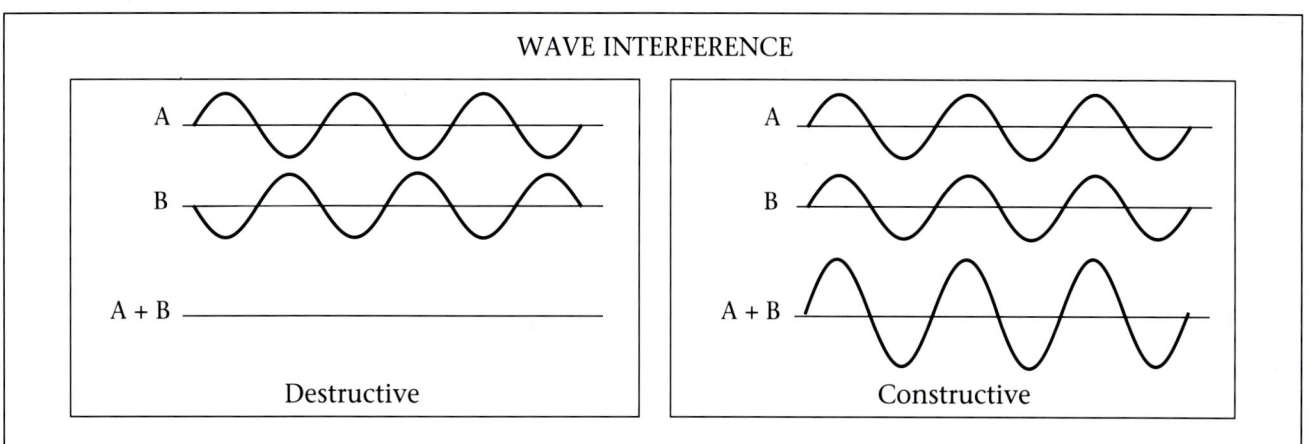

Figure 8.39 *A representation of destructive and constructive interference based on the wave theory of light.*

surface (Fig. 8.40). These ridges do not function by a prismatic effect. About 16% of the incoming light is lost due to scatter from the diffractive elements, 42% is dedicated to distance, and 42% is dedicated to near.

Clinically, the 3M IOL seems to function best in bright light. Some concern has been raised about reports of only about 20/50 near vision in moderate light. Also, the concentric diffractive elements can cause glare and multiple circular images when an oblique light source is encountered.

Several observers have noted that patients with bilateral 3M multifocal IOLs have better visual function than those who have undergone unilat-

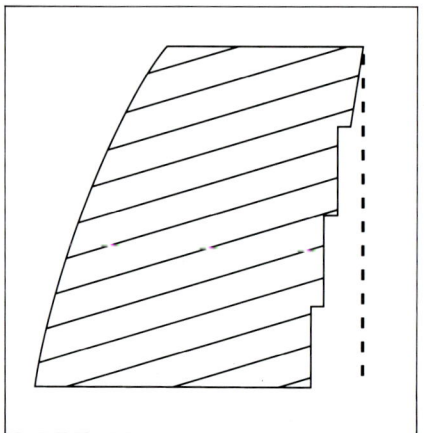
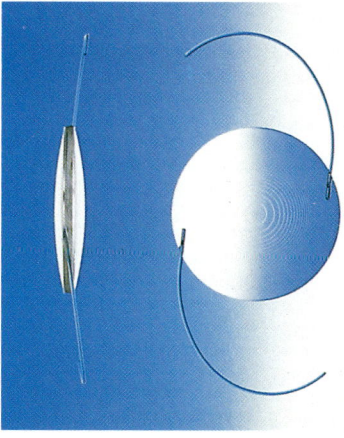

Figure 8.40 *Microridges on the posterior surface of the 3M PC IOL create diffraction* **(left)**. *The 3M Diffractive Multifocal PC IOL* **(right)**.

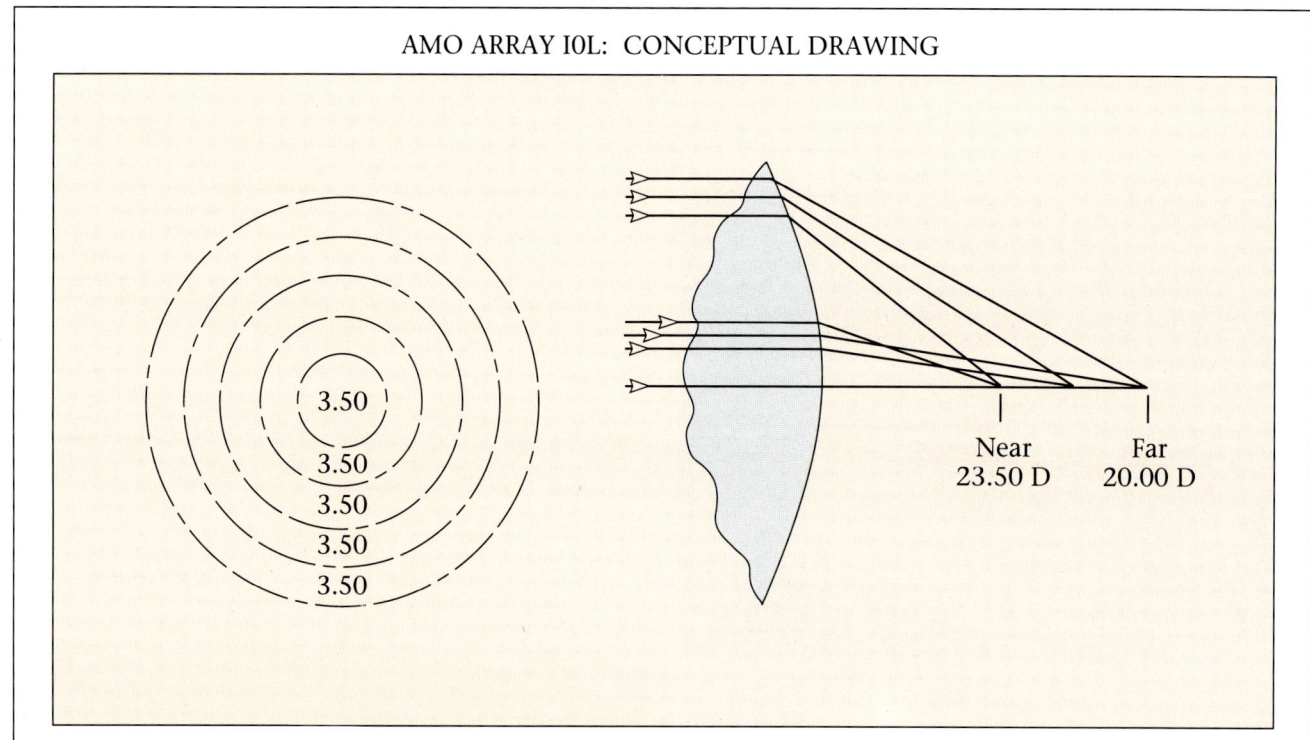
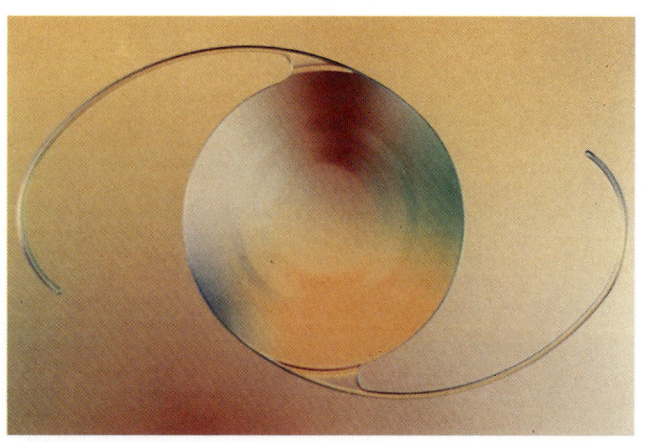

Figure 8.41 *Cross-section view of the AMO Array multifocal PC IOL design* **(top)** *and the IOL* **(bottom)**.

eral implantation. This phenomenon may well relate to the imbalance caused by the increased glare of the multifocal IOL compared to that of a monofocal IOL.

Aspheric

ALLERGAN MEDICAL OPTICS ARRAY MULTIFOCAL IOL

This IOL is composed of a series of five aspheric curves on the front surface of the IOL. Each circular aspheric curve is 0.90 mm wide and encompasses a range of refractive powers from emmetropia to a +3.50 D add (Fig. 8.41). Sixty percent of each curve is dedicated to distance vision. A significant amount of the incoming light is lost due to the transition between the aspheric curves, but no glare would be expected since there are no discontinuities on the surface of the IOL. The first fifty AMO Array Multifocal IOLs were implanted in the United States under an FDA IDE protocol in 1990.

The AMO Array IOL and other multifocal IOLs have been subjected to extensive in vitro optical testing. These tests include:

Resolution Efficiency
Modulation Transfer Function (measures contrast efficiency)
Through Focus Response (measures depth of focus and add power)
Glare Testing

All these tests have been repeated under conditions in which pupil size changes and IOL decentration and tilt were simulated, and the results were compared to a monofocal IOL. This is an example of how optical engineers and IOL designers have spared no effort when attempting to predict the performance of a multifocal IOL.

WRIGHT MEDICAL VARIFOCAL IOL

The Varifocal IOL was the first foldable multifocal IOL ever implanted (Fig.8.42). Ten such IOLs were implanted in the United States as of June 1990, under the auspices of an FDA IDE protocol, and forty more by the end of 1990. One half of the silicone multifocal optic is spherical and dedicated to distance vision. The other half of the IOL has a semicircular portion that is aspheric in

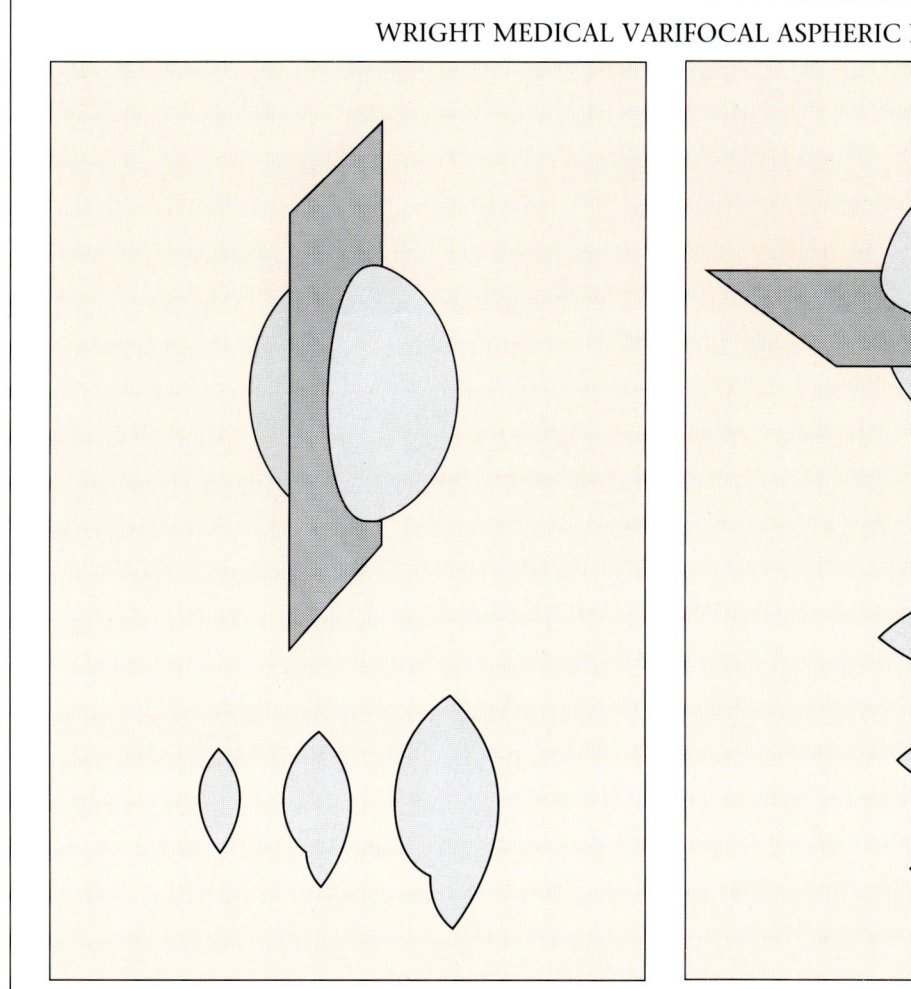
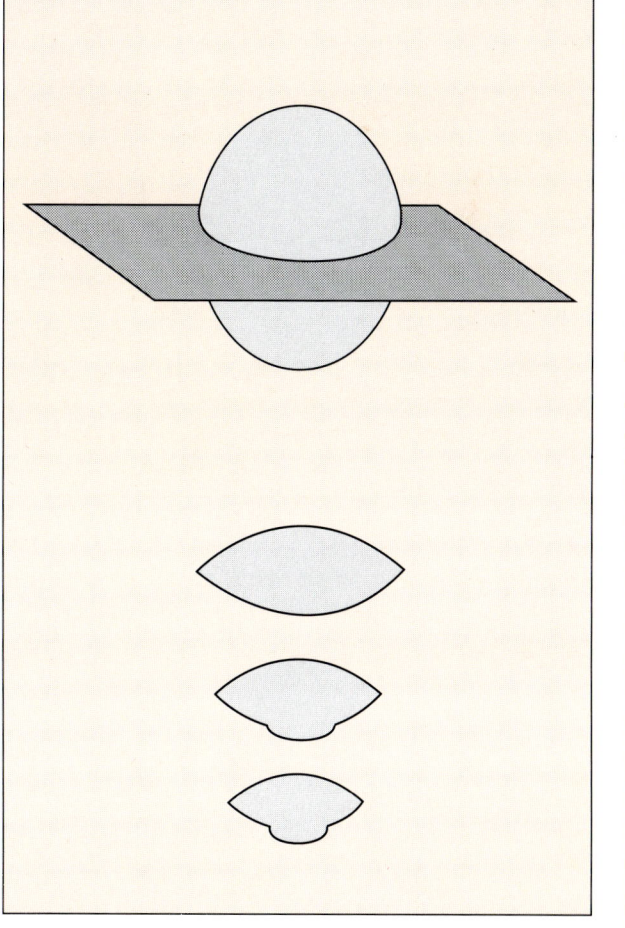

Figure 8.42 *Horizontal cross section* (left) *and vertical cross section* (right) *of the Wright Medical Varifocal PC IOL.*

both the vertical and horizontal directions, creating concentric zones of increasing dioptric power (Figs. 8.42 to 8.44). The peripheral junction of the differently curved surfaces could theoretically cause glare with optic decentration or extremely large pupils.

Holladay performed optical bench testing on various multifocal IOLs early in 1990. The Wright Medical Varifocal IOL demonstrated the best potential of any multifocal IOL tested for distance and near vision at 33 cm (Table 8.45). More clinical experience will demonstrate whether this IOL lives up to the very high expectations for it.

IOPTEX RESEARCH ASPHERIC MULTIFOCAL IOL

This IOL is based on the principle of asphericity as are the Wright Varifocal and the AMO Array IOLs. A central spherical portion of the optic is 1.50 mm in diameter and dedicated to distance. An aspheric zone with an ever decreasing radius of curvature connects the central zone to a more peripheral spherical zone used for reading. This spherical reading zone is connected to a peripheral distance zone by an aspheric segment with its radius becoming progressively longer (Figs. 8.46 and 8.47). There is no optical

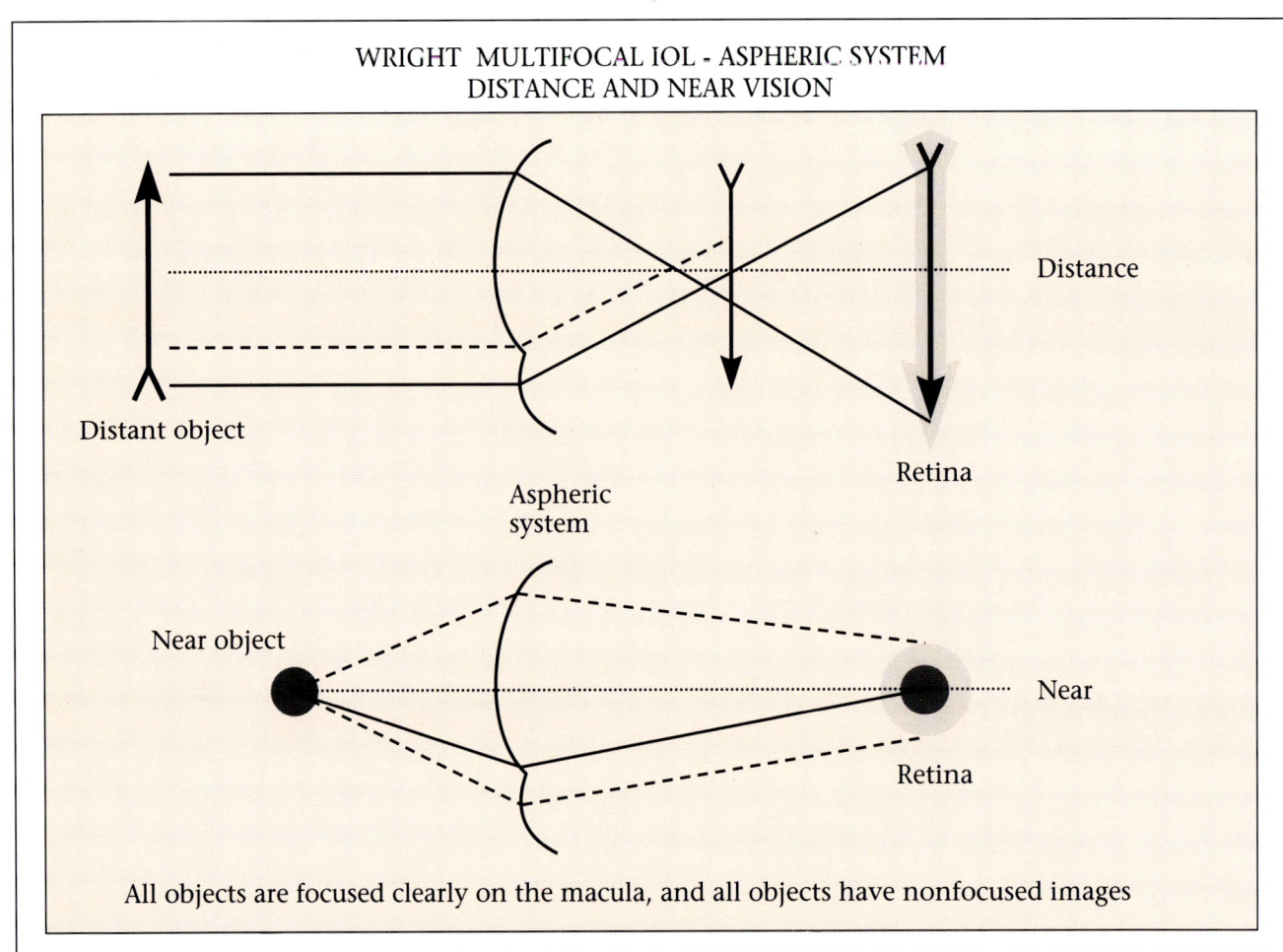

Figure 8.43 *A ray tracing that demonstrates the function of the Wright Medical Varifocal IOL. The spherical portion of the optic focuses distant objects clearly on the macula* (**top**) *and the aspheric portion of the optic serves intermediate and near objects* (**bottom**).

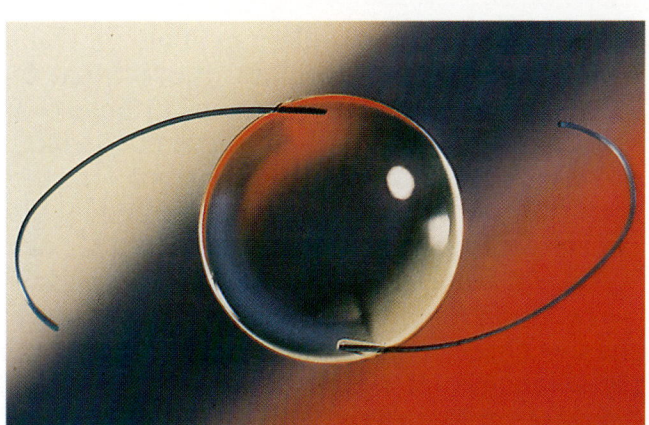

Figure 8.44 *The Wright Medical Varifocal PC IOL, the first foldable multifocal PC IOL.*

Table 8.45
Multifocal IOL MTF Comparison

Resolution Efficiency

Lens	High Contrast Chart	Measured Resolution Efficiency	MTF* 5% Cut-off
Monofocal	20/10	83%	94%
AMO-Array	20/18	74%	56%
Pharmacia-Annular	20/15	66%	53%
3M-Diffraction	20/16	83%	82%
Morcher-Diffraction	20/17	83%	84%
Wright-Aspheric	20/14	74%	63%

*modulation transfer function

Depth-of-Field Measurements

Lens	Defocus to 20/40	Resolution at 33 cm	TFR* at 5%>
Monofocal	1.50 D	20/80	1.00 D
AMO-Array	4.50 D	20/36	4.50 D
Pharmacia-Annular	4.50 D	20/56	4.50 D
3M-Diffraction	3.70 D	20/30	3.50 D
Morcher-Diffraction	3.70 D	20/30	4.00 D
Wright-Aspheric	2.70 D	20/23	3.00 D

*through focus response

discontinuity on the surface of this IOL optic to produce glare.

The initial results of the Ioptex aspheric multifocal IOL were very rewarding. The first patient undergoing cataract surgery with this implant was a 75-year-old woman who six weeks postoperatively was capable of 20/20 uncorrected vision at distance and 20/20 uncorrected at near. This patient's other eye had a monofocal IOL with excellent uncorrected distance acuity of 20/20 and uncorrected near vision of 20/80. Of great significance is that both eyes were correctable to 20/15 vision, and the patient was free of disturbing symptoms such as glare or diplopia (Table 8.48). Very important, also, was the fact that the patient noticed slightly greater "intensity" of vision with the monofocal IOL eye but strongly preferred the multifocal IOL eye when forced to compare the visual function of each eye. The patient could wear bilateral +2.50 D add for near vision without a problem.

The visual function of this patient seems to fit the model predicted by Holladay's data, although the willingness of a patient to accept a very mild decrease in contrast in order to gain improved uncorrected near vision is a subjective response

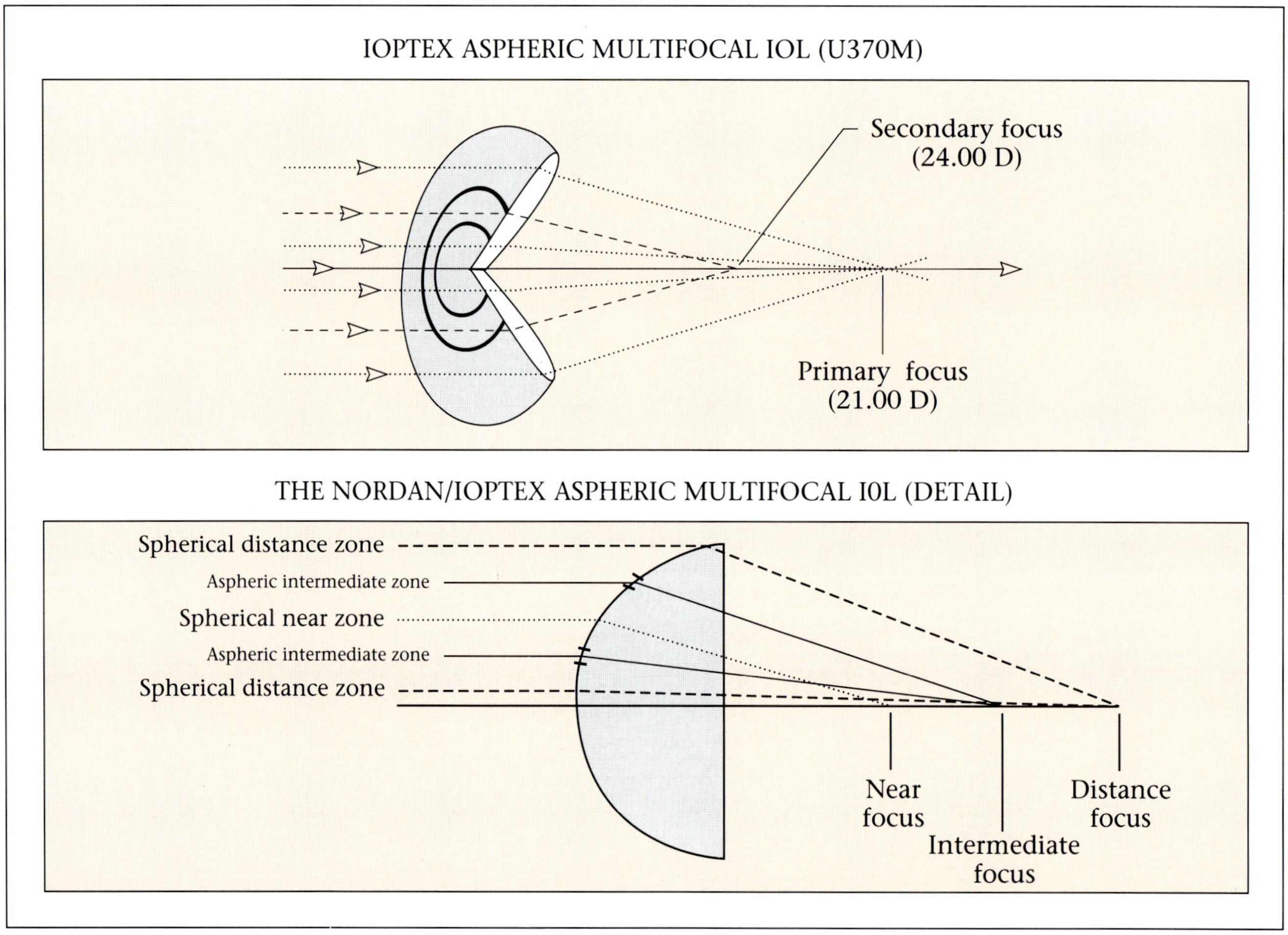

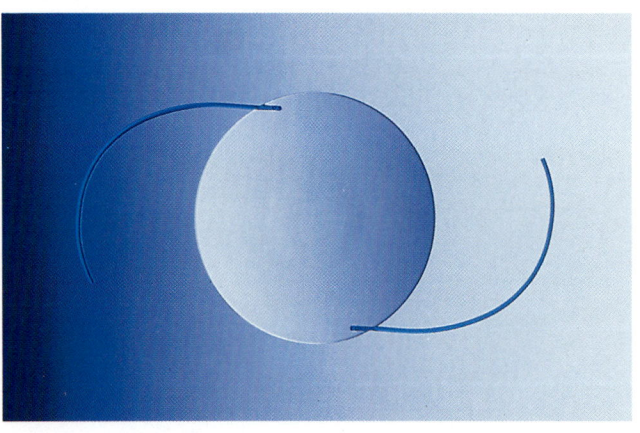

Figure 8.46 *Ioptex Research Aspheric Multifocal PC IOL design* **(top)** *and IOL* **(bottom)**. *There is no discontinuity on the surface of the IOL. The difference in the blue background through the IOL is due to a change in refractive power.*

that cannot be ascertained completely by scientific data. Perhaps a combination monofocal/multifocal IOL will one day provide patients with the most useful uncorrected visual function. At the least, this patient is an example of the advantages of a multifocal IOL.

Conclusion

PC IOLs implanted in the capsular bag have proved to be the procedure of choice for cataract replacement in an uncomplicated procedure. Both ECCE/IOL and phacoemulsification/IOL procedures provide excellent results, and multifocal IOLs may become very useful in the rehabilitation of vision. IOLs with 5.00-mm × 6.00-mm oval PMMA optics have become popular as a means of reducing wound size, but long-term decentration must be considered. IOLs with shorter diameter haptics are better suited for in-the-bag implantation. More than 100,000 foldable silicone IOLs had been implanted by 1990 as well as 100 IOLs with a foldable acrylic optic. Certainly, a 3.80-mm to 4.00-mm incision allows most

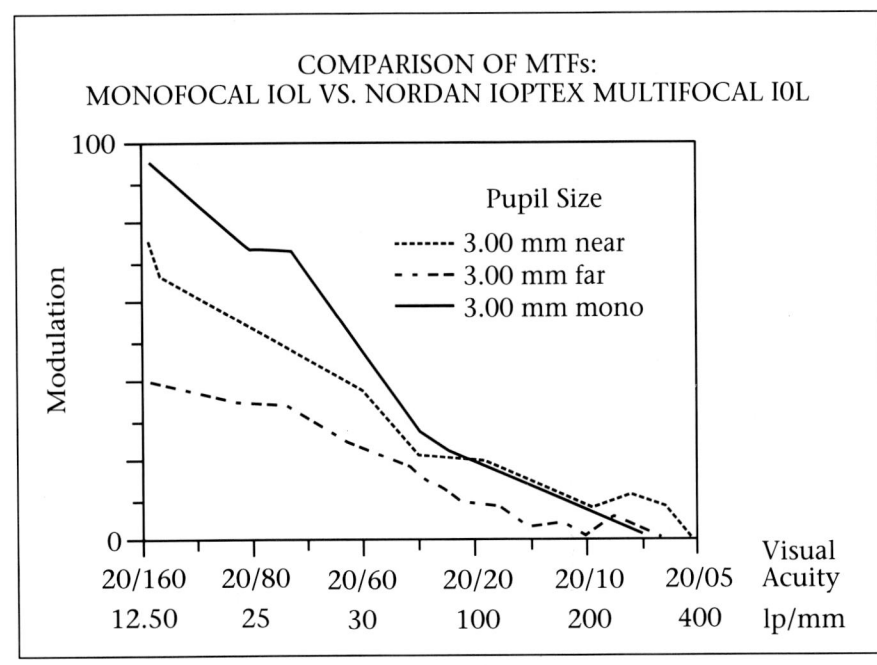

Figure 8.47 *Comparison of the modulation transfer functions of a monofocal PC IOL and an Ioptex Research aspheric multifocal PC IOL.*

Table 8.48
Multifocal/Monofocal IOL Comparison

OD/Multifocal		OS/Monofocal
20/20	Distance visual acuity without correction	20/20
20/15	Distance visual acuity with correction	20/15
20/20–	Near visual acuity without correction	20/80
20/15	Near visual acuity with correction	20/15
Slightly less than monofocal	Contrast	Slightly better than multifocal
Prefers slightly more than monofocal	Patient acceptability	Prefers slightly less than multifocal

A comparison between the eyes of a 75-year-old female with an Ioptex Research Aspheric Multifocal PC IOL in the right eye and a monofocal PC IOL in the left. Both eyes are 20/20 uncorrected at distance and symptom free.

patients undergoing cataract/IOL surgery to achieve earlier visual recovery and to minimize the chance of reduced uncorrected visual acuity from excessive induced or retained astigmatism.

The injectable IOL is still a hope for many, but the highest level of pseudophakos development to date may well be the small incision, multifocal IOL. This chapter has presented important considerations for the cataract/IOL surgeon. IOL optic design and diameter, haptic design, and optic and haptic material are extremely important factors in determining the long-term success of the pseudophakic eye.

Clinical Points to Consider

☛ A well-designed IOL for general use should possess a functional optic that has a diameter of at least 5.00 mm.

☛ The haptic design of a PC IOL should allow for comfortable in-the-bag implantation through a small capsulorhexis and small pupil as well as good centration in the event of asymmetrical implantation or capsular bag contraction.

☛ Multifocal IOLs must provide excellent asymptomatic distance vision and at least 20/40 near vision in order to provide a significant advantage to the patient.

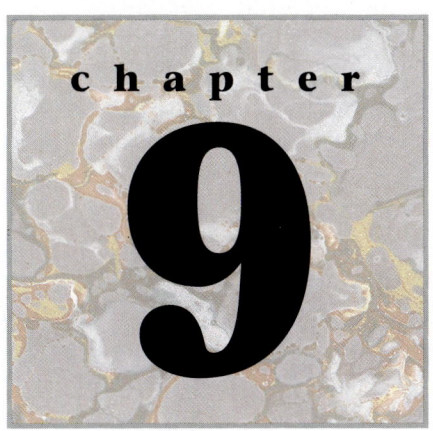

Chapter 9

CAPSULORHEXIS, PC IOL CENTRATION, AND TRANS-SCLERAL PC IOL FIXATION

DAVID APPLE, M.D.   JAMES A. DAVISON, M.D.
LEE T. NORDAN M.D.   W. ANDREW MAXWELL, M.D., Ph. D.

The long-term centration of posterior chamber intraocular lenses (PC IOLs) is of great concern, especially in view of the ever decreasing age of patients undergoing cataract extraction and the need to maintain optimal PC IOL function (Fig. 9.1). Recent PC IOL design changes, such as 5.00 mm × 6.00 mm oval optics, smaller 5.00 mm circular optics, and multifocal IOLs, increase the demand on the surgeon that permanent PC IOL centration be achieved. This chapter will discuss the major determinant of PC IOL centration in uncomplicated cataract IOL surgery, the anterior capsulotomy. Except for exceptional surgical situations, continuous circular capsulorhexis (CCC) has proved to be the preferred method of anterior capsulotomy, assuming that surgical technique is compatible with such a capsulotomy.

Capsulorhexis

CCC is one of the revolutionary innovations of modern cataract surgery. It was presented to the ophthalmic surgical community in 1985 and 1986 (Figs. 9.2 and 9.3) by Calvin Fercho, M.D., John Graether, M.D., Howard Gimbel, M.D., and Thomas Neuhann, M.D. These ophthalmologists were able to use and appreciate CCC because they had developed methods for performing phacoemulsification totally within the capsular bag, i.e., they were not using an iris plane approach in which the superior pole of the cataract is tipped superiorly out of the bag for tip access.

These innovative surgeons realized intuitively that the superiority of capsulorhexis compared to the can-opener capsulotomy was related to its improved and consistent containment of the phacoemulsification process and the implanted IOL. The structural integrity inherent to a capsular bag with a smooth, circular opening in the anterior capsule during and following cataract removal is vastly greater than the structural integrity provided by an irregular capsular margin following a can-opener capsulotomy (Fig. 9.4).

CCC eliminates radial tears of the anterior capsule. These tears are extensions of the "jags"—points of structural vulnerability that tear radially in response to capsular stress in the equatorial zone of the capsular bag—created by the traditional can-opener anterior capsulotomy. They may be contained and rerouted by the numerous microscopic insertions of the zonules (Fig. 9.5).

Anatomy of the Lens and Zonules

It is important to consider the lens-zonule relationship when determining the size and success of an anterior capsulotomy. The diameter of the adult human lens is about 9.50 mm and the ciliary sulcus about 11.00 mm. The zonules extend from the ciliary body and the pars plana to insert on the anterior, equatorial, and posterior surfaces of the lens capsule (see Chapter 10, Fig.10.5). The region of zonular insertion extends about 1.00 mm to 1.50 mm onto the anterior capsular surface and about 0.75 mm onto the posterior capsular surface, leaving a clear anterior capsular zone of about 7.00 mm.

This peripheral ring of zonular insertion helps limit the equatorial and posterior progression of tears originating at the anterior capsulotomy. On the other hand, this zonular insertion zone makes it difficult to obtain a capsulorhexis with a diameter much greater than about 7.00 mm since the direction of the anterior capsule's tearing can be difficult to predict when it encounters the zonules inserting on the anterior capsular surface.

Capsulotomy Methods

There are two basic methods of performing an anterior capsulotomy, can-opener and capsulorhexis. Perhaps, the term anterior *capsulectomy* is more appropriate for this procedure since the central anterior capsule is removed, not merely punctured. Although the entire anterior capsulotomy is usually performed prior to cataract removal and PC IOL insertion, some surgeons perform endocapsular phacoemulsification through a very small initial linear or circular capsulotomy with the remainder of the capsulotomy

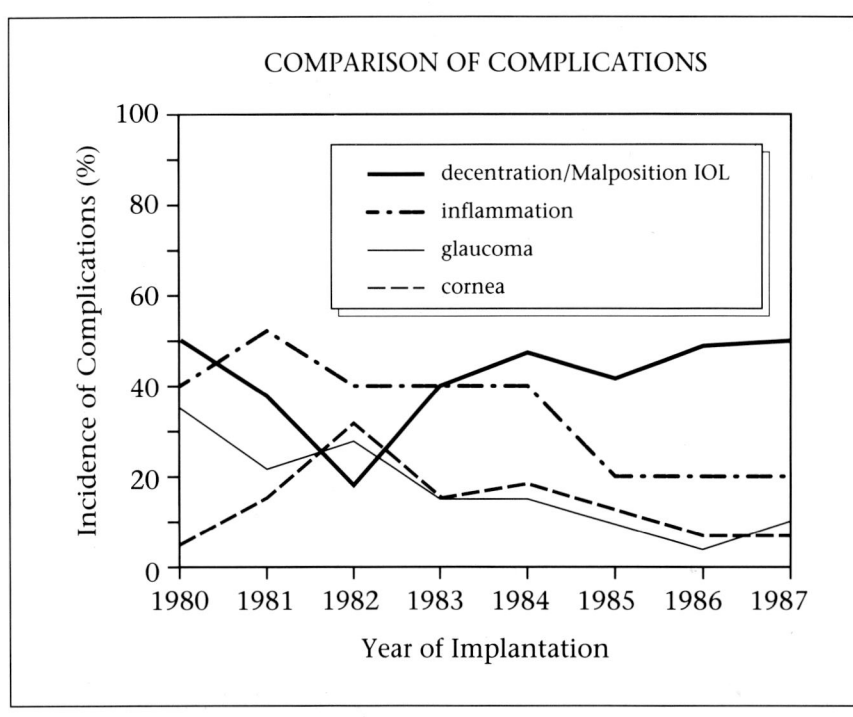

Figure 9.1 *The major types of complications associated with PC IOL explantations evaluated at the Center for Intraocular Lens Research (Charleston, SC; David Apple, M.D., Director)*

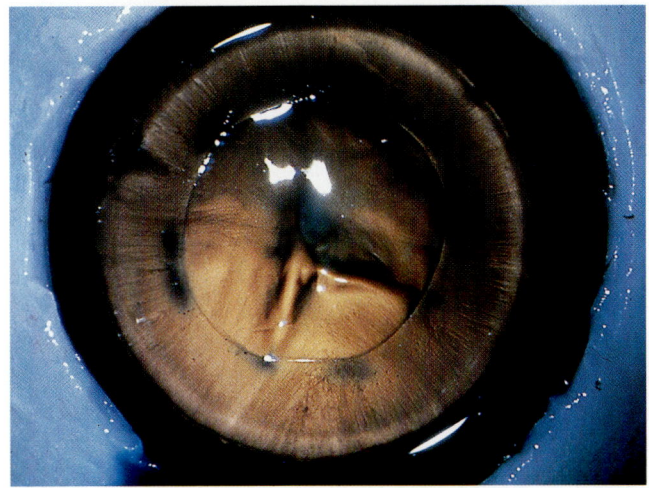

Figure 9.2 *Continuous circular capsulorhexis.*

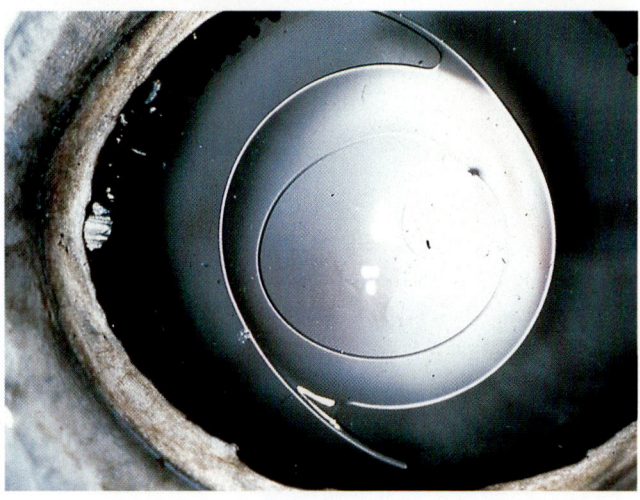

Figure 9.3 *In-the-bag implantation of a PC IOL provides the best chance of long-term IOL centration.*

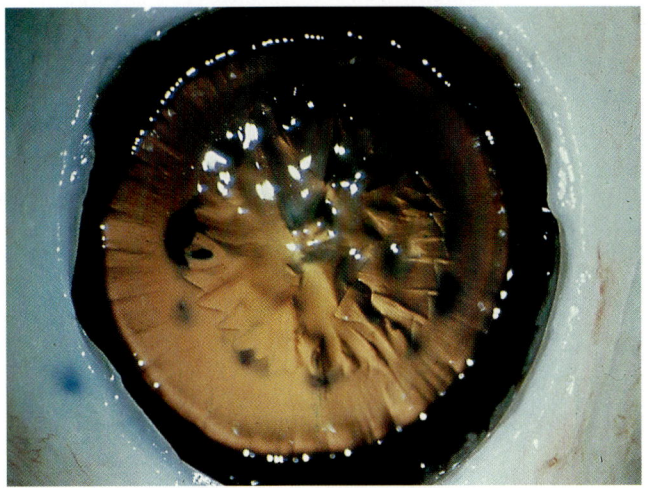

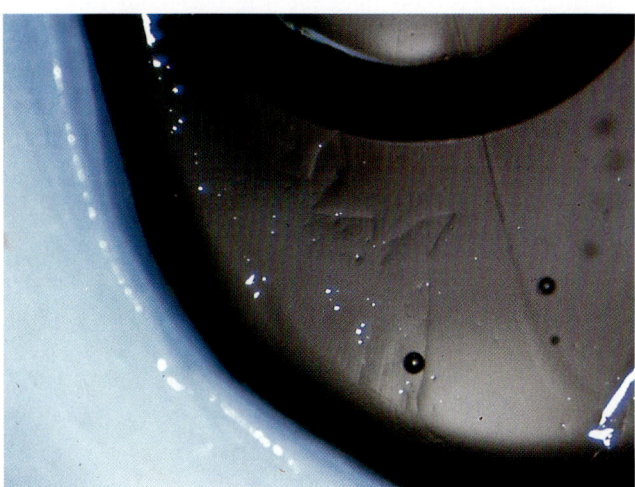

Figure 9.4 **(Left)** *Can-opener capsulotomy.* **(Right)** *An anterior capsular radial tear, following nuclear expression through a can-opener capsulotomy.*

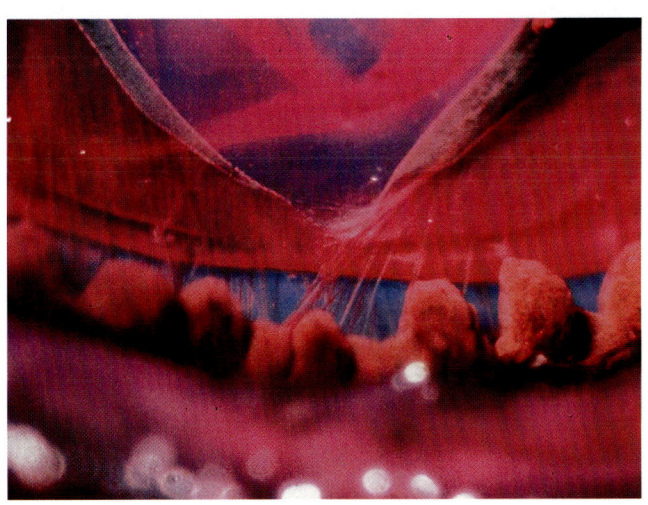

Figure 9.5 *Surgeon's view of human autopsy globe with cornea and iris removed. The anterior capsular radial tear is stopped within the capsular bag equatorial zone.*

performed after PC IOL insertion. The advantages and disadvantages of the can-opener capsulotomy are summarized in Table 9.6.

Can-Opener Capsulotomy

The can-opener method of anterior capsulotomy is performed by connecting multiple punctures of the anterior capsule in a circular or similar pattern. These punctures may be performed with a relatively large 23-gauge cystotome, a smaller 27-gauge needle whose tip is bent backward, or an automated vibrating instrument.

Clinical and postmortem studies of eyes that have undergone extracapsular cataract extraction with implantation of a PC IOL by means of a can-opener anterior capsulotomy indicate that 86% of all can-opener anterior capsulotomies in such circumstances have at least one tear that has progressed to the equator of the capsular bag. These tears are most commonly caused at the time of nuclear expression. Insertion of the zonules at the anterior, equatorial, and posterior aspects of the capsular bag probably limit the progression of these tears.

Continuous Circular Capsulorhexis

CCC may be performed with either a cystotome or a capsulorhexis forceps (Kraff-Utrata), which is used to manipulate the free edge of the anterior capsule in a circular pattern after making a puncture wound. The capsulorhexis tends to "spiral out" or "spiral down", often producing a smaller diameter than intended. A small capsulorhexis is very effective in keeping a PC IOL centered, but the surgeon must be careful not to compromise the safety of the cataract extraction or optical results. ECCE probably requires a capsulorhexis diameter of at least 7.00 mm; this allows for routine nuclear expression after hydrodelineation and usually prevents tearing of the anterior capsule and other surgical complications, the result of increased resistance to nuclear expression caused by the superior portion of the capsulorhexis.

It has been demonstrated in animal studies that the smooth, circular capsular edge of capsulorhexis is significantly more resistant to tearing when stressed by nucleus expression than is the

Table 9.6
Anterior Capsulotomy: Can-Opener Versus Capsulorhexis

	Can-Opener	Capsulorhexis
Advantages	Consistent desired diameter; easily learned	Resistant to tearing
	Facilitates superior nuclear prolapse	Good containment of phacoemulsification
	Easier to use in small pupil cases	Excellent PC IOL centration
	Appropriate for mature and hypermature cataracts with compromised red reflex	Zonular stress may be less than during can-opener capsulotomy
	Viscoelastic not necessary	No capsular tags during I/A
	Removal of 12 o'clock cortex easier	Good support for PC IOL implantation, if posterior capsule broken
	Easier to dial PC IOL into the capsular bag through a large capsulotomy	
Disadvantages	Prone to anterior capsular radial tears	Limits nuclear prolapse; ECCE more difficult
	High zonule stress during procedure	Limits access to superior nucleus during phacoemulsification
	Skip areas with incomplete anterior capsulotomy	More difficult to learn
	IOL dislocation more likely with anterior (pea-podding) and posterior (sunset syndrome) capsular tears	Tendency toward smaller diameter
		Not safe for small pupil cases
	Poor support for PC IOL implantation if posterior capsule broken	Removal of 12 o'clock cortex difficult
	Capsular tags may occlude I/A port during cortex removal	Difficult with compromised red reflex
		Viscoelastic usually necessary
		Tendency for diameter to shrink
		Capsular bag distension syndrome

irregular, angulated edge of a can-opener capsulotomy. Any capsular puncture with an acute angle pointing toward the periphery has the tendency to tear in that direction (see Chapter 13). A 6.00 mm PC IOL optic can be placed through a 4.00 mm diameter capsulorhexis without much difficulty or expectation of creating a capsular tear.

Anterior Capsular Radial Tears

At the same time that CCC was being introduced, other surgeons were beginning to recognize the significance of anterior capsule radial tears as complications. It was recognized that anterior tears are capable of extending and causing posterior capsule tears. Inferior posterior tears are crucial to the initiation of the sunset syndrome, in which the inferior haptic of an IOL has no capsular support and is displaced inferiorly and posteriorly, as is the optic, and becomes embedded in the ciliary body (Fig. 9.7). Of course, when stress is applied to the capsular bag, capsulotomy tears can occur anywhere for 360 degrees during phacoemulsification and nucleus expression.

Critical observations verified that following the nuclear expression step of ECCE, anterior capsular tears most often occur superiorly. Although a superior radial tear of the anterior capsule does not occur in every case of planned ECCE or iris plane phacoemulsification, it routinely allows for nuclear prolapse and the successful completion of most cases. An anterior capsule radial tear is almost always present because prolapse of the superior nuclear pole into the anterior chamber is the essential maneuver common to both iris plane phacoemulsification and the initiation of planned nucleus expression. If prolapse of the nucleus does not create at least one anterior capsule radial tear, the cataract extraction may fail and severe complications may occur.

Repeated anterior prolapse of the superior nuclear pole is essential to iris plane phacoemulsification and its more evolved variation, minimal lift phacoemulsification. Since CCC requires in-the-bag phaco, there is a greatly reduced incidence of intraoperative problems caused by repeated nuclear prolapse (e.g., iris trauma, intraoperative miosis, zonular trauma, and acute intraoperative suprachoroidal hemorrhage).

CCC and phacoemulsification within the capsular bag can provide a structurally competent capsular bag in which to place a posterior chamber IOL. Prior to CCC, single or multiple radial anterior capsule tears were routinely noted in the remaining capsular "bag" after phacoemulsification and ECCE with nucleus expression. Although the term capsular bag has been used for many years to describe the residual capsular shape following ECCE, in reality, the capsular shape was a posterior capsule and a collection of anterior capsular flaps separated by radial anterior capsular tears.

Even with the most conservative iris plane phaco technique, one anterior capsular tear is usually needed. Given a single tear, IOLs can be placed so that the knees of a modified J-loop or C-loop haptic are oriented 90 degrees away from the anterior capsular defect (Fig. 9.8). If the knee of one of the haptics is placed within one clock hour

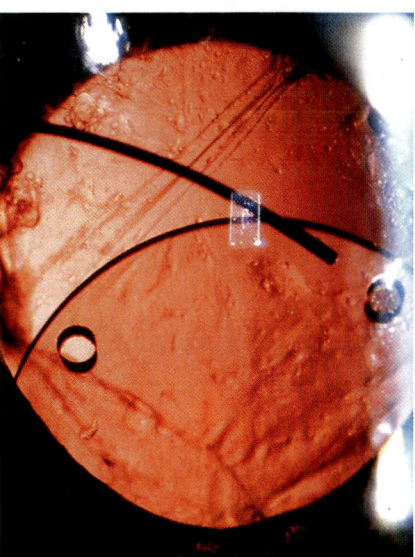

Figure 9.7 *The sunset syndrome may be initiated by an anterior radial tear, but usually requires substantial disruption of zonular fibers, and results in loss of support for the inferior IOL haptic.*

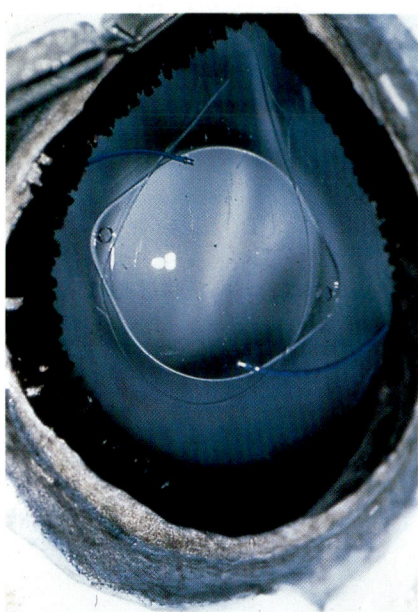

Figure 9.8 *Capsular bag placement is assured by placing the haptics perpendicular to the anterior capsular tear.*

of the capsular defect, it is likely to "pea pod" out of the torn capsular bag at the equator and to reside in the ciliary sulcus or pars plana (Fig. 9.9). This IOL displacement may be visible at surgery, and it may become more obvious as capsular fibrosis squeezes the haptic contained within the capsule and the IOL optic toward the haptic contained more passively at the ciliary sulcus (Fig. 9.10). Even if only one tear is present and the haptic is oriented 90 degrees from this tear, there is still a tendency for late optic displacement toward the anterior capsular defect. This displacement is usually minor and is rarely in a direction away from the defect.

Of course, multiple anterior capsular radial tears, which are more likely to occur during nucleus expression and traditional high lift iris plane phacoemulsification techniques, provide even more of a challenge for the cataract surgeon. Techniques have been developed that allow placement of the IOL within the capsular bag while preventing anterior capsule radial defects. The anterior capsular flaps may unfold to a variable degree, thereby allowing partial extension of the haptic beyond the perimeter of the capsular equatorial ring. Smaller anterior capsular flaps (longer radial tears) allow the furthest extensions while larger flaps (shorter capsular tears) are more effective in restricting peripheral movement. The largest "flap" possible is that which remains after only one anterior capsular radial tear has been created.

Anterior Capsulotomy Considerations

Studies of PC IOL optic decentration have found asymmetric bag/sulcus implantation to be a common cause of IOL optic decentration, and asymmetric implantation has been found in up to 50% of autopsy cases! In most cases, CCC provides results superior to those of the can-opener capsulotomy, although the can-opener method has its place; it is extremely useful when a minimal lift method of phacoemulsification is required to efficiently remove a very firm lens, in which case it may cause less trauma to the corneal endothelium if the surgeon has control of one nucleus for shorter irrigation and phacoemulsification periods than incomplete control of several very firm, relatively large, jagged nuclear fragments for longer irrigation and phacoemulsification periods. A can-opener capsulotomy is also the safest method of anterior capsulotomy in small pupil cases or in cases of mature or hypermature lenses in which the red reflex is obscured so reduced visibility of the anterior capsular edge makes CCC difficult and dangerous.

PC IOL Centration

Optic decentration occurs even with CCC, the result of the interaction between the haptics and the capsular bag. Various forces of capsular fibro-

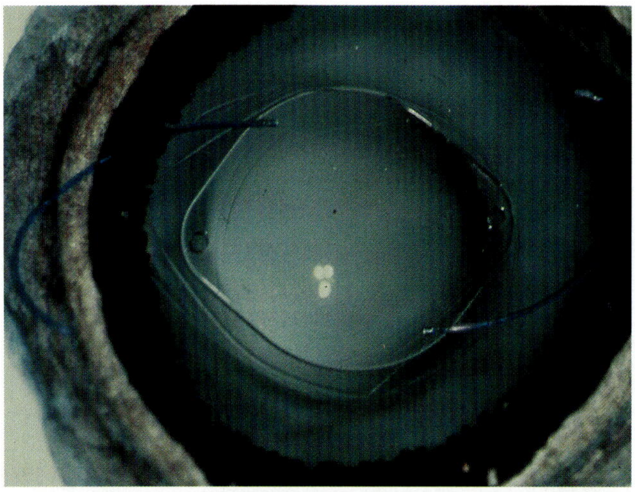

Figure 9.9 The IOL haptic knee "pea pods" out of the defective capsular bag into the ciliary sulcus.

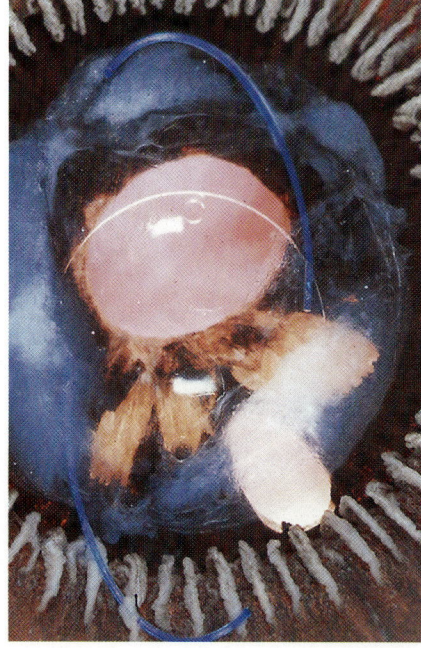

Figure 9.10 *In asymmetric placement, late decentration is made even worse by the forces of capsular fibrosis.*

sis make it difficult to predict if uniform centration will occur. For example, some IOLs are just too big or stiff and will symmetrically or asymmetrically unroll the anterior capsular remnant even in the absence of anterior radial tears. At the other extreme, some IOL haptics are very pliable, thus prone to permanent distortion because of poor memory. The surgeon may be well served to position the PC IOL haptics relative to the capsulorhexis, rather than having a preset idea of optimal haptic position.

Asymmetrical anterior capsule overlap of the optic may occur with both CCC and the can-opener technique. If the edge of the capsulotomy just touches or overlaps the IOL optic for half of its circumference and extends peripherally to it for the other half, a subtle movement of the optic may be caused by the squeezing force of capsular fibrosis (Fig. 9.11). This movement may be significant, depending on the IOL style. Asymmetrical optics, reduced optic diameters, and multifocal optics all present unique structural and optical challenges.

Other less common problems are more likely to occur with CCC than with the can-opener technique. If an optic is overlapped for 360 degrees the capsular bag distension syndrome may occur; in these cases, for unknown reasons, the capsular bag becomes distended by a clear fluid that pushes the IOL forward, producing an artificial myopia. A YAG anterior or posterior capsulotomy will solve this problem. Other problems may become manifest after surgery. The forces of capsular fibrosis can be recruited in a sphincter-like effect, resulting in a reduced capsulectomy diameter. This effect is most pronounced when capsulotomies are too small initially or in cases of pseudoexfoliation syndrome.

CCC Conclusion

These considerations and others indicate that for most patients CCC provides the best compromise for reasonable surgical access to the lens and the best containment of phacoemulsification. CCC also yields a structurally symetrical capsular bag that should reduce long-term IOL complications and improved optical performance. The surgeon may have to alter ECCE technique to accommodate capsulorhexis or change to phacoemulsification, for which capsulorhexis is better suited.

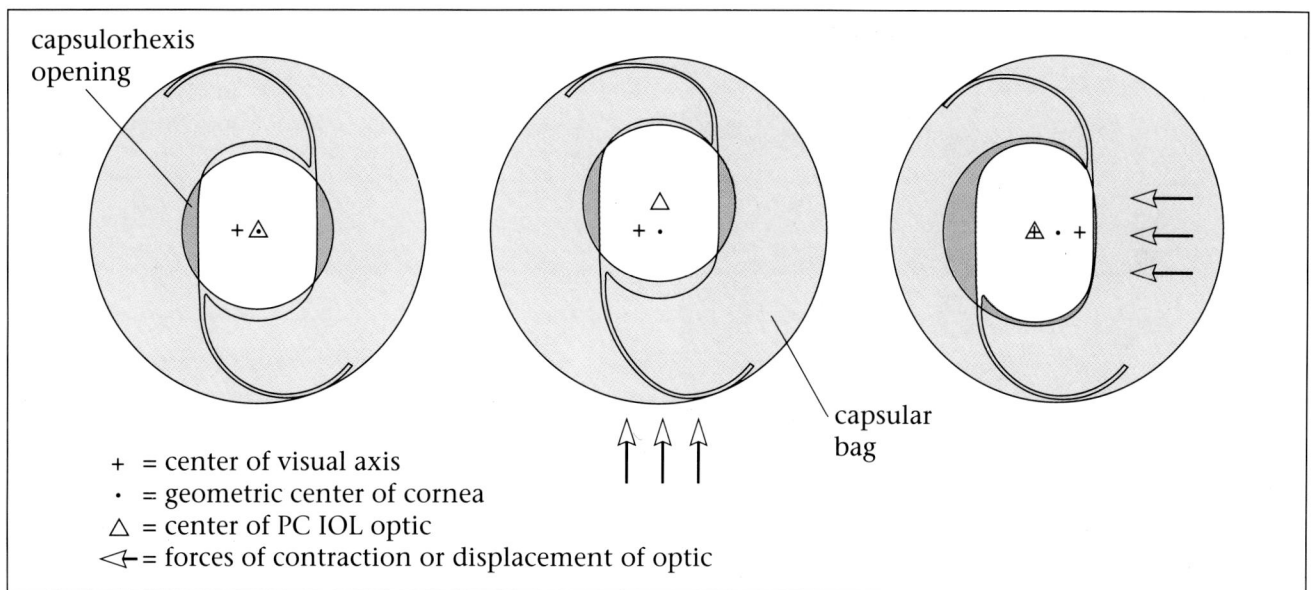

Figure 9.11 *The relationship between an anterior capsulorhexis and an ovoid optic is used to demonstrate factors that may promote centration or cause late decentration of the optic of a PC-IOL. Centration is expected when the capsulorhexis overlaps the optic symmetrically* (left). *If the capsulorhexis is positioned asymetrically relative to the optic, contraction of the capsulorhexis opening may cause late decentration of the optic. Displacement of the optic toward the center of the shrinking opening can occur if the haptics offer no resistance to contracture of the capsular bag* (middle) *or if one edge of the optic is encountered before the other by the shrinking capsulorhexis* (right).

Whatever the adjustments necessary, CCC, the currently preferred anterior capsulotomy method, will provide long-term PC IOL centration and excellent pseudophakic ocular function.

Trans-scleral Fixation of Posterior Chamber Intraocular Lenses

In certain difficult cases, such as traumatic aniridia, peripheral anterior synechiae, and anterior segment neovascularization, fixation of a PC IOL in the ciliary sulcus without the support of the posterior capsule may help rehabilitate the eye (Fig. 9.12). This maneuver requires securing the haptics into position with 10-0 Prolene, usually after performing an anterior vitrectomy. Since the eye is aphakic, the anterior chamber can be inflated with viscoelastic (and removed afterwards by an automated vitrectomy instrument), which is necessary for this implantation technique. Of course, surgical exposure during penetrating keratoplasty (PKP) is excellent. The PC IOL tends to situate itself closer to the retina than it would normally so an IOL of appropriate power must be selected.

Methods

PC IOLs can be secured using sutures on long, straight needles that fit within 27-gauge hollow "guide" needles, as originated by James Lewis, M.D., or with regular, curved corneoscleral spatula needles. Variations of the technique, described by Anthony Mannarino, M.D., and colleagues, offer several advantages (Fig. 9.13).

A PC IOL with Prolene, C-loop haptics is selected and the end of each haptic is blunted by the heat of a dryfield cautery to prevent slippage of the two 10-0 Prolene sutures swaged to straight needles and tied to each haptic. Two 3.00 mm partial thickness scleral incision are made 1.50 mm behind the surgical limbus and 180 degrees from each other. Placing these incisions between the rectus muscles helps minimize the potential involvement of the long posterior-ciliary arteries. During PKP, after excision of the cornea, two 27-gauge needles are inserted through each partial thickness corneal incision into the anterior chamber. These 27-gauge needles act as "guide tubes" for the straight needles of the Prolene sutures attached to the PC IOL haptics.

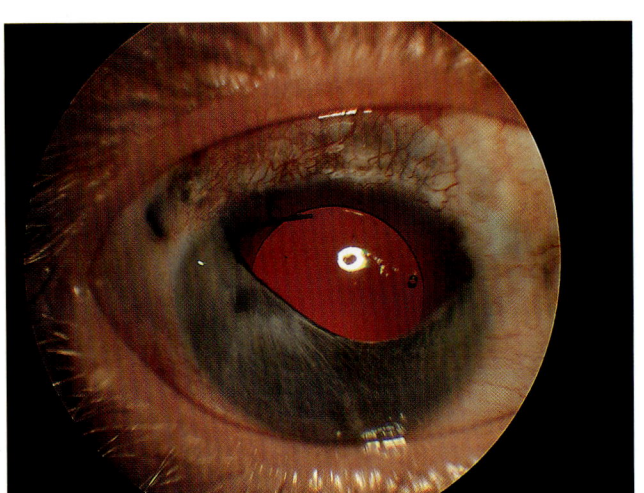

Figure 9.12 *Patient with congenital cataracts who underwent an ICCE with a sector iridectomy. A PC IOL was positioned by trans-scleral fixation after mechanical anterior vitrectomy.*

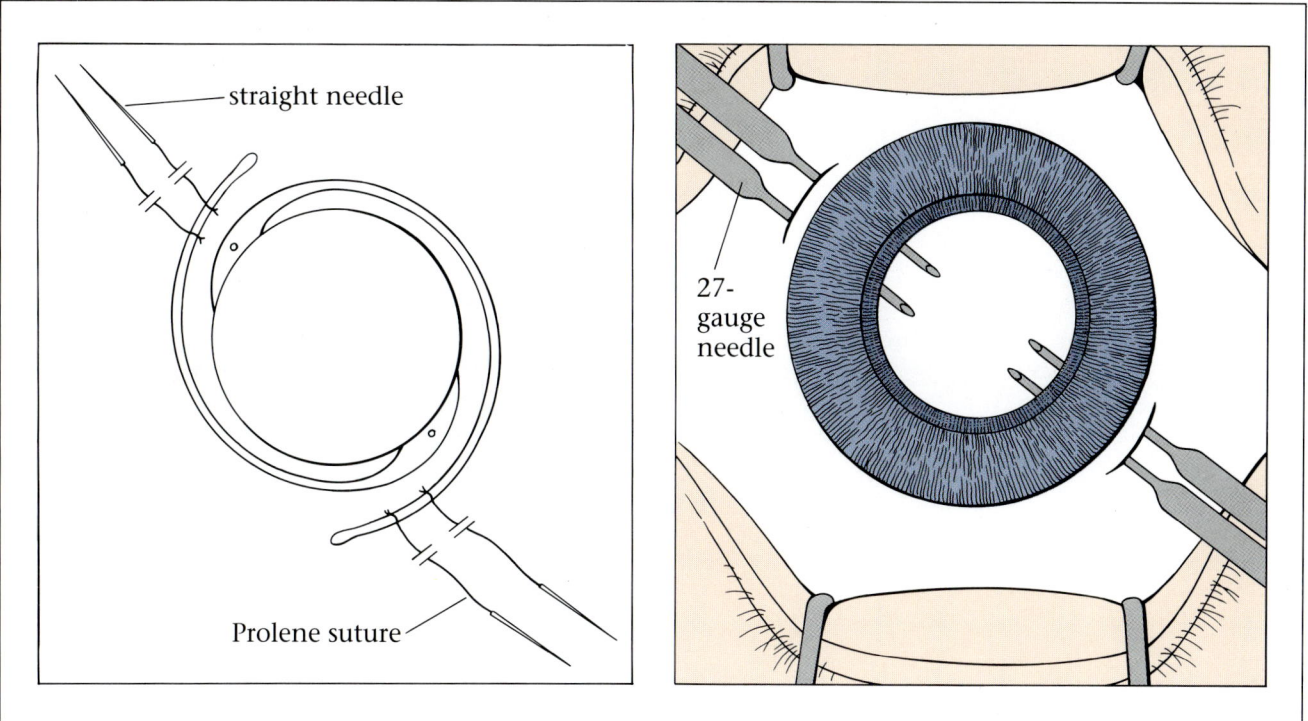
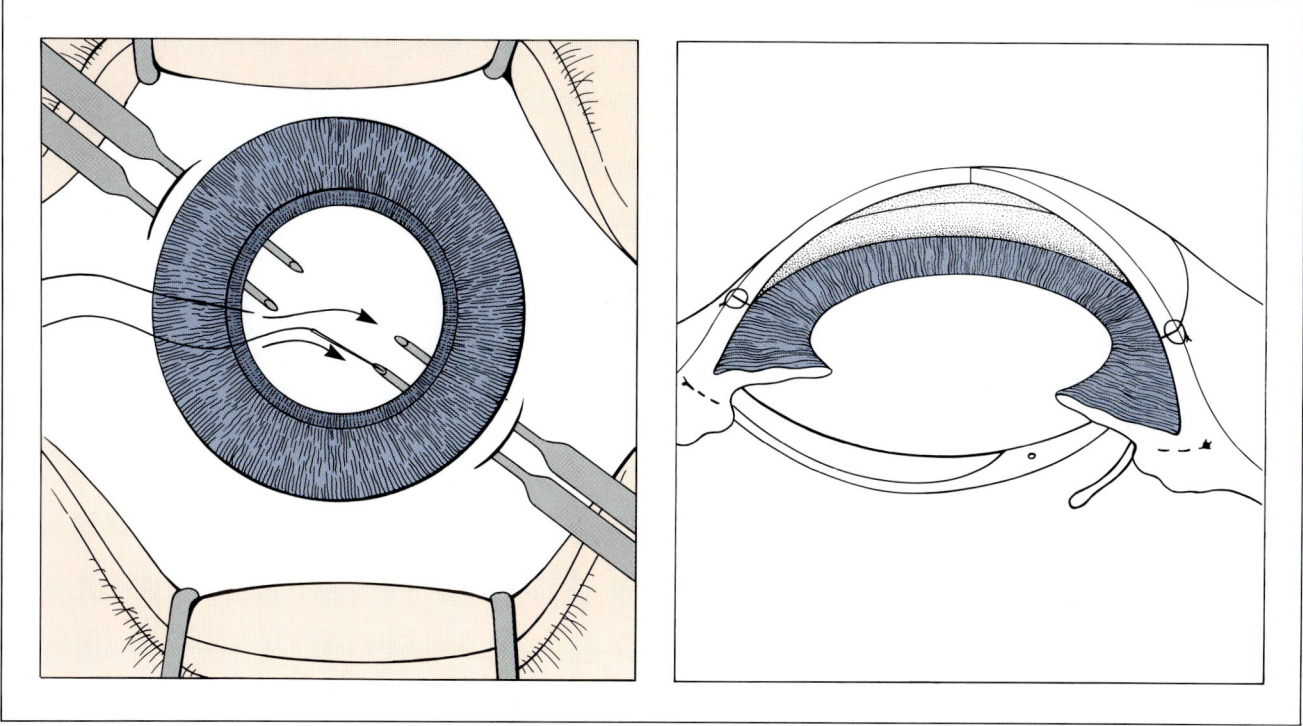

Figure 9.13 *The key steps of trans-scleral fixation of a PC IOL with penetrating keratoplasty.* **(Top)** *The straight needles of the Prolene sutures are guided through the 27- gauge needle.* **(Bottom)** *The PC IOL is suspended in position as the Prolene sutures are snugged and tied to each other in the depth of the scleral incisions.*

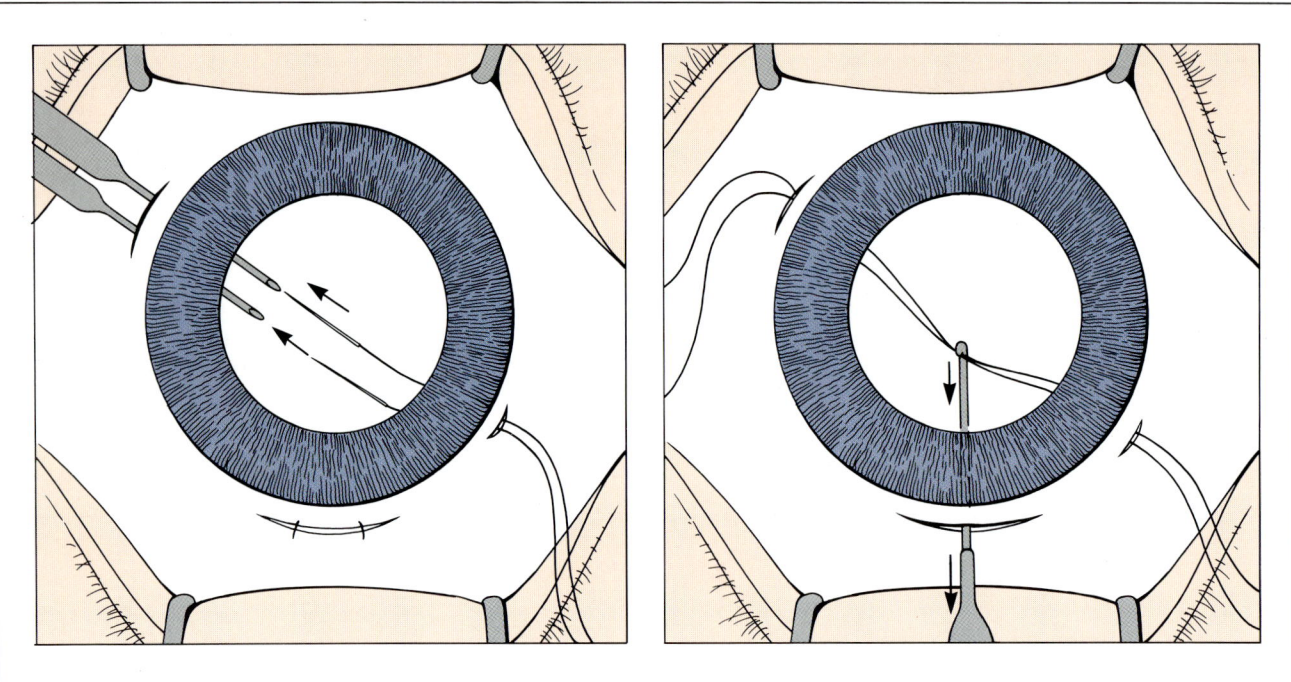
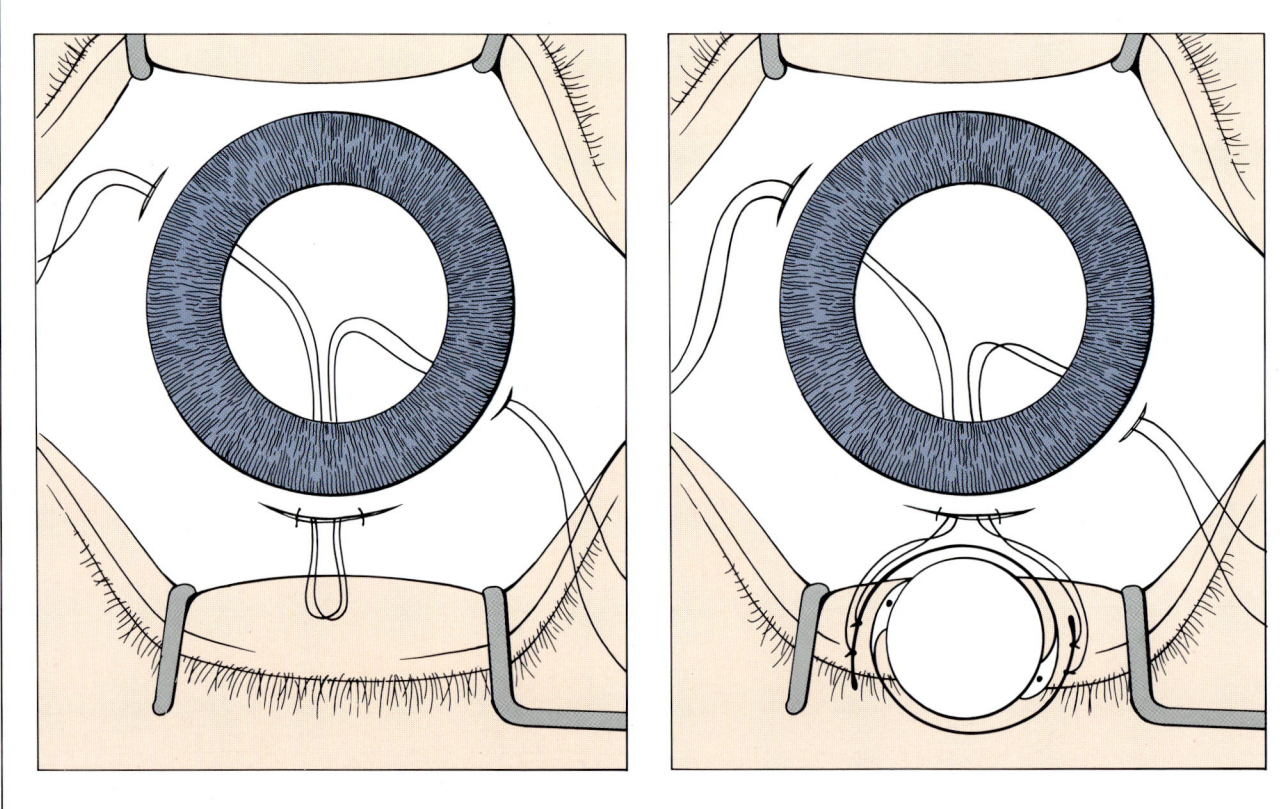

Figure 9.14 *A variation of the method described in Figure 9.13 may be used for obtaining trans-scleral fixation of a PC IOL in an aphakic eye without penetrating keratoplasty.* **(Top left)** *The 27-gauge "guide" needles are inserted across the anterior chamber through the partial thickness scleral incisions.* **(Top right)** *A micro-hook is used to capture the 10-0 Prolene inside the anterior chamber.* **(Bottom left)** *The 10-0 Prolene suture is externalized by means of the micro-hook.* **(Bottom right)** *The 10-0 Prolene suture is cut and tied to the haptics of the PC IOL. The PC IOL is then placed into position as the Prolene sutures are snugged up and tied to each other within the partial thickness scleral incisions.*

The PC IOL is positioned and the Prolene sutures are tied and secured in the depth of the corneal incisions.

If no PKP is planned, two Prolene sutures on straight needles can be introduced from one corneal incision, through the anterior chamber, into two 27-gauge needles that have been inserted into the anterior chamber through the contralateral corneal incision (Fig. 9.14). The Prolene sutures are captured with a collar button and externalized through the corneoscleral incision, which allows for PC IOL implantation. The externalized Prolene sutures are cut and secured to the haptics of the PC IOL. The PC IOL is secured using the method described above (trans-scleral fixation combined with PKP).

An alternate method for suturing a PC IOL into the ciliary sulcus employs two curved corneoscleral spatula needles on 10-0 Prolene, which are introduced into the anterior chamber through partial thickness scleral incisions 1.00 mm from the limbus (Fig. 9.15). The needles indent the iris from beneath and are easily captured there in the anterior chamber by long McPherson forceps, externalized through the superior wound and attached to the PC IOL, as described above.

In both of these methods, the Prolene sutures fixating the PC IOL are tied to each other in the depth of the scleral incision; thus scleral flaps are unnecessary and the chance of providing a pathway for infection is minimized. Also, the four point fixation helps prevent tilting of the PC IOL.

The ciliary sulcus lies perpendicularly beneath the sclera about 0.75 mm behind the surgical limbus. The scleral incisions are placed 1.50 mm behind the surgical limbus when it is necessary to accommodate the oblique entry of a straight needle into the sclera. When sewing a PC IOL into position, it is important to use a C-loop style because the haptics prevent the IOL from tilting by contacting the underside of the iris, and the haptic is relatively straight at the point of Prolene suture fixation. The techniques used for trans-scleral fixation of a PC IOL may be useful in placing "McCannell" sutures to recenter the optic of a displaced PC IOL (Fig. 9.16). Special needle/suture combinations have been developed for this purpose.

Conclusion

If an eye is aphakic, the possibility of anterior chamber IOL implantation should be considered. The visual results tend to be slightly better with an anterior chamber IOL than with a sewn-in PC IOL because of more accurate IOL power selection and simpler implantation. When indicated, though, trans-scleral fixation of a PC IOL into the ciliary sulcus can truly rehabilitate an eye when most hope for recovery has been lost.

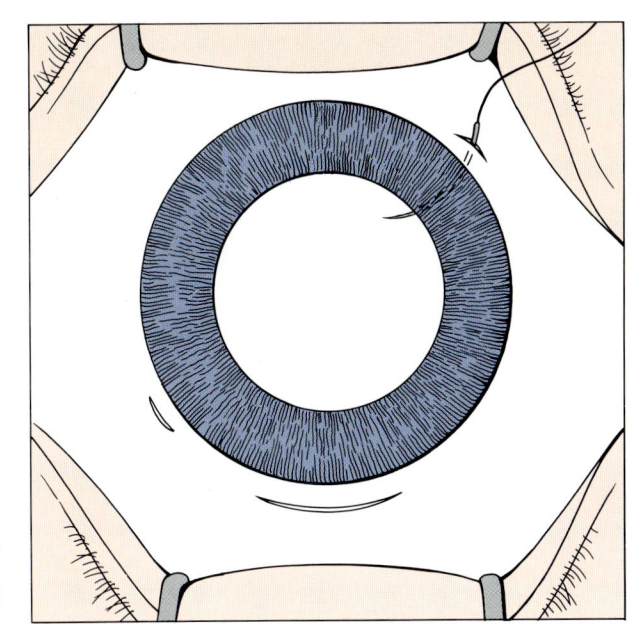 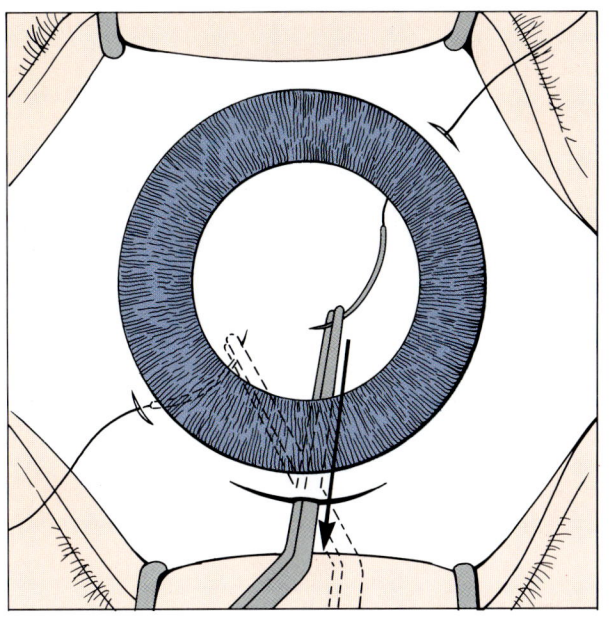

Figure 9.15 (Left) *A method for achieving trans-scleral fixation of a PC IOL using 10-0 Prolene sutures on curved needles, which are placed into the anterior chamber through a partial thickness scleral incision. The point of the needle may be visualized directly in the anterior chamber or its location may be identified by the upward indentation it makes in the iris.* (Right) *A long McPherson forceps grasps the needle and externalizes it through a superior limbal wound or the corneal wound awaiting the donor cornea of penetrating keratoplasty.*

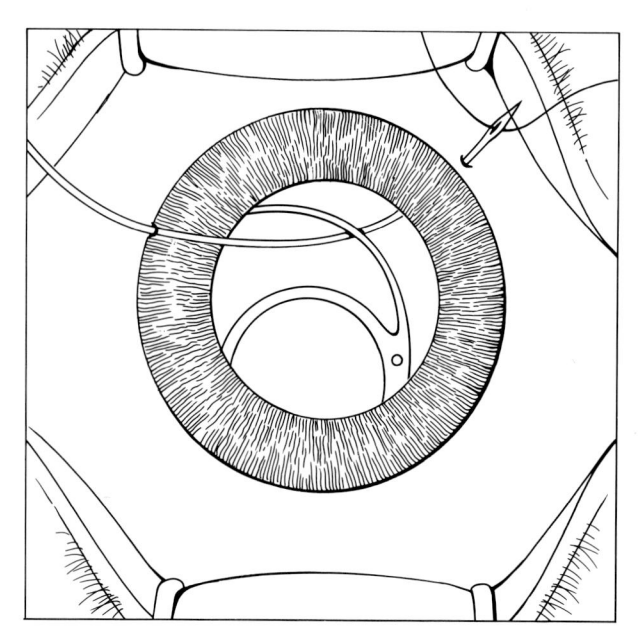
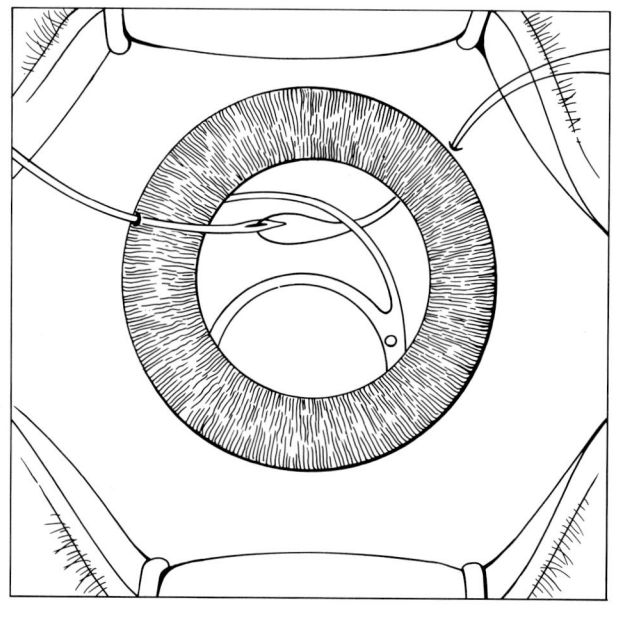
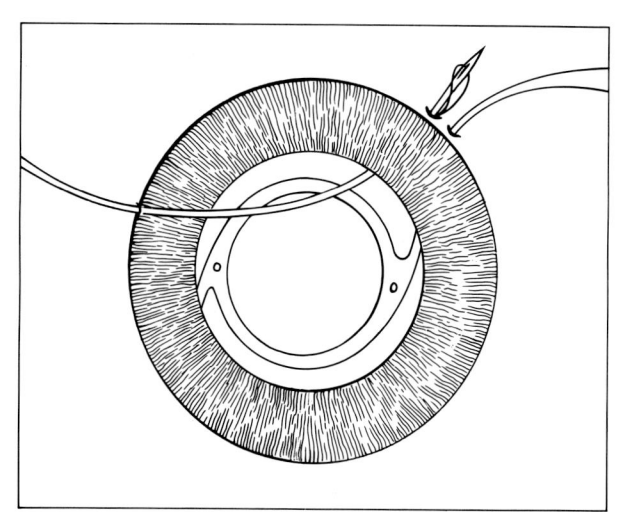
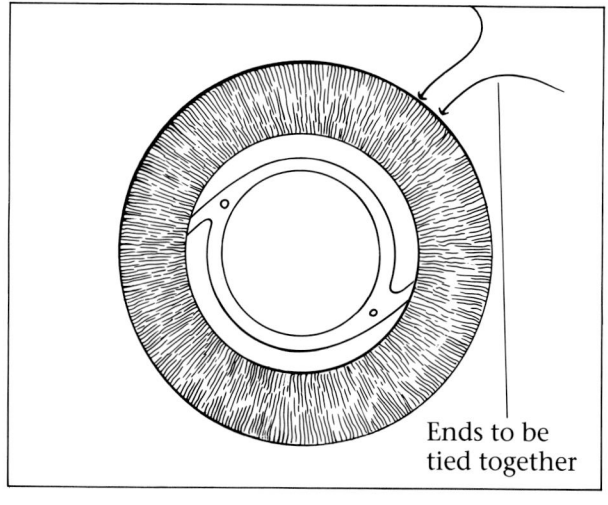

Ends to be tied together

Figure 9.16 (Top and bottom) *Special needle/suture combinations have been developed for placing "McCannell" sutures. These sutures may be used to recenter a displaced PC IOL optic. Either a limbal or a pars plana approach may be used. An example of a limbal approach using an SC-1 needle to recenter the optic of a PC IOL.*

Clinical Points to Consider

- Continuous circular capsulorhexis (CCC) of the anterior capsule provides a symmetrical capsular bag for PC IOL in-the-bag implantation with long-term centration.

- CCC may make ECCE more difficult because it limits prolapse of the superior pole of the nucleus.

- The peripheral rim of the anterior capsule that remains after CCC may serve as an excellent support for PC IOL implantation if the posterior capsule is broken during cataract extraction.

- Trans-scleral fixation of a PC IOL does not always result in excellent optic centration.

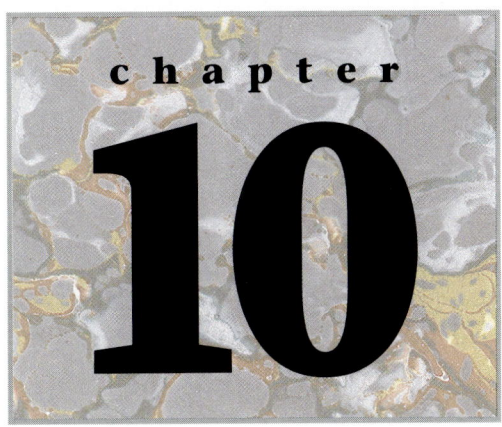

EXTRACAPSULAR CATARACT EXTRACTION

MICHAEL BLUMENTHAL, M.D.   EHUD I. ASSIA, M.D.

Cataract surgery is constantly evolving. Hundreds of technical innovations have been developed and abandoned during its history. To fully understand the advantages of our extracapsular cataract extraction (ECCE) technique, it is important to briefly review the basic principles and technical details of crystalline lens anatomy and physiology.

Surgical Anatomy

Anterior Chamber

The plane of the ciliary ring is located slightly posterior to the lens plane. The zonules, anchored to the ciliary processes, are normally directed slightly posteriorly, creating a constant radial and backward force that stretches the anterior capsule. Under normal conditions the relative anterior-posterior location of the lens does not change significantly when the zonules are either stretched or relaxed. In contrast, during ECCE the zonules have a stable anchorage in the ciliary body, but the anterior-posterior position of the lens is unstable (Fig. 10.1). Fluid escaping from the anterior chamber causes shallowing of the anterior chamber and anterior displacement of the lens. This, in turn, causes a significant increase in the zonular pull, which results in increased capsular radial stretching. Momentary shallowing of the anterior chamber during anterior capsulectomy might result in an uncontrolled tear, often extending to the periphery. Maintaining pressure in the anterior chamber and pushing the lens-zonule diaphragm backward, so it is more posterior than the normal lens position, results in maximal relaxation of the anterior capsule. A collapsed cornea at any stage of the operation might touch the crystalline lens, the intraocular lens (IOL), or an instrument, which could result in irreversible damage to the delicate endothelium. It is, therefore, of utmost importance to keep a deep, stable anterior chamber throughout the operation.

Lens Capsule

The crystalline lens is covered by its capsule, which is a basement membrane produced by the epithelial cells. The capsule behaves as homogeneous material, thickest at the anterior surface and thinnest at the posterior surface. It is now generally accepted that optimal surgical results are obtained when the posterior capsule is preserved and the IOL is firmly implanted in the capsular bag. Implantation of the IOL in the physiologic location of the natural lens is advantageous only if the IOL remains permanently in the bag. A tear in the anterior capsule extending to the equator impairs the integrity and stability of the capsular bag. A minor break in the margin of the capsulectomy significantly lowers its resistance, and relatively little force is sufficient to extend the tear to the equator.

Capsulectomy by the can-opener technique is performed by creating many small tears, each connected to the other. Thus, any individual capsular tear can enlarge and extend to the periphery during nucleus extraction or IOL implantation (Fig. 10.2). In the linear capsulotomy (endocapsular or envelope techniques), a tear toward the periphery is an integral part of the procedure. Both ends of the capsulotomy are directed toward the equator and are not involved in the second step of tearing the anterior capsule (Fig. 10.3). In both cases a "false bag" is created, which corresponds to the high incidence of outward dislocation of at least one loop of the IOL.

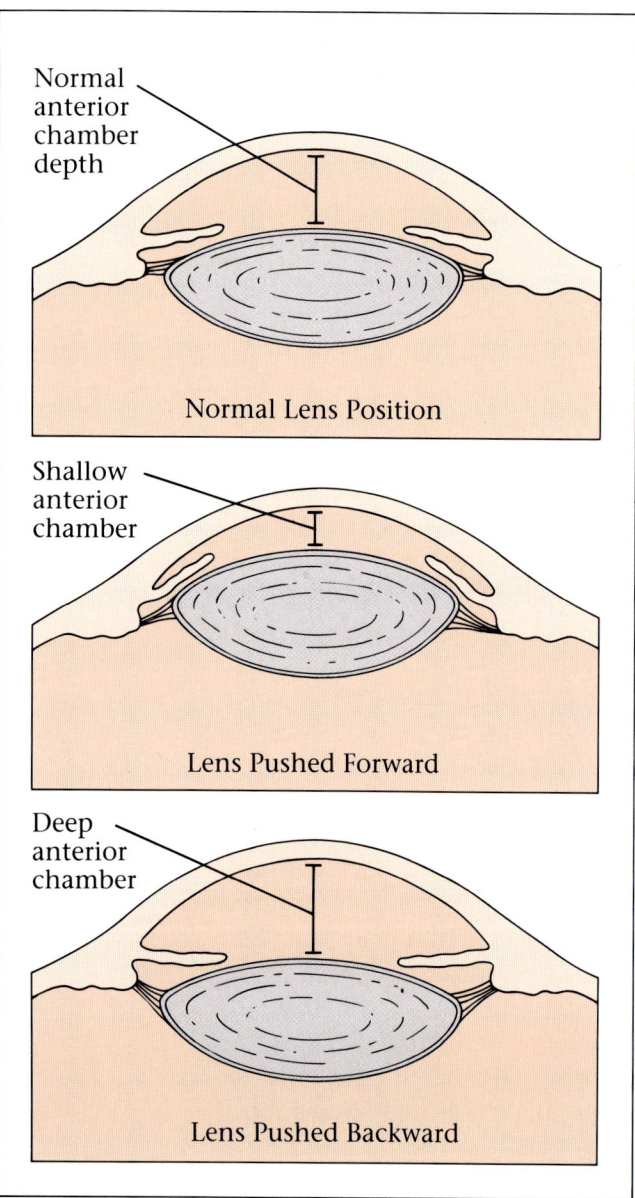

Figure 10.1 *Location of the crystalline lens in the anterior chamber. Normal lens position: the equator is in the plane of the equatorial zonules. Shallow anterior chamber: the lens is dislocated anteriorly with maximal stretch on the anterior capsule. Deep anterior chamber: the lens is dislocated posteriorly with minimal stretch on the anterior capsule.*

To create a "true bag" it is obligatory to perform a round, continuous tear (smooth edges and no breaks). This is done by pulling and tearing one end of the capsulotomy (capsulorhexis) until the "head" and "tail" of the capsulotomy meet. The zonular fibers are attached 1.50 mm to 2.00 mm anterior and central to the equator. A crystalline lens of 10.00 mm has, therefore, only a 6.00-mm to 7.00-mm zonule-free area. When a large capsulectomy (>7.00 mm) is performed, the tear might penetrate the anterior zonular adherence to the capsule. Control of the capsulorhexis is lost if the capsular tear is extended beyond this zonular "frontier." Redirection of the tear to the zonule-free zone requires a second penetration of the zonular frontier, which demands a significantly stronger tearing force and superior skills, especially when the tear is

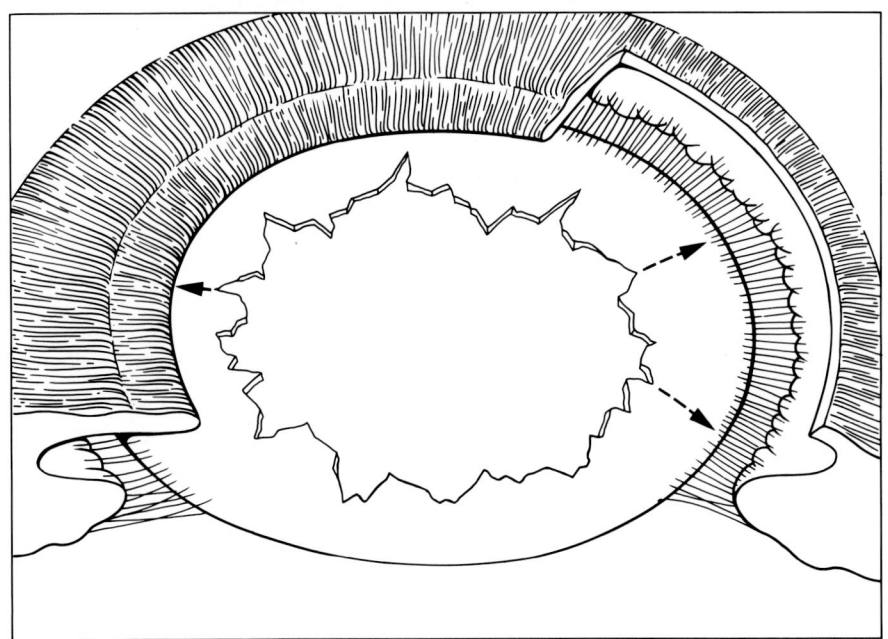

Figure 10.2 *In the can-opener technique, many small tears are created. Any individual tear can enlarge toward the periphery (depending on the direction of forces inflicted during nucleus extraction or IOL implantation).*

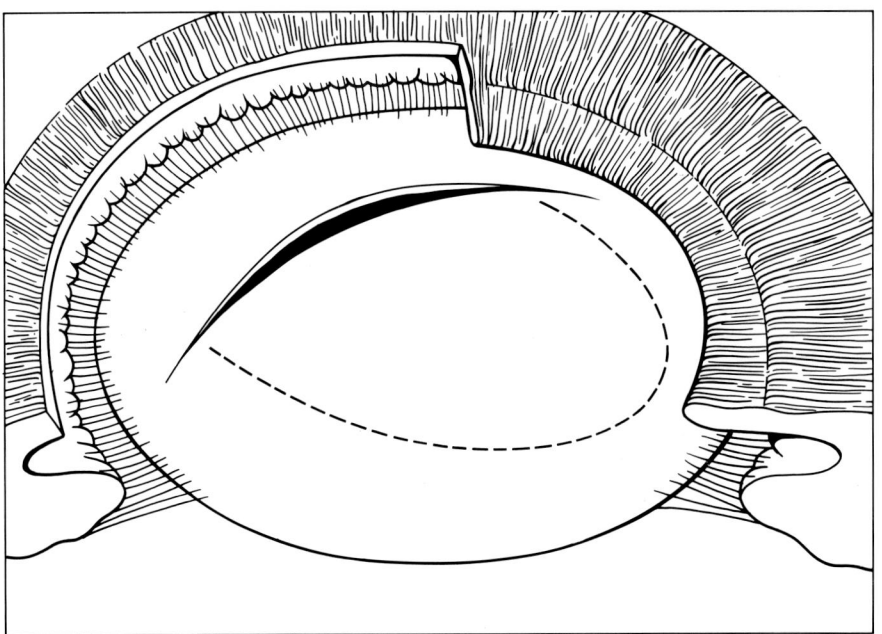

Figure 10.3 *In linear capsulectomy (endocapsular or envelope techniques), a tear toward the periphery is an integral part of the procedure and both ends are directed toward the equator. Second step capsulorhexis (dotted line) does not create a continuous round opening.*

obscured by the iris (Fig. 10.4). On the other hand, a small capsular opening (<5.00 mm) means a much more difficult, sometimes impossible, nucleus expression by external pressure. Application of high external pressure in such cases can result in zonular rupture, vitreous loss, or the nucleus pushing into the vitreous. A successful operation using a round, continuous capsulectomy can be achieved only when combined with techniques that reduce the volume of the nucleus and minimize the stress on the zonules during nucleus delivery.

Crystalline Lens Nucleus

As new lens fibers are constantly formed, the lens volume is continuously increasing. The newly formed fibers in the periphery of the lens compress the older and deeper layers and, together with other aging processes, create a hard, deep core. The traditional division of the lens into a central hard nucleus surrounded by soft cortical fibers is mainly clinical, since there is no distinct border between these two structures. The transition from cortex to hard nucleus is gradual, so there is a large midzone area that exhibits transitional characteristics between the harder nucleus and the softer cortex. Since this intermediate layer engulfs the hard core and clinically behaves as a coat to the nucleus, the preferred term for this layer is *epinucleus*. The clinical anatomy of the lens can be divided as follows (Fig. 10.5):

1. Superficial cortex: soft material (can be aspirated)

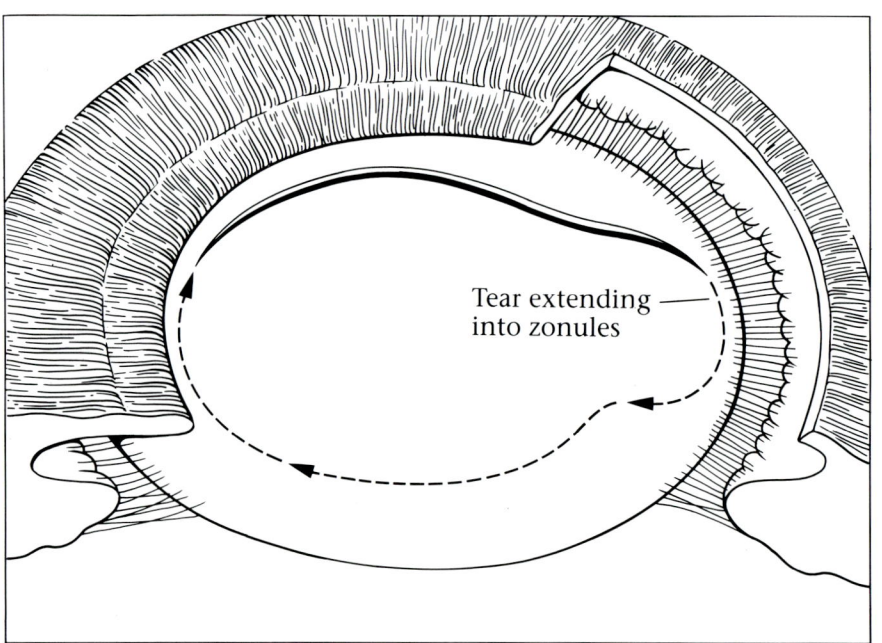

Figure 10.4 *Redirection of a capsular tear extending beyond the zonular frontier requires a significantly stronger force and tearing of some of the anterior zonules.*

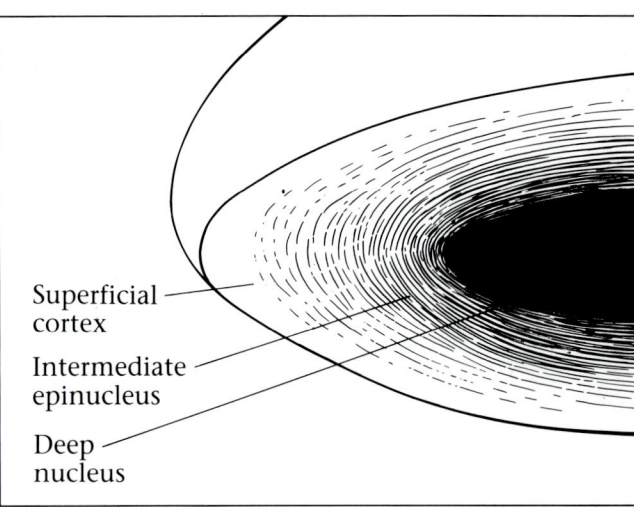
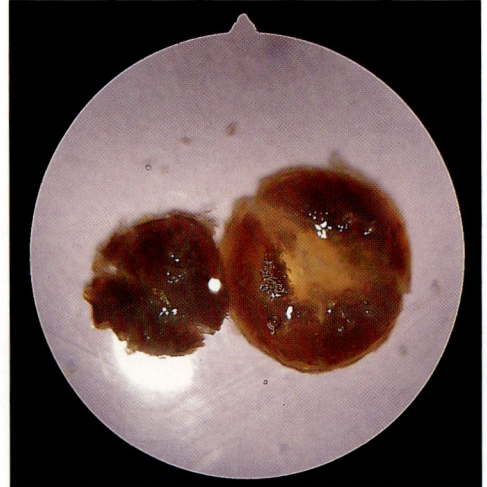

Figure 10.5 (Left) *The anatomic composition of the adult lens: superficial cortex, intermediate epinucleus, and deep, hard nucleus.* **(Right)** *The small, hard nucleus is separated from the epinucleus. This preparation was done on a large nucleus that was removed using the open-system technique without hydroseparation. It is obvious that a much smaller limbal incision is needed to remove the small, hard nucleus that is created by intracapsular hydrodissection. The remaining epinucleus is either squeezed out in one piece or in parts or it is aspirated.*

2. Intermediate epinucleus: semisoft material (can be aspirated or expressed)
3. Deep nucleus: hard core (can be expressed as a whole or in broken parts)

The intermediate properties of the midzone can be used to advantage during the cataract operation. Hydrodissection loosens the adhesions of the fibers between neighboring lamellae. Superficial hydrodissection separates the lens nucleus (including the epinucleus) from the adjacent cortex. Deep hydrodissection combined with mechanical maneuvers will separate the epinucleus from the deeper, hard nucleus, which is smaller than the typical adult nucleus defined by slit lamp examination (Fig. 10.6). After expression of the central hard nucleus, the epinucleus can be squeezed and extracted out of the eye as one anatomic unit, removed in parts, or even aspirated.

Based on the above principles, the steps of my ECCE with IOL implantation include:
1. Maintaining a deep anterior chamber with positive pressure
2. Round, continuous capsulectomy within the zonule-free area
3. Separation of the lens nucleus to epinucleus and hard core
4. Hydroexpression of the hard nucleus through the capsulectomy into the anterior chamber to minimize zonular stress
5. Hydroextraction of the nucleus through the limbal opening under positive pressure (Fig. 10.7).
6. Hydrodissection of the epinucleus and removal by hydroexpression or aspiration.

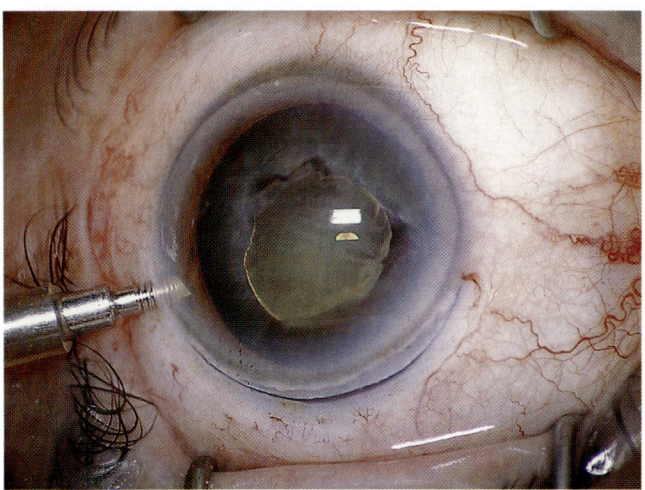

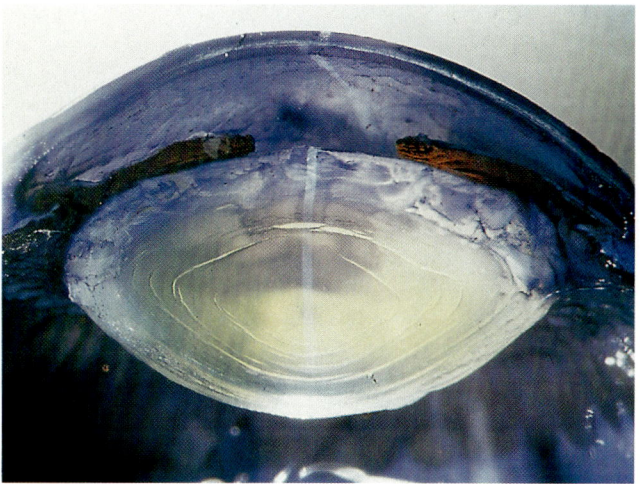

Figure 10.6 (Left) *A hard core nucleus separated from its softer epinucleus—together they are called the adult nucleus.* **(Right)** *Hydrodissection defining the borders between the central hard nucleus, the intermediate epinucleus, and the peripheral cortex. The diameter of the nucleus is reduced from 8.30 mm to 6.50 mm when the hard core is hydroseparated. This photograph was taken from behind the lens so that the ciliary processes are clearly visible.*

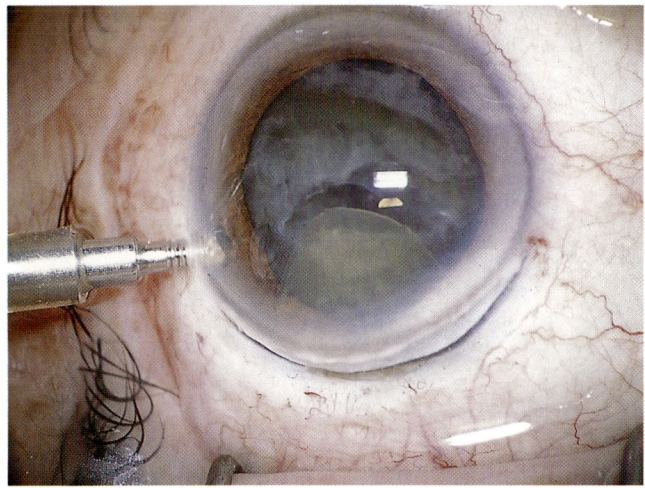

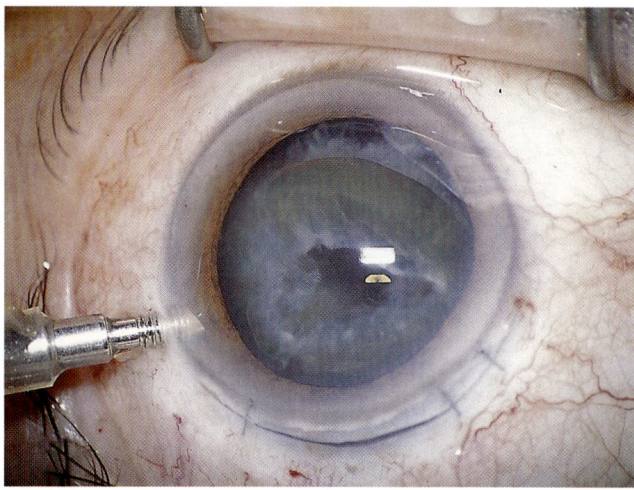

Figure 10.7 (Left) *A hard core nucleus being hydroextracted (expressed) out of the eye.* **(Right)** *The epinucleus remains in the anterior chamber. (Its outside configuration is similar to the adult nucleus.)*

7. Implantation of an IOL in the capsular bag with the anterior chamber formed by positive pressure

8. Suturing the corneal wound under positive, near normal, intraocular pressure

Surgical Procedure

Maintaining the Anterior Chamber

Maintenance of a deep anterior chamber throughout the operation can be achieved by either continuous irrigation with BSS through an anterior chamber maintainer (ACM) or by a viscoelastic. I find that using ACM is more rewarding since it constantly regulates the hydrostatic pressure in the anterior chamber. The pressure is determined by the height of the BSS bottle and the size of the maintainer pore (Fig. 10.8). The 0.90-mm ACM pore is the optimal pore size. Viscoelastic, in most of the cases, can create a deep anterior chamber. However, it is important to realize that viscoelastic often maintains volume, not pressure, and when it escapes through the limbal opening there is no instant volume replacement. Also, viscoelastic and an ACM can be used simultaneously. With low hydrostatic BSS pressure, the viscoelastic will not escape from the anterior chamber. To allow continuous fluid replacement, the ACM is inserted through a separate opening made by a diamond knife 1.00 mm wide, usually at the 2

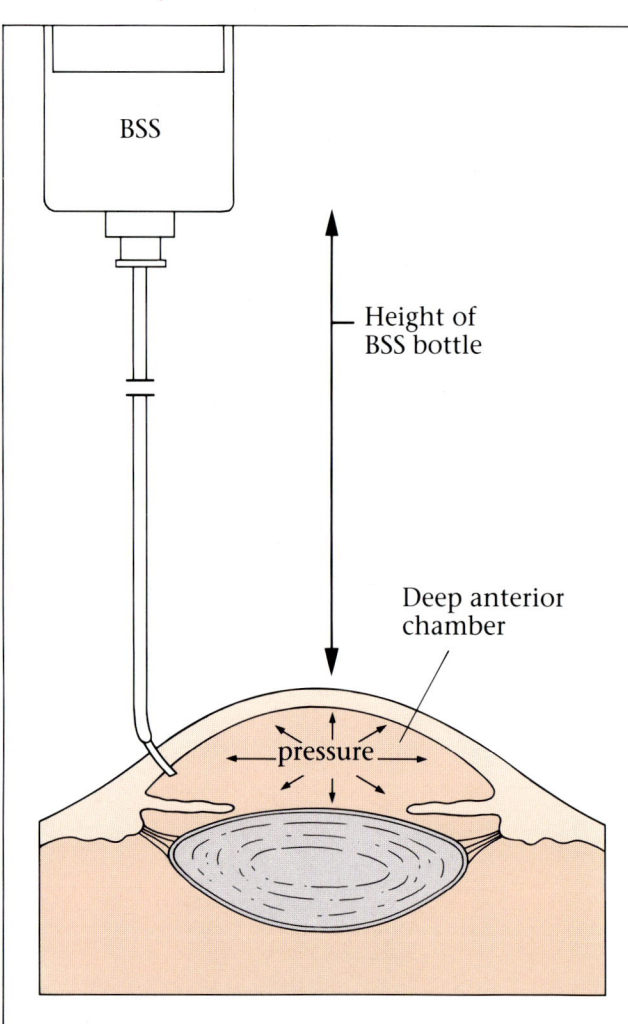

Figure 10.8 *The pressure in the eye is determined by the height of the BSS bottle and the size of the maintainer pore.*

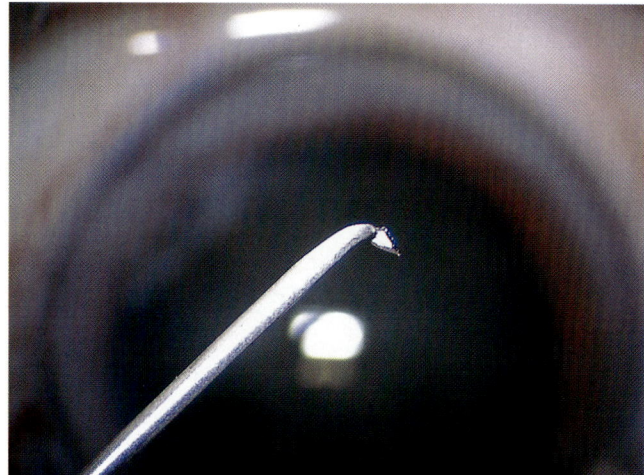

Figure 10.9 *The cystotome is made of a 25- or 27-gauge needle in which the 0.30 mm beveled tip is bent 90 degrees, then twisted an additional 90 degrees so that the cutting edge lies parallel to the axis of the needle.*

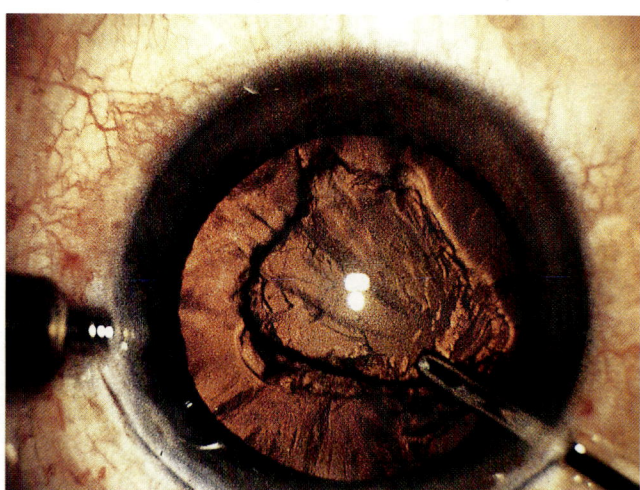

Figure 10.10 *Aspiration of the anterior cortex and epinucleus exposes the anterior surface of the hard core nucleus, which cannot be further aspirated.*

o'clock position. A second perforation at 10 o'clock, or any other place convenient for the surgeon, is used for the capsulotomy needle.

Anterior Capsulectomy

Continuous circular capsulectomy is done by using a bent needle or a cystotome. I prefer a cystotome with a 25- or 27-gauge needle in which the beveled tip, 0.30 mm long, is bent 90 degrees, then twisted an additional 90 degrees so that the cutting edge lies parallel to the axis of the needle (Fig. 10.9). (A disposable cystotome with the same configuration is now available from Visitec). An initial horizontal cut is performed from 2 o'clock to 10 o'clock on the anterior capsule as in the endocapsular technique. One end of the cut is then extended by pressing and pulling the anterior capsule to control the direction of the tear. The running head of the tear is directed to meet the initial cut, thus creating a heart-shaped continuous capsulectomy (endocapsulorhexis). The capsular tear is best evaluated under direct vision in the presence of a bright red reflex. In its absence, one can use other guidelines, such as capsule surface reflex, or one can follow the movement of the free capsule flap induced by the ACM flow.

Hydrodissection of the Nucleus

To separate the epinucleus from the harder core nucleus, it is first necessary to locate their deepest junction. Using a 0.40-mm pore aspiration cannula, the anterior cortical fibers, exposed after the capsulectomy, are aspirated. The semisoft epinucleus, lying under the exposed cortex, is aspirated until the anterior part of the hard nucleus is exposed (Fig. 10.10). Complete separation of the epinucleus from the hard nucleus is then performed by hydrodissection. The cannula is slid superiorly along the hard nucleus and inserted obliquely at the 12 o'clock position into the junction of the epinucleus and the hard core nucleus. BSS, introduced by syringe injection, engulfs the hard nucleus and forms a demarcation line. The cannula is lodged in the newly created space between the epinucleus and the hard nucleus, then introduced smoothly behind the hard nucleus. This is done with fine mechanical sweeps so perpendicular adhesions still present will be broken (Fig. 10.11). These maneuvers isolate the smallest possible hard core nucleus, which is usually small enough to be delivered through the round capsulectomy.

Hydroexpression of the Nucleus to the Anterior Chamber

Delivery of the nucleus through the smaller diameter capsulectomy is accomplished by combined mechanical and hydrostatic pressure. Using the cannula, now located behind the nucleus, fluid is injected together with gentle mechanical manipulations that guide the nucleus anteriorly. The positive pressure in the capsular bag and the anterior chamber pushes the zonule-capsule diaphragm backward and creates a counter force to the resistance induced by the capsulectomy margin. The round capsulectomy changes temporarily into an oval to permit the passage of the nucleus. Viscoelastic in the anterior chamber makes this maneuver less traumatic to the endothelium, because it lubricates the

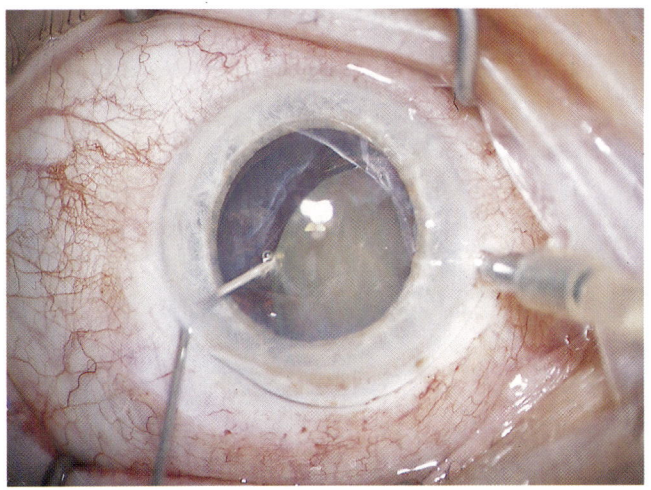

Figure 10.11 *The hydrodissector is introduced behind the hard core nucleus after hydrodissection. Mechanical sweeps break any perpendicular adhesions that are still present.*

nucleus and prevents the ill effects that result from bouncing the nucleus toward the endothelium.

Hydroexpression (Hydroextraction) of the Nucleus

The size of the hard nucleus is evaluated while in the anterior chamber to determine the length of the limbal incision (Fig. 10.12). The incision is performed with a diamond knife while the intraocular pressure (IOP) is maintained at 20 to 25 mm/Hg. Cutting the cornea at near normal pressure allows a smooth and controlled incision for perfect closure of the wound. When the nucleus is engaged at the inner side of the limbal incision, the hydrostatic pressure of the anterior chamber pushes the nucleus out of the eye (Fig. 10.13). Elevation of the BSS bottle can be used to temporarily elevate the IOP and assist in nucleus delivery. In this case there is no need to inflict excessive external force that might distort the globe. Thus, the nucleus has been manually extracted through a relatively small limbal incision, and concomitantly normal IOP has been maintained. In contrast, external pressure to express the nucleus creates very low anterior chamber pressure, and high vitreous pressure, which causes the posterior capsule to be pushed forward by the vitreous body, stretching both the posterior capsule and the zonules.

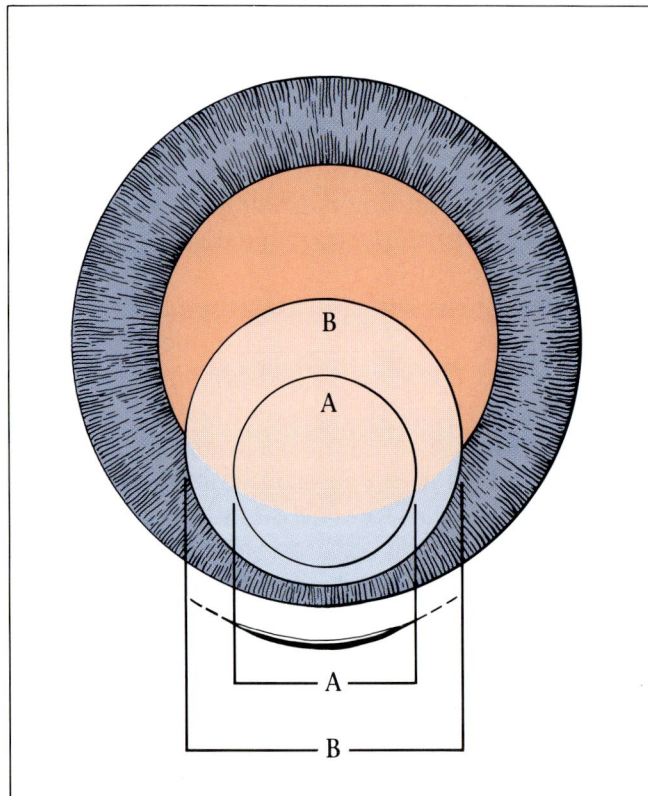

Figure 10.12 *Evaluation of the dimension of the hard nucleus while in the anterior chamber determines the size of the limbal incision.*

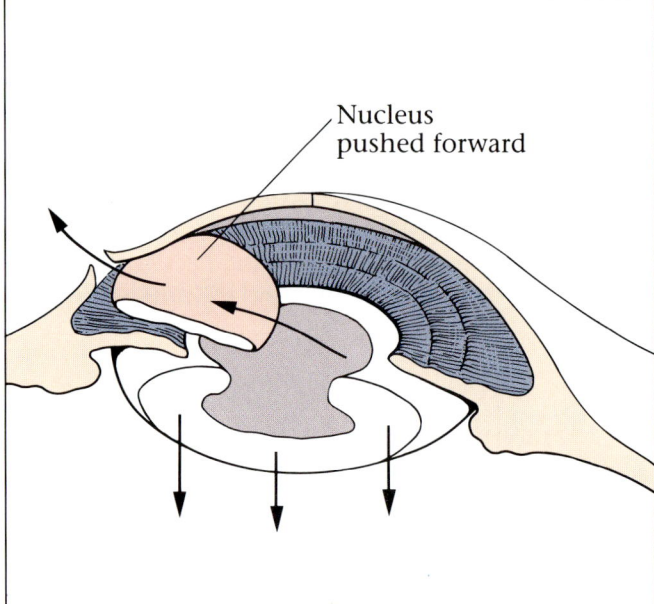

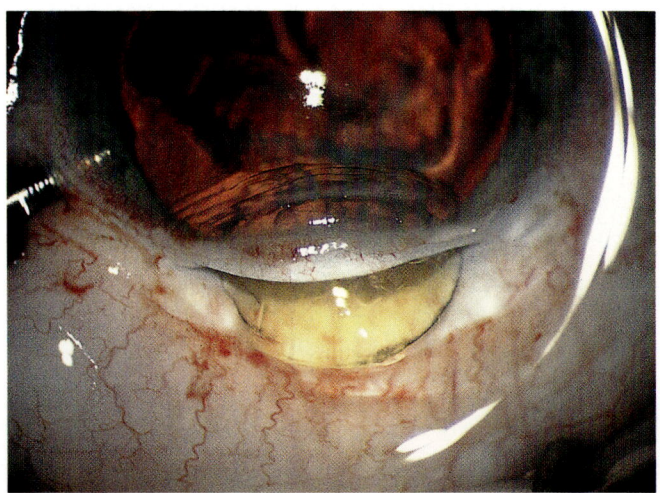

Figure 10.13 *Hydroexpression (hydroextraction) of the nucleus using the closed-system technique.* **(Top)** *The nucleus is pushed forward and the posterior capsule is pushed backward. The position of the capsular bag is stable and the zonules are exposed to minimal stress.* **(Bottom)** *The pressure difference at the limbal opening directs the nucleus out of the eye.*

An additional refinement of this ECCE technique, one that reduces the hard core nucleus into smaller segments by fracturing, can be considered, but technical ability and surgical risk become significant factors. After aspiration of the anterior layers of the cortex and epinucleus, a relatively soft core nucleus can be cut into two or more pieces with either the cystotome or a special cutter (Fig. 10.14). The small nuclear parts are usually too small to adequately occlude the limbal incision, thus hydroexpression is difficult and sometimes impossible. The fractured pieces are best removed by simultaneously filling the anterior chamber with viscoelastic and activating the ACM. The viscoelastic material and the nucleus particles are pushed, in one unit, out of the eye (Fig. 10.15).

Removal of the Epinucleus

The epinucleus, being semisoft, may keep its integrity after the hard core nucleus has been extracted. By maintaining lamellar coherency, its fibers enable the whole epinucleus to be isolated as one unit when hydrodissection occurs between the epinucleus and the cortex. This creates a second junctional demarcation line that facilitates epinucleus hydrodissection using the hydrodynamic properties of the ACM. The relatively soft epinucleus can be squeezed through a small limbal opening and removed in one piece (Fig. 10.16). Isolation of the epinucleus can be assisted by mechanical manipulations using a spatula or a cannula. When hydroextraction of the epinucleus is difficult, it can be aspirated with the 0.40-mm

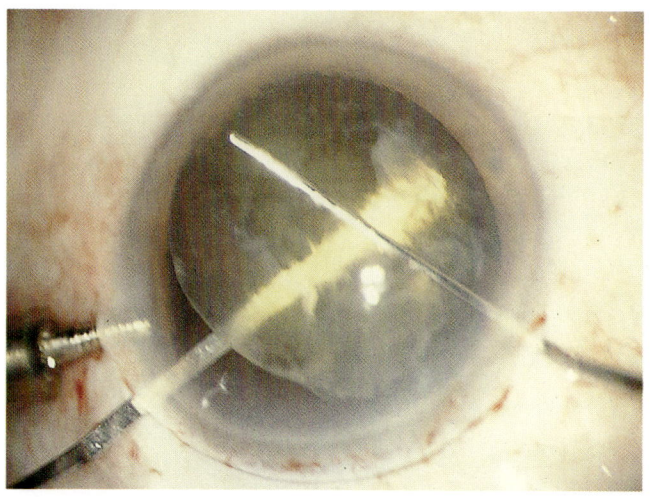

Figure 10.14 *(Left) Fracturing the hard nucleus into smaller pieces. The nucleotome is inserted from the right and located above the nucleus. A spatula is inserted from the left and supports the posterior surface of the nucleus.*

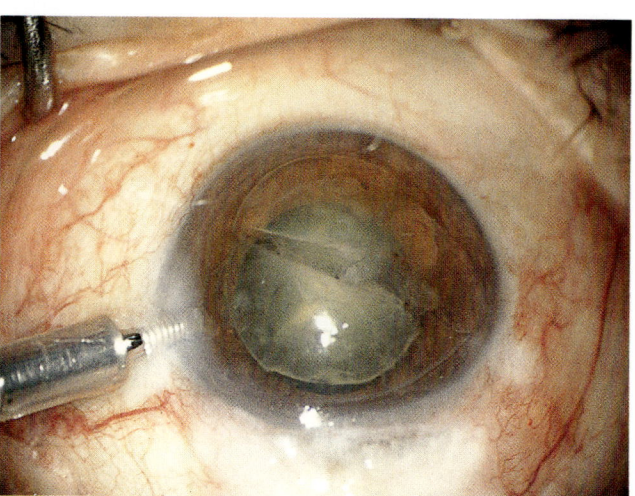

(Right) The nucleus is fractured into two pieces. The diameter of each is half the diameter of the hard core nucleus (3.00 mm to 3.50 mm).

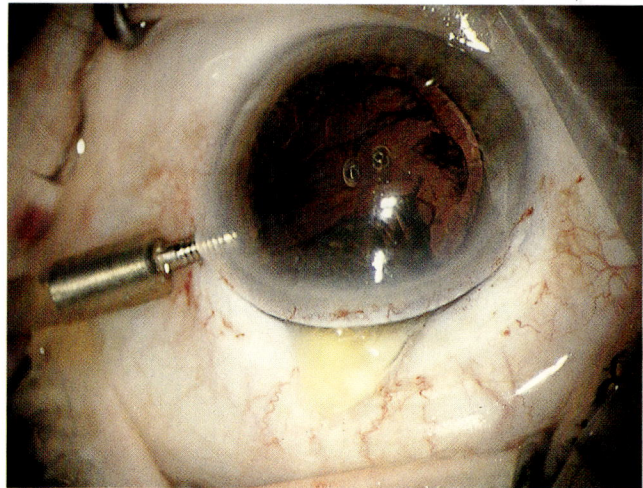

Figure 10.15 *Viscoelastic, including the fractured lens, is pushed out of the eye in one unit.*

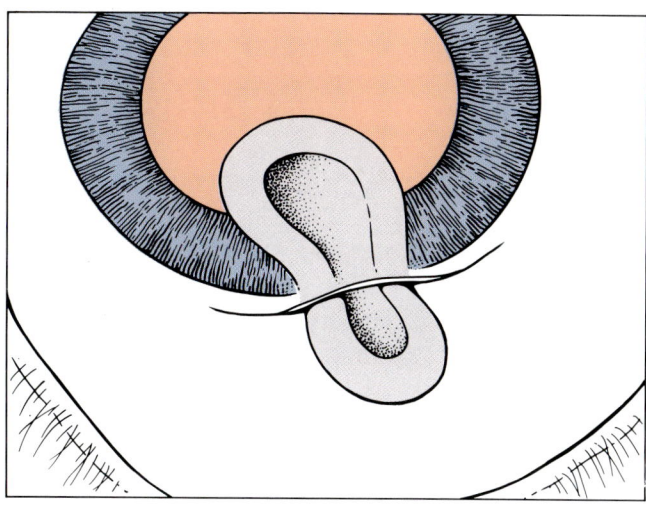

Figure 10.16 *The relatively soft epinucleus can be squeezed through a small limbal opening and removed in one piece.*

pore cannula, even though aspiration is somewhat more difficult than aspiration of the cortical material.

Removal of Cortical Material and Implantation of Intraocular Lens

After the central nucleus and epinucleus have been extracted from the eye, the remaining surgical steps are essentially the same as those of a phaco procedure after phacoemulsification of the nucleus. The remaining cortical lens material is aspirated from the eye by either a hand-held syringe or a mechanical irrigation/aspiration (I/A) unit. An IOL lens is implanted in the bag after injecting viscoelastic into the anterior chamber (Fig. 10.17).

An IOL with a haptic diameter of 12.50 mm is preferred. This haptic measurement allows for in-the-bag implantation without undue stress on the capsular bag and zonules and will provide stability, even if one haptic should inadvertently be placed in the ciliary sulcus. The wound is closed using 10-0 nylon suture (Fig. 10.18), and the viscoelastic removed by aspiration.

Conclusion

ECCE by expression of the central nucleus and epinucleus separately is the most sophisticated method of manual cataract expression. This method allows for the smallest possible wound with a manual ECCE technique, and the anterior chamber maintainer creates the safest conditions possible for cataract removal. Due to its effectiveness, simplicity, and cost, manual ECCE is by far the most commonly used method of cataract removal worldwide.

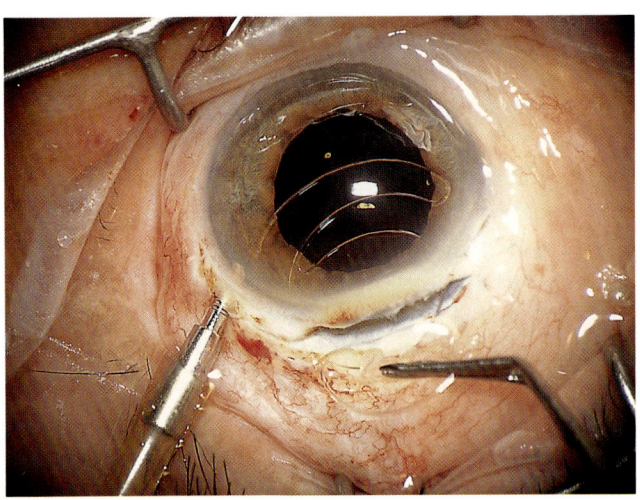

Figure 10.17 *Viscoelastic is injected into the anterior chamber and the IOL is inserted.*

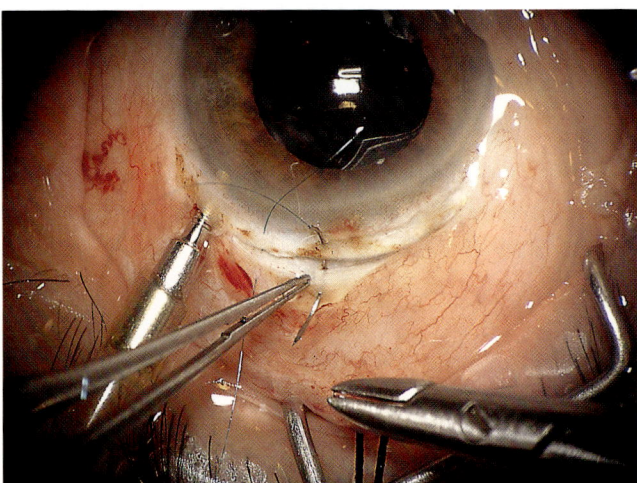

Figure 10.18 *The wound is closed with 10-0 nylon.*

Clinical Points to Consider

☞ An improved ECCE technique should minimize manipulation of the anterior segment.

☞ Maintaining constant pressure of the globe during ECCE has significant advantages.

☞ The choice of wound length for ECCE represents a compromise between expressing the nucleus safely and inducing minimal astigmatism.

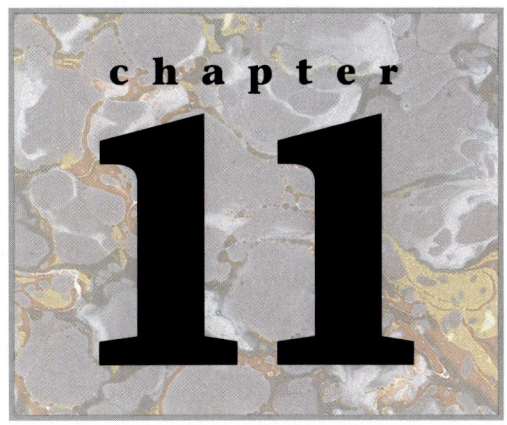

THE MECHANICS OF PHACOEMULSIFICATION

R. BRUCE WALLACE, M.D.   LEE T. NORDAN, M.D.
DONALD FAGEN   B.J. BARWICK

Phacoemulsification in the 1990s is more sophisticated than the phacoemulsification introduced by Charles Kelman, M.D., in the 1970s. Many static functions of the earlier phaco* machines can now be adjusted according to the surgeon's preference (Fig. 11.1). Aspiration vacuum limit, aspiration flow rate, linear control, peristaltic pump, and vacuum pump are examples of phaco machine functions that should be familiar to the surgeon. The modern phaco machine has very specialized technical capabilities that have been created by evolving phaco techniques. These capabilities increase patient benefits but also demand greater surgical skill.

Equipment failure, which is usually related to human error during preoperative setup, can affect the peace of mind and operative performance of even the most seasoned cataract surgeon. Therefore, to perform the best surgery possible under varying conditions, and be able to troubleshoot problems that may arise, the conscientious surgeon should know the principles as well as the mechanical aspects of the phacoemulsification procedure. Now, as before, the surgeon's ability to relate the functions of the phaco machine to intraoperative surgical events vastly improves the chances of a favorable surgical outcome.

This chapter will focus on the mechanics of phacoemulsification and how it can be modified for more efficient, precise surgery. Major topics to be discussed include aspiration and irrigation fluidics, pump styles, and ultrasonic power. The goal of this discussion is to enhance the surgical proficiency of the surgeon through greater understanding of the subjects covered. At the end of the chapter, the various concepts presented will be incorporated into a discussion about the phaco machine and the different factors that influence phacoemulsification surgery.

*The word "phaco" will often be used as an abbreviation for the word "phacoemulsification."

Fluidics

The main factors determining proper hydrodynamics are irrigation, aspiration, and wound size. The goal of proper hydrodynamics during phacoemulsification is to maintain anterior segment anatomy during the exchange of fluid and lens material. The stability of the anatomy helps to reduce trauma to intraocular structures. Stability and the constant pressure of the globe imply that the irrigation and supply of fluid into the anterior chamber will be equal to the aspiration and loss of fluid from the eye (Fig. 11.2).

Irrigation

In most phaco machines, irrigation during phacoemulsification is provided by gravity feed through the space between the titanium phaco tip and the sleeve (Fig. 11.3). The amount of irrigation is determined by the bottle height relative to the patient's eye, by the sleeve diameter, and, most importantly, by the loss of fluid from the eye because the gravity system is passive and can

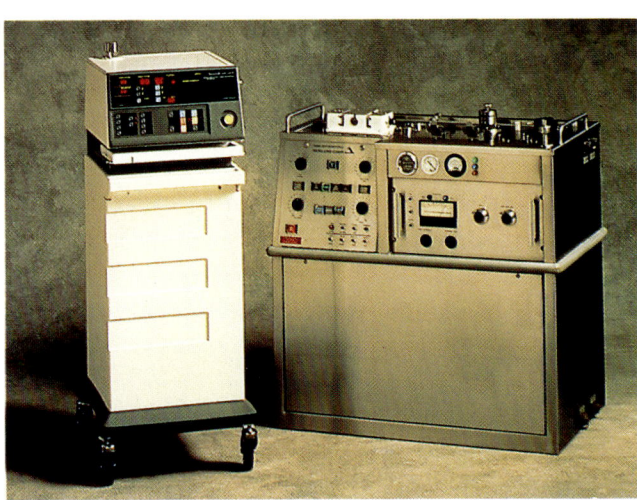

Figure 11.1 *The bulky Kelman phacoemulsification machine of the 1970s, manufactured by Cavitron, and the Series 10,000-Master, 1989, produced by Alcon Laboratories (formerly Cooper Vision).*

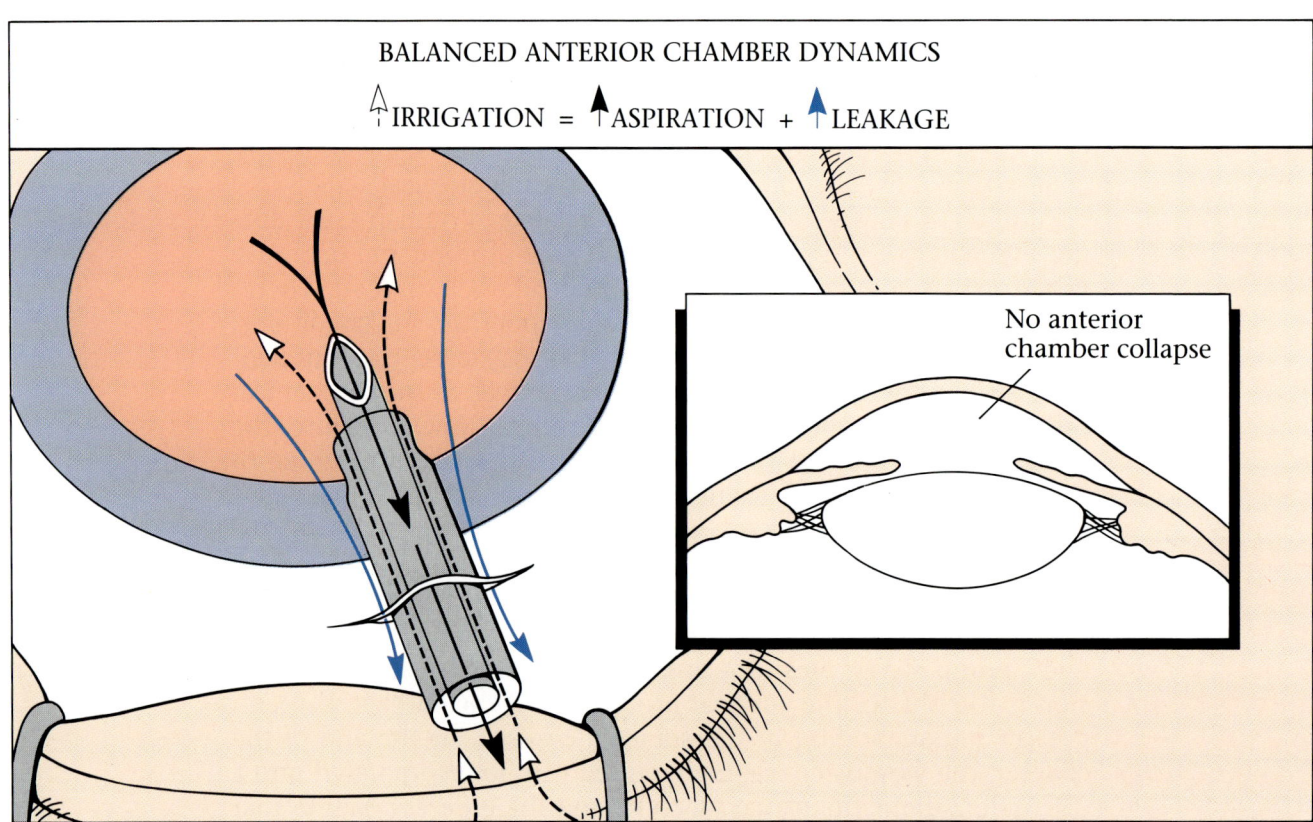

Figure 11.2 (Above) *Balanced irrigation, aspiration of fluid, and wound leakage prevent anterior chamber collapse and breaking of the posterior capsule with the phaco tip. In this example, the flow into the anterior chamber is matched by the flow out due to aspiration and leakage of fluid, resulting in a stable anterior chamber.*

provide fluid only after the anterior chamber pressure has been reduced. A tight wound can limit irrigation if the space between the flexible sleeve and the phaco tip is compromised when manipulating the handpiece (see Fig. 11.2). This problem is not present with a rigid sleeve, although such a sleeve is not generally used because contact with the rapidly vibrating phaco tip can cause serious overheating problems and tip damage if the sleeve is metallic. Excessive leakage between the rigid sleeve and the wound can also occur. Most phaco surgeons use a shelved incision to reduce iris prolapse and create an efficient wound, although some fluid will, and should, always leak through the wound. Entering the anterior chamber with an appropriate size keratome, i.e., 3.00 mm to 3.20 mm, facilitates proper irrigation.

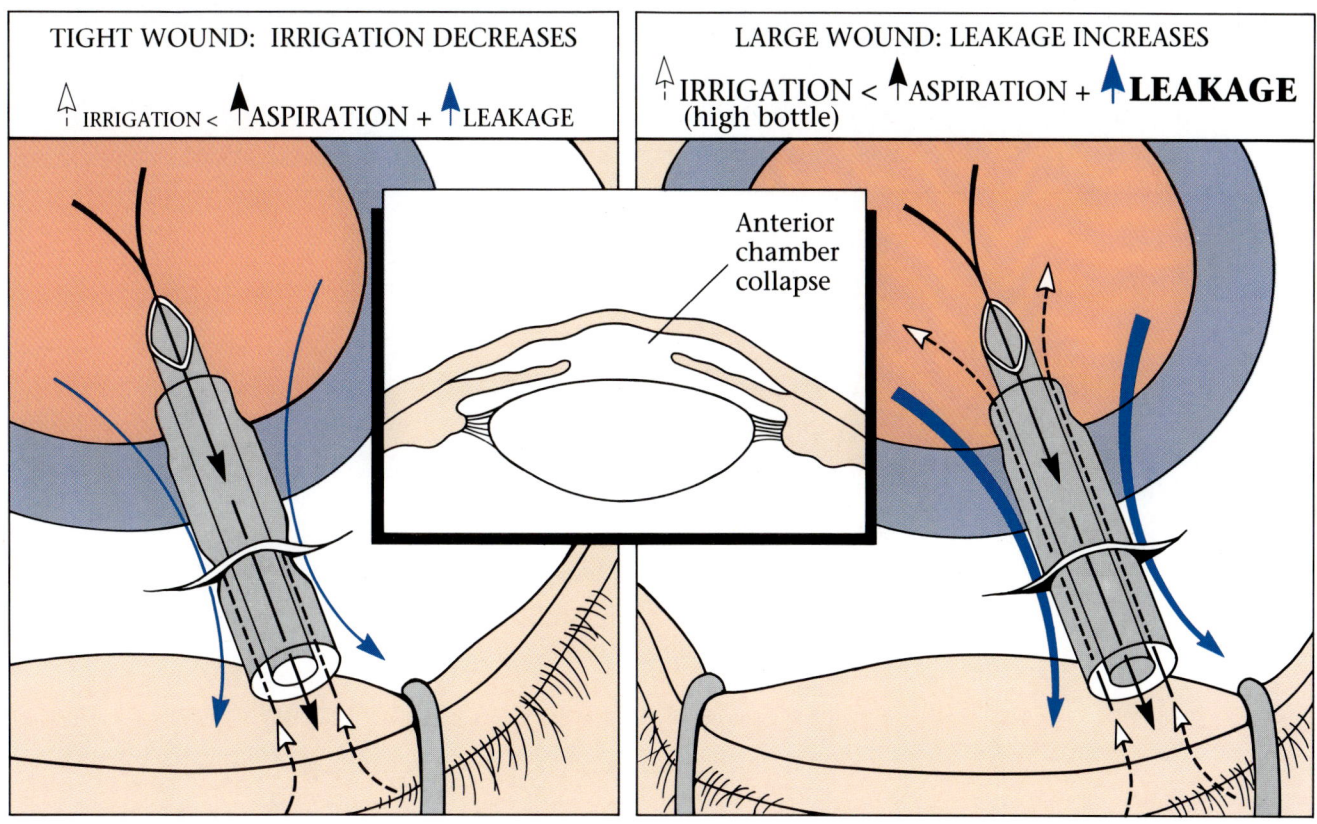

(Figure 11.2 cont.) (Left) *During aspiration the anterior chamber collapses sporadically. This occurs because the wound is too tight and the irrigation inflow is compromised when the irrigation sleeve is narrowed against the side of the wound.* **(Right)** *The anterior chamber is collapsing continually because the wound is too large, causing an inappropriate amount of fluid to leak from the anterior chamber.*

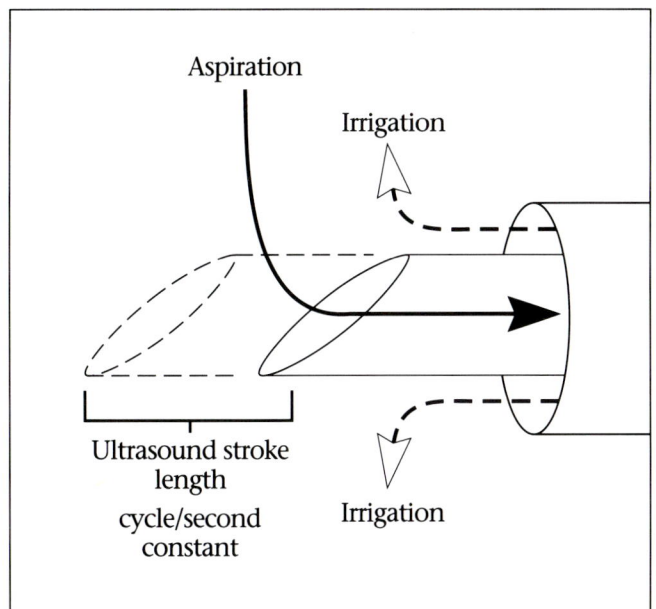

Figure 11.3 *Phaco tip and irrigation sleeve construction provide for aspiration through the center of the titanium phaco tip and irrigation along its outer surface. The ultrasound power available to emulsify a cataract is provided by the titanium phaco tip, which vibrates at a constant frequency. A change in power is achieved by varying the longitudinal stroke length of the tip.*

SURGICAL REHABILITATION OF VISION

The irrigation bottle during phaco is usually placed between 65 cm to 75 cm above the eye. The eye should be at the same level above the floor as the pump (cassette) of the phaco machine. Merely raising the bottle will not cure the problem of anterior chamber collapse caused by an excessively large wound, since irrigation and leakage are increased concomitantly by the increased force created by the higher bottle (see Fig. 11.2).

Aspiration

The precise and efficient aspiration of lens and fluid during phaco is a major reason for using the equipment and a major determinant of surgical success. Aspiration is defined as the evacuation of fluid through a closed system. During the last two decades, many of the improvements in cataract extraction by phaco relate to finer control of the aspiration system during phacoemulsification of the nucleus and to cortical clean-up by mechanized irrigation and aspiration (I/A). Two important concepts concerning aspiration are *flow rate* and *vacuum level*.

Flow rate is the quantity of fluid per minute pulled from the eye through the instrument tip and irrigation tubing. Flow rate is measured in cubic centimeters per minute (cc/min) and is dependent on the level of vacuum created in the

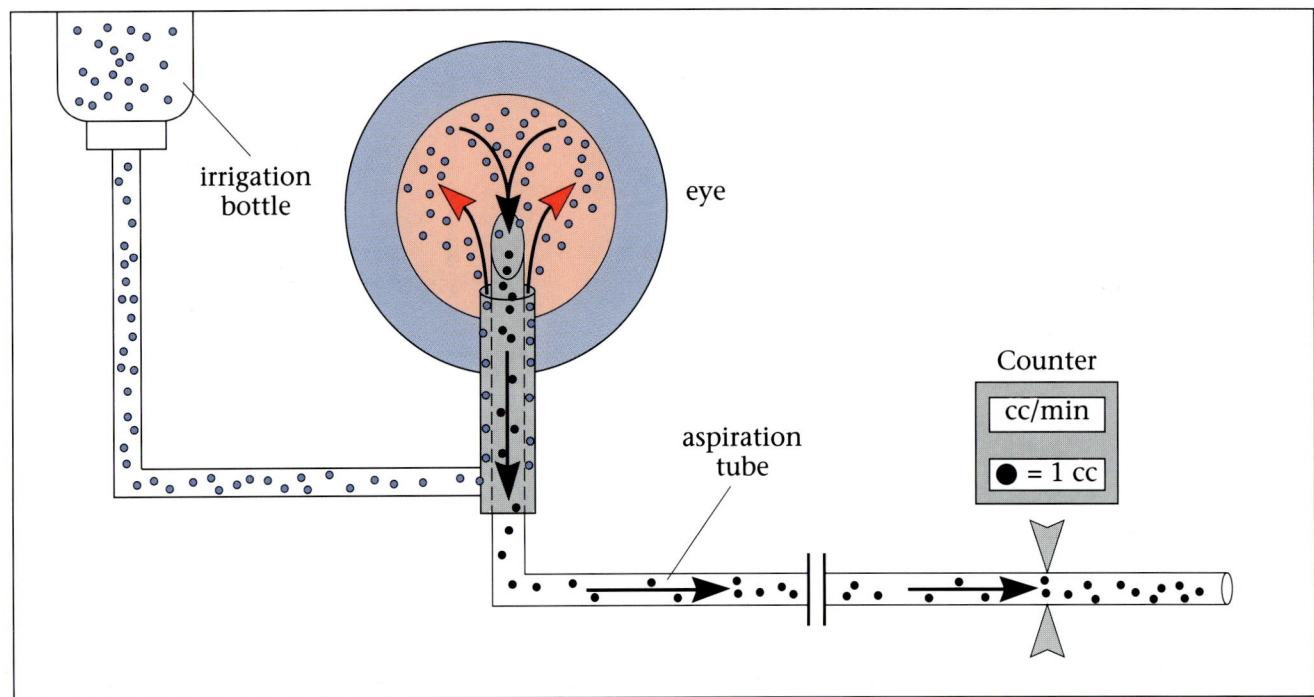

Figure 11.4 *Flow rate is the quantity of fluid removed from the eye per minute and is usually measured in cubic centimeters per minute (cc/min).*

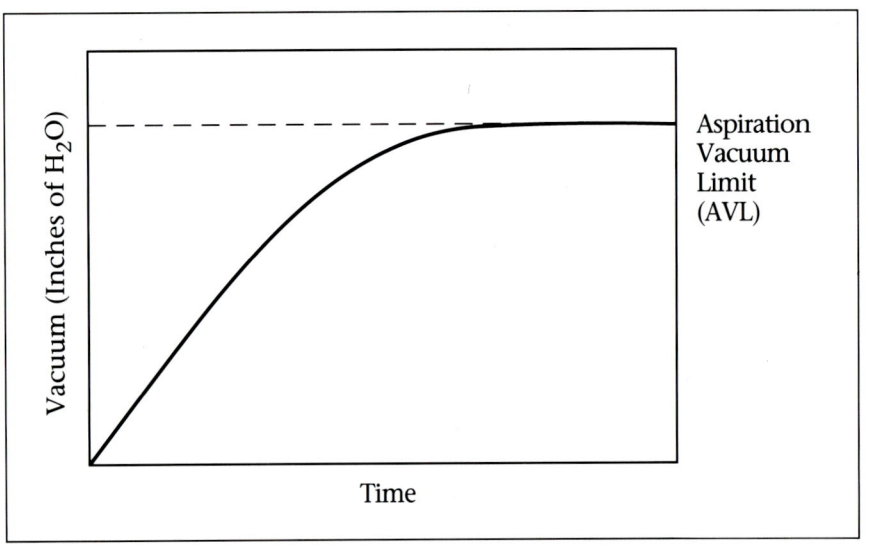

Figure 11.5 *The same level of vacuum is created regardless of whether fluid is removed from a closed vessel quickly or slowly. The flow rate determines how quickly a certain level of vacuum is achieved, but the vacuum level is determined by the efficiency of the vacuum pump and by the pressure created by the external environment (atmosphere).*

aspiration tubing by the aspiration pump as well as the surface area of the port of the irrigation tip (Fig. 11.4). Flow rate determines the *rate of rise* of the aspiration vacuum when the aspiration port is occluded. In other words, the more quickly the fluid is pulled from the aspiration tube, the more quickly the vacuum is created. Remember, the rate of rise of the vacuum is independent of the absolute limit of the vacuum level that can be created (Fig. 11.5).

Vacuum level is the difference in pressure between atmospheric pressure and the pressure inside the aspiration tubing (Fig. 11.6). This difference in pressure is created by the aspiration pump acting on the fluid inside the aspiration tubing and is commonly called *suction*. Vacuum is measured in inches of H_2O or millimeters of mercury (mm Hg), which represent the weight (i.e., the height) a column of fluid rises when a partial vacuum is created in the aspiration line.

Vacuum as well as pressure are actually measures of the total molecular activity inside a closed container. A partial vacuum is created when this activity is less than that of the environment and vice versa for pressure (Fig. 11.7). (A total vacuum is never achieved because there is always some molecular activity.) Both pressure and vacuum are measured in the same units.

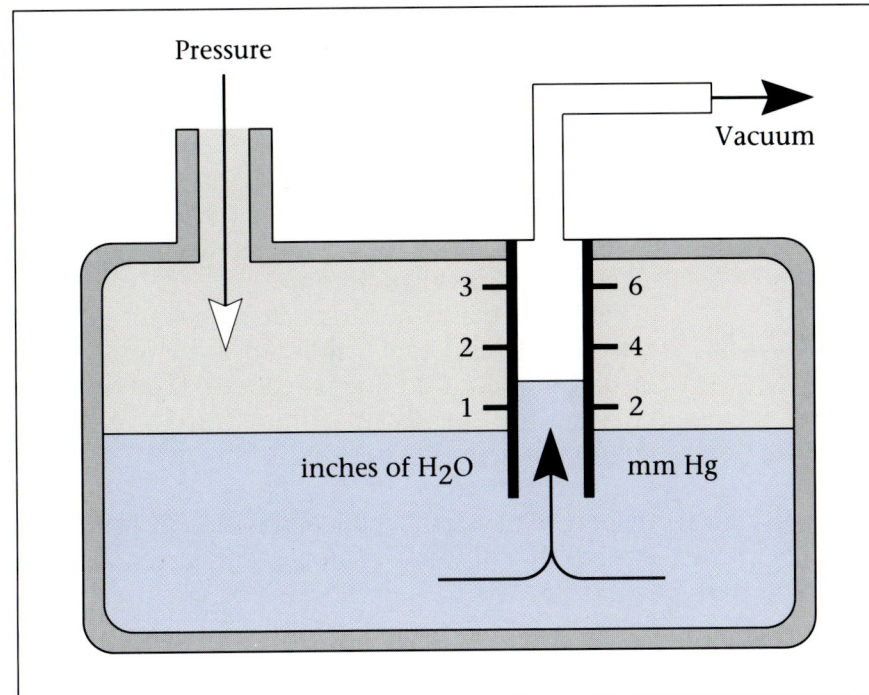

Figure 11.6 *The reduction in pressure inside the aspiration line allows the atmospheric pressure to push a column of fluid into the aspiration line. The height of this column of fluid is the measure of vacuum level achieved.*

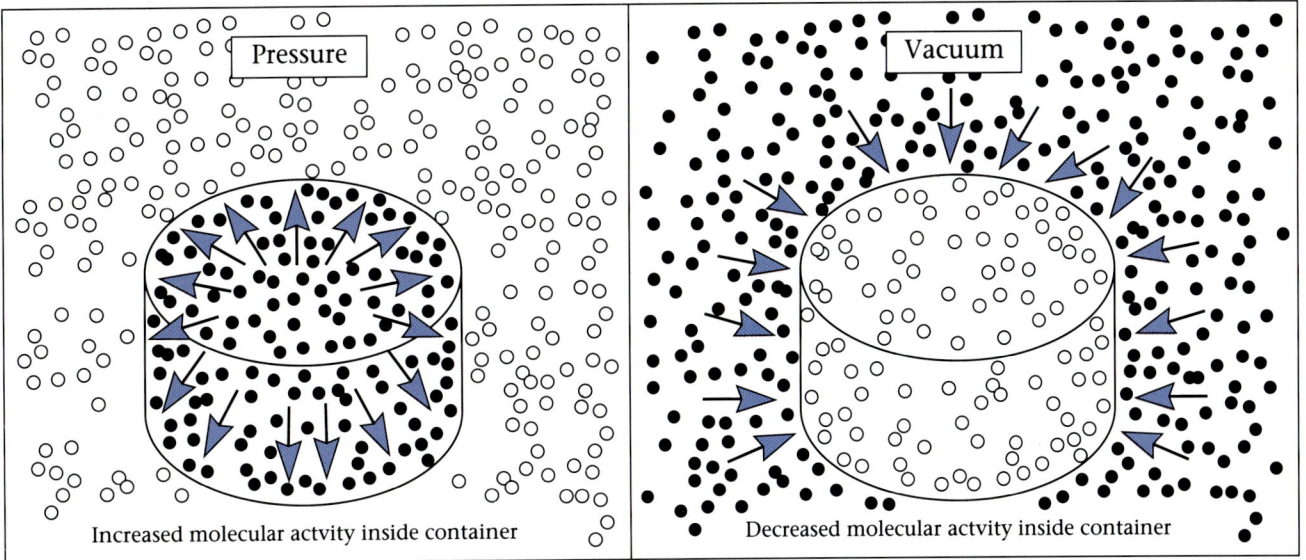

Figure 11.7 *Pressure is created when the sum of the molecular energy in a fluid inside a container is greater per surface area than the sum of the molecular energy of the environment, which pushes in the opposite direction on that same surface area. A partial vacuum is created when the sum of the molecular energy of the fluid per surface area is less than that of the environment.*

Intraocular pressure is measured in mm Hg. This signifies that a column of mercury, up to a given number of millimeters high, could be placed on the cornea (supported by the pressure of the aqueous) without indentation of the cornea. This column of mercury is analogous to the rising column of fluid that is pushed by the atmosphere when a vacuum is created in the aspiration line.

Prolonged occlusion of the aspiration port causes a sharp increase in vacuum level as the fluid is evacuated by the pump. Some phaco machines have a sound system that provides the surgeon with audio feedback that changes as the vacuum level increases or decreases.

In a clinical situation, the degree of occlusion of the aspiration port is constantly changing as lens material creates occlusion and is then aspirated into the tubing, only to have more lens material create occlusion again. A higher vacuum level will be created at an aspiration port with a smaller area than at a port with a larger area (Fig. 11.8). This concept is illustrated by the following equation:

$$\text{Port Vacuum (mm Hg/mm}^2\text{)} = \frac{\text{Vacuum Created (mm Hg)}}{\text{Port Area (mm}^2\text{)}}$$

The vacuum level created at the port varies inversely to the area (or diameter) of the port. Therefore, it should not be surprising to find that the standard vacuum level obtained with the 1.00-mm diameter port of the phaco tip is in the range of 45 mm Hg to 50 mm Hg and the standard vacuum level obtained with the 0.30 mm diameter port of the I/A tip is in the range of 450 mm Hg. The surface area of the phaco tip port, 0.80 mm^2, is about ten times that of the I/A tip port, 0.07 mm^2. The vacuum level's highest limit is determined by the efficiency of the aspiration pump and the surrounding atmospheric pressure.

The phaco unit is capable of producing vacuum levels outside the recommended ranges for use with certain handpieces and tip combinations. Therefore, a safety mechanism is built into the instrument to limit the vacuum to a predetermined maximum level. When the phaco tip is introduced into the eye and engages nuclear or cortical material, the tip lumen is occluded and a build-up of vacuum begins to take place in the handpiece and in the tubing between the tip and the pump. The strength of vacuum continues to increase until a limit is reached. Even though the peristaltic pump continues to run and create a much greater vacuum, the control system automatically limits the vacuum to the level selected by bleeding air or fluid into the aspiration line. This process is called *venting*.

Venting fluid rather than air allows for a faster rise time to full vacuum because the amount of air in the aspiration line is reduced; thus the phaco machine spends less time stretching an air column and applies the energy directly to achieving vacuum (Fig. 11.9). The result is a more responsive system, reduced chance of mini-collapse of the anterior chamber, and faster vacuum rise time.

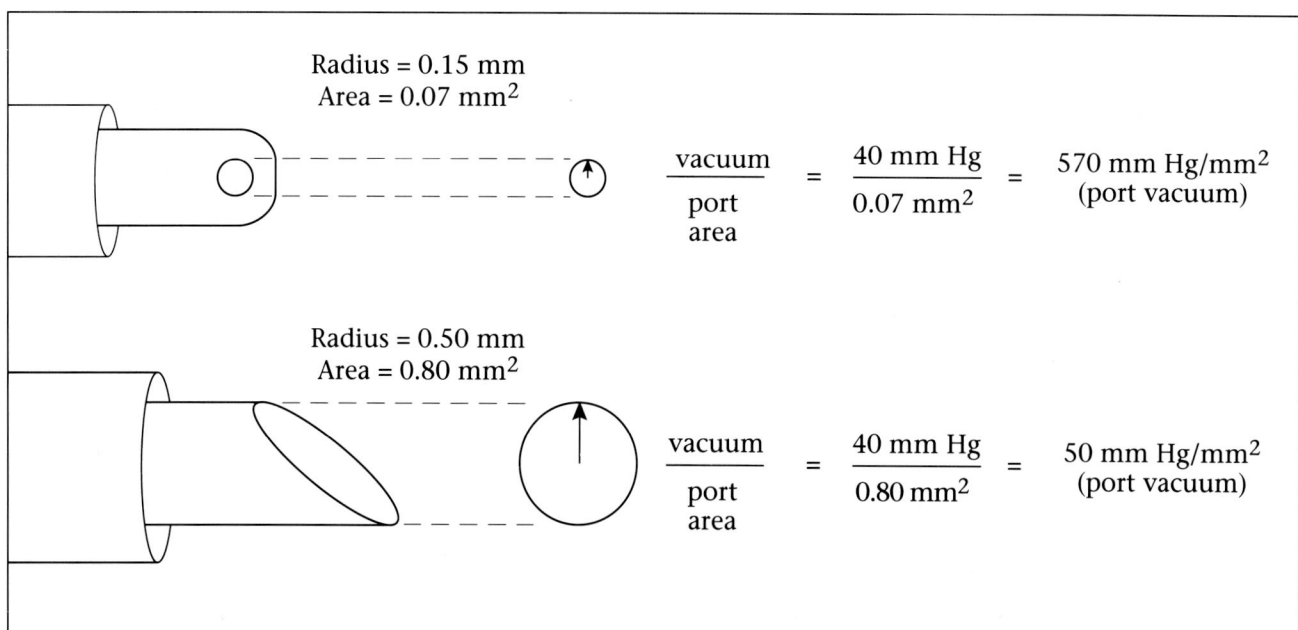

Figure 11.8 *A smaller diameter aspiration port provides higher aspiration vacuum per square millimeter than a larger diameter port using the same aspiration vacuum. Of course, the aspiration tip port size must remain large enough to accept cortical material. (The most commonly used aspiration tip for automated cortical clean up during cataract extraction is one with a 0.30 mm diameter port.)*

Pumps

Aspiration capability in current phaco equipment is provided by either a peristaltic or a vacuum pump. The performance characteristics of each will be described.

Peristaltic

A peristaltic pump creates aspiration by advancing fluid through a tube that is wound tightly around a "humped" rotating wheel (Fig. 11.10). The shape and speed of the wheel as well as the diameter of the tubing determine the volume of fluid moved per unit of time. Therefore, a peri-

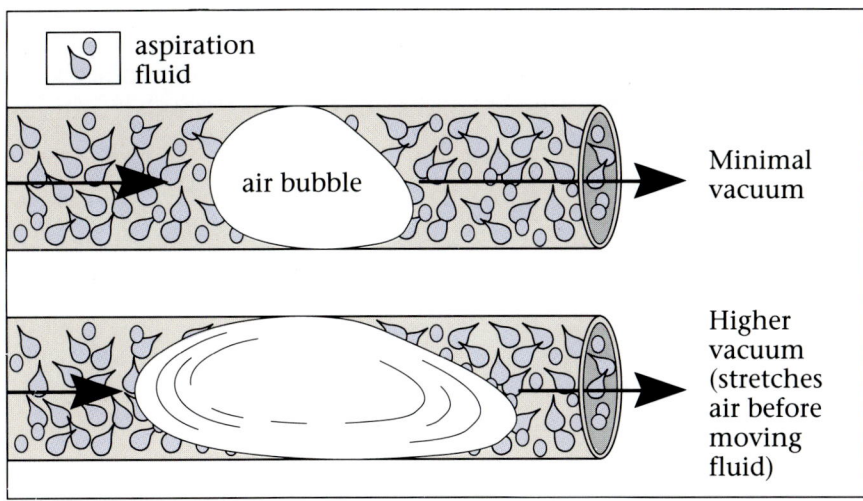

Figure 11.9 *Controlling aspiration vacuum levels by venting fluid rather than air into the aspiration line reduces minicollapse of the anterior chamber and allows for shorter vacuum rise times.*

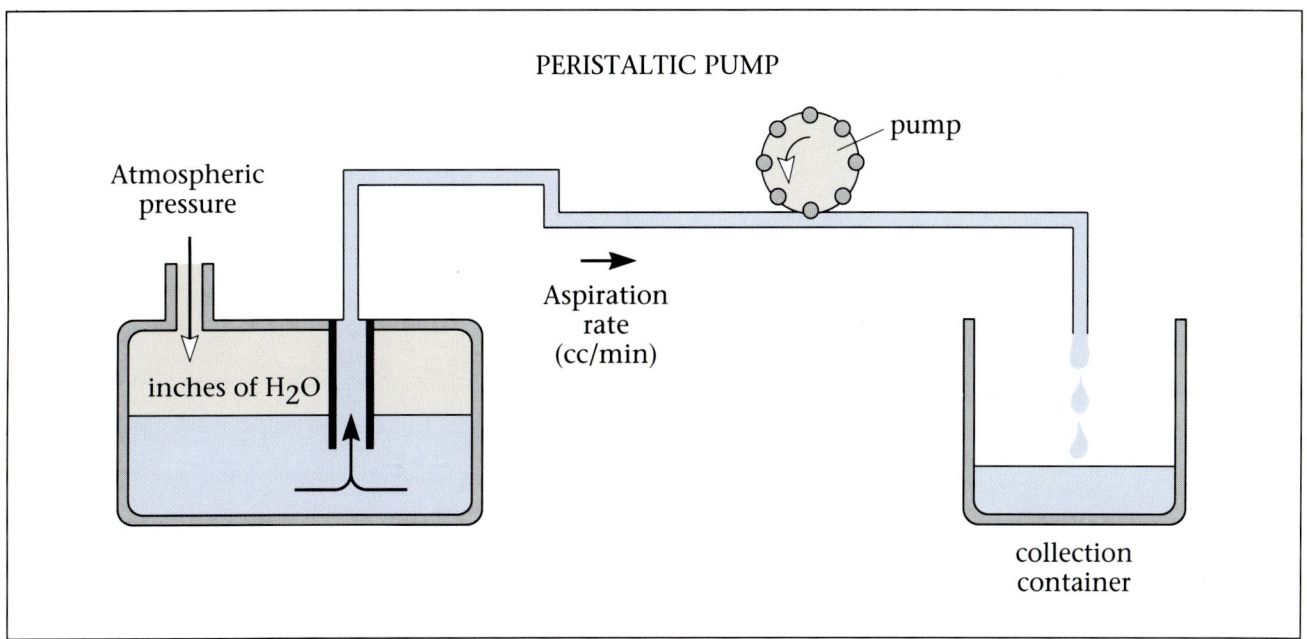

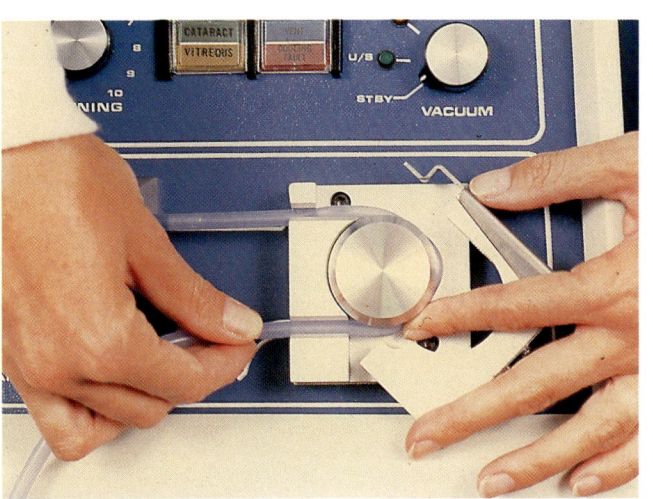

Figure 11.10 (Above) *The mechanics of aspiration created by a peristaltic pump in a phaco machine.* **(Left)** *Aspiration tubing being loaded around the rotation wheel of a peristaltic pump of a Cooper Vision 8000 phaco machine. Some phaco machines accept a cassette to which the irrigation and aspiration lines are permanently attached. This cassette is easily loaded into the phaco machine, much like loading a tape into a VCR, and engages the irrigation and aspiration lines automatically.*

staltic pump is a form of volumetric pump. With a peristaltic pump, flow rate depends on pump speed when the tip is not occluded. Aspiration vacuum builds when the tip is partially or totally occluded, and, once again, the rate of rise of the vacuum depends on the pump speed.

A good analogy for the function of a peristaltic pump would relate to the winding of a garden hose around a handle-operated spool. When the hose is free, the speed at which the hose wraps around the spool (flow rate) is determined by the handle's speed of rotation. If someone holds the hose at its free end (occlusion), a new resistance force (vacuum) gradually develops, increasing as the handle is rotated and the hose is stretched further. The speed of the hose winding around the spool decreases if the resistance affects the speed of the handle (pump). Once this resistance is released (loss of occlusion), the speed of the hose (flow rate) once again returns to normal (Fig. 11.11).

The vacuum level limit and the flow rate (vacuum rate of rise) can be adjusted independently on newer phaco machines with peristaltic pumps.

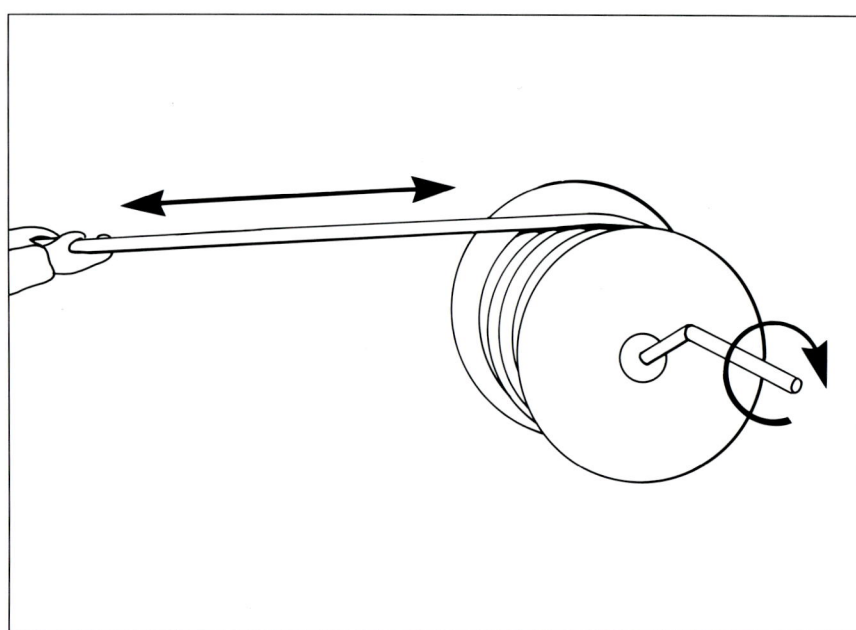

Figure 11.11 *Winding a garden hose around a spool illustrates well how a peristaltic aspiration pump functions.*

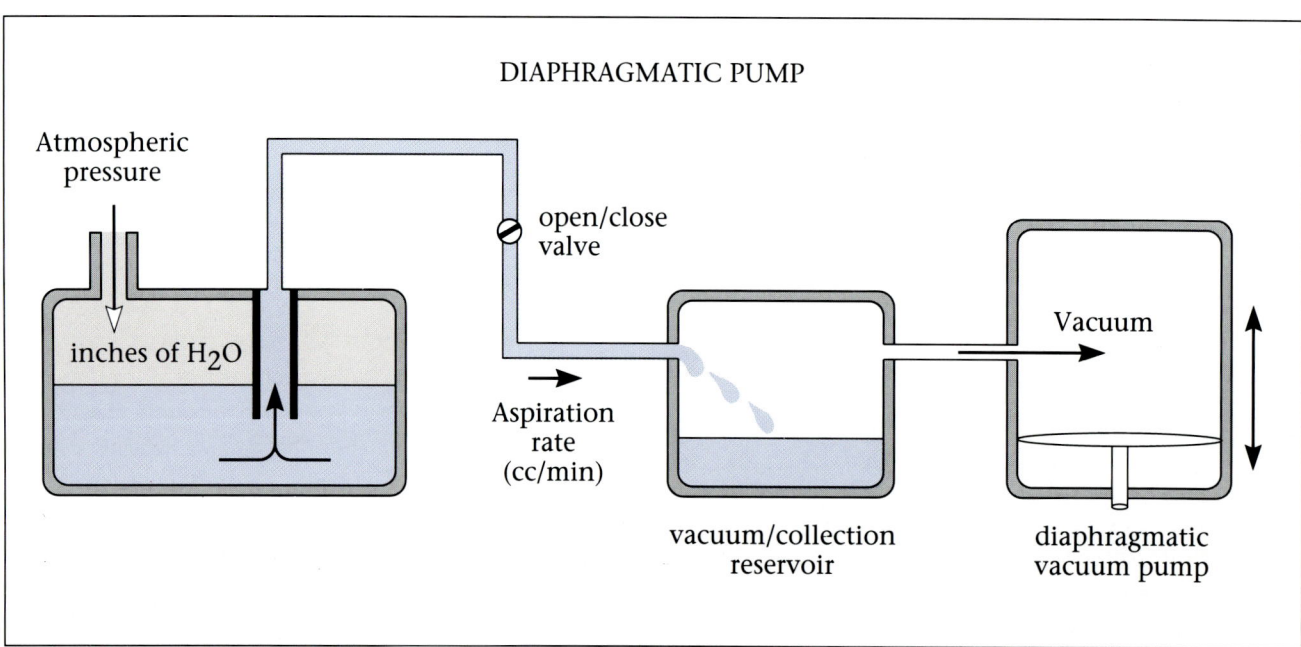

Figure 11.12 *The functional details of a diaphragmatic aspiration pump.*

The vacuum level can be adjusted by setting the transducer to allow for venting at a certain limit. The flow rate is determined by setting a limit to the rotation speed of the peristaltic pump. Also, if the surgeon desires, both the vacuum limit and the flow rate can be varied by *linear control*, which is the instantaneous change of each parameter by depression of the foot pedal.

However, linear control applies to either vacuum limit or to flow rate, not both at the same time. In other words, vacuum level limit can be kept constant while the flow rate is modulated with linear control, or the flow rate can be kept constant while the vacuum level is modulated with linear control. These combinations can greatly affect surgical capability and will be discussed later in the chapter.

Vacuum

The evacuation of air from a closed container by a vacuum pump can be used to form a vacuum reservoir. This vacuum reservoir creates a flow in the aspiration tubing that is similar to the flow of fluid being sucked through a straw. The two styles of vacuum pumps are *diaphragmatic* or *Venturi*.

A diaphragmatic pump uses a moveable diaphragm to force air through a one-way valve, thus creating a partial vacuum inside a closed container (Fig. 11.12). The vacuum level varies indirectly with the volume of the reservoir, directly with the efficiency of the diaphragm pump (i.e., leaks), and directly with the ambient atmospheric pressure.

A Venturi pump uses a flow of gas, rather than a diaphragm, to create the partial vacuum inside the reservoir (Fig. 11.13). Since flowing gas exerts less pressure perpendicular to its path of movement than parallel to its path of movement (Bernoulli's Law), air can be evacuated from a container by exposing it perpendicularly to this flow. The velocity of the flowing gas is increased tremendously by the Venturi effect, which states that gas flowing under constant pressure increases its velocity when the aperture narrows. The greater the velocity of the flowing gas, the greater the vacuum level obtained inside the container.

The volume of the vacuum reservoir in either a diaphragmatic or a Venturi phaco pump must be small enough to create a useable vacuum but large enough to accommodate the fluid aspirated from the eye during the procedure without necessitating a container change. Experience has shown this volume to be about 250 cc to 500 cc. The flow rate is directly linked to the vacuum level. In a vacuum pump system, there is no true linear control of the vacuum because vacuum is always present in the reservoir.

Vacuum pumps have a continuous source of suction available in the reservoir, which is capable of creating flow in the tubing whenever the controlling valve is activated. Peristaltic pumps, on the other hand, create flow only when the pump wheel rotates. Both systems require at least partial tip occlusion for aspiration vacuum to develop inside the handpiece and the adjacent tubing.

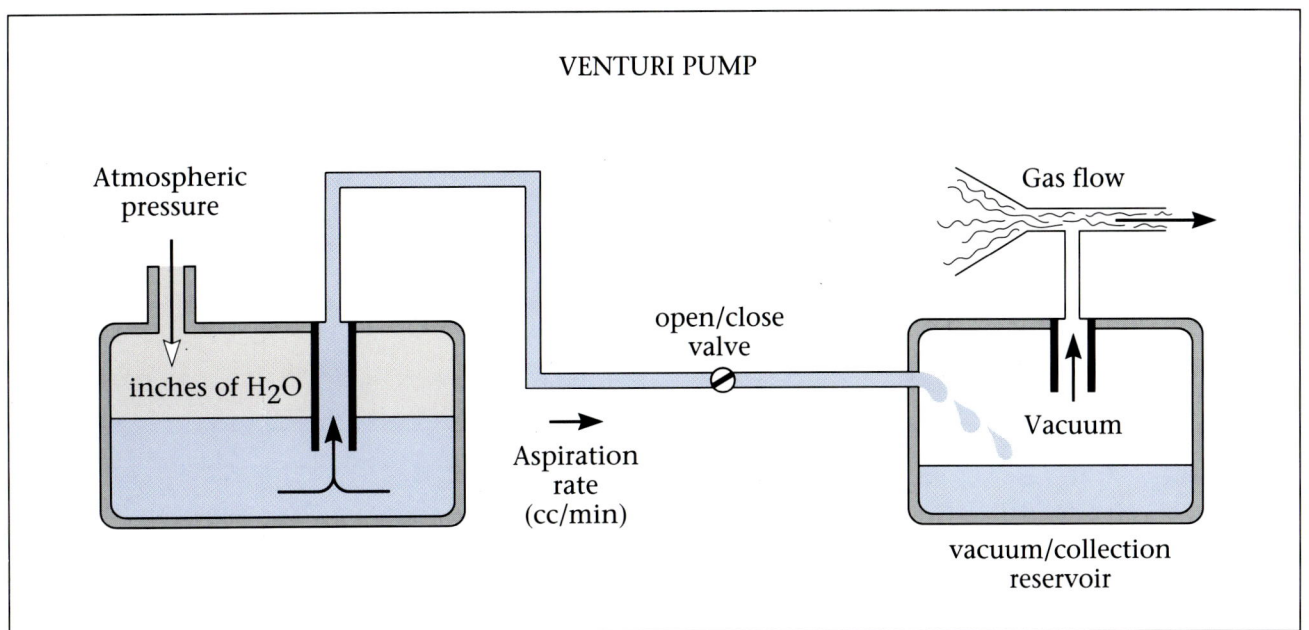

Figure 11.13 *The functional details of a Venturi aspiration pump.*

These pump characteristics, combined with other factors, such as phaco tip design, can greatly influence surgical performance. The next portion of this chapter will discuss handpiece function, phaco power, foot pedal function, and phaco tip design and their clinical application.

Ultrasonic Handpiece

The phaco handpiece when attached to the phaco tip, imparts energy to the tip, causing it to stroke (vibrate). This energy and motion are transmitted to the nucleus of the cataract, which is then emulsified (liquefied) and removed from the eye by aspiration through the center of the tip or by a separate aspiration device. Modern phaco handpieces are light and small enough for the surgeon's comfort and they are autoclavable so that they can now be sterilized between cases. It is also important that the surgeon have a simple procedure for attaching the tip and irrigation sleeve to the handpiece.

The titanium phaco tip vibrates by varying its dimensions in the longitudinal direction, not side-to-side. Current phaco machines use vibration frequencies in the range of 28,000 to 60,000 cycles per second (28 to 60 hertz). Two methods have been used to create this vibration—*magnetostrictive* and *piezoelectric*.

Magnetostrictive refers to a series of soft metallic wafers that are bound together in such a way that they cause vibration of the tip when they are deformed by the electrical energy supplied by the console (Fig. 11.14).

Piezoelectric refers to the presence of a highly refined crystal that vibrates at a given frequency when excited by electrical energy. Virtually all modern phaco handpieces are piezoelectric because of their simplicity, efficiency, and light weight (Fig. 11.15). Current piezoelectric hand-

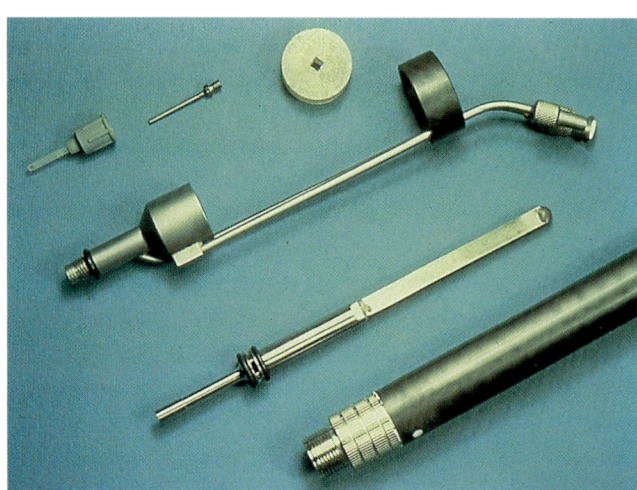

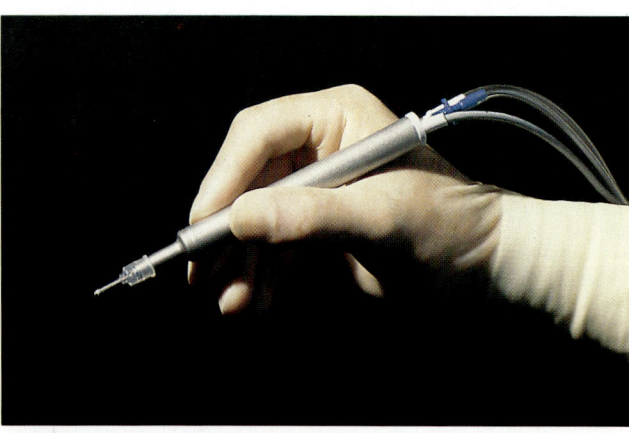

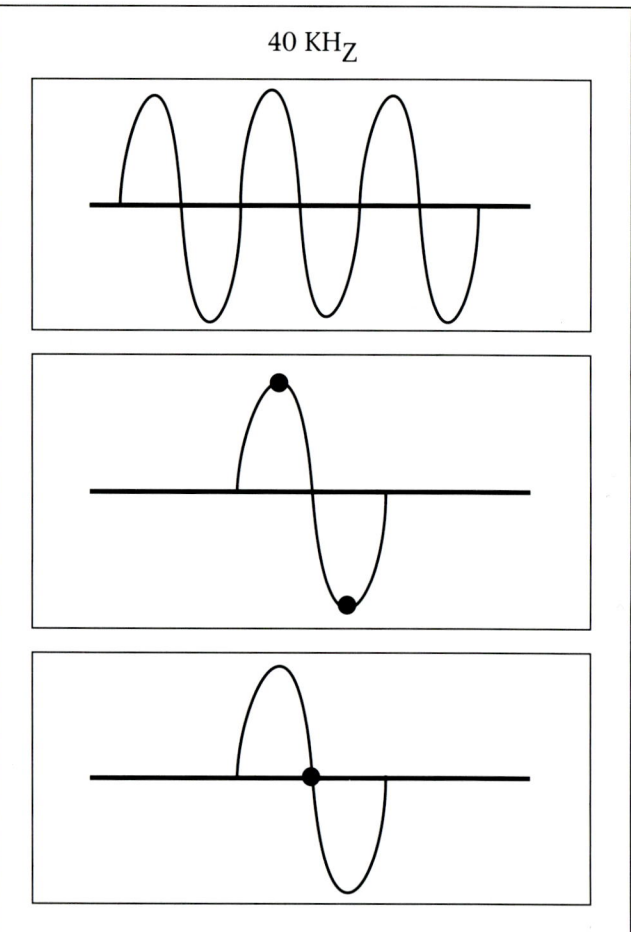

Figure 11.14 (Upper Left) *The components of a Cooper Vision magnetostrictive ultrasound phaco handpiece.* **(Lower Left)** *A modern slim Alcon Laboratory (fomerly Cooper Vision) piezoelectric ultrasound phaco handpiece held in the surgical position.* **(Right)** *(Top) The energy output delivered by a phaco tip has a sinosoidal distribution, although clinically the energy seems constant. (Middle) Energy production depends on movement of the phaco tip; maximal energy is produced when the tip achieves greatest velocity. (Lower) No energy is produced when the phaco tip is not moving while reversing direction at the end of a stroke.*

pieces, however, may need replacing after six to twelve months of constant use and autoclaving.

Phaco Power

Phaco *power* is an important concept because it relates directly to surgical performance. Power is defined as work per unit of time, and may be expressed algebraically:

$$\text{Work} = \text{Force} \times \text{Distance}$$
$$\text{Power} = \frac{\text{Work}}{\text{Time}}$$

Therefore,

$$\text{Power} = \frac{\text{Force} \times \text{Distance}}{\text{Time}}$$

Since the frequency of vibration (force) remains constant, more power can be generated by increasing the stroke length (distance) of the tip (see Fig. 11.3). This increase in power is correlated to the movement of the foot pedal, giving the surgeon linear control of phaco power in either a continuous or pulse mode.

There is a difference, however, between setting the ultrasound power limit at 70% and achieving 70% ultrasound with the limit set at 100%. The foot pedal excursion will encompass the total range of ultrasound power chosen, but the surgeon's ability to regulate the power will be different. Thus, a phaco machine that has a 70% ultrasound limit allows the surgeon greater control because even though the pedal moves the same distance as it would on a machine with a 100% ultrasound limit, smaller increments in phaco power can be achieved (Fig. 11.15).

Foot Pedal Function

The surgeon's ability to satisfactorily use the sophisticated functions of a phaco machine depend on the foot pedal (Fig. 11.16). The foot pedal is the intermediary between the surgeon's desires and the phaco machine's actions. The foot pedal creates the "rhythm" of the procedure by establishing the lag time between the surgeon's foot and the events in the anterior chamber. The pedal's ergonomic design, the excursion distance, and the "feel" of the stops between various phaco machine functions are important aspects of the foot pedal because they affect the surgeon's performance.

The foot pedal has four positions (including *foot-position 0* or standby) that are attained progressively as the foot pedal is depressed from the

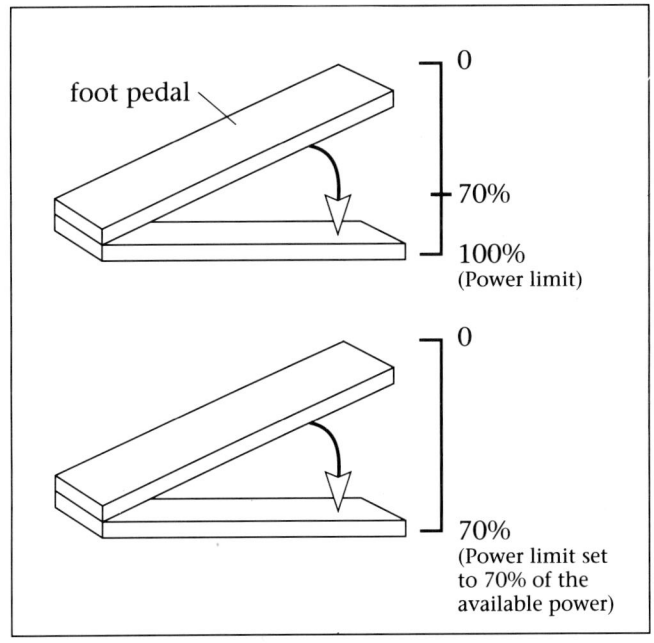

Figure 11.15 *A foot pedal that produces 70% phaco power at full excursion affords the surgeon more control than a foot pedal with 100% power at full excursion but depressed to the 70% power level.*

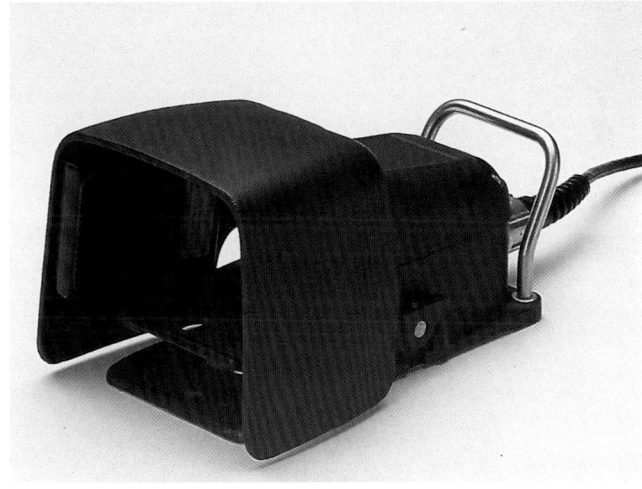

Figure 11.16 *A phaco foot pedal.*

initial position (Table 11.17). Depressing the pedal to *foot-position 1* from *foot-position 0* starts irrigation by activating a solenoid switch that opens a pinch valve around the irrigation line. The rate of irrigation is determined by gravity and the loss of fluid from the anterior segment. The surgeon should remember that *foot-position 1* can function as a "safe haven" during a surgical case because the irrigation mode allows for a formed anterior chamber without ongoing aspiration or phacoemulsification. In *foot-position 1* the surgeon can suspend the action of a procedure and plan the next move.

With most modern phaco machines, under certain conditions, aspiration flow rate (rate of rise), aspiration vacuum level, and/or phacoemulsification power may be controlled in either an "all or none" manner (panel mode) or in a linear manner (surgeon control). An ascending audio tone may be available to indicate a rising aspiration vacuum level. Regardless, the increase in phaco power is easily noticed by the increasing buzz and action of the phaco tip.

Phacoemulsification Tip Design

Presently all phaco tips are made of titanium and most are approximately 0.90 mm in diameter. The irrigation sleeve increases the diameter of the functional tip to about 1.60 mm. Titanium is a good material for this task because it is inert and durable, maintains geometric stability, and is capable of vibrating at a given frequency without metal fatigue. High quality phaco tips can be used for about 10 to 15 cases but are often supplied as disposable items.

The phaco tip has a bevel of 15, 30, or 45 degrees (Fig. 11.18). A compromise between the better occlusion capability of the 15-degree tip and the better cutting ability of the 45-degree tip is found in the 30-degree tip. Occlusion of the tip is a major factor because emulsification and aspiration of nuclear material cannot occur without the nucleus in contact with the tip (the phenomenon of *followability*). The factors that promote occlusion and followability are a more perpendicular tip, increased wall thickness of the tip, low ultrasound power, and high aspiration (Table 11.19). A high degree of followability is desired during the early phases of phaco when the mass of the nucleus is large and there is no danger of encountering the lens capsule. Low followability may be very desirable when working within the capsular bag—the 45-degree tip combined with a low aspiration rate has gained popularity for this use.

In the earlier days of phaco, 45-degree tips were necessary to allow sculpting of a hard nucleus because the power and aspiration delivered to the tip was limited. Nowadays there is

Table 11.17
The Phaco Foot Pedal

Position	Function	
0 (Standby)	Irrigation	OFF
	Aspiration	OFF
	Phacoemulsification	OFF
1	Irrigation	ON
	Aspiration	OFF
	Phacoemulsification	OFF
2	Irrigation	ON
	Aspiration	ON
	Phacoemulsification	OFF
3	Irrigation	ON
	Aspiration	ON
	Phacoemulsification (or vitrectomy instrument)	ON

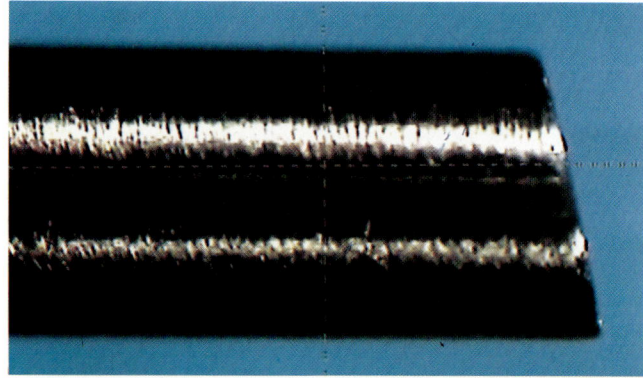
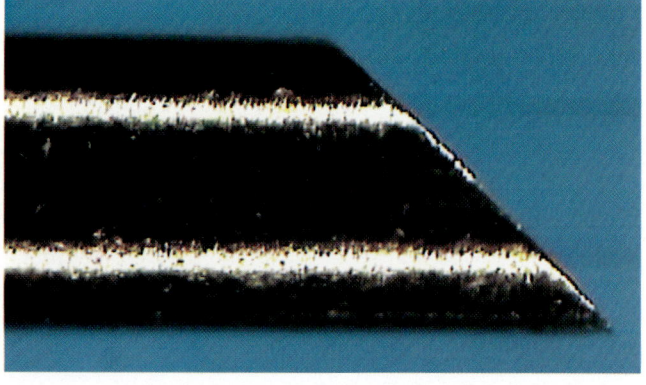

Figure 11.18 *A high magnification photograph of a 15-degree* (**top**) *and 45-degree* (**bottom**) *titanium phaco tip.*

enough power to sculpt almost any nucleus, but the issues of control and safety loom larger as more surgeons perform phaco within the capsular bag. Phaco tips that measure only 0.50 mm in diameter have been developed for endocapsular phaco, and some surgeons use the irrigation source as a second instrument so that creation of only two very small (1.00 mm) incisions are needed for entry into the anterior chamber. The Optical Micro Systems Astro Tip and the Alcon ultrasound I/A tips combine the power of phaco with the safety of I/A.

Automated Anterior Vitrectomy

The phaco surgeon must be prepared to perform an anterior vitrectomy using an automated vitrectomy unit (i.e., AVIT, Ocutome). In many cases of posterior capsule rupture and vitreous loss, an anterior vitrectomy can remove vitreous to below the level of the iris. If even a small rim of anterior or posterior capsule remains, a posterior chamber intraocular lens (IOL) can be implanted into the ciliary sulcus. One of the advantages of capsulorhexis is the presence of a rim of anterior capsule, which can nicely support the haptics of a posterior chamber IOL even in the event of posterior capsule rupture. Automated anterior vitrectomy during phacoemulsification is considered in detail in Chapter 17.

Desires and Reality: A Personal Perspective

Up to now, the mechanics of phaco equipment have been discussed. At this point, however, it would seem valuable to correlate this theoretical and mechanical information with the surgeon's task of performing the best cataract/IOL procedure possible. Not all phaco surgeons will agree with the following opinions but, hopefully, they will consider the concepts discussed.

Phacoemulsification Pumps

As stated before, vacuum pumps have a constant source of vacuum available in order to create flow, unlike peristaltic pumps, which create flow only when the pump wheel turns. With a peristaltic pump there is a lag time between depressing the pedal and overcoming the inertia of the nonrotating pump; however, a vacuum pump using a 500 cc reservoir, for example, has a much more difficult time overcoming the inertia of the column of fluid in the aspiration line. Thus, compared to the vacuum system, a peristaltic pump is more responsive to the anterior segment surgeon's need for aspiration with a shorter response time, a faster rate of vacuum rise, and a higher vacuum level limit. When the vacuum pump system is "cranked up" to create a short response time with a 50 cc reservoir, for example, there is a tendency for the aspiration to overshoot, that is, not cease instantaneously when the foot pedal is released, as would occur when the peristaltic pump stops turning.

Also, the diaphragmatic pump is less durable and occupies more space than the peristaltic pump. A Venturi system requires an external source of gas to function, such as a large tank of nitrous oxide or a hose linked to a wall source of nitrous oxide. For these reasons, the vacuum systems have not become the more popular form of phaco pump. The peristaltic pump has remained the standard for the anterior segment surgeon. The vacuum pumps continue to be the favorite for surgeons performing surgery on the vitreous because of their ability to control the build-up of low aspiration vacuum. Modern high-powered phaco units, only a little larger than a telephone console, are now available (Fig. 11.20). Of course, surgeons will adapt to either system.

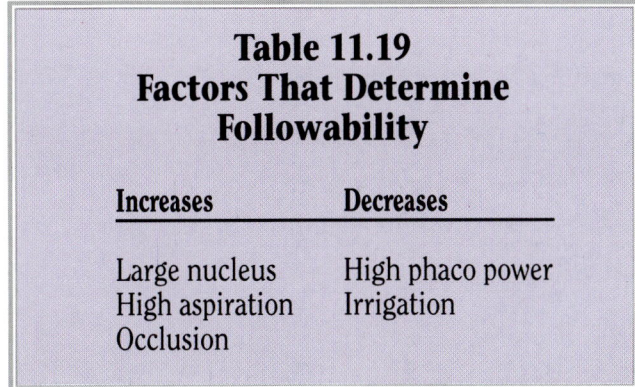

**Table 11.19
Factors That Determine Followability**

Increases	Decreases
Large nucleus	High phaco power
High aspiration	Irrigation
Occlusion	

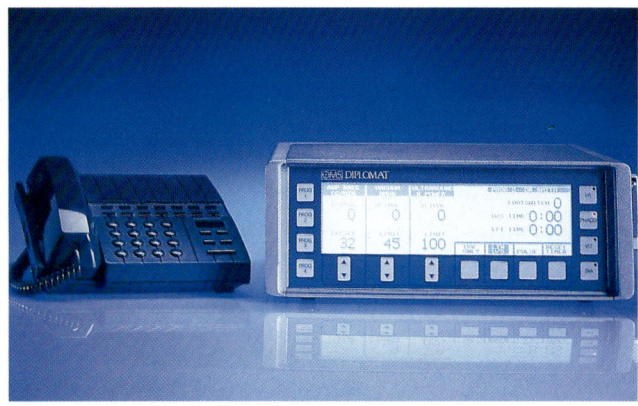

Figure 11.20 *An Optical Micro Systems (OMS) Diplomate peristaltic pump phaco is similar in size to a telephone console.*

Power and Aspiration

Table 11.21 depicts the various capabilities possessed by the ideal phaco machine. The ideal phaco machine would have the ability to respond to various demands during the phaco procedure. Consider the concepts presented in Table 11.19. The surgeon wishing to create a large degree of followability would need high vacuum during the sculpting phase in order to counteract the increased vibration of the nucleus caused by the increased phaco power necessary for effective emulsification. While working in the bag, however, a low rate of rise of aspiration vacuum would allow the surgeon to remain near the capsular bag and make it less likely that the capsule will follow into the tip. A hard nucleus in the bag requires a low rate of rise with higher phaco power. The reverse, a low phaco power with a high rate of rise, while theoretically possible, does not allow the surgeon enough response time to avoid rupturing the capsular bag.

Perhaps phaco machines of the future will have several modes that can be accessed by a foot switch so that the surgeon can easily transfer between the "sculpting" and the "in the capsular bag" modes (Fig. 11.22). Another possibility is a phaco machine with the ability to provide linear phaco and linear aspiration flow rate simultaneously, which would enable greater aspiration to become available for increased followability as more phaco power is needed. Because low levels of phaco power would be correlated with low levels of aspiration, there would be a greater degree of safety while working in the capsular bag. Presently, phaco power is linear and the aspiration level can be adjusted but remains at that level thereafter.

Clinical experience has demonstrated that when the endothelium of the cornea suffers detrimental effects during a routine phacoemulsification procedure, it is because of the location and quantity of irrigation, not the amount of ultrasound. Of course, the cases that require large amounts of ultrasound usually involve a more difficult procedure with varied locations of the phaco tip in relation to the endothelium. A phaco surgeon's dilemma arises from the desire to work in the capsular bag as far away from the endothelium as possible, even though a denser nucleus will require about two to three times the irrigation volume than is required by tilting the same nucleus into the iris plane and finishing the case more quickly. Ultimately, personal experience and good judgement must guide each surgeon in the quest for improved results.

In recent years, several phaco machine manufacturers have begun to indicate both a *running* and a *cumulative* phaco time. Running phaco time reflects the total time that the phaco mode of the ultrasonic handpiece is in operation at all, whether it be 1% or 100%. Older phaco machines and those used in panel control are on 100% or are off, unlike linear control, which allows for partial phaco power. Cumulative display of energy (CDE) time is the algebraic summation of the phaco power in linear control and expresses this total of phaco energy as though it were achieved by activation of 100% phaco power (Fig. 11.23). The surgeon can then get a feel for the "average" phaco power used during a case, even though various aspects of the nuclear phaco require different amounts of phaco power.

For example, the procedure represented in Figure 11.23 required a total phaco time of one minute and 35 seconds at various linear phaco power settings. However, this one minute and 35 seconds of varying phaco power was the equivalent of 48 seconds at 100% phaco power (Fig. 11.24). Dividing the CDE time by the running phaco time

$$\frac{48 \text{ seconds}}{95 \text{ seconds}} = 0.50$$

indicates an average phaco power of 50%.

Table 11.21
Power and Aspiration

Portion of Procedure	Vacuum Level Limit	Aspiration Rate of Rise	Phaco Power
Sculpting (large mass, danger low)	High	High	High
In the capsular bag (near capsule, danger high)	Low	Low	Low
Cortical aspiration	High	Moderate	

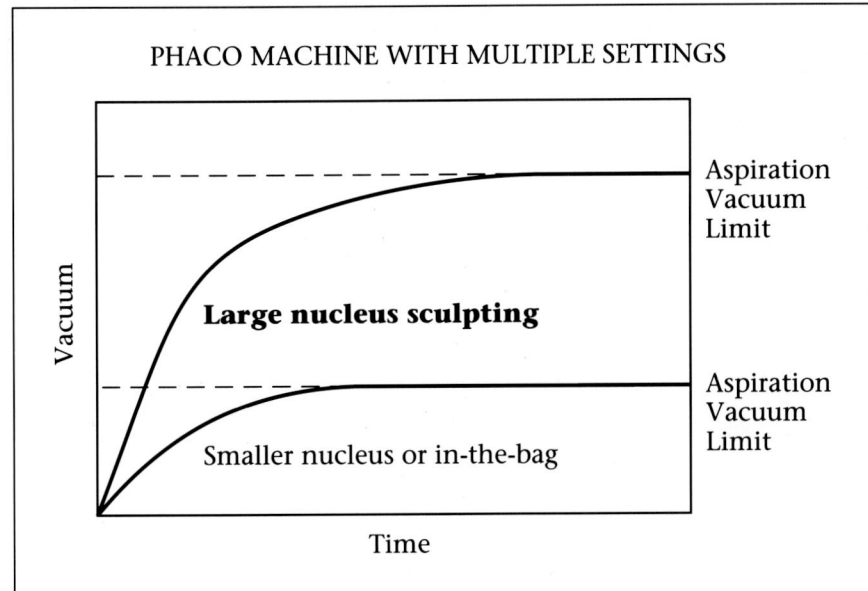

Figure 11.22 *A phaco machine that would provide multiple aspiration rates of rise at the touch of a foot switch during phacoemulsification of the nucleus would be very valuable for removal of the nucleus in the capsular bag.*

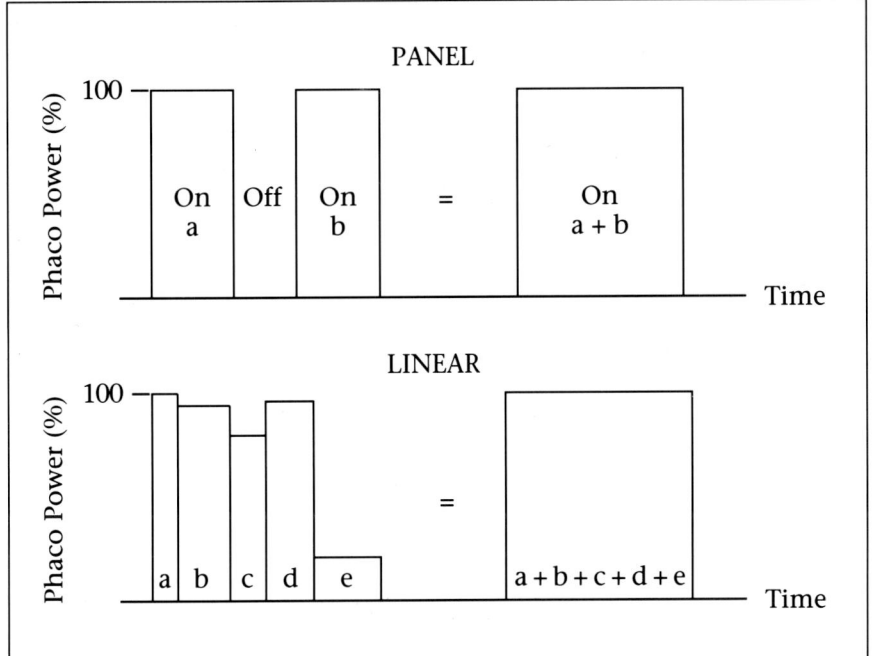

Figure 11.23 *Running ultrasound time equals cumulative display of energy (CDE) ultrasound time only when the linear ultrasound mode is employed at 100% power. When the linear ultrasound mode is used at less than 100% power, the CDE time will always be less than the running time. The running time measures the duration that the ultrasound mode was activated at any level, and the CDE time measures the total amount of ultrasound energy as though it were applied at 100% power.*

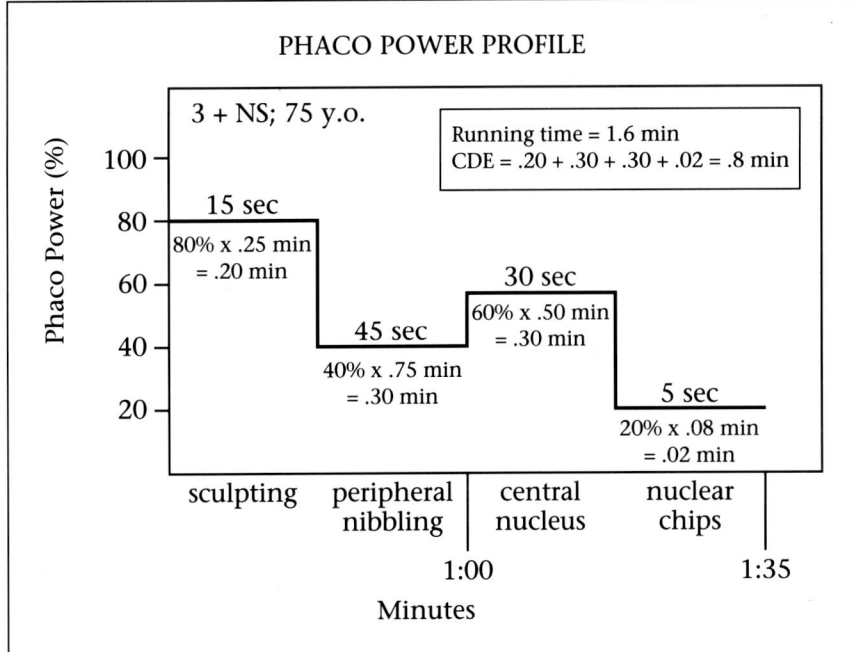

Figure 11.24 *An example of linear phaco. This is an "average" phaco case, showing the ultrasound time necessary to perform the various aspects of phacoemulsification of the nucleus. Ninety-five seconds of ultrasound time is the running ultrasound time. The CDE ultrasound times for each portion of the procedure are calculated.*

The Future

We owe a great deal to the innovators who have provided us with the dependable, effective phaco machines available today. Phaco enables the surgeon to remove a cataract while working in a hydrodynamically stable system with a fully formed anterior chamber. Currently, three factors make phaco the most sophisticated form of cataract extraction: lack of tissue manipulation, constant intraocular pressure, and better astigmatism control due to the small wound. Even if the ultrasound component of the phaco machine is replaced by a more efficient modality, such as laser, the surgical skills and decision-making abilities required by phaco will greatly benefit patients and surgeons in the future.

Clinical Points to Consider

- It is necessary to have a solid understanding of fluidics, including irrigation, aspiration, and anterior chamber depth when doing phacoemulsification.

- The phaco surgeon should be familiar with the differences between a peristaltic pump and a vacuum pump.

- A comparison between the running phaco time and the CDE time may indicate trends in a surgeon's phacoemulsification technique.

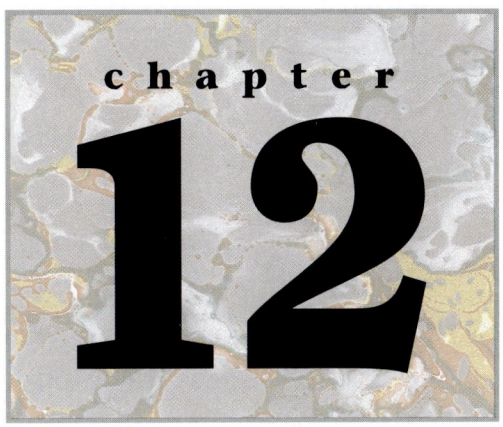

THE PHACOEMULSIFICATION PROCEDURE

LEE T. NORDAN, M.D.   W. ANDREW MAXWELL, M.D., Ph.D.

Cataract removal by phacoemulsification is a specialized form of extracapsular cataract extraction (ECCE) that emulsifies the nucleus instead of expressing it, as is required in ECCE; otherwise, phacoemulsification and standard ECCE are generally the same. Phaco's smaller wound offers several advantages, including maintenance of a pressurized globe throughout the procedure, less chance of choroidal effusion or suprachoroidal hemorrhage, faster patient rehabilitation, and better uncorrected postoperative visual acuity because of less surgically induced astigmatism.

Since the goal of cataract/intraocular lens (IOL) surgery is the best possible uncorrected vision, the surgeon must minimize significant pre-existing astigmatism. The surgeon should not be satisfied with a cataract/IOL procedure that preserves 3.00 D of against-the-rule astigmatism and leaves the patient with 20/80 uncorrected visual acuity, even though the surgeon can claim to have created no new astigmatism.

Patients who undergo phaco and foldable IOL implantation with a 4.00 mm wound and single horizontal suture closure usually achieve their final, stable refraction in one to two weeks. The standard ECCE requires six to eight weeks before sutures can be cut, if necessary, and then another four weeks or so for stabilization of the refraction. Thus, it is not surprising that a large amount of energy has been spent improving and simplifying phaco techniques as well as refining foldable IOL technology and implantation methods.

Many excellent methods of performing cataract removal/IOL implantation using phaco have been devised. Furthermore, surgeons develop unique nuances while performing the general steps. This introduction is designed to help the phaco surgeon understand the basic steps of phaco and gain an appreciation of often underestimated factors such as operating room setup, patient head position, and draping. These general steps can then be melded into a smooth, consistent surgical phaco technique.

Each step of the phaco procedure depends on successful completion of the preceding ones; thus, a systematic approach is necessary to achieve consistently good results. This chapter introduces the phaco procedure using our surgical technique (we both are right-handed). This standardized outline provides a valuable basis for comparison with clinical cases, which often challenge the creativity of the surgeon.

At the least, this chapter should provide several key ideas to convince the ECCE surgeon that phaco provides significant advantages for the patient and that it can be approached in a systematic, controlled fashion. Because conversion from ECCE to phacoemulsification requires new surgical skills, it is emotionally as well as technically very difficult; the surgeon knows that a poor result obtained while learning phaco could have been avoided if an ECCE had been performed.

We hope that this brief view of phacoemulsification will assist the cataract surgeon in converting to phacoemulsification or improving current phaco technique. Phacoemulsification, small incision IOLs, and astigmatism control are the factors that allow patients to achieve best corrected visual acuity in the shortest possible time. The surgeon's efforts to learn phacoemulsification should be well rewarded.

Outline of Phacoemulsification

Preoperative Preparation

Patient's keratometry and IOL power

OPERATING ROOM SETUP
Equipment, patient and staff location
Microscope position and pedal position
Irrigation bottle height

Patient Preparation
Preoperative ocular medication (antibiotics, dilating, and anti-inflammatory agents)
Preoperative intravenous medication
Retrobulbar block
Ocular pressure-lowering device
Facial nerve block
Blood pressure check
Patient position
Sterile ocular prep
Draping

Surgical Procedure
WOUND AND CAPSULOTOMY
Blepharostasis
Globe fixation sutures
Limbal peritomy
Wetfield cautery
Scleral flap wound
Side-port wound
Entrance into the anterior chamber
Viscoelastic
Capsulorhexis

CATARACT REMOVAL
Hydrodissection
Phacoemulsification
   Sculpting of nucleus
   In-the-bag
   Iris plane
      Nuclear prolapse
Cortical aspiration
Viscoelastic
Wound enlargement

IOL IMPLANTATION

WOUND CLOSURE
Initial wound closure
Viscoelastic removal
Suture adjustment
Keratometry
Final wound closure
Subconjunctival antibiotics
Conjunctiva repositioned

POSTOPERATIVE REGIMEN
Topical medications (antibiotics and anti-inflammatory)
Patch and protective (Fox) shield
Antiglaucoma medication
Postoperative instructions
Return appointment

Preoperative Preparation

The surgeon should know the patient's *keratometry* and *IOL power*. Wound size and location are based on preoperative astigmatism. Wound length and orientation are determined preoperatively to minimize postoperative astigmatism. According to Table 12.1, a 4.00 mm wound can be used to maintain low preoperative astigmatism, wound recession to correct with-the-rule astigmatism, and astigmatic keratotomy or wound recession to correct against-the-rule astigmatism.

Operating Room Setup
Proper operating room setup facilitates safe and efficient staff and equipment performance (Fig. 12.2):

The *phacoemulsification machine* is to the right and rear of the surgeon. For maximum control, the phaco machine tubing and the phaco handpiece cord run parallel to the surgeon's right

Table 12.1 ASTIGMATISM CORRECTION TECHNIQUES
Cataract Extraction
(Surgeon's View)

Pre-op Astigmatism			
A 0-1.50 D	1. Small wound = 4.00 mm (80%)		
B With-the-Rule Oblique (13%)	1. 1.75 – 3.50 D, 6.00 mm wound recession (10%)	2. 3.75 – 6.00 D, 8-10 mm wound recession (2%)	3. 6.25 – 10.00 D, 12.00 mm wound recession (1%)
C Against-the-Rule (7%)	1. 1.75 – 2.50 D (4%) OZ = 7.00 mm, width = 3.50 mm	2. 2.75 – 4.00 D (2%) OZ = 7.00, 9.00 mm, width = 3.00 mm	3. 4.25 – 10.0 D (1%) lateral wound recession

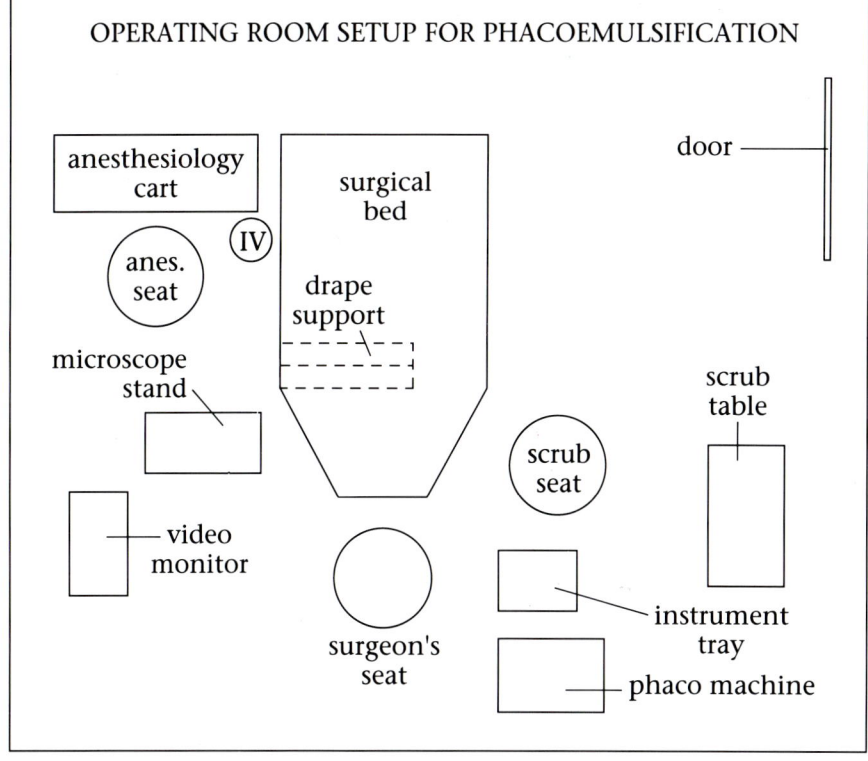

Figure 12.2 *The operating room setup for phacoemulsification.*

SURGICAL REHABILITATION OF VISION

lower arm. This will prevent interference with the movements of the handpiece. The cord and tubing do not cross the instrument tray because instruments can easily be knocked to the floor.

The *microscope* is positioned with a 15-degree tilt of the ocular end toward the surgeon, which allows for a red reflex and enough clearance to prevent the phaco handpiece from hitting the surgeon's chest. The oculars of the microscope are set to the appropriate power and pupillary distance for the surgeon and scrub nurse.

The *irrigation bottle* is positioned 69 cm above the cassette or pump; the cassette and the eye are at the same height (39 inches) above the floor (Fig. 12.3). The bottle height is determined by the distance from the fluid level of the drip chamber to the patient's eye.

The microscope stand, anesthesiology equipment, and video monitor are in the proper position. The seats for the surgeon and scrub nurse are set to the proper height.

The *phaco pedal* is to the surgeon's left, the microscope pedal to the surgeon's right, and the wetfield cautery pedal in the middle. This arrangement is best because the microscope demands finer control than the phaco pedal and is used by the dominant foot. The *phaco power* is set at 70% of maximum in the linear control mode.

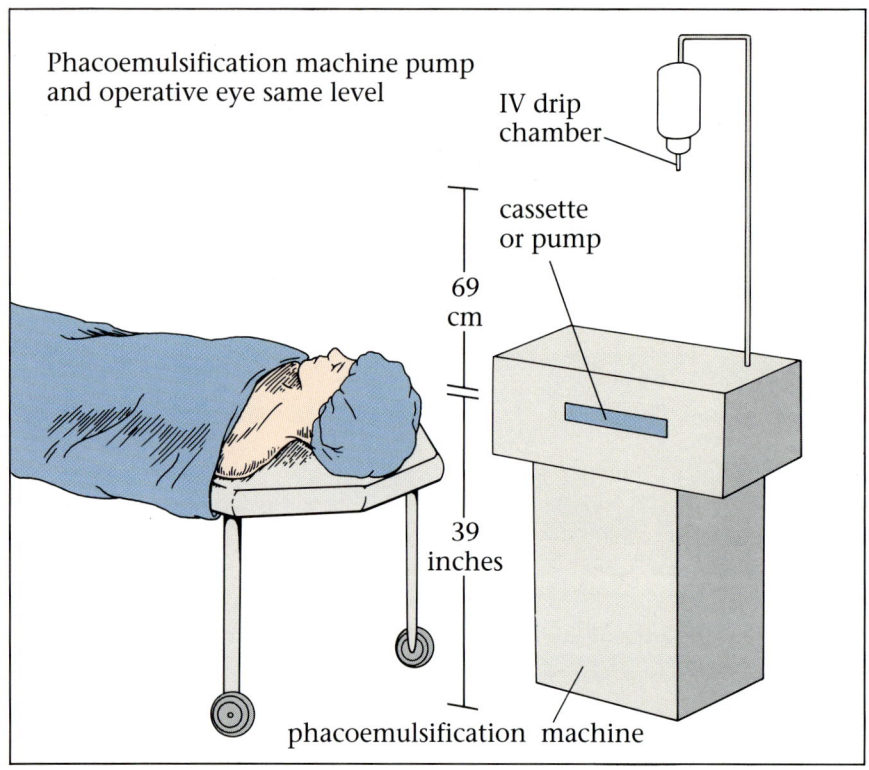

Figure 12.3 *The pump of the phaco machine should be at the same height as the patient's eye.*

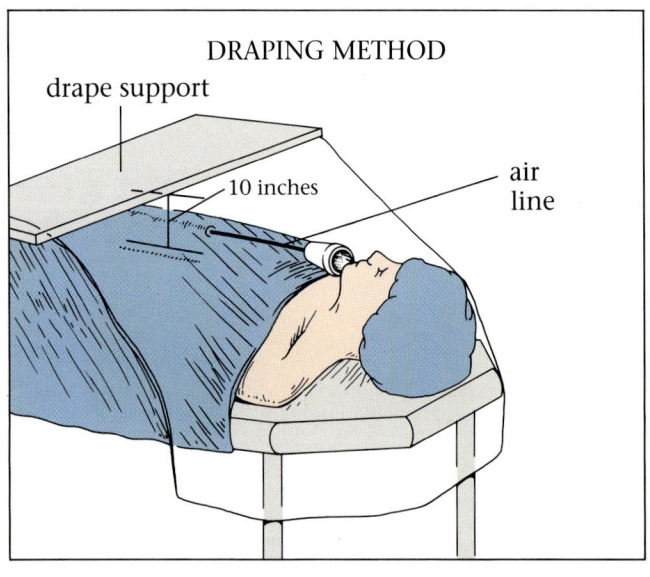

Figure 12.4 *Phacoemulsification draping method allows easy access to the patient's airway.*

Patient Preparation

Preoperative *antibiotics* (Tobrex or Polytrim) and *dilating agents* (Cyclogyl 2% and Neo-Synephrine 10%) are administered to the operative eye three times at five minute intervals.

Intravenous sedation is accomplished using a combination of a narcotic agent, such as a fentanyl derivative (Sublimaze), and a sedative amnestic such as midazolam (Versed).

A *retrobulbar block* consisting of 4 cc of a 50/50 mixture of Xylocaine 2% and Marcaine 0.5%, is given using a long (1¼ inch) 27-gauge needle.

An *ocular pressure lowering device*, set at 30 mm Hg, is used for six minutes to lower intraocular pressure.

The *facial nerve block* is accomplished by the Nadbath technique, using 5 cc of the retrobulbar anesthetic mixture and a short (⅝ inch) 25-gauge needle.

The anesthesiologist must insure that the *systolic blood pressure* does not exceed 160 mm Hg.

The patient is brought into the operating room and the bed is made flat. A neck support is provided so the patient's head is tilted back slightly. The patient's lateral canthus is 39 inches above the floor; a mark on the microscope stand or a yardstick simplifies positioning the patient. A pillow is placed under the patient's knees to reduce back discomfort.

The *ocular prep* is done with alternating scrubs of Betadine solution and normal saline. If necessary, ultrasound pachymetry is performed before the prep.

Head and lap drapes are applied. As the *ocular drape* (1060 plastic drape 3M) is positioned (Fig. 12.4), the lashes are everted and the lids are spread. The 1060 ocular drape is held in place by a nonsterile support or Mayo stand, which is eight to 10 inches above the patient's chin. This permits the anesthesiologist access to the patient's airway and prevents the patient from feeling confined.

Supplemental air is delivered under the 1060 ocular drape via a Styrofoam cup or 50 cc syringe attached to an air line. A nasal cannula is not used because air delivered through it can dry out the nasal mucosa, causing the patient to twitch or rub the nose and, secondarily, move the eye.

The 1060 ocular drape is pinched together just below the lower lid to provide an attachment point for the inferior rectus suture. The sterile plastic drape should capture the everted lashes. Flaps, created by horizontal and vertical incisions made with Wescott scissors, allow the lid speculum to fold the 1060 drape easily into the superior and inferior lid fornices (Fig. 12.5) and isolate the lid margins from the operative field.

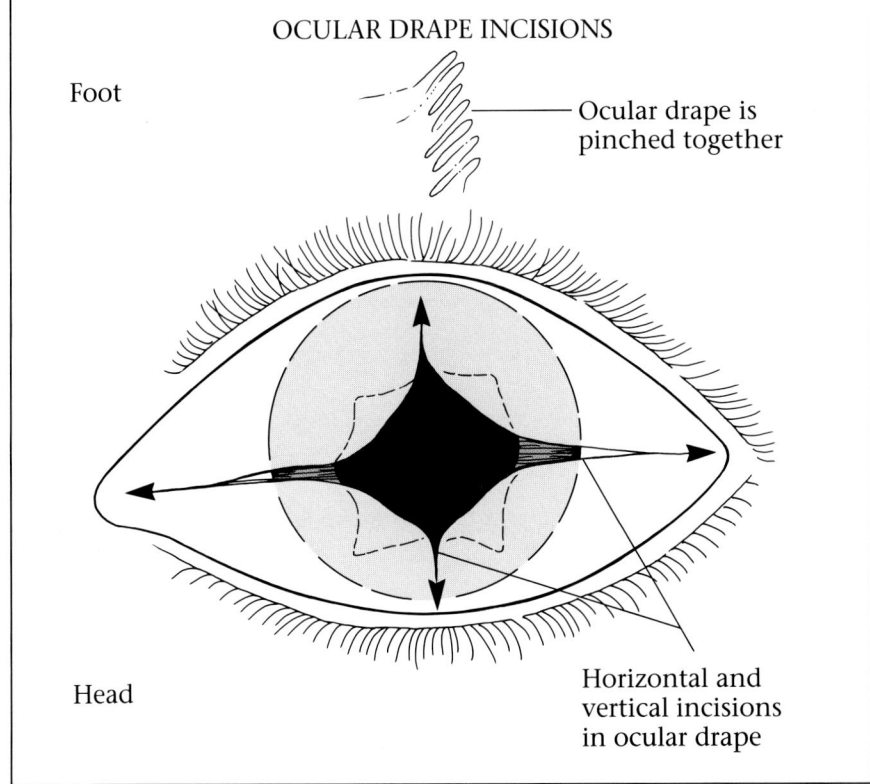

Figure 12.5 *Ocular drapes.*

Surgical Procedure

Wound and Capsulotomy

Blepharostasis is achieved with a Kratz-Barraquer lid speculum. The absence of a crossbar affords the surgeon maximum freedom of movement with the phaco handpiece.

The microscope is moved into position.

An astigmatic keratotomy is performed, if necessary.

Fixation sutures, 6-0 silk with small spatula needles, are placed into the episclera or under the rectus muscle tendon, superiorly and inferiorly, with the aid of a microscope. The globe is tilted slightly away from the surgeon to maximize exposure of the superior limbal area.

The inferior rectus suture is placed 4.00 mm to 6.00 mm from the limbus. The superior rectus suture is placed 6.00 mm to 10.00 mm from the limbus and must be back far enough from the limbus to create an inferior tilt of the globe. The rectus sutures are anchored to the plastic drape by mosquito hemostats.

The fixation sutures may be placed "on axis" of the steeper meridian in order to rotate the globe to allow for surgery at 12 o'clock.

A *limbal peritomy* is performed with a small version of Wescott scissors. Wetfield cautery is used to control localized bleeding.

A corneoscleral incision (perpendicular to the surface) of the desired length is made 1.50 mm behind the posterior border of the limbus and dissected into clear cornea using a trifacet diamond blade. The globe is fixated by Colibri forceps held in the left hand, which grasp the episclera just to the left of the incision.

A *scleral flap wound* is created using the same trifacet diamond blade (Fig. 12.6). The scleral flap's angle of dissection is slightly anterior, not parallel, to the iris. This insures entry into the anterior chamber at least 0.50 mm to 1.00 mm in front of the iris root near Schwalbe's line.

A *side-port incision* for the "second" left hand instrument is created 80 degrees to the left of the primary incision using a 30-degree Alcon blade.

The Alcon 3.20-mm keratome enters the *anterior chamber* through the superior wound but only three-quarters of the way up the blade to avoid an excessively large wound. A *viscoelastic* (Viscoat) is injected slowly into the anterior chamber.

A *capsulorhexis* of the anterior capsule is performed (Fig. 12.7). A cystotome punctures the anterior capsule, and a capsular flap is created by either the cystotome or a radial and a circumferential incision with Vannas scissors. Kraff-Utrata forceps perform the capsulorhexis by grasping the flap and regrasping the anterior capsule as often as necessary. A continuous, circular capsulorhexis helps insure in-the-bag IOL placement and excellent long-term centration.

Cataract Removal

PHACOEMULSIFICATION

Hydrodissection of the nucleus is attempted with a 27-gauge needle on a BSS syringe (Fig. 12.8). Hydrodissection separates the central nucleus from the peripheral cortex and allows the nucleus to be rotated in the bag during phacoemulsification.

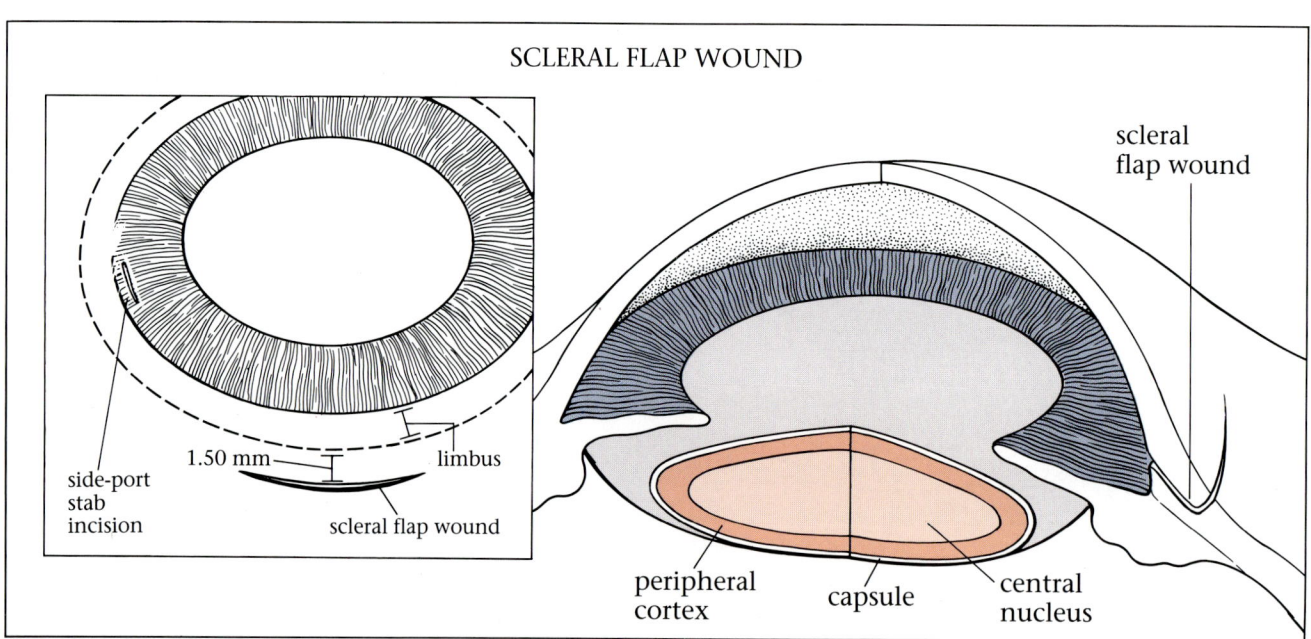

Figure 12.6 *Scleral flap wound.*

STRATEGIC DECISION

At this point in the procedure, the surgeon should determine the strategy that will obviate possible difficulties. The decision depends on the success or failure of hydrodissection, hardness of the nucleus, and pupil size: If hydrodissection has been successful and the pupil is at least 6.00 mm, in-the-bag phaco should be initiated. If the nucleus has been hydrodissected, rotation and control of the nucleus should be easier. Also, hydrodissection increases safety by providing a layer of fluid between the nucleus and the underlying cortex.

If hydrodissection has been unsuccessful and the pupil is small, the nucleus should be dislocated and prolapsed into the iris plane for phacoemulsification. If the patient has a small pupil, in-the-bag phaco should be avoided because a broken posterior capsule could be difficult to handle with such limited visibility.

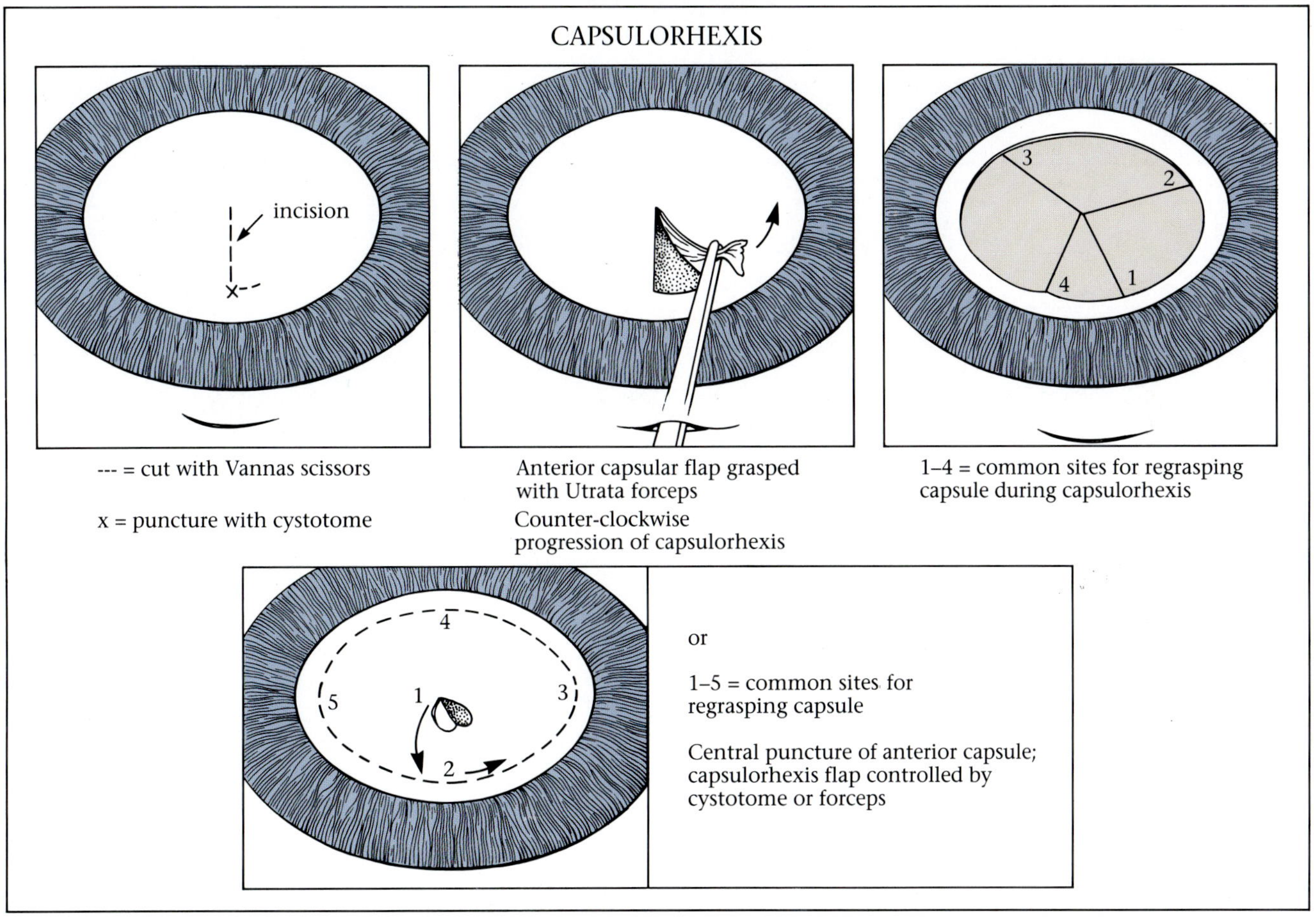

Figure 12.7 *A 6.00 mm capsulorhexis.*

Figure 12.8 *Hydrodissection.*

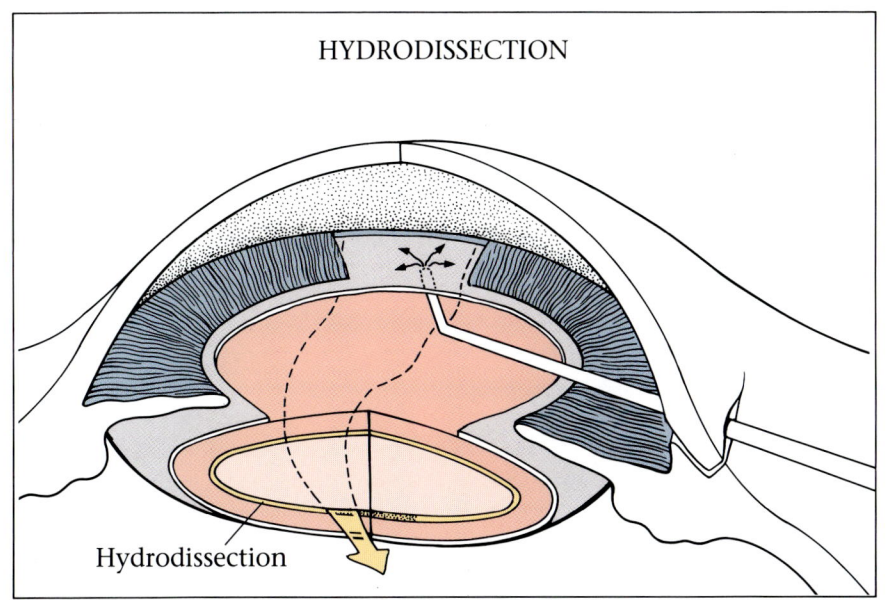

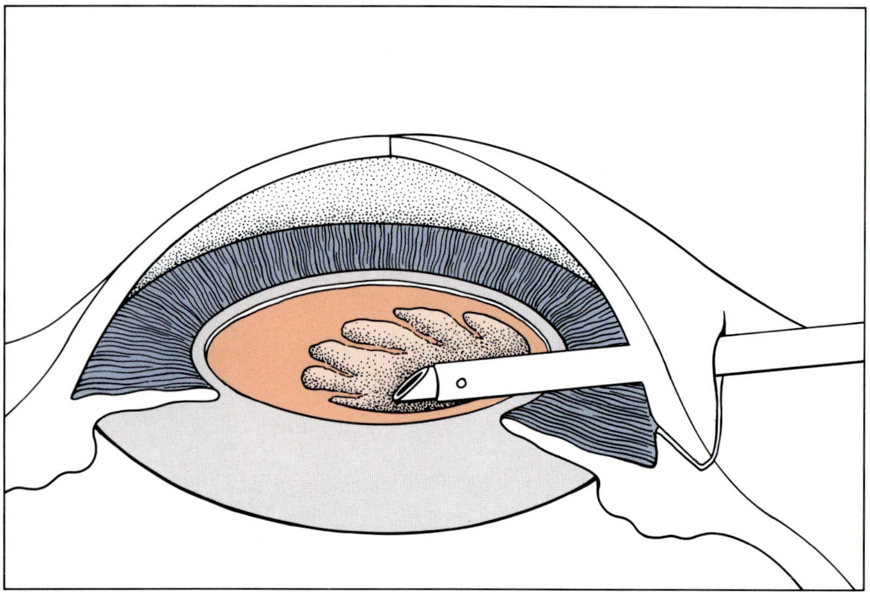

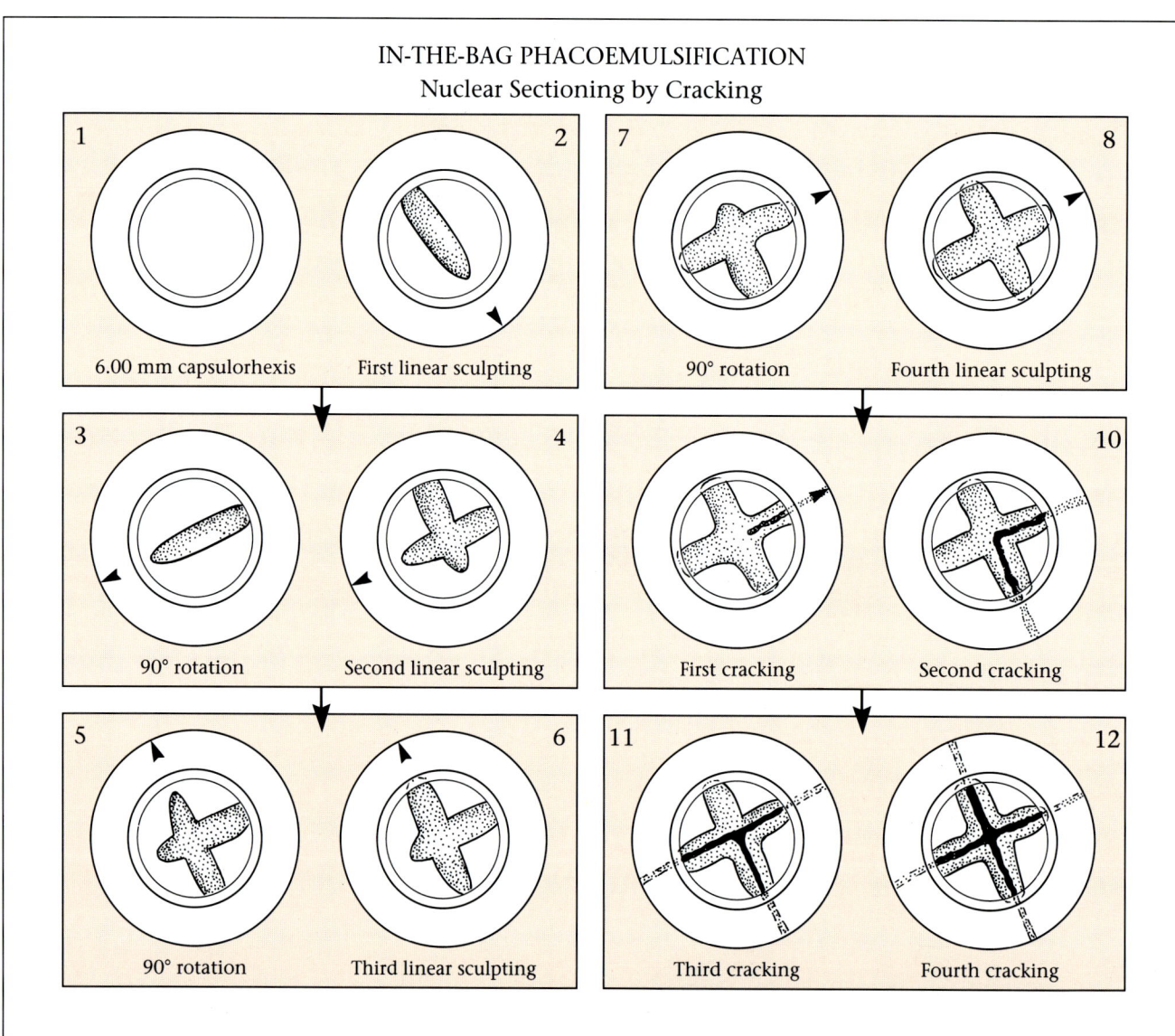

Figure 12.9 *Phacoemulsification begins with sculpting of the nucleus.*

Figure 12.10 *The sequence of deeply sculpted "crosses" and nuclear cracking that convert the remaining nucleus into four pieces during in-the-bag phaco.*

A very hard nucleus calls for phacoemulsification at the iris plane since the case will take about one to one and one-half minutes of phaco time compared to three to four minutes with an in-the-bag approach. Phaco time per se is not of concern but rather the prolonged irrigation and the tear in the capsulorhexis at the 12 o'clock position that will be created by nuclear prolapse. Thus the surgeon may have to compromise (create a tear in the capsulorhexis) when choosing iris plane phaco.

Sculpting. The phaco machine is in the irrigation mode, *not* the ultrasound mode, to avoid accidentally phacoemulsifying the iris while inserting the phaco tip into the anterior chamber.

The phaco tip is introduced into the anterior chamber through the 12 o'clock wound. During its introduction into the anterior chamber, the phaco tip is rotated 90 degrees to 180 degrees to avoid iris capture. The tip is rotated to its normal position, and when the surgeon is ready to begin phaco the machine is changed to the ultrasound mode.

When possible, for maximum control, the phaco handpiece is held like a pencil in the right hand, with the second and third fingers of the left hand pressed against the handpiece.

The first step of phacoemulsification is nuclear sculpting. The phaco power is raised or lowered, as necessary. With a hard nucleus, extensive sculpting is performed; with a soft nucleus, moderate sculpting is performed.

After sculpting, nucleus dislocation (rotation within the capsular bag) is accomplished with the spatula (0.50-mm cylodialysis spatula) in the left hand through the side port.

Phacoemulsification of the nucleus continues, either by an in-the-bag technique or nucleus prolapse to the iris plane (Fig. 12.9).

In-the-Bag Phacoemulsification. This requires nuclear occlusion of the phaco port after sculpting and peripheral nibbling has left the nuclear plate in the bag. Occlusion can be accomplished using either the *cross* method of John Shepard, M.D., in which deep sculpting (Fig. 12.10) enables effective nuclear cracking (Fig. 12.11), or the *inverted tip* method, in which a 45-degree phaco

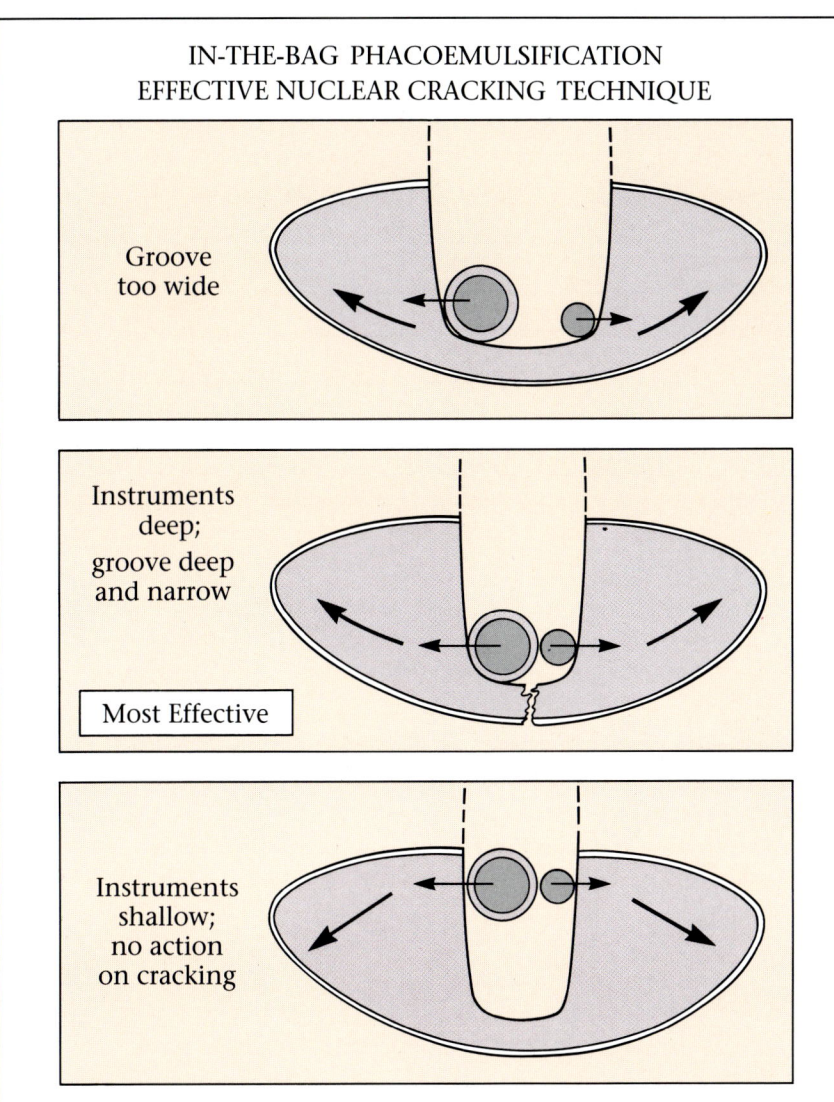

Figure 12.11 *The spatula and phaco tip must be placed at the bottom of a narrowly sculpted "cross" furrow to easily crack the nucleus.*

tip is rotated upside down, so the nuclear plate can occlude the phaco tip and be lifted and emulsified (Fig. 12.12), allowing for safer phacoemulsification. Both of these methods are designed to provide occlusion points so that the phaco tip can function effectively.

Iris Plane Phacoemulsification. Nucleus prolapse is accomplished as follows (Fig. 12.13):

1. The spatula of the left hand limits the upward movement of the inferior pole of the nucleus after it has been dislocated (free to rotate within the capsular bag) using the spatula.

2. The phaco tip is retracted toward the wound as irrigation is stopped by the surgeon transitioning from *foot-position 1* to *foot-position 0*.

3. The phaco tip is used to capture the superior pole of the nucleus as it moves upward.

4. The spatula of the left hand is moved to support the nucleus from the side.

5. The phaco tip is repositioned below the superior pole of the nucleus and irrigation is resumed, cleaving the nucleus from the cortex.

6. Iris plane phaco is accomplished by removing a peripheral sector of the nucleus at 12 o'clock, rotating the nucleus with the spatula, and then removing the next sector. The central

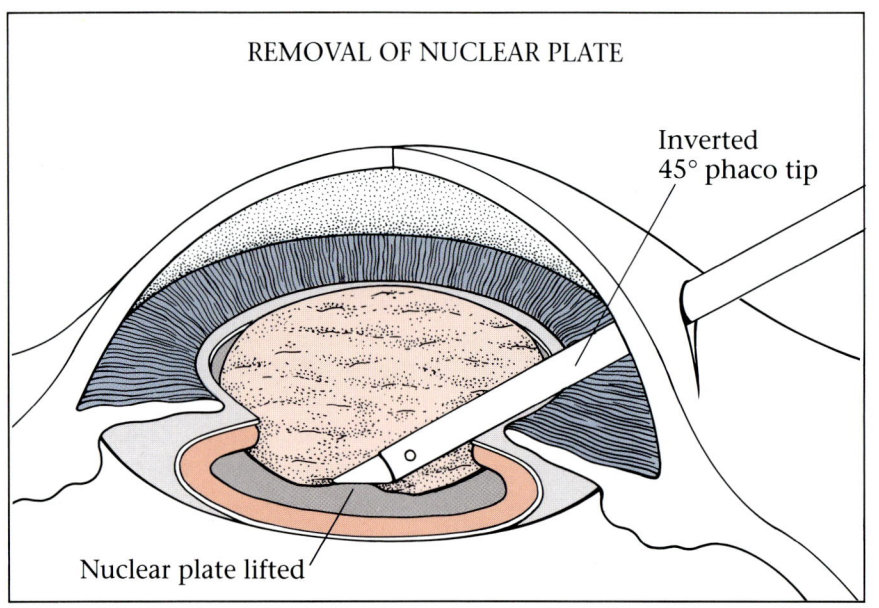

Figure 12.12 *During in-the-bag phaco, a 30- or 45-degree phaco tip can be inverted to gain occlusion of the port and elevate the nuclear bowl by aspiration.*

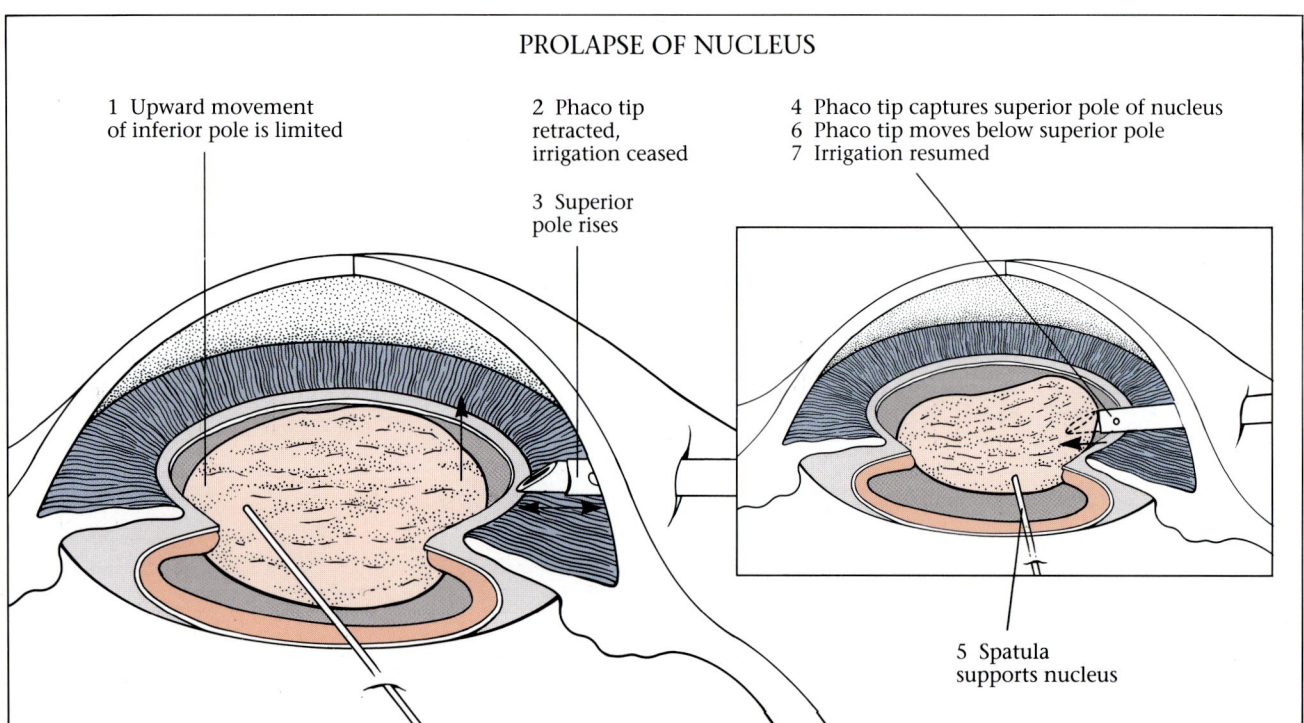

Figure 12.13 *Prolapse of the nucleus.*

nucleus is removed last. The phaco tip should not stray far from the 12 o'clock location in search of nucleus; rather the nucleus should be aspirated toward the phaco tip (Fig. 12.14).

CORTICAL ASPIRATION

Cortical aspiration is accomplished using an irrigation/aspiration (I/A) tip with a 0.30 mm diameter port. Aspiration begins in the 11 o'clock to 1 o'clock area. Initial circumferential movements and only moderate aspiration levels insure efficient cortical removal. The aspiration port is oriented upward or sideways. A curved I/A tip may be useful for removal of cortical material at 12 o'clock. The phaco machine allows linear control of the aspiration flow rate (Fig. 12.15).

The posterior lens capsule is polished with a Terry Squeegee, as necessary, or vacuumed with the I/A tip if the phaco machine has a capsule-vacuum setting. Viscoelastic is injected into the anterior chamber. The wound is enlarged with the keratome (Fig. 12.16).

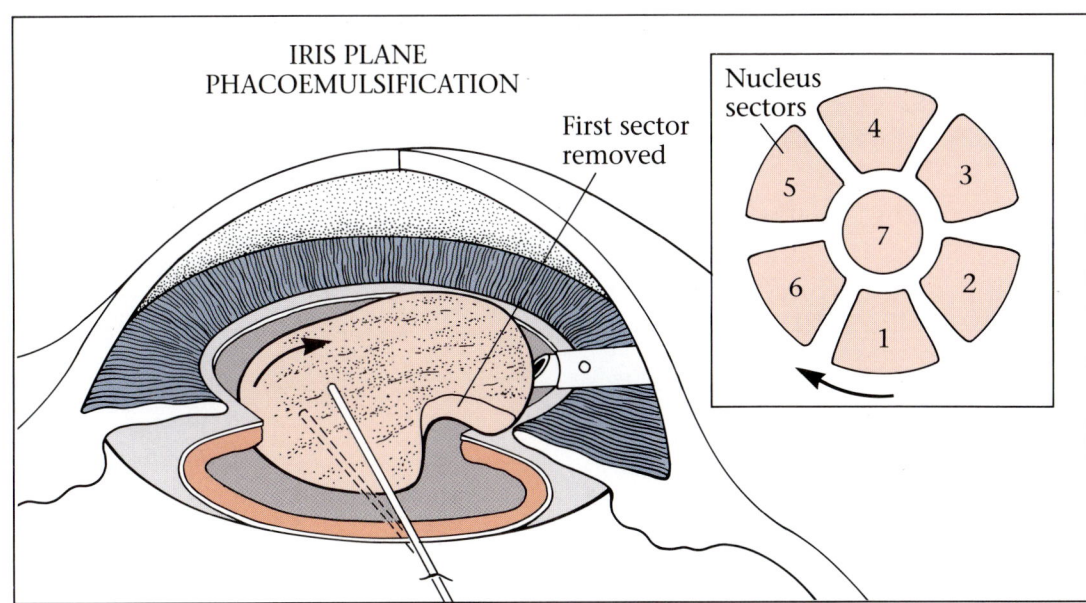

Figure 12.14 *Iris plane phacoemulsification.*

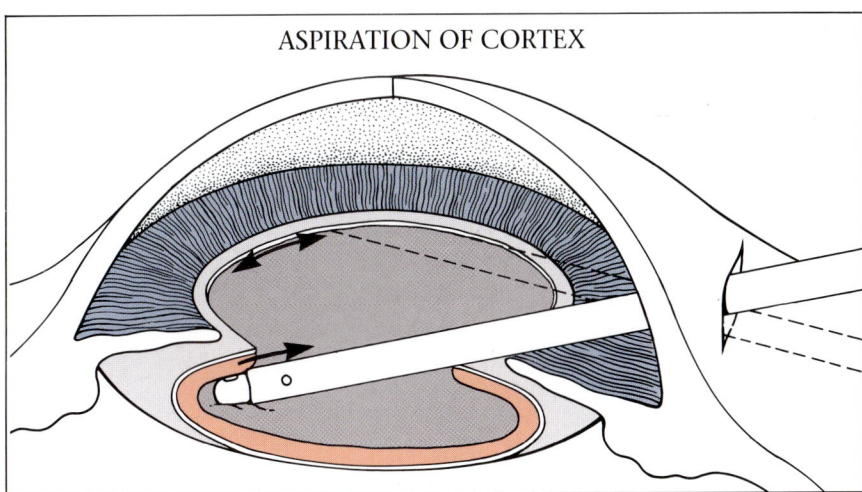

Figure 12.15 *Aspiration of the cortex.*

Intraocular Lens Implantation

The posterior chamber IOL is inspected, irrigated with BSS, inserted through the wound, and placed into the capsular bag (Fig. 12.17) as follows:

1. The IOL optic is held with long McPherson forceps in the right hand and the inferior haptic is placed into the bag at 6 o'clock. The anterior aspect of the wound is grasped by Colibri forceps held in the left hand.
2. The distal tip of the superior haptic is grasped with the long McPherson forceps of the right hand, and the left hand places a capsular bag locator over the optic of the IOL and into the capsular bag at 2 o'clock.
3. The right hand rotates the superior haptic clockwise, which forces it into the bag *under* the capsular bag locator.

An atraumatic technique that assures total in-the-bag placement of both haptics is especially important when the pupil becomes smaller than the capsulorhexis. If the PC IOL is dialed into position, the superior haptic may remain in the ciliary sulcus rather than enter the bag.

4. A Sinskey hook is used to engage the crotch between the inferior haptic and the IOL optic, which has now moved to 8 o'clock, and the IOL is centered with a slight clockwise movement.

Wound Closure

Initial wound closure is accomplished using 10-0 nylon suture.

For a 6.00-mm wound, a five-bite running pattern may be used with the first suture bite taken in the wound. The first throw of the knot is made (Fig. 12.18) using a double rather than a triple

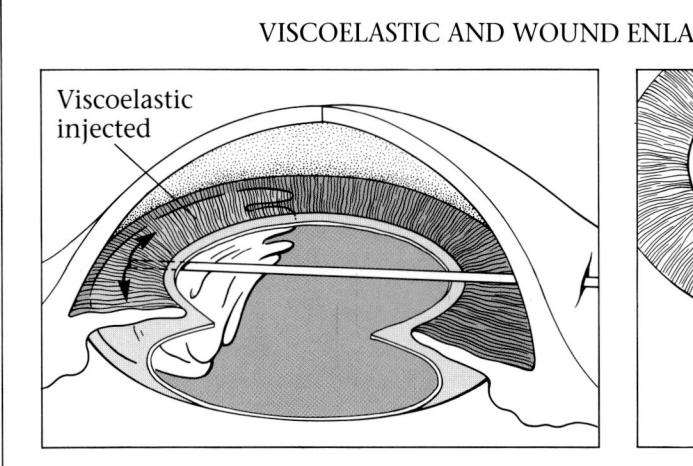
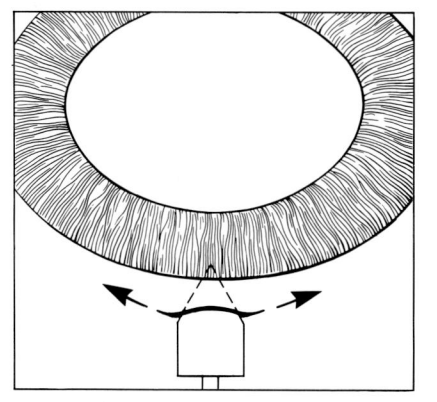

Figure 12.16 *Viscoelastic is injected into the anterior chamber and the wound enlarged with the keratome.*

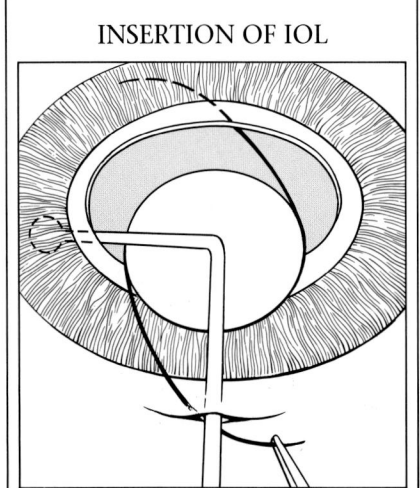

Figure 12.17 *Intraocular lens implantation.*

throw in the wound because it is easier to adjust after viscoelastic removal. Alternatively, a 6.00-mm wound may be closed using the infinity suture (see Chapter 20) or radial sutures at each end with a horizontal suture in between.

A 4.00-mm wound is closed with a single horizontal suture or a single X-pattern.

The Viscoat is removed from the anterior chamber by I/A, which must be set to the maximum power. The BSS bottle is lowered from 69 cm to 55 cm.

Suture tension is adjusted. The anterior chamber is inflated to normal intraocular pressure using BSS and verified by indenting the cornea with a dry surgical sponge. Keratometry is performed to insure slight with-the-rule astigmatism. Suture tension is readjusted, if necessary. Using scissors, the knot is tied and cut flush with the scleral surface.

Antibiotics (Ancef; Nebcin) and a steroid (Solumedrol) are applied topically near the wound and subconjunctivally inferiorly with a short 25-gauge needle.

The conjunctiva is repositioned and secured at 10 o'clock and 2 o'clock by wetfield cautery. The lid speculum is removed.

Postoperative Regimen

Maxitrol ointment, then a semipressure dressing and Fox shield are placed on the eye. Neptazane, 50 mg PO, is given before discharge. The patient is given an appointment for the next day and instructed to call if severe pain is experienced.

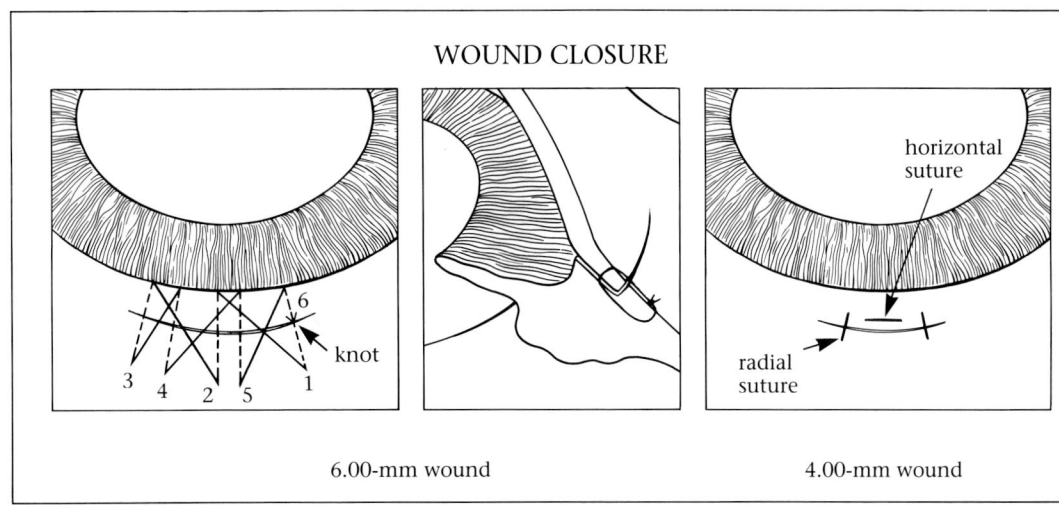

Figure 12.18 *Wound closure technique depends on wound length.*

Clinical Points to Consider

☞ The patient's preoperative corneal astigmatism should determine the location and length of the phacoemulsification incision.

☞ Proper operating room setup and patient position and fixation of the globe so it tilts away from the surgeon are necessary for successful phacoemulsification.

☞ The phaco surgeon should be able to easily prolapse the nucleus and perform iris plane phaco if problems occur during in-the-bag phaco.

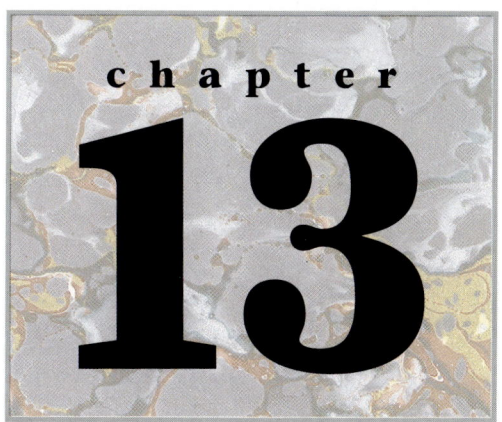

Cataract Removal by Phacoemulsification

JAMES A. DAVISON, M.D.

Within a short span of time in the mid 1980s, several lectures on the process now known as capsulorhexis (Fig. 13.1) were presented by Cal Fercho, M.D., Howard Gimbel, M.D., John Graether, M.D., and Thomas Neuhann, M.D. These experienced surgeons, whose findings were subsequently published, realized the advantages of performing phacoemulsification completely within the capsular bag as well as how an architecturally perfect capsular bag (Fig. 13.2) benefits intraocular lens (IOL) fixation and centration.

Although these surgeons were able to emulsify the nucleus within the capsular bag using a can-opener capsulotomy, they were often frustrated by anterior capsular radial tears. To create a stronger anterior capsular edge that would resist the troublesome tear extensions and eliminate anterior capsular remnants, they tried various methods, including thermal capsule-cutting cautery. Clearly, there was a need to develop a way to preserve an intact anterior capsular remnant consistently during and after phacoemulsification. Some surgeons who performed planned extracapsular cataract extraction (ECCE) also realized the importance of an intact capsular bag, although nucleus expression necessarily disrupted the structural integrity of the capsular bag.

The capsular bag had been traditionally, if rather loosely, defined as whatever capsular structure remained for possible IOL fixation after ECCE, regardless of type. With the introduction of capsulorhexis, this definition was refined and expanded to include the symmetrical capsular structure that remained after partial anterior capsulectomy by continuous tear circular capsulotomy. The new emulsification process, involving an inferior nuclear attack within the architecturally improved capsular bag after a smooth, small central anterior capsulectomy, has become known as capsular bag phacoemulsification, a form of *in situ* phacoemulsification.

Even earlier, T. Hara, M.D., and T. Hara, M.D., were carrying out important pioneering work, developing subcapsular and intracapsular phacoemulsification. Gindi and colleagues had described an endocapsular surgical technique in elegant photographic detail. In most early endophacoemulsification techniques, the cataract was emulsified within a relatively intact lens capsule. Only a small entry perforation, a true capsulotomy, was made in the most supero-anterior capsule, and no anterior capsulectomy was performed. Other methods employed a small superior anterior capsulectomy. The central anterior capsule was retained during emulsification and, depending on the technique, perhaps left intact after IOL insertion. Pars plana techniques of endocapsular surgery had also been pioneered by Girard, Wilson, and Parel but were never commonly used by the cataract/IOL surgeon.

As of the late 1980s, the popular term *endophacoemulsification* not only referred to a specific surgical technique performed through a small capsular *puncture* but also served as a designation for a number of other phacoemulsification techniques. Actually, only a micropuncture technique should be regarded as true endophacoemulsification. Phaco accomplished under an anterior capsular flap after a small superior anterior *capsulotomy* (intercapsular phacoemulsification) and surgery within the capsular bag after a small central anterior *capsulectomy* (capsular-bag phacoemulsification)

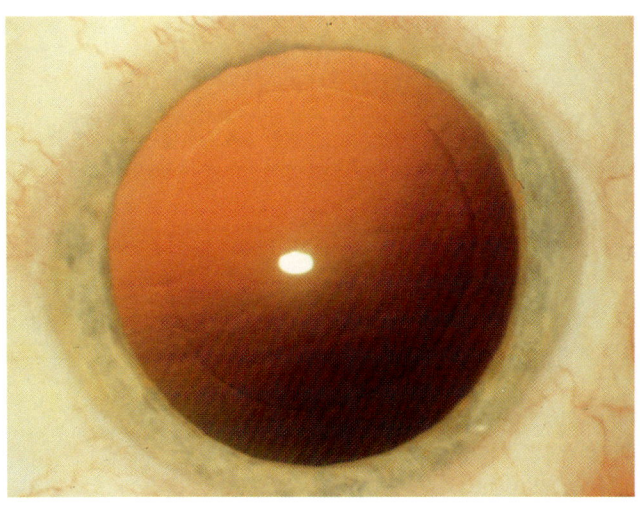

Figure 13.1 *Capsulorhexis anterior capsulotomy as performed by Thomas Neuhann, M.D. Note the perfect circular nature of the capsulorhexis opening.*

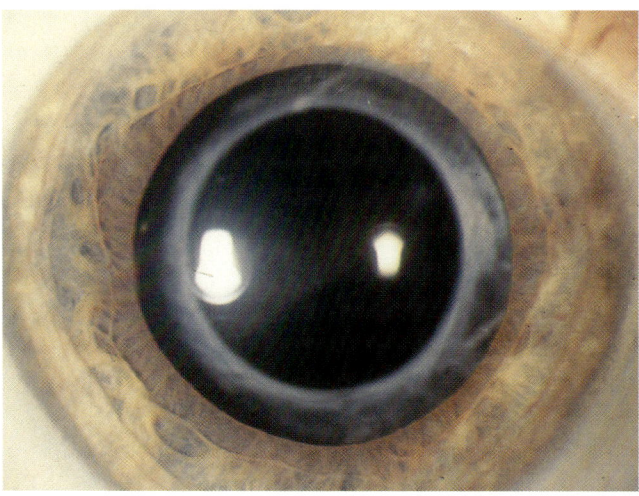

Figure 13.2 *A perfect capsulorhexis opening embraces and centers a posterior chamber lens.*

Table 13.3
Location Specific
Phacoemulsification Techniques

I. Anterior chamber—nucleus prolapsed entirely into anterior chamber

II. Iris plane—superior pole of nucleus prolapsed slightly above iris plane (includes minimal-lift technique)

III. In situ
  A. Capsular bag—central anterior capsulectomy before phacoemulsification
  B. Intercapsular—central anterior capsulectomy after phacoemulsification or no anterior capsulectomy
  C. Pars plana approach—equatorial capsulotomy
  D. Endocapsular—micropuncture of anterior capsule

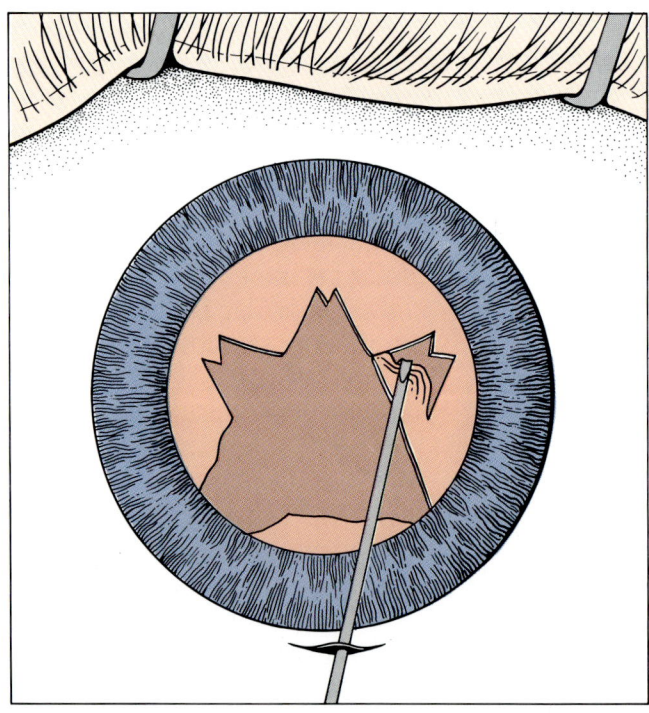

Figure 13.4 *Smaller tears are used to expand the anterior capsular defect to make anterior chamber nuclear prolapse possible.*

should be considered as subcategories of in situ phaco; that is, phaco is accomplished within the capsular bag but the lens capsule has been substantially altered by the surgical process.

Two other location-specific phacoemulsification procedures—anterior chamber and iris plane phacoemulsification—already existed when these new forms of in situ phacoemulsification emerged (Table 13.3). These firmly established methods required relocation of the nucleus either into the anterior chamber or to the iris plane for the emulsification process.

The earlier phaco techniques, anterior chamber phacoemulsification and iris plane phacoemulsification, require a large anterior capsulectomy. This allows for partial or complete prolapse of the nucleus from the capsular bag, which permits manipulation of the nucleus into a relatively safe place for exposure to the phacoemulsification tip. These large capsulectomies are created by connecting a series of fairly large multiple peripheral capsulotomy tears (Figs. 13.4 to 13.8). Any remaining anterior capsular flap tissue is usually viewed as an obstacle and an inconvenience. An

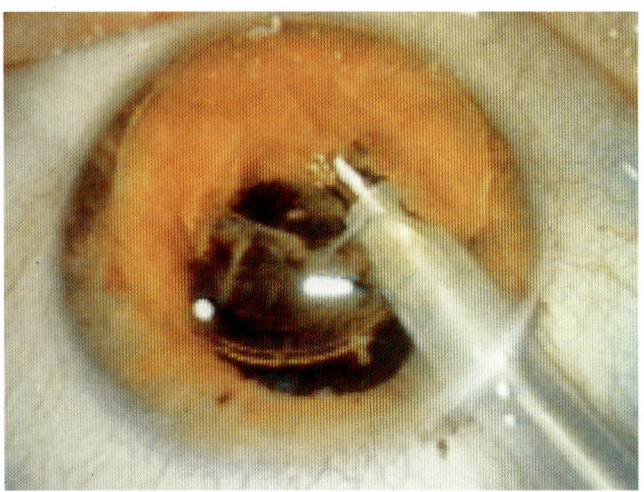

Figure 13.5 *The large anterior capsulotomy allows nuclear prolapse so phacoemulsification can be efficiently accomplished in the anterior chamber.*

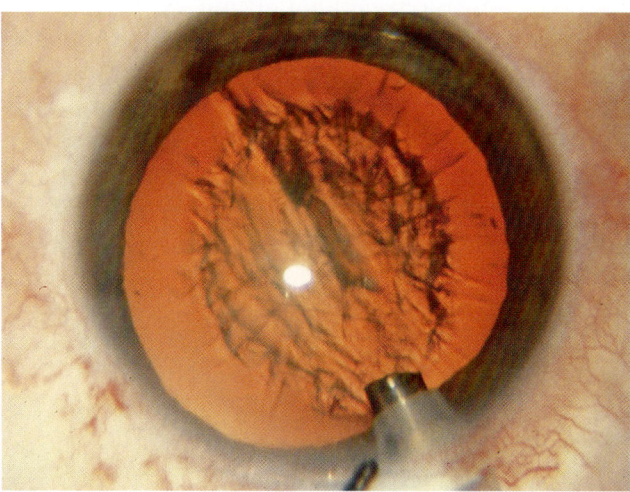

Figure 13.6 *Multiple tear can-opener anterior capsulotomy comprised of 35 to 50 small tears. For a minimal-lift technique, the capsulotomy is smaller than that traditionally recommended for the classic iris plane method, is slightly oval, and will leave more generous anterior capsular flaps.*

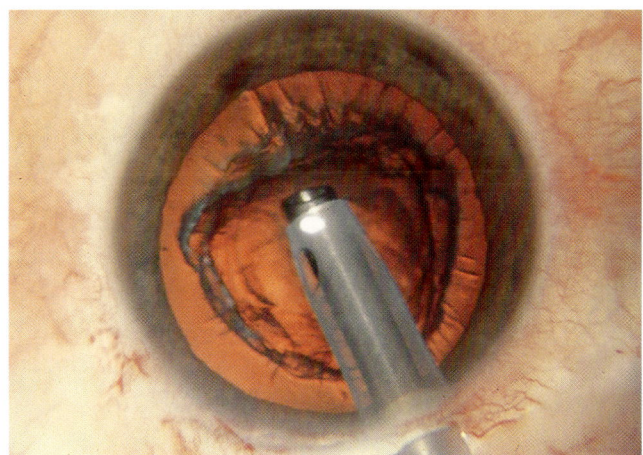

Figure 13.7 *Central sculpting is accomplished with the 15-degree phacoemulsification tip.*

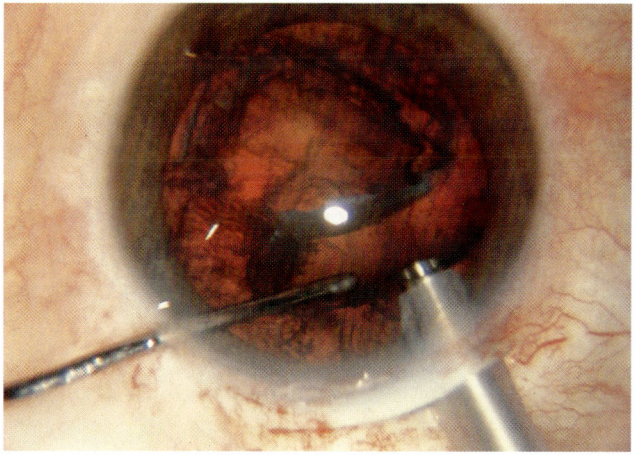

Figure 13.8 *After the anterior peripheral superior rim is emulsified, the nucleus is allowed to drop back. It is rotated by the cyclodialysis spatula so about two or three new clock hours of nuclear rim are presented to the phaco tip access zone superiorly. The prolapse maneuver is repeated so the new superior pole will present itself just as it had initially. Emulsification proceeds, exposing new rim tissue with each rotation.*

intact capsular bag is not important in anterior chamber IOL implantation, nor when a posterior chamber IOL is placed in the ciliary sulcus. In ciliary sulcus fixation, the posterior capsule is only needed to help stabilize the IOL and keep it from falling posteriorly. Remaining anterior tissue may actually contribute to asymmetric bag-sulcus haptic positioning and IOL decentration. A large capsulectomy provides good access for phacoemulsification, but any hope of a structurally competent, three-dimensional capsular bag is sacrificed during nuclear prolapse.

Another group of techniques is transitional in both an evolutionary and anatomic sense. For the most part, phacoemulsification was accomplished within the capsular bag, but the anterior capsule was still torn in many cases when the nucleus was manipulated. This manipulation was less than the complete relocation (prolapse) of the nucleus into the anterior chamber dictated by the earlier methods of phacoemulsification, but it was more than that required by the newer in situ techniques.

Surgeons who desired capsular bag fixation of IOLs but did not know about capsulorhexis, practiced transitional phacoemulsification techniques. The minimal-lift bimanual technique, a modification of the iris plane method, and the more advanced roundel technique, which attacks the 6 o'clock position of the nucleus, are good examples (Fig. 13.9). The anterior capsulotomy techniques used for the roundel and minimal lift have two points in common: the anterior capsulectomies are small (about 5.50 mm in diameter) and comprised of relatively central, very small, multiple capsulotomy tears (Figs. 13.10 and 13.11).

These transitional phaco techniques were an improvement over the earlier methods, but they were imperfect. The objective of performing phacoemulsification entirely within the capsular bag was largely, but not entirely, accomplished, i.e., the maintenance of a perfect capsular bag was not uniformly achieved since single or multiple anterior capsular radial tears developed frequently with either method. These tears occurred superi-

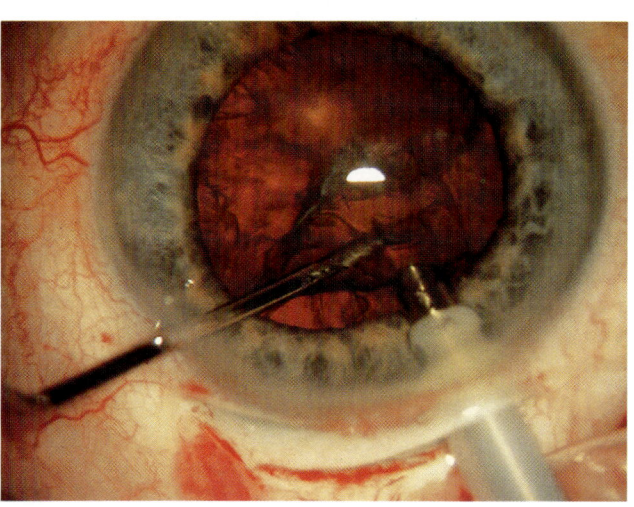

Figure 13.9 *Peripheral nuclear thinning while being only slightly elevated is the hallmark of the minimal-left method.*

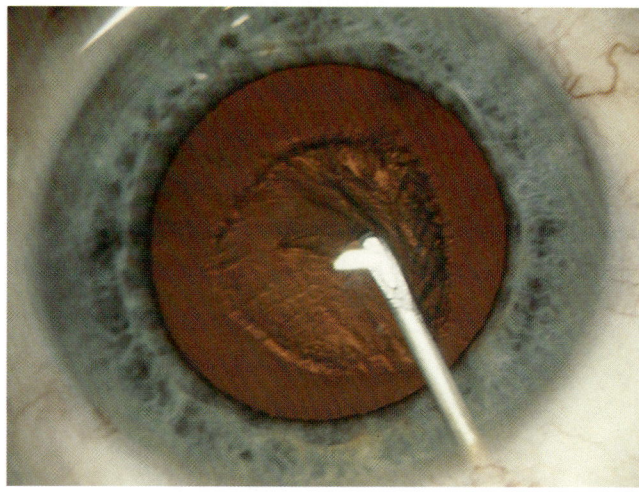

Figure 13.10 *A 5.50 mm slightly eccentric, but basically round, anterior capsulotomy.*

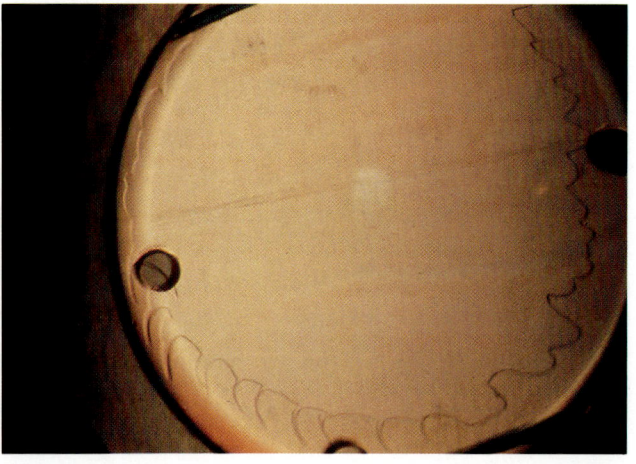

Figure 13.11 *Anterior capsulotomy featured in the roundel phaco technique of T. Hara, M.D. Note that even though the capsulotomy consists of a multiple tear pattern, no anterior radial equatorial tears exist.*

orly as a result of the minimal-lift method because this procedure requires attack of the superior nuclear rim (Figs. 13.12 and 13.13). The tears occurred inferiorly with the roundel technique because of inferior nuclear attack as an initiating component of nuclear rim debulking and removal (Fig. 13.14). These capsular bag configurations led to fairly stable and relatively symmetrical capsular bag fixation (Fig. 13.15), but even with appropriate positioning, a trend persisted toward

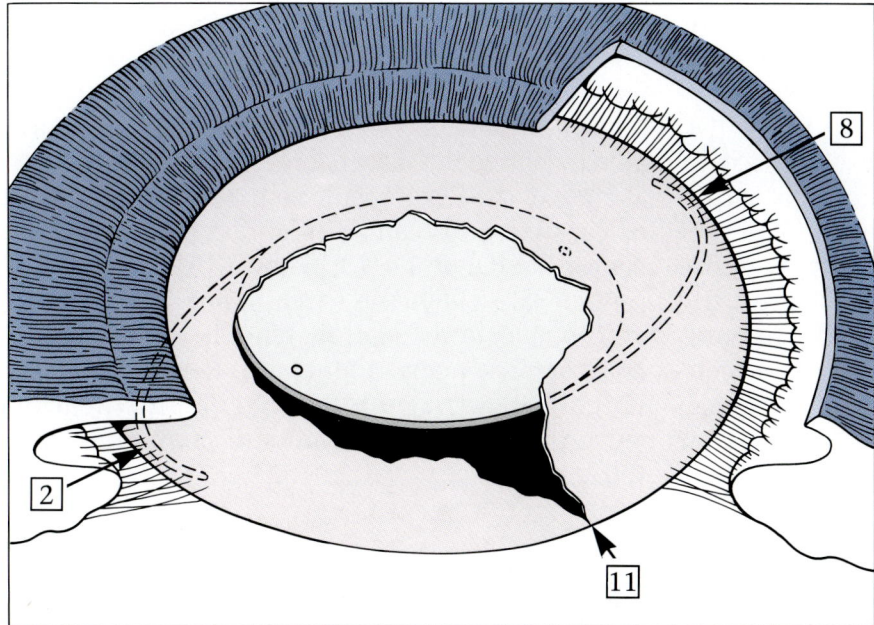

Figure 13.12 *A modified J-loop IOL is placed with loops positioned 90 degrees away from the tear at the 11 o'clock position and contained within the 2 o'clock and 8 o'clock capsular bag positions.*

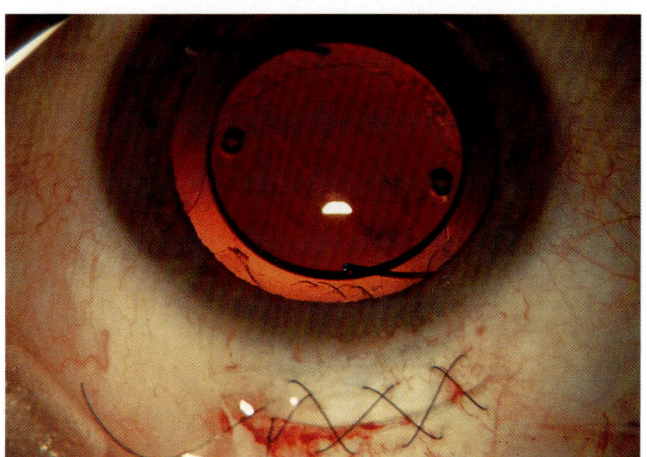

Figure 13.13 *Anterior radial tears at 11 o'clock and 2 o'clock positions.*

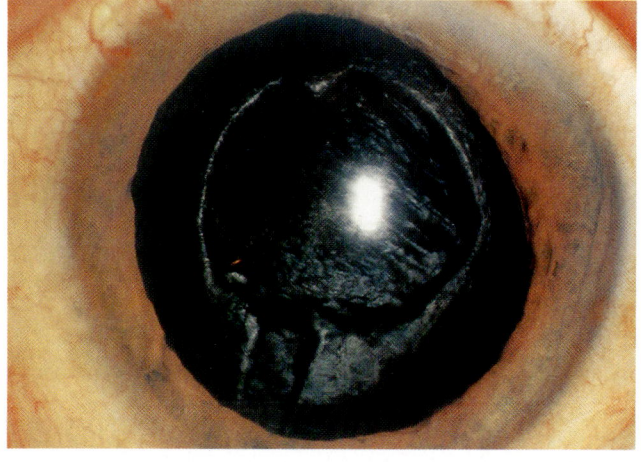

Figure 13.14 *A single anterior capsular radial tear has occurred inferiorly in the roundel phacoemulsification technique.*

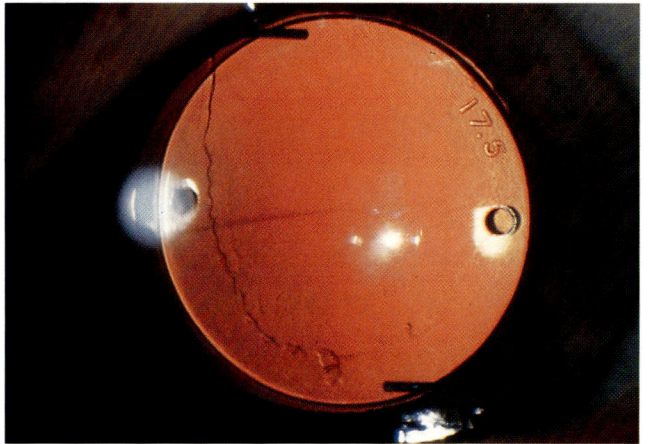

Figure 13.15 *Anterior radial tear present at the 11 o'clock position, but the IOL is well centered and contained within the capsular bag.*

minor, usually subclinical, late optic decentration toward the anterior capsular defect (Fig. 13.16).

Some of the transitional phacoemulsification surgeons shared a problem similar to that of their colleagues who employed nucleus expression; they practiced *mismatch* phacoemulsification IOL implantation, and there were many of us who unknowingly practiced this transitional technique. David Apple, M.D., and colleagues have shown in their pioneering clinicopathologic studies that the most common problem in ECCE IOL surgery may result from the surgeon mismatching one of the two classical large anterior capsulotomy phacoemulsification methods or one of the nucleus expression techniques with the desire for capsular bag IOL fixation. Many times the result of this mismatching is asymmetric bag-sulcus haptic placement and resultant optic decentration. IOL haptic knees are placed under small anterior capsular flap remnants that remain after doing procedures requiring large anterior capsulectomies and nucleus prolapse. Oversized rigid IOLs with posterior optic angulation contribute to the tendency for anterior capsular flap remnants to unfold, allowing the haptic knee to escape into the ciliary sulcus. Sometimes the unfolding is incomplete, and the knee migrates toward the sulcus while the peripheral haptic is still contained by the partially unfolded flap (Fig. 13.17). Some of these decentration problems were solved by the long C-shaped haptic IOL design of William Simcoe, M.D. These haptics are able to bridge the defects created in the equatorial zone of the lens capsule so that adjacent anterior capsular flaps can be recruited to support and center the IOL (Figs. 13.18 and 13.19).

As of late 1989, the three major location-specific phacoemulsification schools were anterior chamber, iris plane, and in situ. Most of the individualized variations of phacoemulsification within these categories are still commonly used today.

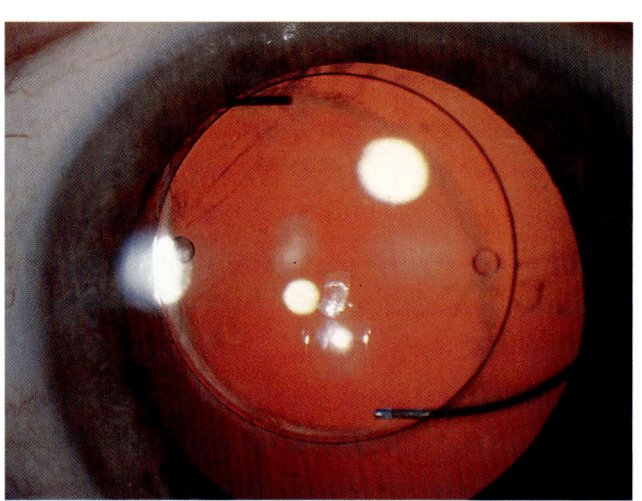

Figure 13.16 *The IOL optic is decentered 1.00 mm to 1.50 mm superiorly despite haptic location within the capsular bag. Subtle superior optic migration is not infrequent with a superior anterior capsular radial tear, but it is clinically acceptable in most circumstances.*

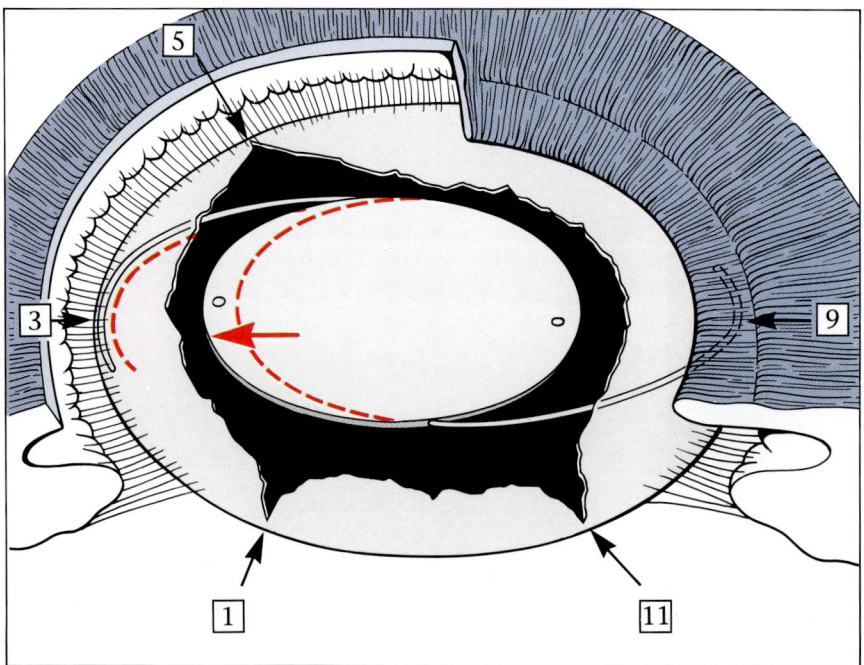

Figure 13.17 *Anterior radial tears exist at the 11 o'clock, 1 o'clock, and 5 o'clock positions. There is no symmetrical support for the modified J-loop IOL within what is left of the capsular bag. The optic will ultimately decenter toward the 3 o'clock position because of the asymmetrical capsular support.*

In Situ Phacoemulsification

Many different forms of in situ phacoemulsification have evolved subsequent to capsulorhexis. The almost innumerable variations fall into one of the two previously mentioned subcategories—capsular bag or intercapsular phacoemulsification—depending on the disposition of the anterior capsule.

Capsular Bag Phacoemulsification

In capsular bag phacoemulsification strategy, the final optical anterior capsulectomy is created by capsulorhexis before phacoemulsification is accomplished entirely within the capsular bag. The nucleus is removed by dividing it into smaller components. This removal involves a physical separation of the nuclear fibers that comprise the posterior central and peripheral nuclear plate. Separation is accomplished either through folding over and fracturing the deep midperipheral nuclear plate by suction of the peripheral anterior nuclear remnant or through bimanual separation of the entire nuclear bowl into quarters or smaller pieces. Separation of the nuclear fibers created by either method results in a fracture-like appearance in the full thickness of the deep nuclear plate. Howard Gimbel, M.D., and John Shepherd, M.D., were the first to introduce and popularize bimanual posterior central nuclear separation techniques. Gimbel's popular divide-and-conquer endolenticular surgery and Shepherd's in situ

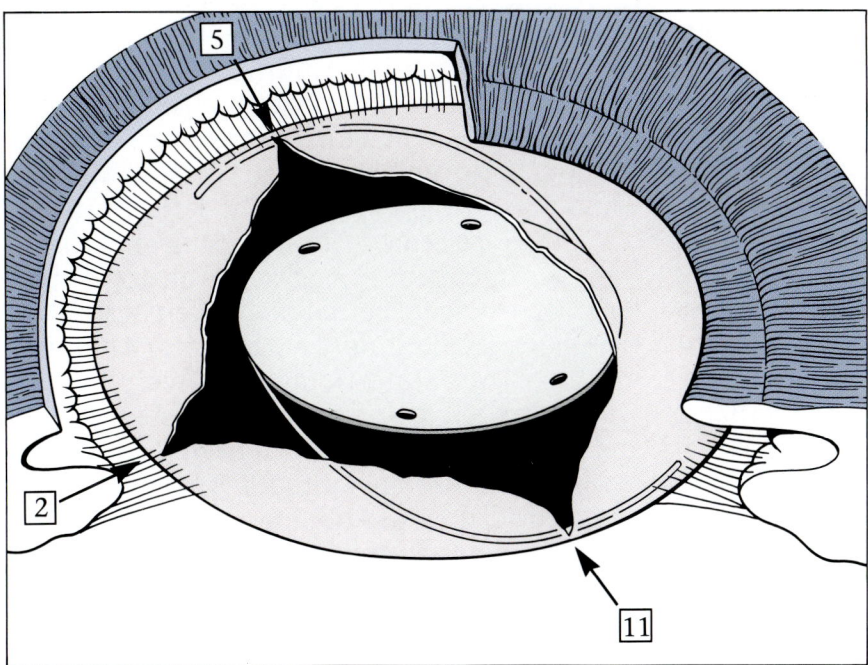

Figure 13.18 *The long loops of the Simcoe style lens bridge the anterior radial defects present in the equatorial zone and use adjacent anterior capsular structures to provide stable fixation for the IOL optic.*

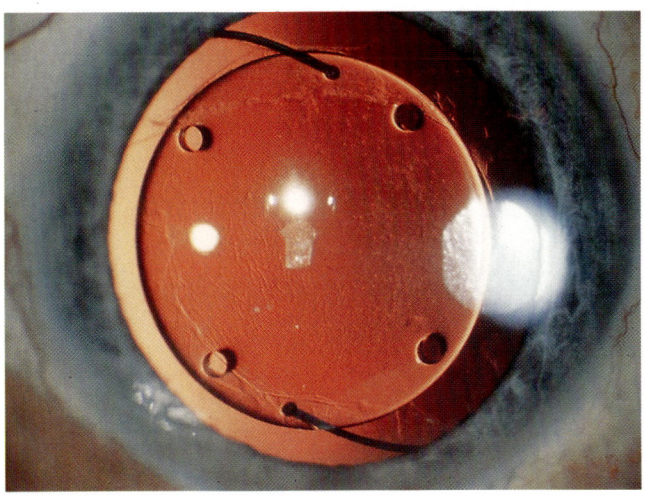

Figure 13.19 *Clinical photograph of Simcoe style IOL in place within the capsular bag with two anterior radial tears present at the 10 o'clock and 5 o'clock positions.*

fracture surgery are the basis for subsequent derivations of this technique (Figs. 13.20 and 13.21).

Phacoemulsification within the capsular bag is my preferred technique (I use it for almost 100% of my cases), and it will be analyzed in this chapter. This efficient, very safe technique is appealing for two reasons. First, there is the relative physical containment of a safe, bimanual emulsification process. Second, a relatively inert, architecturally perfect, three-dimensional capsular envelope is preserved, which facilitates placement of the IOL. The traditional capsular complications (posterior rupture or anterior radial tear) are now extremely rare.

Intercapsular Phacoemulsification

In intercapsular phacoemulsification, a small superior anterior capsulectomy or capsulotomy is created and the lens emulsified between the anterior and posterior capsules (Fig. 13.22). The final optical anterior capsulectomy may or may not be created at some point after phacoemulsification (Figs. 13.23 and 13.24).

The physical barrier effect offered by emulsification under the anterior capsule may be advantageous in cases of zonular trauma and vitreous in the anterior chamber. However, single-instrument intercapsular techniques, at least in my experience, seem to be more difficult than two-handed surgical methods. Further, endothelial cell survival after intercapsular phaco has not been shown to be superior to that following capsular bag techniques that employ a 5.50 mm capsulorhexis. In its current evolutionary state, the two most apparent and frequent disadvantages of intercapsular phacoemulsification are posterior capsular rupture and anterior radial capsular tears that extend into the capsular bag equatorial zone.

Anatomic Considerations

Several special circumstances lend themselves to cataract removal by the minimal-lift superior nuclear rim prolapse technique. With a minimal-lift technique, suction is applied at the superior nuclear rim from the outside in so that peripheral capsular aspiration is less likely to occur. This minimal-lift technique should be used if extensive inferior zonular weakness exists (e.g., post-trauma). Extreme cases of pseudoexfoliation or advanced age can cause surprising general zonular laxity. In such a case, if the cataract is 3+ to 4+ brownish hard, I feel that it is simply safer and more efficient to fall back on the minimal-lift superior nuclear prolapse technique.

Phacoemulsification within the capsular bag is by definition ultrasonic dissection and removal of the lens nucleus in situ. The purpose of the dissection is to remove the cataractous nucleus while preserving a structurally perfect capsular bag for IOL placement. To accomplish this dissection, it is important to analyze the anatomy of the lens; that is, conceptualize the lens as having three vertical zones within its 4.00 mm height—thin superficial, relatively thicker (approximately two-thirds thickness) midlevel, and thin deep—with all three having central and peripheral horizontal latitudes. The great advantage provided by positioning nuclear fragments for phacoemulsification not only centrally in the X and Y planes but also in a central location vertically *within* the capsular bag is very appealing.

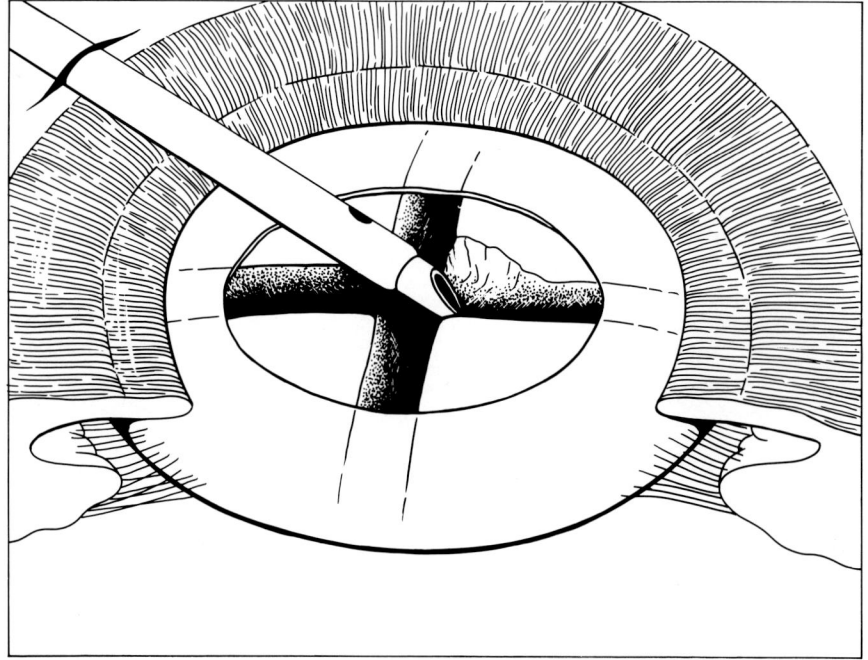

Figure 13.20 *In situ phacoemulsification method of John Shepherd, M.D. The peripheral nucleus is divided into four segments, and the surgeon may choose to emulsify either inferior nuclear quadrant.*

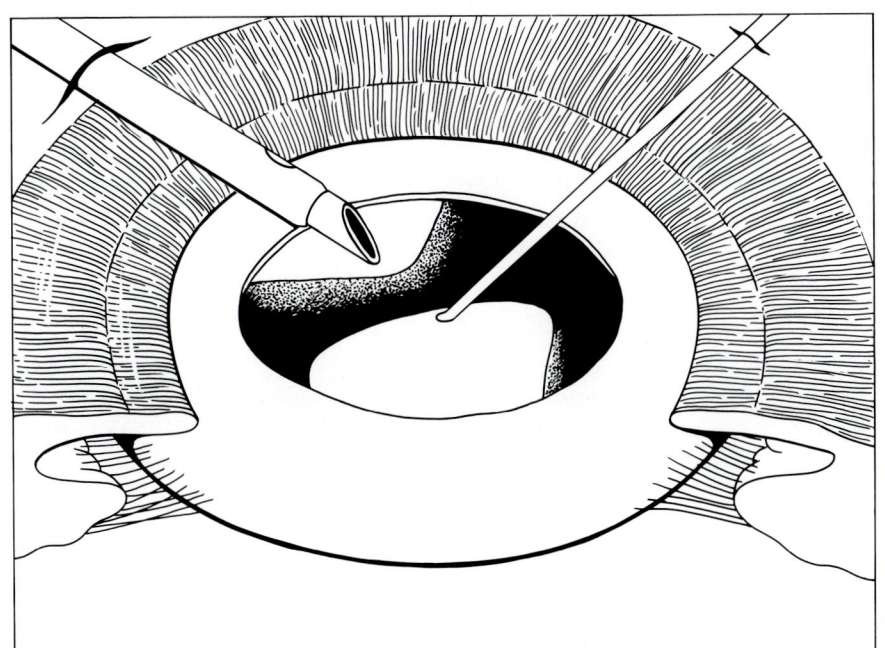

Figure 13.21 *After the inferior nuclear segment is withdrawn, the two superior ones can be rotated into an accessible inferior position.*

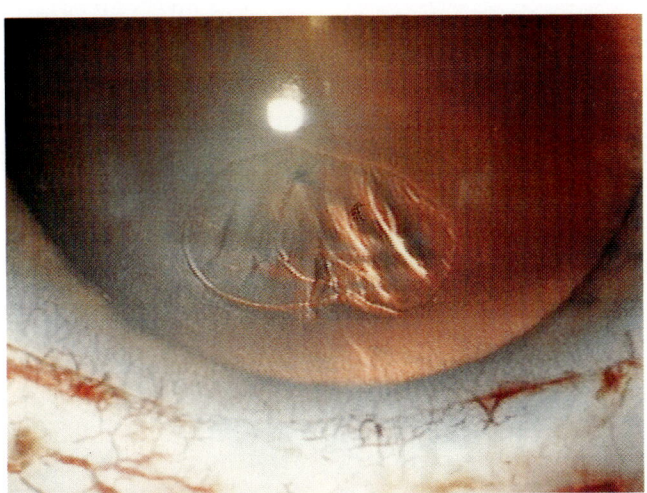

Figure 13.22 *A small eccentric continuous tear anterior capsulotomy provides nuclear access during intercapsular cataract extraction but has less tendency for anterior radial tear extension than a straight line or hatch mark capsulotomy. Linear capsulotomies tend to allow anterior radial tear extensions to the equator, but continuous tears, even when ovoid, resist such extensions.*

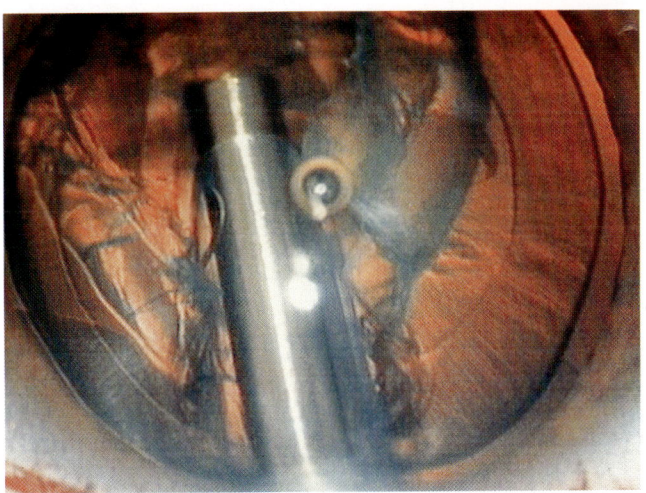

Figure 13.23 *The zones of nuclear hydrodissection are particularly visible as nucleus removal progresses in intercapsular phacoemulsification. It is particularly important that the posterior nucleus be held amply above the posterior capsular surface because neither the phacoemulsification tip aperture nor its furthest posterior projection are visible.*

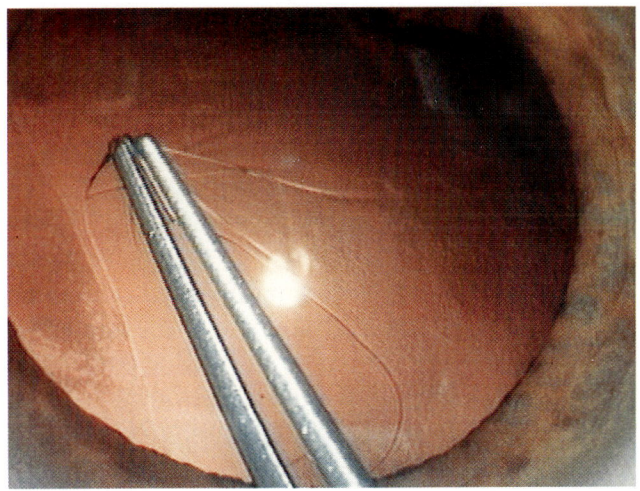

Figure 13.24 *After nucleus and cortex removal, an optical anterior capsulotomy can be performed as an extension of the original mini-capsulorhexis. Although not perfectly circular, the final capsulorhexis opening will result in excellent capsular bag fixation while protecting the corneal endothelium from direct emulsification energy.*

The previously mentioned techniques of anterior chamber phaco and nuclear prolapse in iris plane phaco rely on substantial three-dimensional movement and manipulation of the entire nucleus, enabling the phaco tip to remain relatively stationary at or above the iris plane, as new sections of nucleus are repeatedly presented to it. Nuclear material is removed by driving the phaco tip through the presenting nuclear material. The superficial, midlevel, and deep peripheral portions of the lens are presented to the tip by vertical nucleus relocation and manipulation.

In some of the in situ phacoemulsification techniques (intercapsular or true endocapsular), a second instrument cannot help control the lens or lens fragments in a more central position away from the posterior capsule.

Principles of Phacoemulsification

To successfully employ any of the strategies for ultrasonic dissection of the nucleus within the capsular bag, three basic phacoemulsification principles must be applied in a meticulously detailed fashion.

I. Tip Function Isolation. The tip has three application modes: manipulation, cutting, and suction (aspiration).

In the manipulation mode, the tip is used simply as an instrument to push, pull, or move the nucleus or nuclear fragments. Using the cyclodialysis spatula in the opposite hand, the lens nucleus can be rotated or the posterior fibers separated, resulting in the desired fracture in the posterior nuclear bowl.

In the cutting mode, nuclear material is shaved away but the phacoemulsification tip is not permitted to become occluded. With a 45-degree tip, material can be shaved relatively close to the capsule. This tip design lessens the danger of drawing the capsule in with uncontrolled occlusion and aspiration because the cutting action occurs only at the end and forward edges of the tip while aspiration of particulate dust occurs away from it. On the other hand, efficient simultaneous phaco and aspiration of a large nuclear fragment is possible only when the aperture of the phaco tip is at least partially occluded. Thus, cutting and suction are isolated by the design of the phacoemulsification tip and the operative manipulations.

In the suction mode, the phacoemulsification tip is deliberately occluded by nuclear material. When occlusion occurs, vacuum starts to build and becomes an important factor in the progression of the operation. Prior to occlusion, establishment of significant vacuum across the tip aperture does not develop. Notwithstanding emulsification energy, the major operative dynamic principle in the nonoccluded state is aspiration flow. During the cutting process, flow rate is high and vacuum is low. When the tip is occluded, however, the opposite situation is created. Flow rate drops and vacuum builds. Formed nuclear material can then be slowly drawn into the tip. In lenses of any firmness, aspiration of formed material is facilitated by brief taps of the foot pedal to obtain extremely low phaco power, perhaps only 10% to 20% of the maximum. With soft nuclei, almost no emulsification power is needed. Peripheral occluded aspiration efforts generally are not applied when the tip is close to the capsule. Rather, the peripheral material is drawn centrally, not only by slow aspiration but also by a central movement of the tip itself. In this way, peripheral nuclear material can be aspirated when the tip is in a safer central location.

II. Nuclear Division. The nucleus can be divided into more manageable portions for attack by the phaco tip in suction mode. The fracturing process results in multiple nuclear fragments whose central surfaces can be engaged by the suction of the occluded phaco tip. Vacuum creates a temporary adhesion, enabling the fragment to be drawn into a relatively safe central zone in the middle of the capsular bag for emulsification and aspiration. Centralization of the active emulsification and aspiration process is essential in order to safely remove the lens substance through a 5.50 mm opening in the anterior capsule and can be accomplished by bimanual tearing or fracturing of posterior nuclear fibers. Division can also be accomplished by folding over and breaking off peripheral anterior and midlevel nuclear wedges with suction after thinning of the deeper nuclear plate. Bimanual separation works better with most lenses firm enough to prevent a cyclodialysis spatula from easily sinking through the remaining nucleus. Peripheral nuclear collapse and wedge aspiration work well in very soft nuclei.

III. Nuclear Rotation. Inferior nuclear attack is required in all cases since successful, uniform, convenient superior access is denied by the generous intact anterior capsular remnant left after capsulorhexis. The segment of the nucleus to be acted on by the phaco tip is rotated to an inferior position (i.e., below the 3 o'clock to 9 o'clock axis), if not already in that position, regardless of the action desired. Cutting, suction, manipulation, bimanual segmentation (cracking), wedge fracture, and rotation maneuvers involving the phaco tip are all accomplished predominantly in the inferior position.

For successful cataract surgery, these phacoemulsification principles need to be complemented by meticulous capsulorhexis, cortical aspiration, IOL implantation, wound construction, and closure. All cataract removal techniques need optimal operating room equipment setup and assignment of surgical personnel.

Phacoemulsification Surgical Procedure

The purpose of the following sections is to outline the important details of capsular bag phacoemulsification surgical techniques (Table 13.25). Each detail is of critical importance and no step should be taken without the successful completion of the previous one. The surgeon must be obsessed with detail and accuracy; everything from the subtle to the obvious must be appreciated or the operation will be unnecessarily difficult and the risk of failure increased. Understanding the concepts associated with these details helps make capsular bag phacoemulsification an understandable, safe, and efficient surgical procedure.

Setup for Phacoemulsification

A high-quality microscope with a footswitch-operated X-Y adjustment platform and focus-zoom control is essential for capsular bag phacoemulsification. A total power of 10× to 15× is required for capsulorhexis and nucleus dissection. Much of phacoemulsification is done at midlevel magnification because it enables the surgeon to be aware of what is going on at the phaco tip as well as the rest of the posterior chamber. Sometimes higher magnification is needed for capsulorhexis and wound construction. In order to comfortably and efficiently look down slightly at the operative field, most surgeons select a 175-mm objective lens and traditionally angled optics, although this varies among surgeons.

I am six-feet-two-inches tall and have a long back. A 250-mm objective lens plus a microscope ocular capable of variable angle configurations with the ocular accessory mounted upside down enables me to sit tall and comfortably without having to flex my neck or back (Fig. 13.26). While operating, I keep my upper arms at my sides, look straight ahead, and do not hunch over. This upright position allows me to use my arms and hands comfortably. My legs and feet are free to move and operate the foot controls

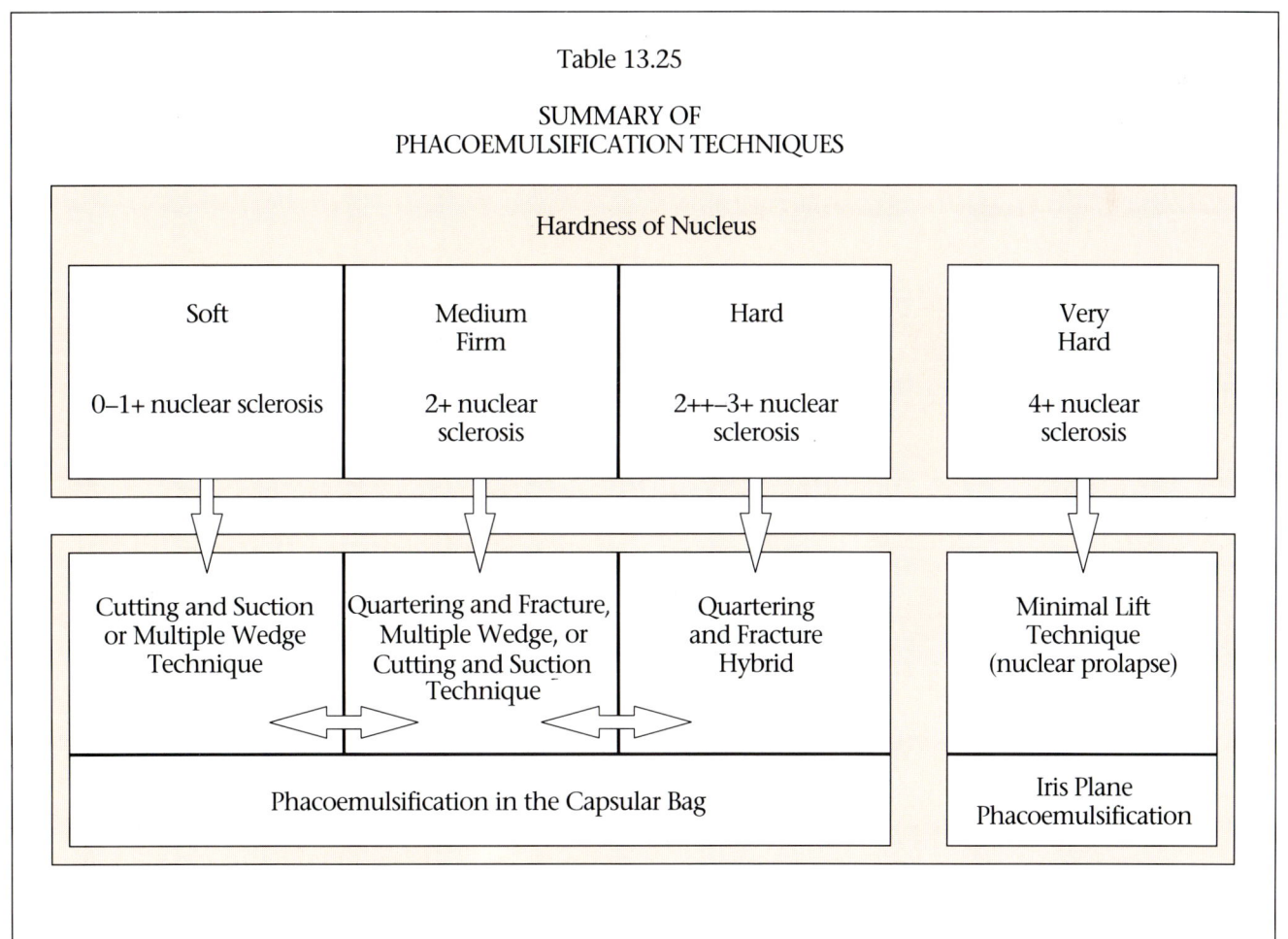

Table 13.25

SUMMARY OF PHACOEMULSIFICATION TECHNIQUES

Hardness of Nucleus			
Soft	Medium Firm	Hard	Very Hard
0–1+ nuclear sclerosis	2+ nuclear sclerosis	2++–3+ nuclear sclerosis	4+ nuclear sclerosis
Cutting and Suction or Multiple Wedge Technique	Quartering and Fracture, Multiple Wedge, or Cutting and Suction Technique	Quartering and Fracture Hybrid	Minimal Lift Technique (nuclear prolapse)
Phacoemulsification in the Capsular Bag			Iris Plane Phacoemulsification

because they are not needed to balance or support my upper body.

A high-quality, reliable phacoemulsification machine with foot switch-operated linear control phacoemulsification and suction is necessary for successful surgery. Linear control is used at all times. The 45-degree ultrasonic tip is ideal for isolating and facilitating the cutting, suction, and manipulation functions. To accomplish these functions safely, I change some of the machine's standard factory preset settings. When using the Alcon Ten Thousand Series machine, I increase the vacuum to 101 mm Hg from 47 mm Hg during phacoemulsification but reduce the flow rate to 17 cc/min versus the preset rate of 25 cc/min. The reduced flow rate has several advantages. The operation proceeds a little slower and in a more controlled fashion, the likelihood of capsular aspiration at the end stages of phacoemulsification is reduced, and diaphragmatic movements of the iris and posterior capsule are not as obvious. The increased vacuum is helpful in sucking formed material into the tip; the tip will become occluded by any firm flat nuclear plate when presented to the aperture, and brief taps of low power emulsification energy will eat into the plate usually without having to further increase the vacuum setting. I prefer the 45-degree tip, although most surgeons who practice capsular bag phacoemulsification use the preset factory settings and a 30-degree tip.

The surgeon should wear tennis shoes or similar footwear because the soft soles heighten awareness of pedal position and facilitate the fine movements

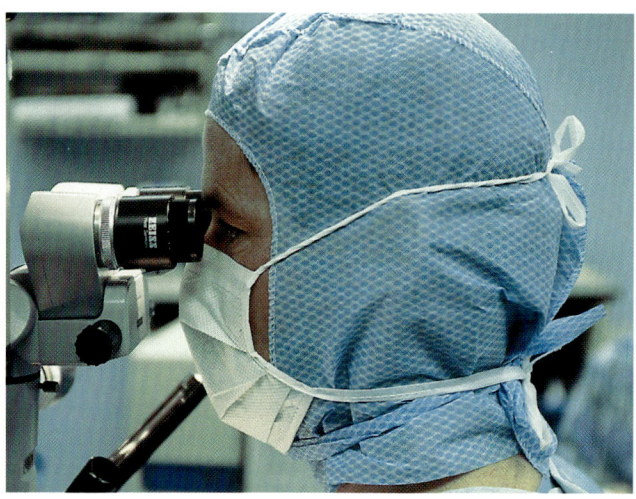

Figure 13.26 *I look straight ahead without flexing my cervical spine. The microscope oculars are mounted upside down so I get a little extra height.*

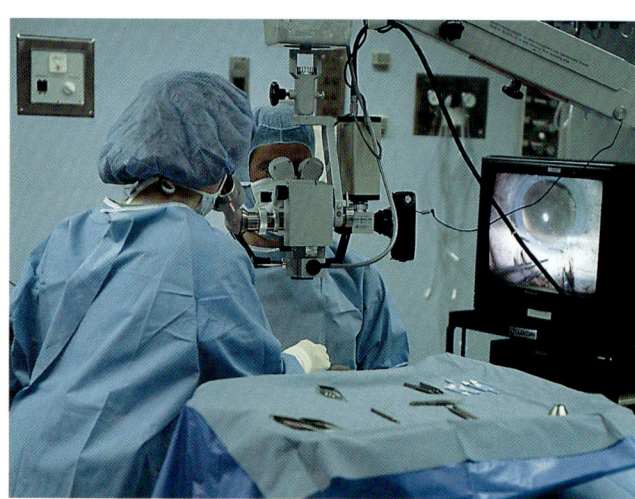

Figure 13.27 *The videomonitor enables the scrub nurse, circulating nurse, and anesthesiologist to have a close-up view of the surgery.*

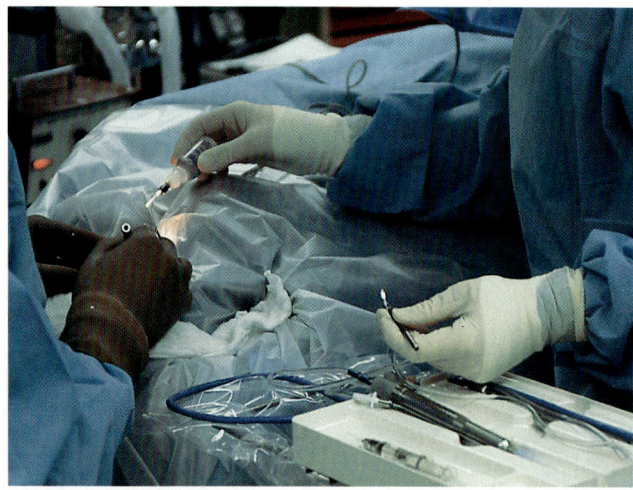

Figure 13.28 *Almost no difference in height exists between the patient's eye and the instrument tray.*

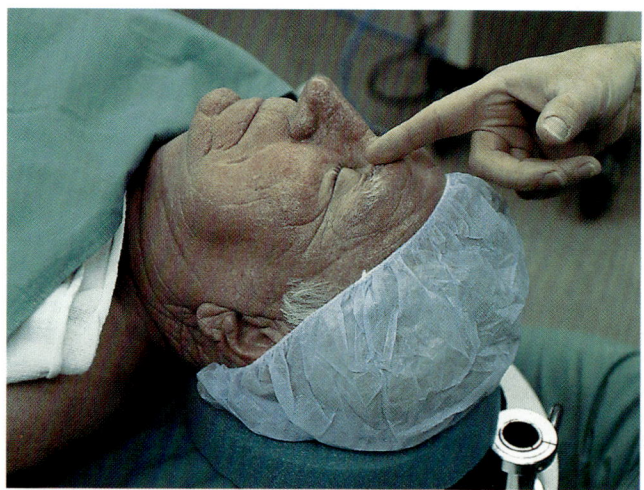

Figure 13.29 *Steep brows may require a slight neck extension for good phaco tip access. Do not overcompensate. It is easier for a patient to extend the neck than to flex it during surgery.*

required for this procedure. I use my right foot for the microscope control rather than for the phacoemulsification foot switch control because I feel it is a more complex function. I usually make about fifty adjustments on the microscope pedal during an operation.

The surgical suite should be arranged so everyone on the surgical team is easily aware of each other. The surgeon, sitting at the head of the table, should be able to communicate with everyone in the room and hear every sound coming from the patient, the phacoemulsification machine, and the surrounding personnel. The surgeon's peripheral vision will help monitor much of the activity. The anesthesiologist or nurse anesthetist should sit at the patient's left so all anesthesia equipment is isolated and independent from the surgical machinery. The scrub nurse should have access to the phacoemulsification machine tray, Mayo stand, and back table. The circulating nurse can perform important machine programming functions while doing required paperwork and being available to bring needed items into the surgical field. A videomonitor facilitates the staff's awareness of the surgical situation (Fig. 13.27).

The patient should be comfortable, with arms and head supported and bladder empty. The operative eye should be at the appropriate level relative to the phacoemulsification machine, as determined by the operator's manual. Calibration of required parameters, such as bottle height and suction, are based on this height. Most settings are calibrated with the eye at the same height as the aspiration pump. All of the machine's programmed parameters must be correct. The accessory instrument tray is usually at the same height as the eye and aspiration pump so instruments can be passed horizontally with no vertical arm movement (Fig. 13.28). The patient should face the ceiling with the neck comfortable. A prominent brow necessitates extending the neck slightly (Fig. 13.29).

Face position is extremely important. Remember, during surgery it is easier for a patient to hyperextend the neck than to flex it. A neck support incorporated into the headrest is of great value. The nonoperative eye is covered with a Fox shield to prevent the drapes inadvertently touching it during surgery. I use a Chan wrist rest with a breathing bar overhead (Fig. 13.30). It keeps the drape off the patient's face and also permits efficient oxygen delivery. The breathing bar is not used if the phaco wound must be placed at the side. The wrist rest is more appropriately called a "water trough." My wrists never touch it, but it keeps BSS from running onto the foot pedals.

A paper drape is positioned before applying the transparent 3M incise plastic drape. The edges of the drape should not cause tissue to bunch centrally toward the eye. It is important to avoid redundancy of skin and drape at the upper lid and brow. To prevent the paper drape from interfering with phacoemulsification tip movement, the nasal edge of the drape should be applied no closer to the operative eye than the midline of the nose, the inferior edge is brought down and applied well away from the inferior orbital rim, and the superior edge is applied above the brow. The phacoemulsification handpiece will actually pivot on the brow and extra draping material will only increase height, awkwardness, and instability. The 3M incise drape is then applied, retracting the lashes and opening the eye. Wetting the cornea

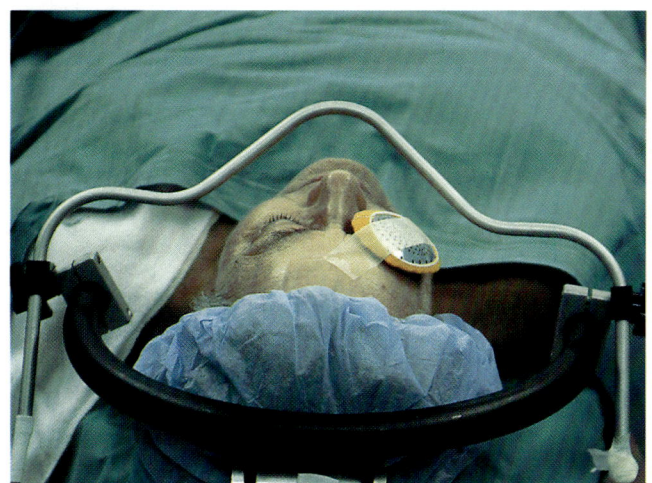

Figure 13.30 *The wrist rest (water trough) is in place with the perforated breathing bar above. The head is turned slightly toward the nonoperative eye, which is covered by a Fox shield.*

just before this step helps prevent corneal abrasions. A horizontal incision is then made in the drape, joined by vertical upper and lower incisions to better conform the drape opening to the intrapalpebral fissure. An open, widened wire speculum (Kratz-Barraquer) is put in place.

Depending on anatomy and exposure, fixation sutures may be placed on the globe above and below, using 4-0 silk with a taper needle. Kirby forceps are used to grasp the rectus muscle insertion so as not to traumatize the levator complex. Inferiorly, the fixation suture may be placed through the insertion of the inferior rectus. The fixation sutures should be placed at these positions to give the globe a slight tilt away from the surgeon to make wound dissection easier. The sutures are stabilized by a small hemostat above and a large Serrafine clip

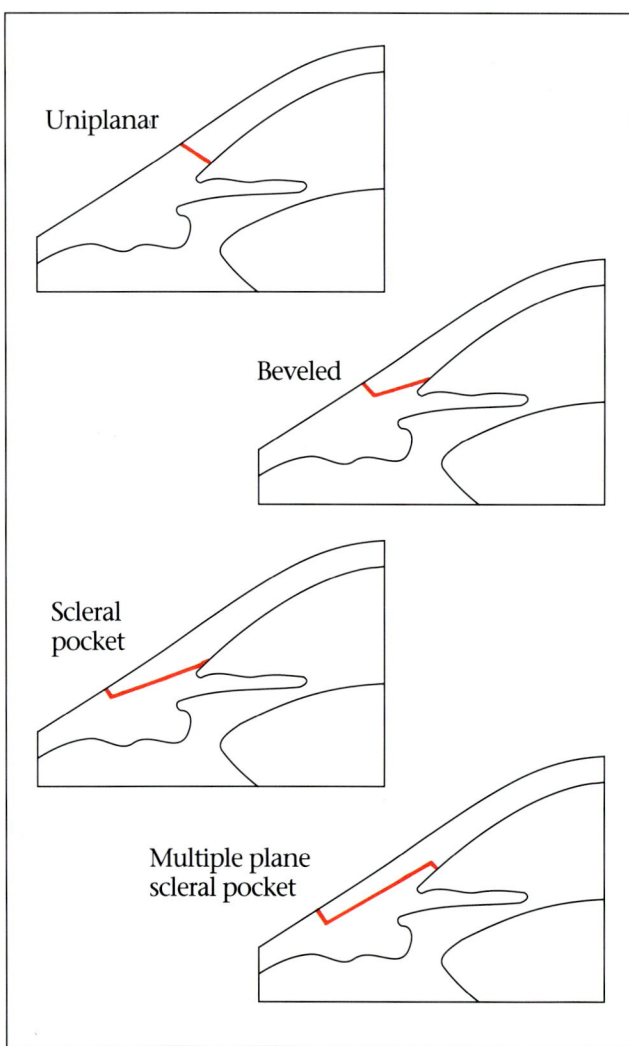

Figure 13.31 *Incision evolution can be traced from the uniplanar corneal incision to the very posterior exaggerated triplanar self-sealing scleral pocket incision. Actually, the extremes depicted are probably never achieved, but this conceptualization may help the surgeon visualize the appropriate planes. The anterior beveled and traditional scleral pocket incisions are intermediate stages in the evolution of phacoemulsification wounds.*

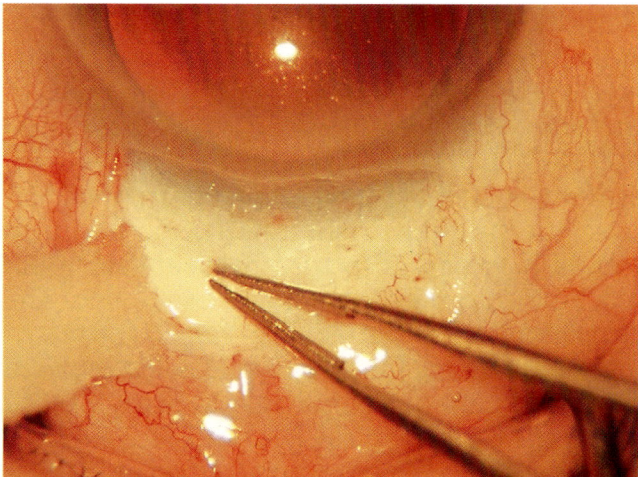

Figure 13.32 *Bipolar cautery is applied lightly to the sclera, tracing the larger vessels, potentially the most troublesome.*

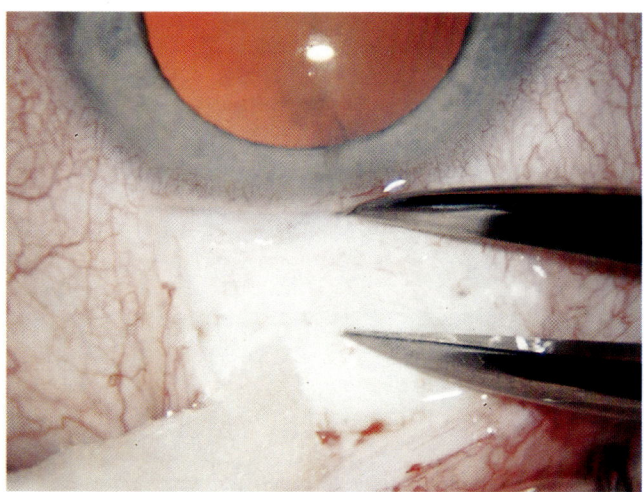

Figure 13.33 *A caliper is set at 3.00 mm and marks the distance of the incision from the conjunctival limbus.*

below. The Serrafine clip is secured to the occlusive plastic drape that is pinched together below the lower lid to create a fixation point. A lap towel is used to soak up BSS.

The phaco machine should be tested and ready, and all other equipment in the room made ready for use.

Wound Construction

Incisions, when viewed through the microscope, appear two-dimensional (Fig. 13.31). Successful phaco/IOL incisions, however, all have a common three-dimensional pattern, i.e., there are three distinct surgical planes created. The surgeon is actually constructing a wound as opposed to making an incision.

The importance of a perfect wound cannot be overstated. It is the gateway to the entire operation. A well-constructed wound can be closed by virtually any method, including without sutures, with good results. A poorly constructed wound, regardless of how well it is closed, can be the source of astigmatism, filtration, irritation, hemorrhage, corneal trauma, iris trauma, or worse.

A scleral pocket incision is less likely to create irritation and induce astigmatism than more anterior incisions. Properly accomplished, the modern triplanar scleral pocket incision is virtually self-sealing, retains aqueous in the anterior chamber and rejects blood that may seep from the peripheral portions of the incisions, and is distant enough from the visual axis so as not to induce significant early or allow late keratometric astigmatism. Innumerable personal variations in this incision pattern exist.

A fornix-based conjunctival miniflap is created. A very light wetfield cautery is applied to blanch most of the surface and deeper vessels. Tracing the larger vessels with the cautery is more efficient and less destructive to tissue than sweeping from side to side (Fig. 13.32). Excessive cautery is avoided.

I find that for 6.00 mm biconvex optics, a straight measured incision of 5.50 mm is adequate. There is possibly some scleral fiber compression and perhaps even disruption of the wound extremes, but this caliper setting is sufficient. I find that I must set it on 4.00 mm to obtain an adequate folded silicone IOL incision. To improve exposure and stabilization, the eye may be grasped at 3 o'clock and 9 o'clock with a Penn Anderson forceps, although this is usually not necessary. A caliper is used to mark the distance of the incision from the anterior aspect of the limbus, 3.00 mm (Fig. 13.33). It is important to measure this distance each time because there is a tendency for "corneal creep" to occur with scleral incisions.

A No. 57 Beaver blade is positioned at a right angle to the sclera. The incision is started by drawing a straight line 3.00 mm from the limbus. Very little pressure is used during this initial scratch, which penetrates the sclera to approximately one-third depth. The appropriate incision length is confirmed (Fig. 13.34). The incision is deepened to two-thirds depth with the blade, which is still held at a right angle to the sclera. The angle of the blade is then changed slightly (Fig. 13.35). The blade is pushed toward the cornea, not drawn as before. This helps establish

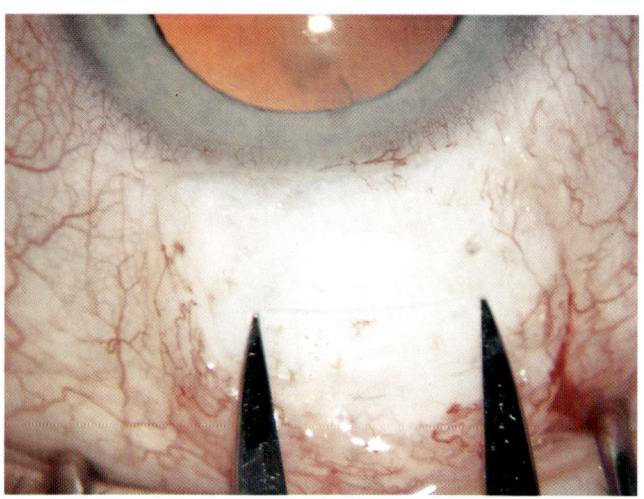

Figure 13.34 *The caliper confirms that the scleral incision is 5.50 mm long.*

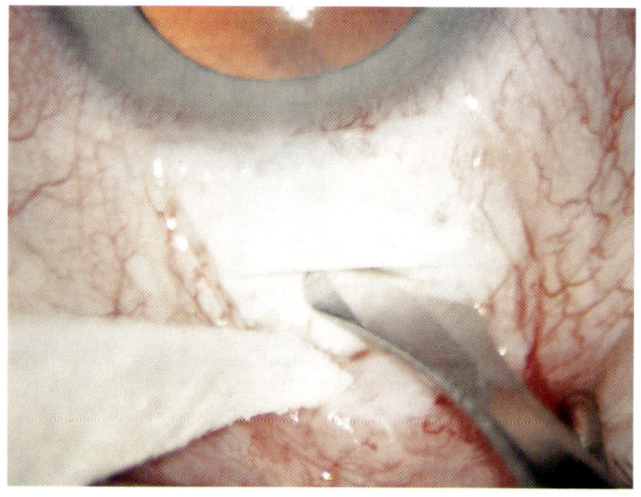

Figure 13.35 *Scleral dissection proceeds with the No. 57 Beaver blade under direct visualization. The sclera is carefully grooved to at least half thickness depth and then just a little bit more.*

the appropriate plane for the bed of the incision. The depth of the incision and the thickness of the flap should be monitored frequently as the blade starts to elevate scleral fibers.

The incision is carried forward for about 0.50 mm to 1.00 mm by the No. 57 blade at approximately two-thirds to one-half depth (Fig. 13.36). Actually, the depth usually shallows to one-half. A thin flap may develop if attention to accurate depth is not focused during these initial steps. An Alcon crescent knife or an angled Grieshaber round blade is then used to dissect further forward in the sclera. This blade engages the advancing dissection plane where the No. 57 blade stopped (Fig. 13.37). A slight lifting motion is used in an attempt to make the incision a little shallower when dissecting forward with this blade. This shallowing is needed, in part, because the radius of curvature of the cornea is shorter than that of the sclera, with the transition occurring at the limbus. Frequent drying (Fig. 13.38) of the sclera facilitates visualization.

By the time the edge of the blade can be seen emerging into clear cornea at the limbal vascular

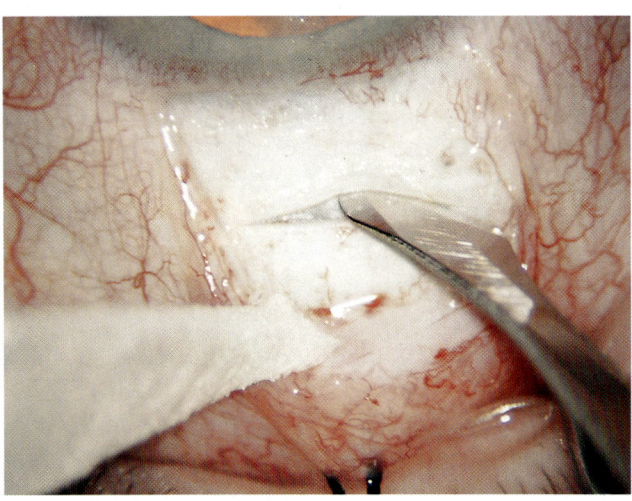

Figure 13.36 *The angle of the No. 57 Beaver blade is changed slightly. The blade is pushed forward toward the cornea, dissecting scleral fibers in almost blunt fashion.*

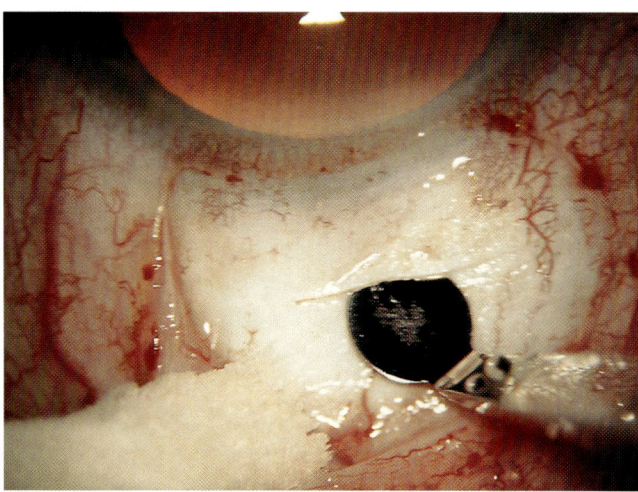

Figure 13.37 *The round blade continues the established incisional plane.*

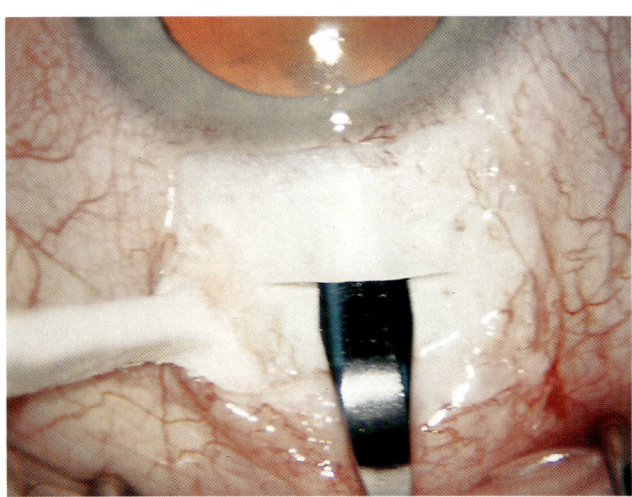

Figure 13.38 *The depth of the scleral dissection can be monitored more accurately by frequently looking at the scleral fibers and the wound after they have been dried while the blade is lifted slightly, tenting the sclera.*

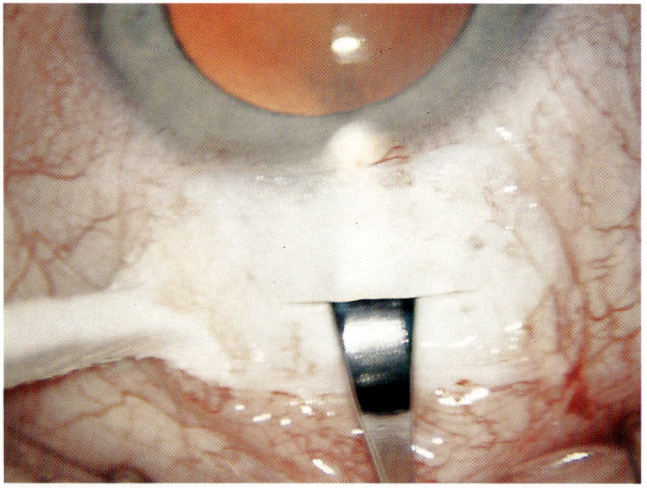

Figure 13.39 *The forward dissection stops as the blade enters clear cornea at about one-half depth.*

arcade, the incision will have shallowed to approximately one-third to one-half depth (Fig. 13.39). The conscious attempt to shallow the incision helps prevent premature entry into the anterior chamber (Fig. 13.40). I prefer steel, but many excellent phaco surgeons employ a trifacet diamond blade for both the scleral groove and dissection.

The incisional plane then changes and becomes parallel with the iris. Entry in this iris-parallel fashion is accomplished with a 3.20-mm keratome (Figs. 13. 41 to 13.43). This final change of planes at the cornea protects the iris from direct trauma and prolapse. More important, it forms a substantial internal peripheral corneal flap that acts as a valve, sealing aqueous in and blood out of the anterior chamber. This lessens the importance of the traditional suture closure. Extremely poor visualization during phacoemulsification will be encountered if wound entry is too corneal, since substantial distortion of the cornea makes it very difficult to visualize the surgical process.

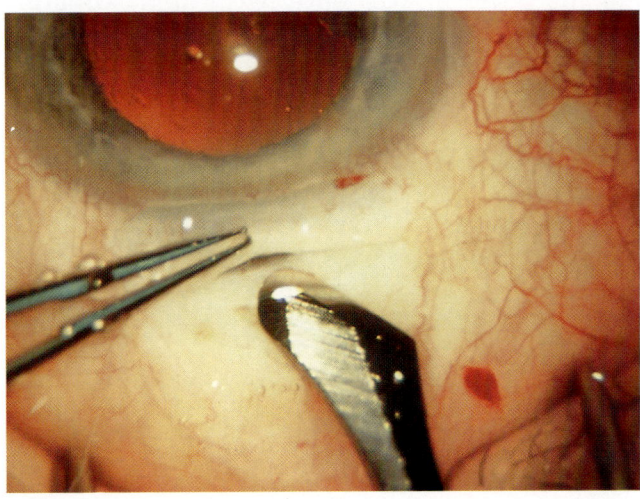

Figure 13.40 *Premature entry has occurred even though this wound was grooved 2.00 mm from the limbus. It is actually easier to start the incision further back and establish an appropriate scleral dissection plane.*

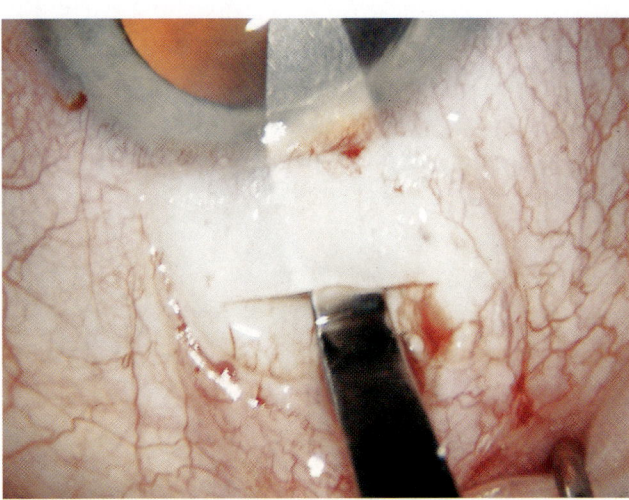

Figure 13.41 *The keratome has pierced Descemet's membrane just central to the limbal arcade, but this eye is short and has a small, thick cornea.*

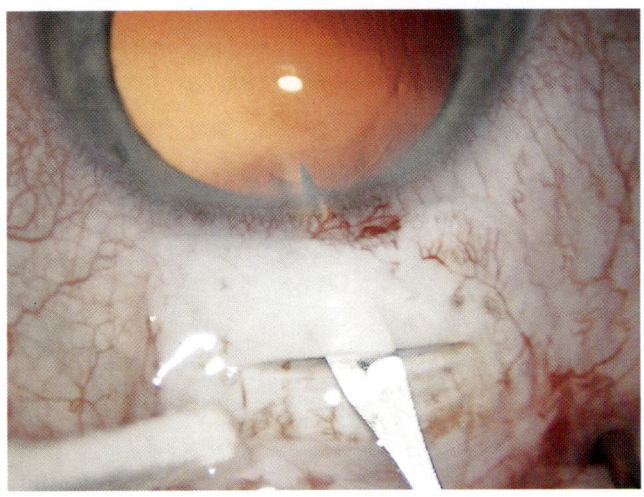

Figure 13.42 *Descemet's level trauma is seen after phacoemulsification. The wound can be extended with the keratome or a sharp blade.*

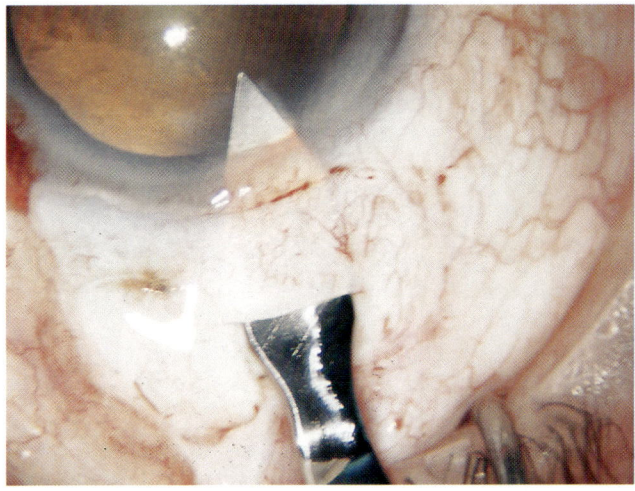

Figure 13.43 *A better, more peripheral Descemet's level entry is seen just central to the limbal vascular arcade. Linear Descemet's fold shows well on the surface of the keratome.*

The eye is entered through clear cornea near the limbus by a stab incision using a 22.50-degree disposable blade at the 1:30 clock-hour position (Fig. 13.45). A polished-down 0.50-mm cyclodialysis spatula (about 0.40 mm wide) and 30-gauge blunt cannula will be introduced through this incision.

Anterior Capsulotomy

Ideally, an anterior capsulotomy should be central and circular, in order to provide the most favorable optical condition. This enables the remaining capsular bag to provide the most symmetrical structural support, which is important early and even more important late because of capsular fibrosis and the relentless force of capsular contraction. If the IOL optic is covered by the anterior capsule on one side and not the other, late decentration may occur due to hammocking of the optic by the anterior capsular edge if it is close to the optic. The optic may be squeezed in any direction by the progressive adhesion of the anterior and posterior flaps.

The perfect size of the anterior capsulotomy is open to debate. Because of late postoperative decentration possibilities, I think it should either cover or not cover the entire peripheral optic symmetrically. My preference is to slightly overlap the anterior IOL optic with approximately 0.25 mm of the anterior capsular remnant. I

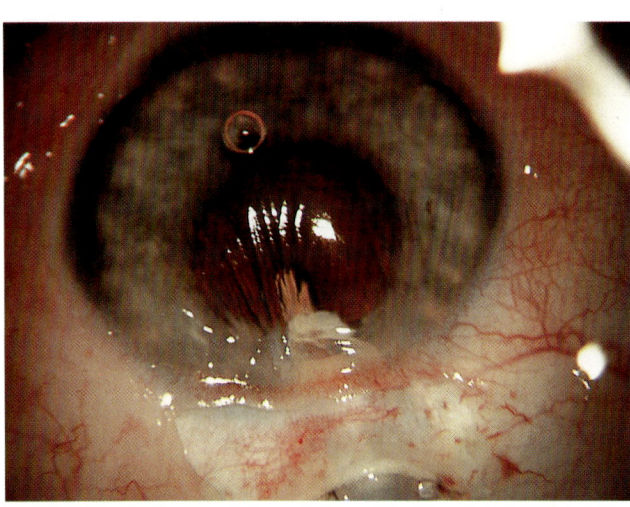

Figure 13.44 *Dangerously compromised visualization from corneal distortion is apparent. In small eyes, Descemet's entry should be further peripheral, perhaps peripheral to the arcade.*

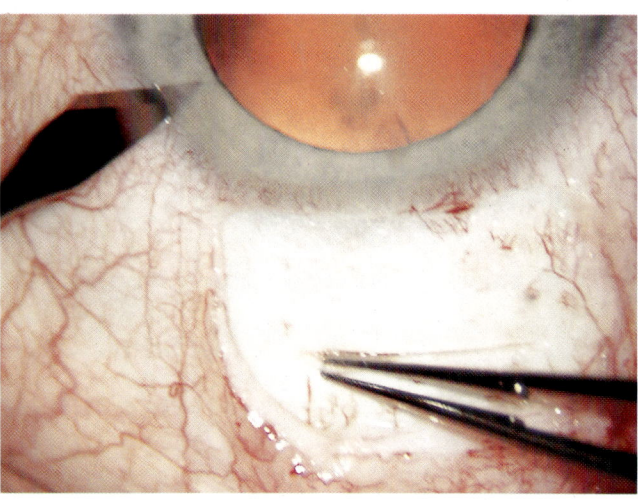

Figure 13.45 *The 0.12 forceps are grasped in the right hand and full thickness entry accomplished into the anterior chamber with a 22.5-degree disposable super blade held in the left hand. The entry is not parallel with the iris but aims at the pars plana 180 degrees away.*

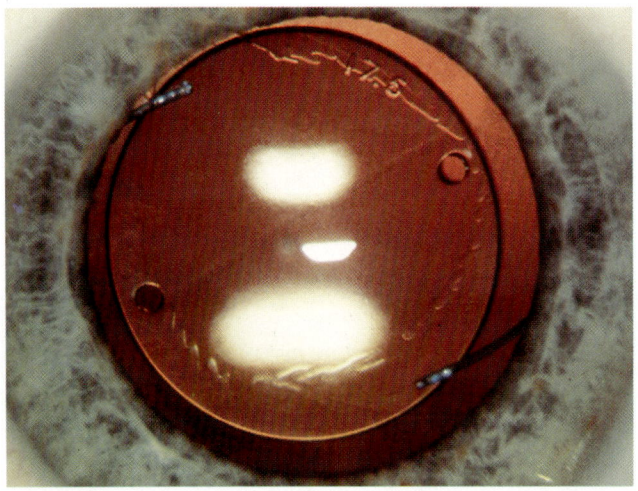

Figure 13.46 *The size of an anterior capsulotomy seems satisfactory just after surgery. Note the anterior radial capsular tear at the 11 o'clock position.*

believe this overlap provides symmetrical structural support, good long-term optic centration, and it may even help reduce edge glare.

If the capsulotomy is too small, surgery will be unnecessarily difficult, resulting in increased risk to both the anterior capsular remnant and posterior capsule, and also eventual optical problems. As capsular fibrosis occurs, the size of the opening in the anterior capsule may stay as originally created or it may get a little smaller (Figs. 13.46 and 13.47). It will never get larger. Anterior capsulotomy shrinkage is made worse by capsulorhexis because of a sphincter-like recruitment effect that appears to develop as the anterior capsular remnant undergoes the contraction of epithelial cell fibrosis (Fig. 13.48). The anterior capsulotomy can become incredibly small in rare cases of pseudoexfoliation even if it is created with the correct dimension. The forces of progressive capsular fibrosis can drastically shrink the opening because of the lack of counteracting zonular traction in these extreme cases (Fig. 13.49). A larger can-opener may actually be better in extreme cases.

Ultrasonic removal or cryopexy of the anterior capsular epithelial cells in pseudoexfoliation cases may be particularly helpful in preventing this complication, which could ultimately result in a dislocated IOL within the detached capsular bag. Eradication of these cells may also reduce the number of cases in which an exaggerated epithelial cell response creates a proteinaceous glue-

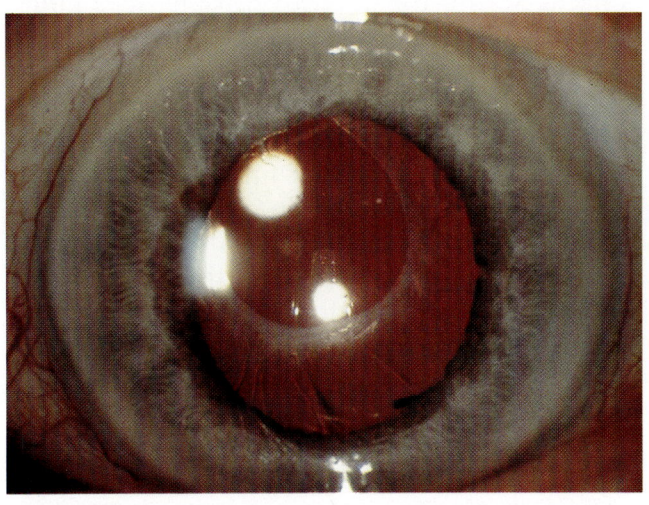

Figure 13.47 *After several years, the anterior capsular opening may shrink substantially, drawing the opening toward an eccentric anterior capsular defect.*

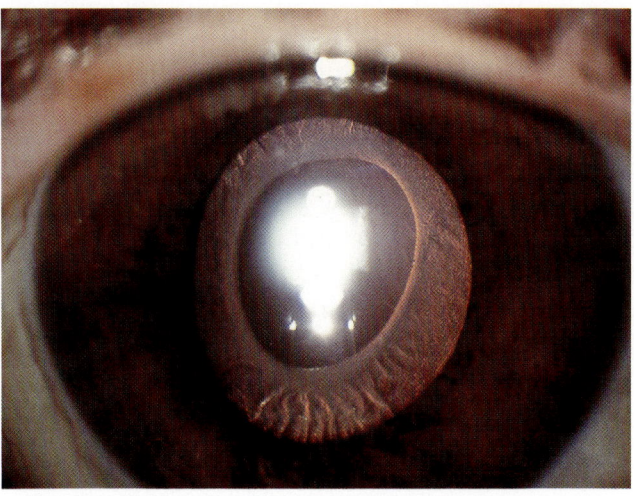

Figure 13.48 *The anterior capsular opening was larger when originally created. As capsular fibrosis progressed, a sphincter-like effect seemed to be present in some of the anterior capsular remnants created by capsulorhexis.*

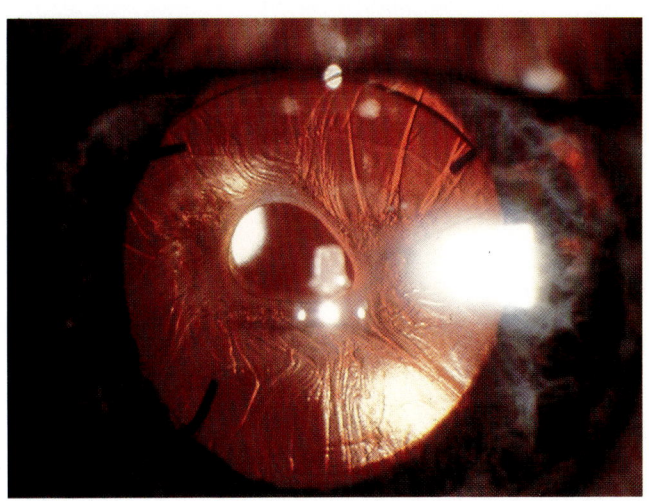

Figure 13.49 *This eye has extremely loose zonular attachments with pseudoexfoliation, which do not counteract the normal forces of progressive capsular fibrosis. The unopposed forces excessively contract the capsule, converting a 6.50 mm anterior capsulotomy into one that is 2.00 × 3.00 mm. Obvious pseudophacodonesis is present as the 7.00 mm IOL with curled haptics wobbles with every eye motion.*

sheen at the edge of the capsulorhexis, further reducing the functional visual area of the IOL optic (Fig. 13.50).

Again, if approximately one-quarter or more of the optic is left uncovered, the edge of the capsulorhexis may hammock the optic edge and slightly decenter as capsular fibrosis occurs. Capsular contraction influence on the IOL optic may cause this subtle, late decentering tendency to be exaggerated if the IOL haptics are soft. Firm haptics probably help resist the asymmetric fibrotic forces on the optic. Clinically significant optic decentration is unlikely with slightly asymmetric capsulorhexis or asymmetric IOL optics. Difficulties might be more likely if both asymmetries occurred in the same case.

As a general rule, the anterior capsule should overlap the peripheral optic about 0.25 mm all the way around its perimeter *at the time of surgery*. If a 6.00-mm optic IOL is being used, a 5.50-mm continuous tear circular capsulotomy should be fashioned. Capsular fibrosis will generally increase this coverage by another 0.25 mm. If the capsulorhexis is the correct size at surgery, this reduction in size secondary to fibrotic contraction is usually not optically significant. Perfect capsular openings are more critical in younger patients with larger pupils or those in whom multifocal lenses have been implanted. Some of the advantages of a 7.00-mm lens will be lost if the anterior capsular opening is only 5.00 mm in diameter. The peripheral focusing zone of a multifocal lens may be rendered optically noncontributory by too small a capsular opening.

ANTERIOR CAPSULOTOMY SURGICAL TECHNIQUE

When performing the anterior capsulotomy, the rectus sutures should be released and the anterior chamber filled with enough viscoelastic to maintain a taut flat capsular surface. This pressure will prevent troublesome wrinkles that may develop while the capsulotomy is being scribed. The capsulotomy is begun by puncturing the anterior capsule with a 25-gauge needle, which has been bent 90 degrees at its tip and about 30 degrees where it inserts into the hub (Fig. 13.51). After the needle is plunged into the anterior capsule, it is pulled parallel to the desired position of the final capsulectomy. One of two patterns will form, either a triangle flap or a simple curvilinear incision without a flap. When trying to produce a perfect circular anterior capsulotomy, I find the triangle flap easier to manipulate. The linear pattern is a little more difficult because I usually must sweep around the initiation point with the final capsulotomy tear or the superior aspect of the anterior capsulotomy might end up a little small. A triangular flap is more easily produced if the bent portion of the needle is fairly long, perhaps 0.50 mm.

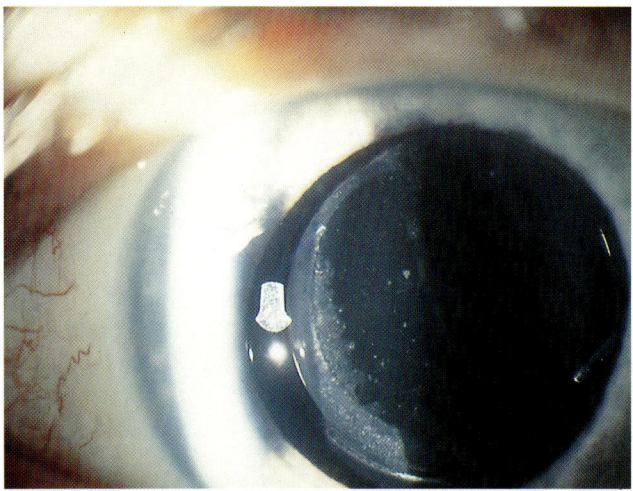

Figure 13.50 *Proteinaceous debris is present on the surface of some IOLs after capsulorhexis, thereby reducing the functional visual area of the IOL. These deposits are probably a product of inflammation from lens epithelial cell/IOL interaction.*

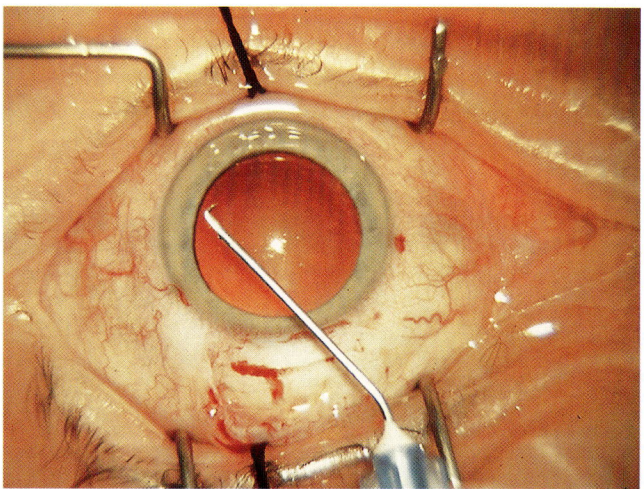

Figure 13.51 *To create an anterior capsulotomy, a 25-gauge needle has been bent in two places. The bend at the tip is made at a 90-degree angle with a sharp corner to facilitate manipulation of the anterior capsular flap. A gentle bend is created at the base so that the handle may be held like a pencil.*

Triangle Flap Initiation. The needle punctures the anterior capsule and the full depth of the bent portion is left within the lens. The needle is pulled slightly toward its shaft to create the small flap of anterior capsular tissue (Fig. 13.52). After the flap has been identified, the dragging stops and the needle is used to curl the flap over onto the remaining intact capsular tissue (Fig. 13.53). Then a series of linked small capsular tears, which will form the radius of the anterior capsulotomy, are easily formed and simultaneously linked together by pulling from the center toward the periphery in radial fashion (Figs. 13.54 to 13.56). Attention is returned to the initial flap. The needle engages this curled flap very lightly and starts to drag it around so the outer edge forms the anterior capsulotomy. The capsular edge formed by the linked small tears now forms the radius of

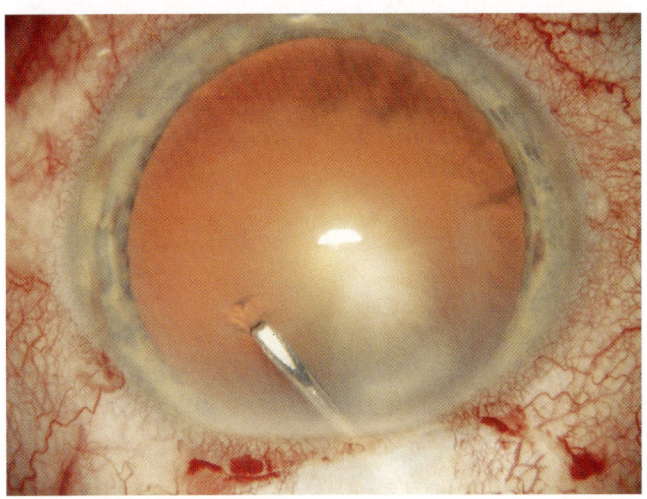

Figure 13.52 *A vertical puncture is created with the bent 0.50 mm portion of the 25-gauge needle. With the needle still at full depth, the point is dragged toward the shaft, creating a small triangular flap.*

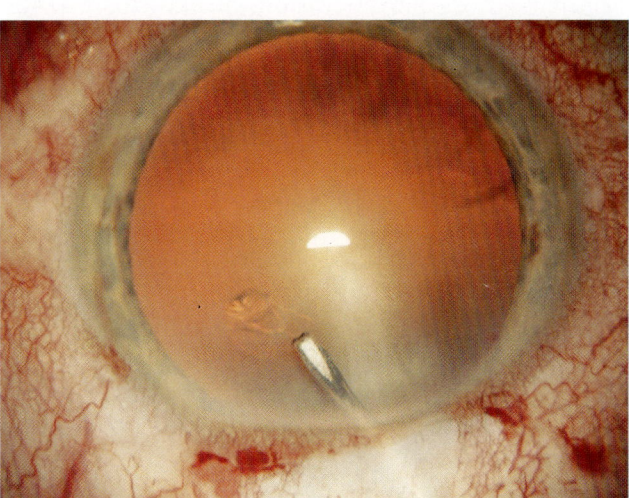

Figure 13.53 *The triangular flap is curled over onto the surface of the remaining anterior capsule.*

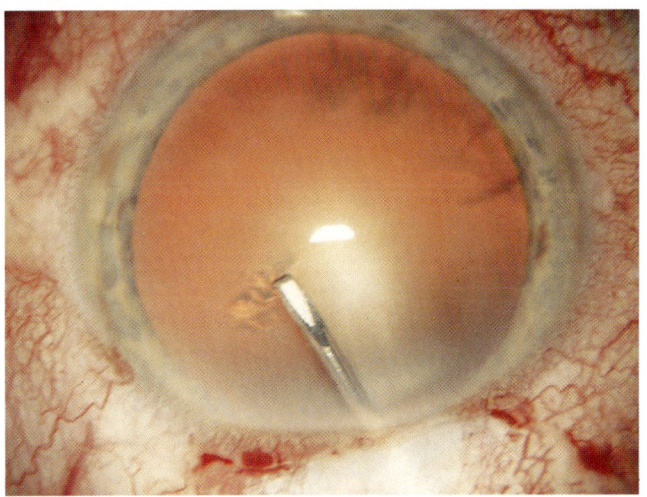

Figure 13.54 *Small linked tears are made in the anterior capsule by stroking from center to periphery in radial fashion.*

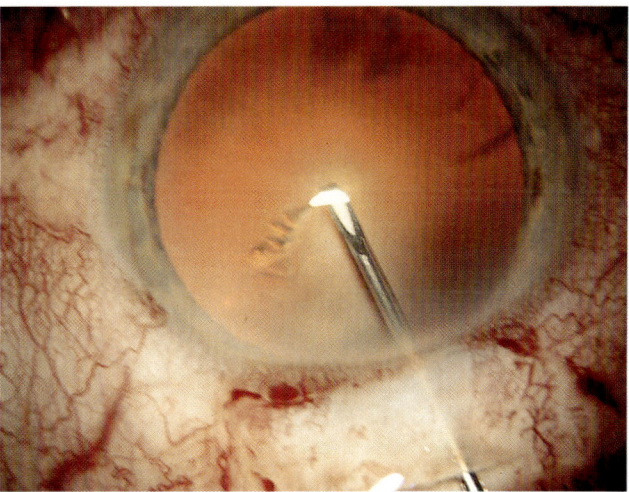

Figure 13.55 *Several more tears are created.*

the circle that will become the anterior capsulotomy (Fig. 13.57). The center of the circle is the pivot point for the creation of the capsulotomy. This rotation around the pivot point helps the capsulotomy to be continously curved in pupil parallel fashion at all times. The needle is constantly repositioned so it is never more than 2.00 mm from the active tearing point (Figs. 13.58 and 13.59). It is important to "erase" the initiation point with the last movement of the needle by having the final tear of the anterior capsule originate more peripherally than its finish. (Figs. 13.60 and 13.61).

Incisional Initiation Pattern. At times, even with a perfect 90-degree acute angle bend and a long penetrating segment, a triangular flap will not develop. A simple incision becomes obvious within the first millimeter of the initiation point. The incision is then dragged in a pupil-parallel curved fashion for several millimeters (Fig. 13.62). Linked small tears are again created to the future center of the capsulotomy circle (Fig. 13.63). The radius formed by the linked tears forms one side of a large triangle flap and the initiating incision forms another. The apex can be turned over and the outer capsular edge dragged to form the anterior capsulotomy just as in the small triangular initiation pattern (Figs. 13.64 and 13.65).

If a pupil-parallel curvilinear pattern strays toward the periphery, a straight line capsulotomy will start to develop and may get lost among the

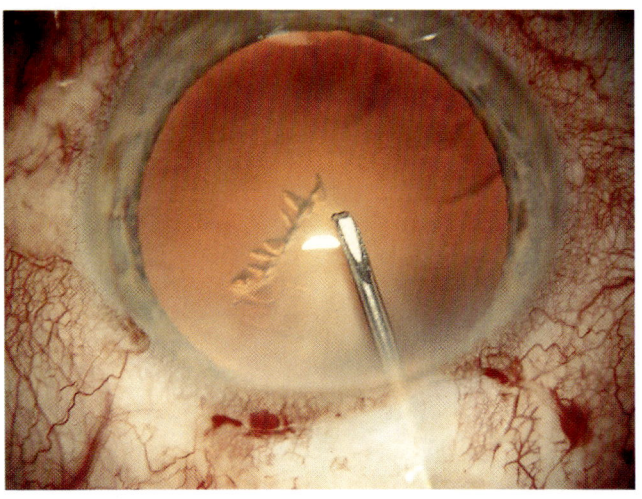

Figure 13.56 *The linked tears extend to the center of the future capsulorhexis.*

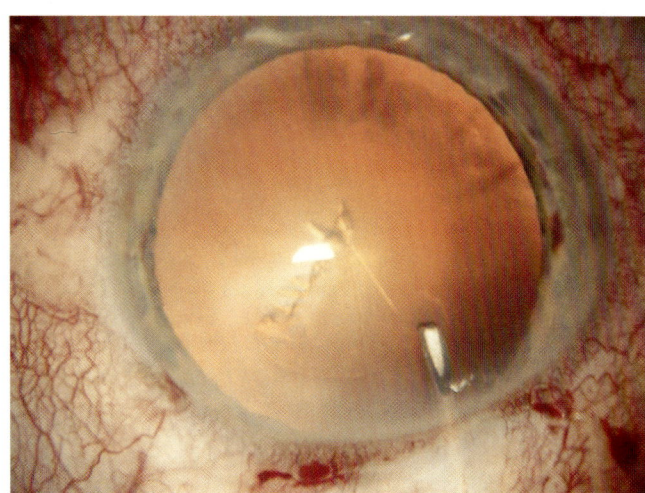

Figure 13.57 *The initial triangular flap is held lightly and pulled in a pupil parallel manner. The linked tears have formed one side of a new larger triangular flap, which will be rotated around the capsulorhexis center.*

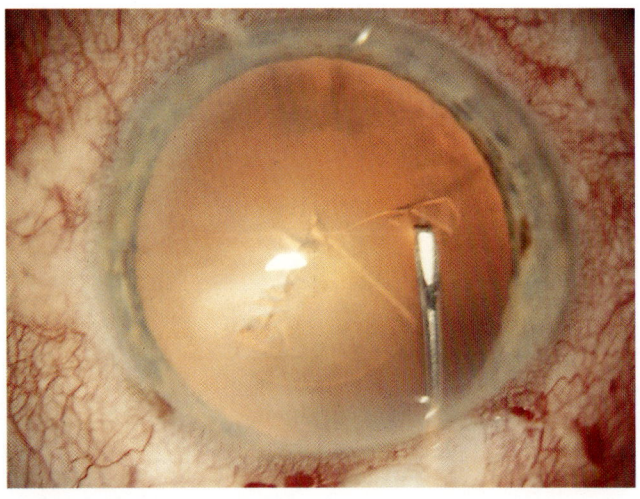

Figure 13.58 *The anterior capsular tear is formed as the triangular flap pivots around the center.*

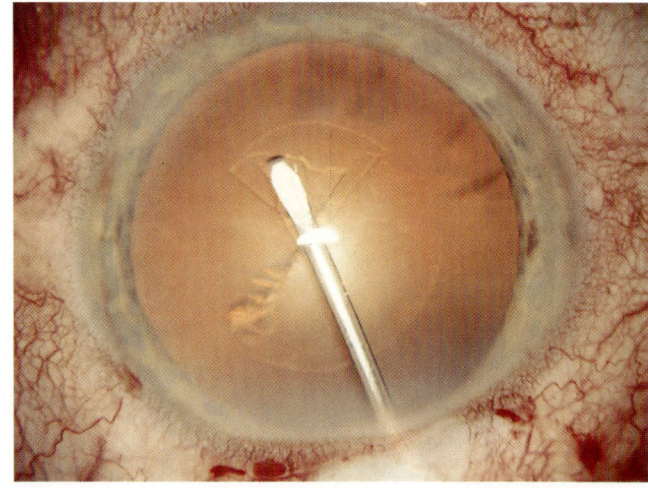

Figure 13.59 *The needle pushes very lightly and is never further than 2.00 mm from the active, developing tear.*

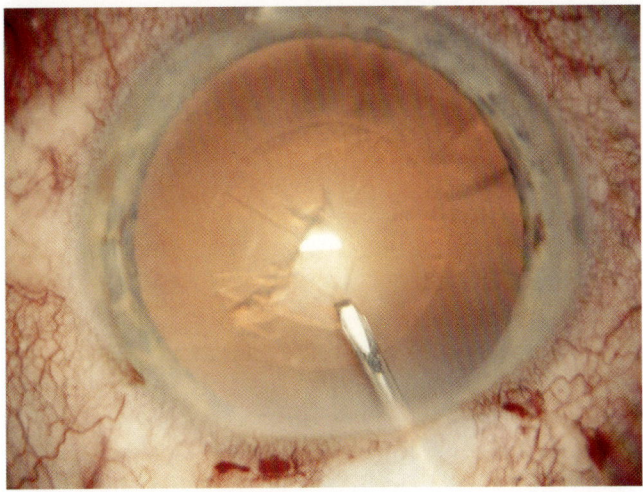

Figure 13.60 *The finishing tear will be just peripheral to the starting point.*

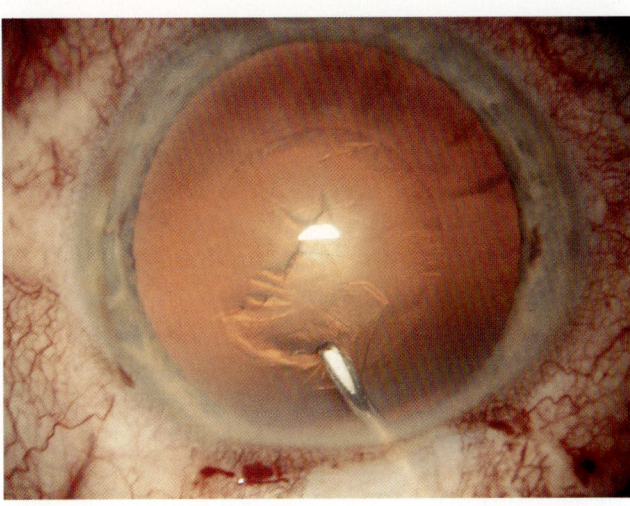

Figure 13.61 *To create a continuous clean edge, the flap is grasped very close to the active tear at the finish.*

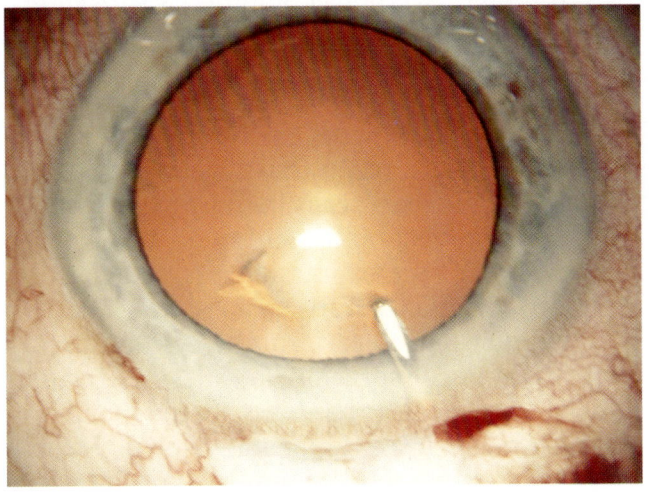

Figure 13.62 *A linear incision has developed in the anterior capsule. A triangular flap is not present.*

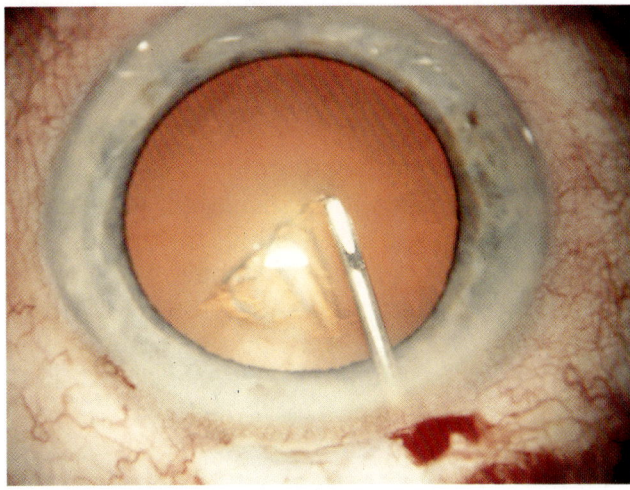

Figure 13.63 *Multiple, linked, small anterior capsular tears extend to the center of the intended capsulorhexis.*

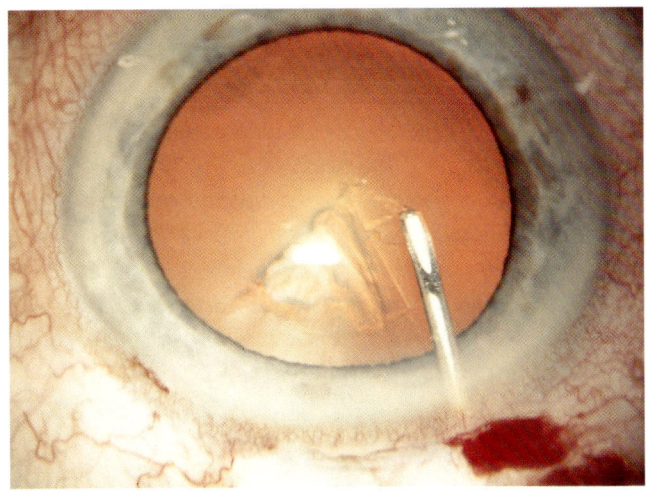

Figure 13.64 *The larger capsular flap is gathered and the capsulorhexis tear continued.*

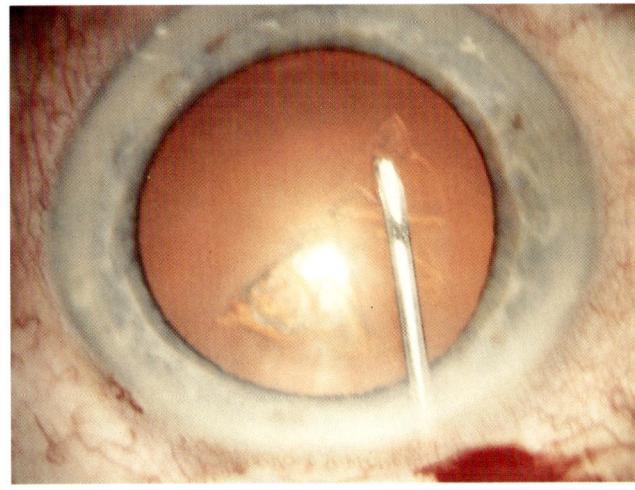

Figure 13.65 *The capsulorhexis is created as it is in the small triangle technique, making sure to erase the starting point.*

zonular fibers in the equatorial zone. This may result in a capsulotomy that gets lost among the zonular fibers in the equatorial zone. Sometimes these can be saved (Fig. 13.66), but at other times it is better to reinitiate a capsulorhexis at another location and incise the capsule in the other direction or bring a can-opener pattern around from the initiation to the weak spot. Frequent directional over-compensation of the capsular tear may be evident in initial capsulorhexis attempts (Fig. 13.67). It is of no consequence and is certainly better than losing control of this capsular tear at the region of zonule insertion and beyond or making the capsulotomy too small and ending up with anterior radial tears to the equator.

Capsulorhexis in children is difficult because pediatric anterior capsules are tough, thus more difficult to tear well, and pediatric tissues are tremendously elastic—the scleras are spongy and the lenses soft. These features contribute to increased vitreous pressure and a situation in which the gelatinous lens nucleus tends to self-express while the anterior capsulotomy is being made. These factors cause the capsulotomy to extend peripherally more than desired, making it difficult to control. The surgeon should make sure to start in an exaggerated central position, perhaps imagining a final goal of a 4.00-mm anterior capsulotomy. The capsulotomy will spiral out to at least 5.50 mm on its own, and the finish will easily erase the starting point.

Capsulorhexis is an excellent technique, but it is not the best for all situations. At times, when visualization is extremely difficult, such as with a totally white, partially liquid cataract, when anticipating a minimal-lift technique, or in case of extreme zonular weakness in pseudoexfoliation, a can-opener capsulotomy gives the best results with the least risk (Fig. 13.68).

Hydrodissection

The incision is enlarged with the 3.00-mm keratome (Beaver 5520) (Fig. 13.69), and the 22-gauge cannula is reintroduced while still on the viscoelastic syringe. Approximately half the viscoelastic is removed and used later during IOL insertion. Remember, the anterior chamber had been overfilled to accomplish the anterior capsulotomy; removing some viscoelastic helps prevent iris prolapse and makes hydrodissection easier.

BSS is injected under the anterior capsular remnant as superiorly as possible at the left, right (Fig. 13.70), and inferior quarters. A curved cannula can be used to dissect at the 11 o'clock position, but this is rarely necessary. Frequently, one of these injections will dissect posteriorly. Posterior hydrodissection is not necessary at this point for these methods, but peripheral equatorial dissection is easily obtained.

Nuclear Strategy

A specific nuclear management strategy should be selected. The surgeon must decide whether to use one of three basic capsular bag techniques or a minimal-lift technique. Although the need to perform a nucleus expression or intracapsular cataract extraction is rare, it does arise and it is good to know how to perform these procedures as well. Patient cooperation, pupil size, zonular integrity, and nuclear hardness should all be considered when devising an operative plan. Flexibility and experience are the keys to knowing which technique to perform.

If the patient tends to be less than perfectly cooperative and the nucleus is quite firm, I consider the minimal-lift technique since it is faster and generally not as exacting as the capsular bag methods. Depending on lens hardness, zonular integrity, and patient cooperation, if the pupil is

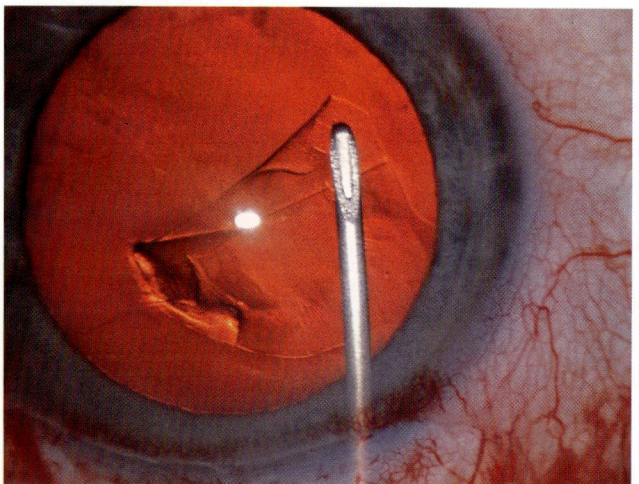

Figure 13.66 *The anterior capsulotomy did not parallel the pupil for very long but extended to the 10 o'clock position into the anterior equatorial zone. Some of the anterior zonular insertion was involved. No anterior radial tear is present, but the capsular bag has undergone significant structural change as a result of the excursion into the equatorial zone. Late optic decentration may be the result of such an extremely asymmetrical capsulorhexis.*

4.00 mm or smaller, I may perform a sector iridectomy and a can-opener capsulotomy with a combination of the minimal-lift and capsular bag method. One disadvantage of the minimal-lift method is the single anterior radial capsular tear, which is almost always produced at the 11 o'clock position. This relatively small, usually subclinical, complication can be accepted easily if the minimal-lift technique will substantially reduce the risk of clinically significant complications (Figs. 13.71 to 13.73). (The minimal-lift technique is an excellent and very safe technique. It should be used in some difficult circumstances and is probably one of the best methods with which to begin learning phacoemulsification.)

If the inferior zonules have developed a localized one or two clock hour defect, capsular bag phacoemulsification can be attempted, with aspiration activity directed toward the stronger quadrant and away from the defect. A minimal-lift variation may be needed during the later stages of emulsification to prevent inadvertent capsular aspiration. Capsular aspiration is less likely early because the capsule is actually protected by the bulk and shape of the remaining nucleus. If the superior zonule has a focal defect, both inferior quadrants will still be available for standard capsular bag phacoemulsification. A minimal-lift variation should be avoided late in this setting because of the flaccidity and potential aspiration of the superior capsule at its zonular defect.

Among the capsular bag variations a fair amount

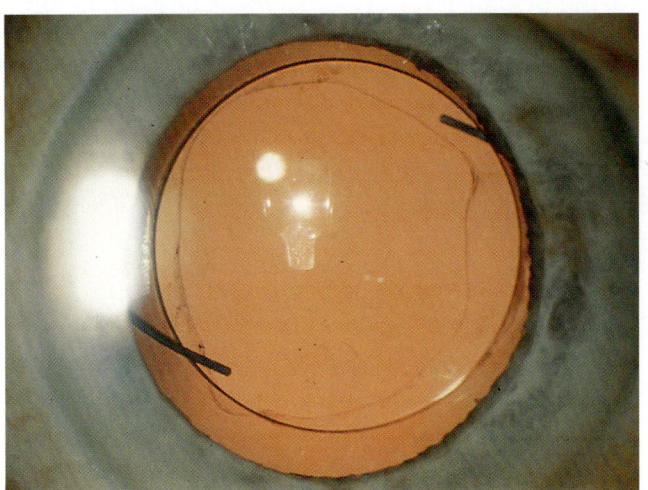

Figure 13.67 *A wavering of the capsular edge is apparent from capsulorhexis tear "oversteer," but, on the whole, this capsulotomy looks structurally sound and contains the IOL well.*

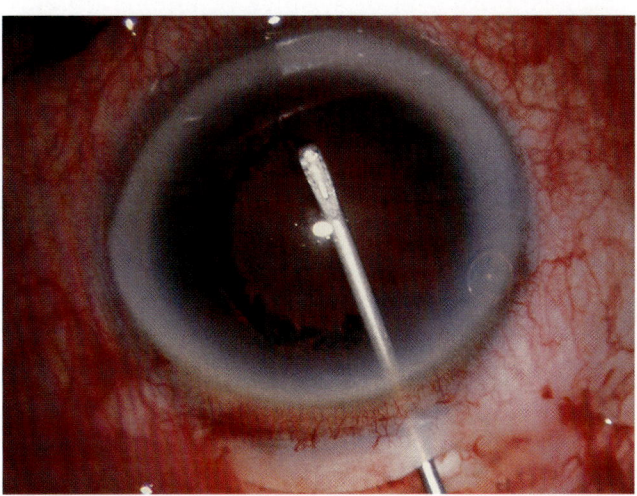

Figure 13.68 *A very dense, firm cataract in a patient with a fairly small eye and prominent arcus senilis presents a good opportunity to employ a multiple tear anterior capsulotomy.*

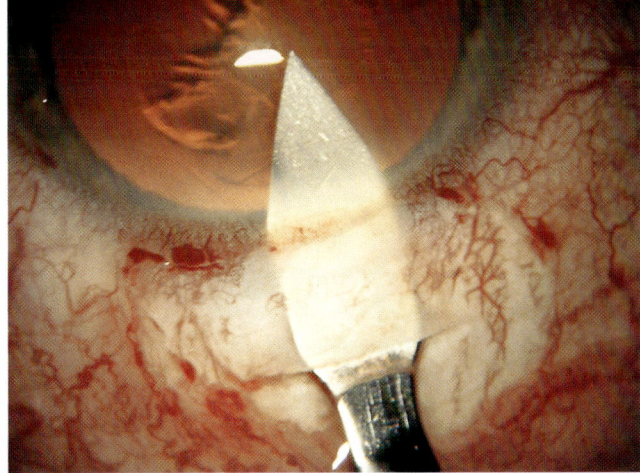

Figure 13.69 *The keratome (Beaver 5520) is placed in the plane of the incision it started just before the anterior capsulotomy. It is driven further into the anterior chamber parallel to the iris, making sure that its point has not engaged the iris or corneal endothelium.*

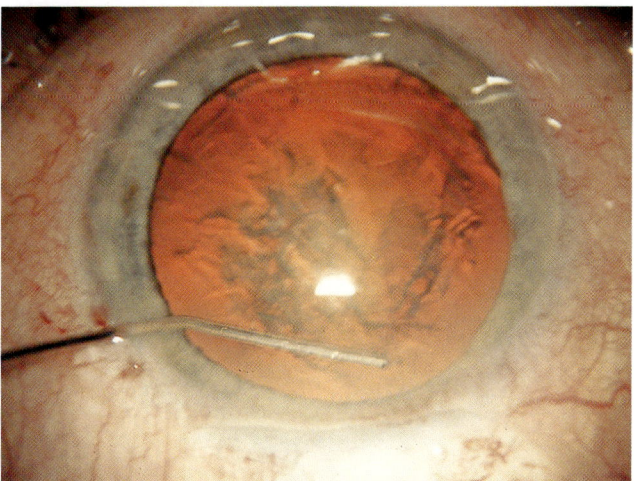

Figure 13.70 *Hydrodissection is accomplished with a 30-gauge cannula placed through the superior incision. The cannula may be placed through the stab incision to dissect a soft nucleus from above.*

of overlap exists; thus, in most cases, two or even three techniques can be selected. Additionally, various features of one strategy are often integrated into another as the individual case unfolds. This allows the surgeon a great deal of flexibility when encountering various clinical circumstances (Table 13.74 and Fig. 13.75).

Initial Phacoemulsification Steps

Certain initial steps are common to all phacoemulsification surgery. The machine must be tested and ready. Back-up handpieces, foot pedals, packs, tips, and tubing are essential. An entire back-up machine is ideal. The surgeon must know the complex control panel functions and mechanics of the machine intimately in order to direct troubleshooting efforts, solve problems quickly and, if needed, be able to resolve technical problems for the circulating nurse.

To start, receive the handpiece from the scrub nurse. The test chamber cap should be in place so a last-minute check can be done (Fig. 13.76). The irrigation and aspiration (I/A) lines should be firmly attached to the phaco unit. A catastrophe may occur if the irrigation line falls off during phacoemulsification. The ultrasonic energy should be turned on. At 80% energy, it should sound like a "normal" 80%. If it sounds weak or variable, the tightness of the tip should be checked and the unit retuned; if necessary, the tips or handpieces should be changed. The foot pedal should be working properly. The silicone sleeve should be checked to make sure the correct amount of tip shows and to insure that it is not defective.

If placed, the patient's rectus sutures should be loosened appropriately so the eye is free to move during phaco. The surgeon's mask should be tight so the oculars do not fog. The surgeon's head, trunk, shoulders, arms, hands, legs, and feet

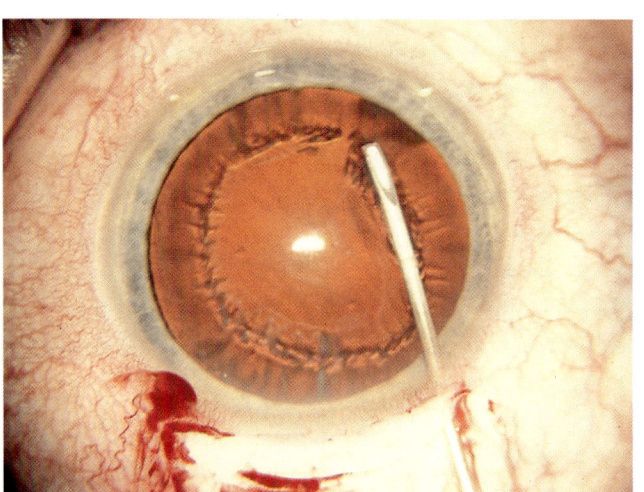

Figure 13.71 *For minimal-lift phacoemulsification, a can-opener capsulotomy is created with the opening slightly eccentric toward the 11 o'clock position. The eccentricity of the capsulotomy facilitates formation of the anterior capsule radial tear usually necessary for the minimal lift technique.*

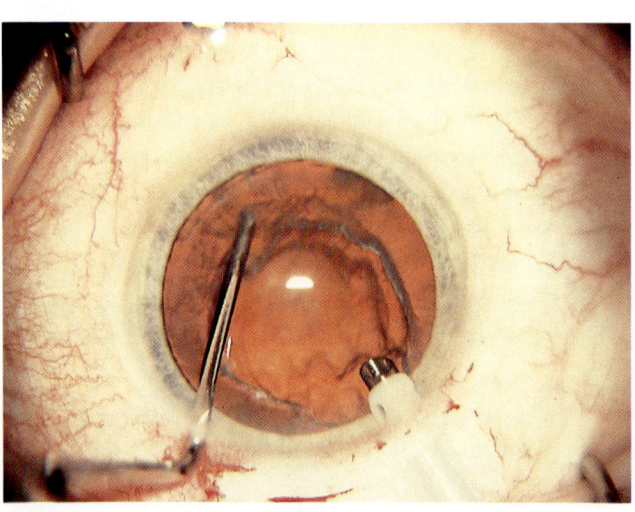

Figure 13.72 *The superior anterior rim has been reduced and the nucleus has fallen back. It is then dislocated with the cyclodialysis spatula and rotated clockwise a couple of clock hours.*

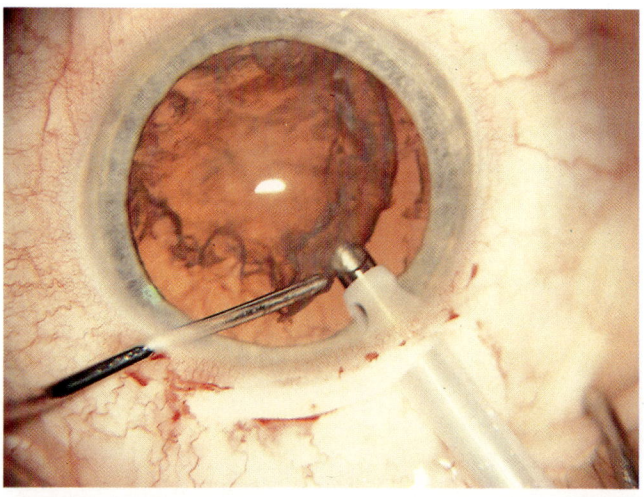

Figure 13.73 *As the peripheral anterior nuclear volume is reduced, more of the anterior and midlevel nuclear rim can be removed with greater safety as it is transferred to a safer, more central position.*

should be comfortable, with the lower legs extended slightly so that delicate movements can be made with the feet without losing balance or moving the rest of the body.

Grasp the scleral flap with the 0.12-mm forceps and lift slightly as the phaco tip is inserted into the anterior chamber. The tip should be bevel down (Fig. 13.77) and infusion should be on *foot-position 1*. *Foot-position 0* can be used if the anterior chamber is still slightly overfilled with viscoelastic. This approach creates the least trauma to Descemet's membrane and the iris. If the iris is traumatized now, it will have a greater tendency to prolapse later. Rotate the tip to a bevel-up position, and briefly tap the pedal into *foot-position 2* to aspirate the remaining viscoelastic and the anterior capsule remnant.

The handpiece, supported by both the right and left hands, should move in a controlled yet versatile fashion. The right and left hands, fingers, and arms work together as a single unit. The right and left index fingers guide the tip. The left index finger may be positioned on either the left side or the top of the phaco handle. The wire and tubes that exit the handpiece should be draped over the right forearm so no traction or gravity can be transmitted from them to the handpiece.

Sculpting should begin in a shallow fashion, using fairly low power. Unnecessarily high power can create turbulence beneath the iris; this ultrasonic trauma can cause significant immediate loss of pupil size and make the rest of the operation difficult. Without permitting the tip to become occluded, nuclear material should be shaved away, the amount and pattern depending on nuclear hardness and the ultimate strategy being used.

As sculpting descends further into the midnuclear level, an irritating reflex may appear as the microscope light reflects back from the surface of

Table 13.74 Summary of Phacoemulsification Strategies

HARDNESS OF NUCLEUS (NUCLEAR SCLEROSIS)

Phacoemulsification in the Capsular Bag			Iris Plane Phaco
Soft	Firm	Hard	Very hard
0 to 1+ C & S MWT	2+ Hybrid MWT C & S	2++ to 3+ Hybrid	4+ MLT

C & S = cutting and suction
MWT = multiple wedge technique
Hybrid = quartering and fracture hybrid
MLT = minimal-lift technique

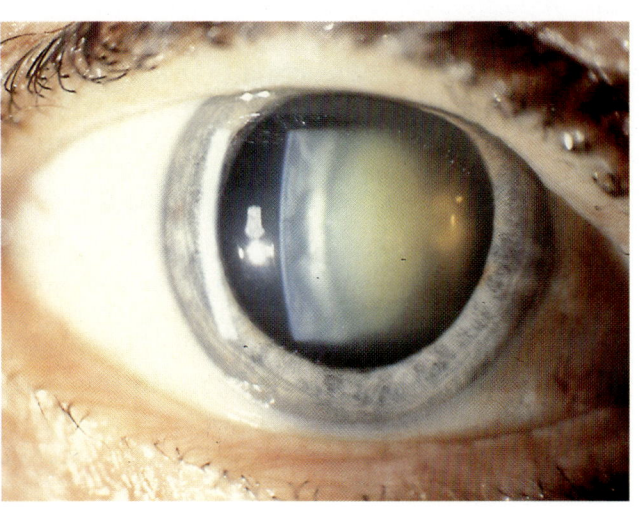

Figure 13.75 *This cataract has a 2+ central firmness and a generous surrounding pillow of softer nucleus and cortex. Any phacoemulsification method will work well in these eyes. This type of cataract is ideal for the beginning phacoemulsification surgeon and should be sought for technique expansion and improvement.*

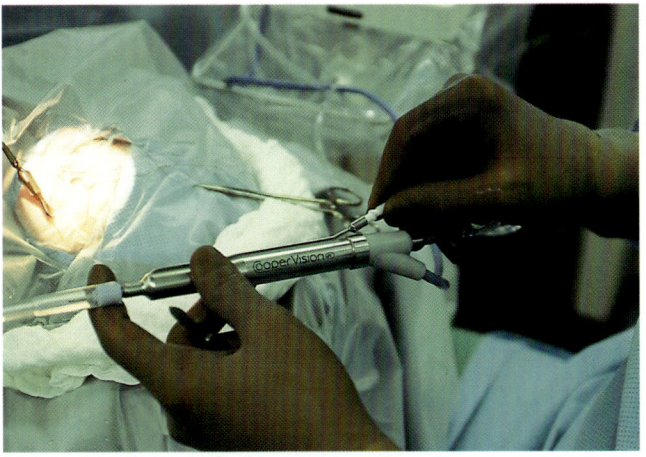

Figure 13.76 *After the handpiece has been tuned, the surgeon makes sure the irrigation and aspiration tubing is firmly attached while listening to the phacoemulsification tip vibrate. Poor sound indicates a need to retighten the tip and retune it before surgery is begun. Marginal tip performance does not improve as the operation proceeds; it usually gets worse. Loss of the irrigation line during surgery could be catastrophic.*

pooled BSS (Fig. 13.78). This is most likely to occur in eyes that have deep orbits. The reflex is confusing, but if the fluid covers a portion of the peripheral cornea, a dangerous loss of depth perception may occur. Ribbons of precut gelfoam may be placed in one or both fornices to drain excess fluid.

The need to change phaco tip orientation and the ability to finely manipulate nuclear material is characteristic of all capsular bag techniques. Tip rotation is generated by a change in finger and wrist position. Thus, when the right side of the interior nuclear bowl is shaved, the handpiece is rotated so the bevel is open to the left, i.e., it faces the evacuated nuclear center (Fig. 13.79), and when the tip shaves the left nuclear interior surface, the wrist and fingers rotate the tip so the bevel is open to the right. The wrist and forearm can only rotate so much before the action becomes awkward and tip control becomes less than optimal. The hands and fingers must be periodically repositioned to maintain fine control of the handpiece.

When performing dissection of deeper or more superior nucleus, the tip is aimed more posteriorly as the left hand index finger creates fulcrums to stabilize this movement (Fig. 13.80).

It is safest to use a 45-degree angled tip for capsular bag nuclear dissection. As the tip is angled deeper into the nuclear bowl, its functional angle of attack steepens. When phacoemulsification begins, the tip's angle of attack is flat and parallel to the horizontal plane of the lens. In this early stage, it is easy to see the entire aperture of the tip as it shaves the nucleus. As the tip descends vertically, the aperture's visibility is reduced because the overhang of the anterior aspect of the tip obscures the view. This critical image is lost earlier with the 30-degree tip and even earlier with the 15-degree tip (Fig. 13.81).

The visibility of the aperture and the separation of emulsification energy and suction made possible by the 45-degree tip is especially important when cutting the postero-inferior grooves during hybrid fracture quartering phacoemulsification. The adjacent nuclear tissue on the right and left side of the grooves, which has not been cut, provides few clues to the depth of the ongoing cut of the tip within the central grooves. Thus, it is not only easy to cut too deep, but full suction might be applied inadvertently to the posterior capsule if 15- or 30-degree tips are used (Fig. 13.82).

When both hands are employed during dissection, the right hand guides the phacoemulsification tip and the left manipulates the cyclodialysis spatula (Fig. 13.83). The little finger and ring finger of either hand are stabilized by contact with the patient's forehead.

Capsular Bag Phacoemulsification: Strategy Selection

I. Soft Nuclei. Soft nuclei have very little yellowing. They may not even have much whitish central change. Younger patients with posterior subcapsular changes make up the bulk of patients with these cataracts. A basic cutting, suction, peripheral nuclear collapse technique is usually preferred to initiate the phacoemulsification process. The multiple wedge strategy may also be needed, either as a second choice or in combination with the cutting and suction technique.

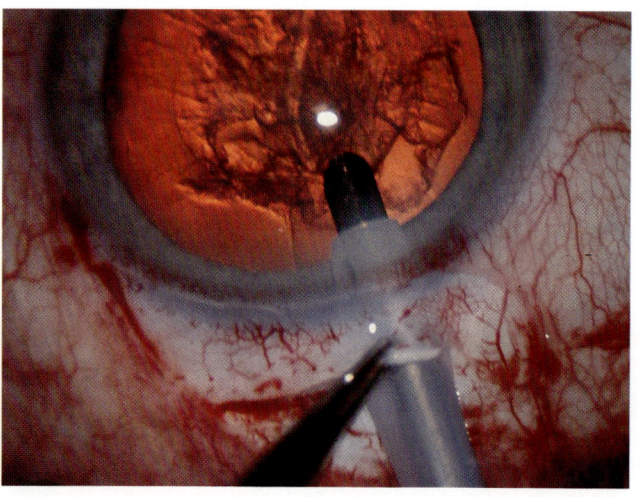

Figure 13.77 *The phacoemulsification tip is inserted upside down and then turned bevel up while in* foot-position 1. *The surgeon should be careful not to disturb Descemet's membrane.*

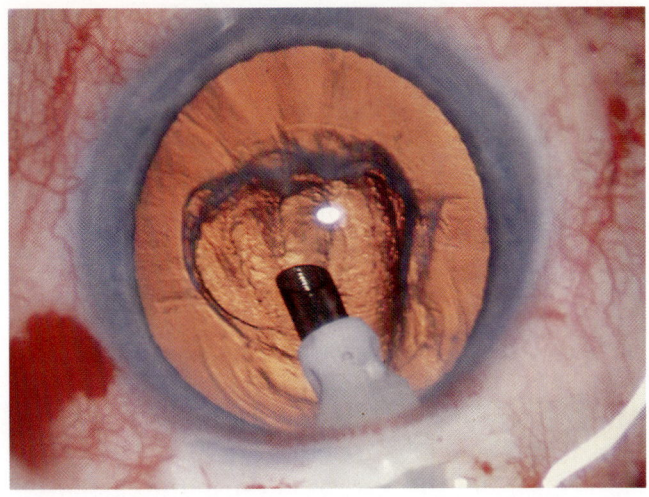

Figure 13.78 *Initial sculpting almost completed in a fairly soft lens. If too much sculpting is done, the periphery will be too thin for effective manipulation. Note that a troublesome fluid pool has accumulated and causes an irritating reflex.*

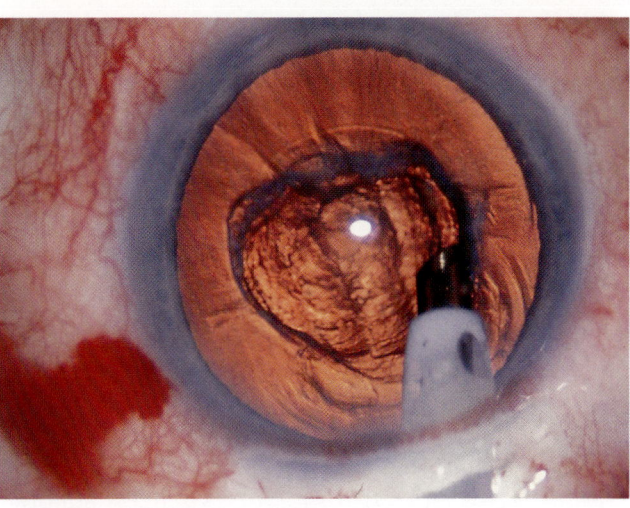

Figure 13.79 *Side sculpting is accomplished with a gentle rotation of the tip, which allows the bevel to stay toward the central cavity created by previous nuclear sculpting.*

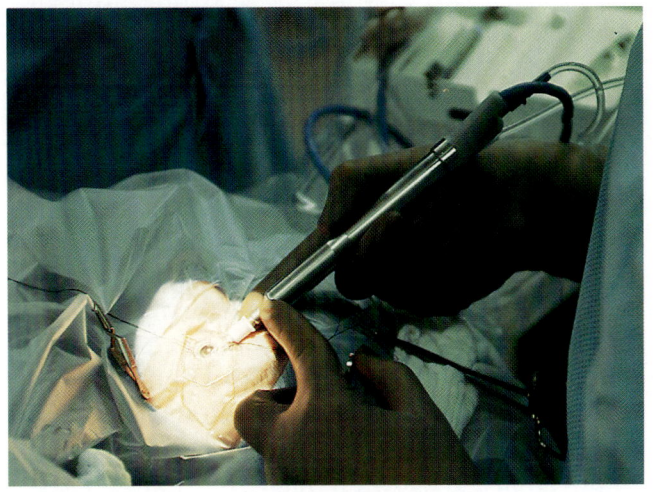

Figure 13.80 *The deepest emulsification is accomplished easily. Even though the right hand is not supported by the forehead, it is stabilized by the left hand through the tips of the index fingers.*

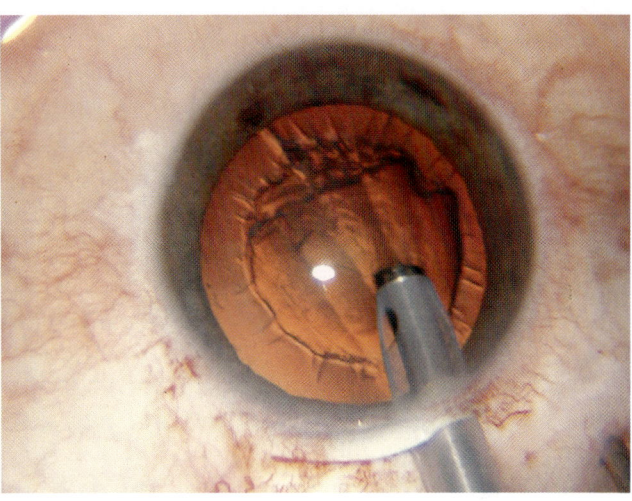

Figure 13.81 *A 30-degree phacoemulsification tip allows for easy occlusion but poor visualization of deeper shaving maneuvers.*

Figure 13.82 *As emulsification proceeds, the 15- or 30-degree tip has a greater chance of inadvertently aspirating the posterior capsule because its tip aperture is almost facing the capsule's concave surface.*

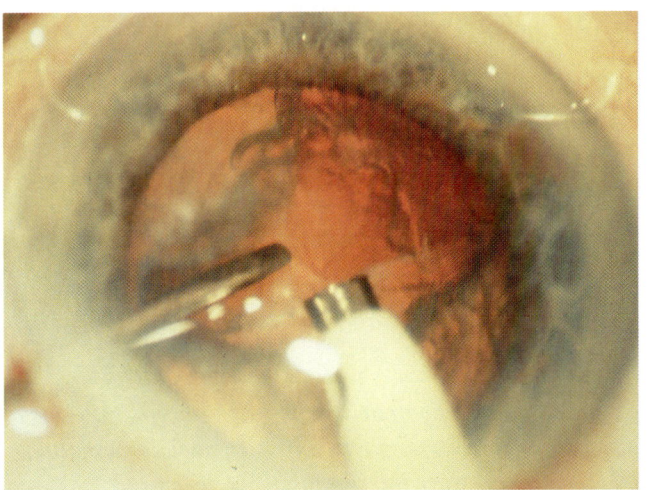

II. Medium Firm Nuclei. Nuclei of 1+ to 2+ medium firmness are characterized by a mostly whitish, minimally yellow central nuclear change. These lenses have enough nuclear firmness so that easy manipulation is possible, yet they have a generous soft peripheral nucleus that blends with the cortex. The softness permits neat hydrodissection, and leaves a generous peripheral cortical pillow, which protects the capsule. These lenses are the easiest on which to operate and should be sought by the beginner.

Virtually any technique can be used. I prefer a hybrid nuclear fracture and quartering strategy. The posterior nuclear cracking has been adapted from both the Gimbel and Shepherd versions. Posterior nuclear quartering has been integrated into the cutting and suction method used for softer lenses, enabling easy and efficient emulsification of firmer cataracts.

If I am unable to fracture or if I get only incomplete clefting, I can then convert to my preferred secondary technique, the multiple wedge strategy. The phacoemulsification tip may be turned over and occluded as in the cutting and suction method. The multiple wedge or cutting and suction techniques can be used to initiate the phacoemulsification process if the surgeon is uncomfortable with nuclear fracture and quartering.

III. Hard Nuclei. Nuclei of 2++ to 3+ hardness will have a yellowish gold to goldish brown quality, or they may be chalk white with very little yellow-brown. These nuclei are larger and have less soft peripheral substance.

In my hands, the hybrid fracture and quartering strategy is the safest and most efficient for these nuclei. The cutting and suction and multiple wedge techniques are extremely inefficient here. They also require tearing of the peripheral nucleus to accomplish safer, more central aspiration. This tearing action cannot be performed safely in hard nuclei; a bimanual fracture is necessary.

IV. Very Hard Nuclei. Nuclei of 4+ hardness are reddish brown or brownish. Nuclei this hard are encountered very infrequently in the modern ophthalmic surgical practice. Hydrodissection is unnecessary in these cases because the nucleus is completely loose from its peripheral attachments at this point. In fact, it tends to move too easily.

A minimal-lift technique is the safest and most efficient strategy for these lenses. I use a can-opener capsulotomy, which is displaced slightly superiorly because the superior nucleus will be prolapsed into the iris plane. A single superior anterior radial capsular tear will allow the prolapse. Before that, while the lens is in situ, in the capsular bag, as much nuclear material as possible must be removed by nuclear sculpting. Thinning is accomplished by rotating the nucleus in the bag before it is prolapsed, which allows access to the entire central nucleus for phacoemulsification.

The soft nucleus techniques will not work in these situations. A hybrid quartering techique can be employed but lens firmness and poor followability of nuclear material when the tip is occluded make it extremely tedious. Prolonged actual and measured phaco times combined with heightened surgeon anxiety produce increased

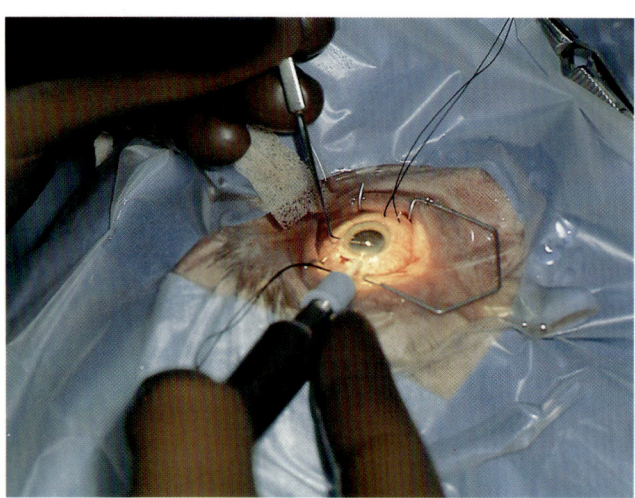

Figure 13.83 *A view of the surgeon's hands and fingers from over his right shoulder.*

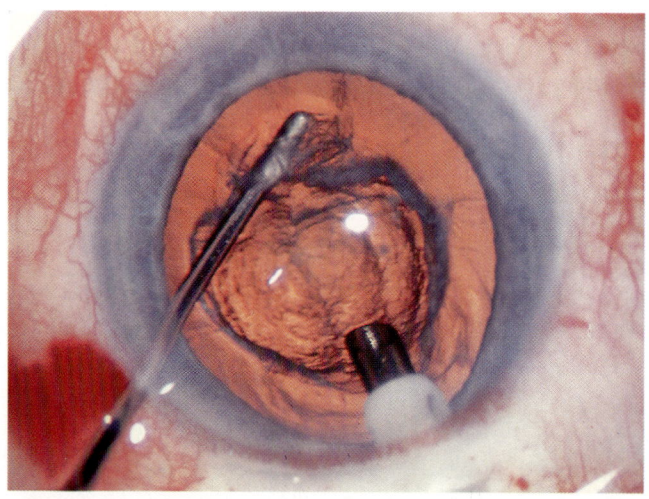

Figure 13.84 *If hydrodissection is incomplete, nucleus dislocation can be completed with a cyclodialysis spatula by applying pressure inferior to the nuclear rim.*

risk for capsular aspiration or corneal endothelial trauma.

Selected Surgical Strategies

I. SOFT NUCLEI: CUTTING AND SUCTION TECHNIQUE

The phacoemulsification procedure used for soft nuclei has four basic steps:

1. Central sculpting
2. Debulking the inferior equatorial nucleus
3. Posterior nuclear thinning, inward collapse, and aspiration of the remaining equatorial nucleus
4. Removal of the central posterior nuclear disc

Central Sculpting. With the infusion on, the 45-degree phaco tip is introduced bevel down so it does not traumatize the iris. After the bevel is turned up, sculpting begins. The tip should not be driven so deeply that the lumen becomes filled with nuclear material. During central sculpting, this material is shaved from the nuclear surface and the aspirated material is completely separated from the remaining nucleus.

It is easier to see and avoid inadvertent occlusion by turning the tip on its side when emulsifying the sides of the peripheral nucleus. The tip should "bank" within the sulcus being created in the peripheral nuclear bowl, like a bobsled moving along a sloped track. The 45-degree tip's functional angle of attack is shallow during the first few passes, becoming steeper with subsequent passes.

Before removing most of the peripheral nucleus, the cyclodialysis spatula loosens the nucleus by gently moving it and detaching it from the cortex. The loosening can be completed by a posterior stirring motion at three points of contact (Figs. 13.84 to 13.86). The surgeon should be especially careful not to sink the spatula through soft lenses. Good hydrodissection is very important with soft nuclei, especially in the area of the superior nucleus, which can be difficult to attack by the phaco tip. In very soft lenses, hydrodissection of the superior nucleus can be accomplished by inserting the 30-gauge cannula through the stab incision and directing its stream under the supero-anterior capsular border. Alternatively, a curved cannula can be used. At times, the superior nuclear material can be effectively accessed only by progressively teasing it inferiorly in hand-over-hand fashion with the phaco tip and spatula. Usually this can be most easily accomplished after the inferior nucleus has been removed. This allows the central superior portion to descend without resistance as the teasing process progresses.

As deeper nuclear material is emulsified, the ultrasonic tip's functional angle of attack is gradually increased. The chance of inadvertent occlusion and posterior capsular damage also increases. This is especially true if the tip is driven from superior to inferior along the posterior nuclear surface because the area just emulsified is hidden by the shaft of the ultrasonic tip and cannot be seen. With the 45-degree tip, the aperture can be identified when thinning the posterior nucleus, even at the steepest angle of attack. This is especially critical in soft nuclei where softer, more homogeneous material seems to leap into the tip if it is almost occluded.

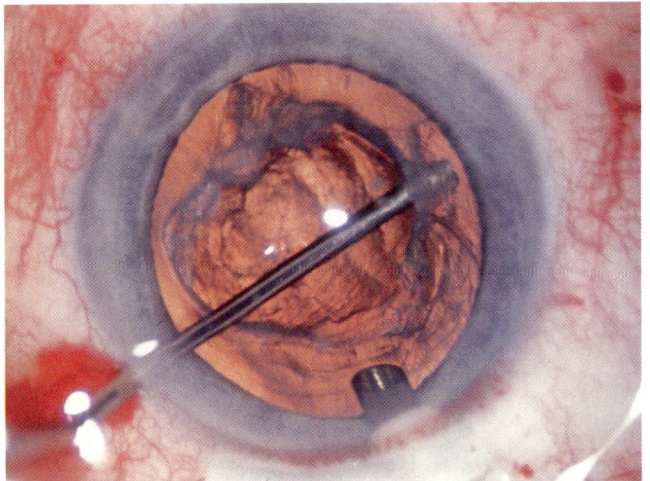

Figure 13.85 *With soft lenses, great care must be taken not to sink through the nucleus into the posterior capsule during nuclear dislocation maneuvers.*

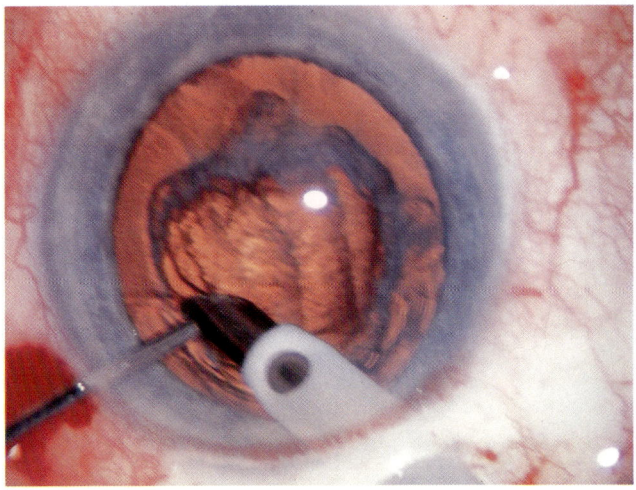

Figure 13.86 *Dislocation of the superior nucleus can be accomplished with gentle infero-posterior pressure from the phaco tip* (foot-position 1).

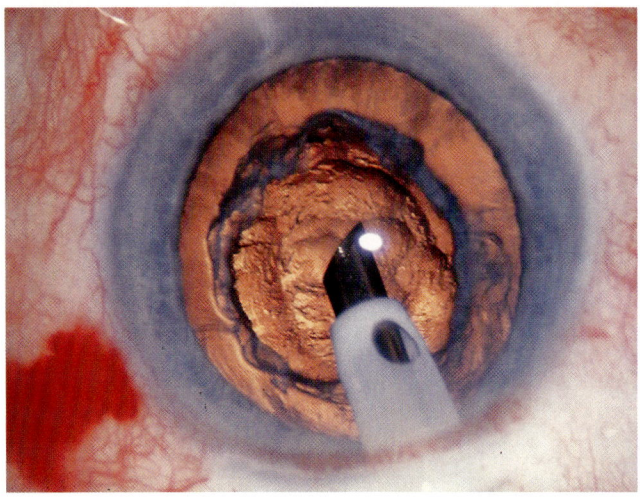

Figure 13.87 *Deeper midperipheral nuclear thinning is accomplished after the nucleus is loosened completely with the cyclodialysis spatula. The tip is on its side so the surgeon can see the exact depth of the cut as it made.*

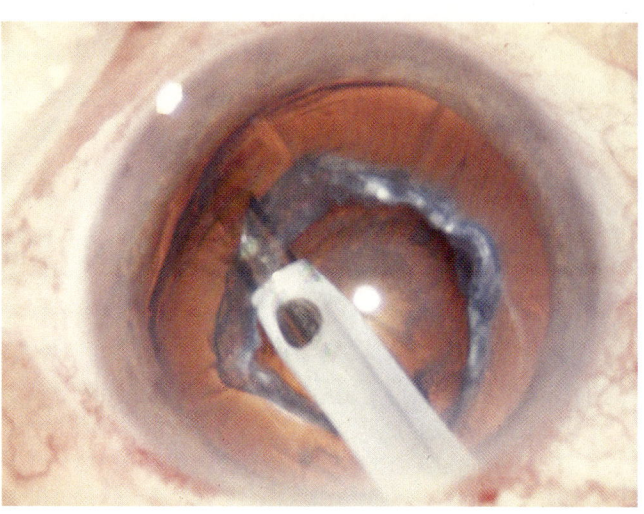

Figure 13.88 *The maximum possible phacoemulsification energy has been reduced to 60% with the machine in the linear mode. Brief taps of very low power of phaco energy will cause one section of soft nuclear rim to fold.*

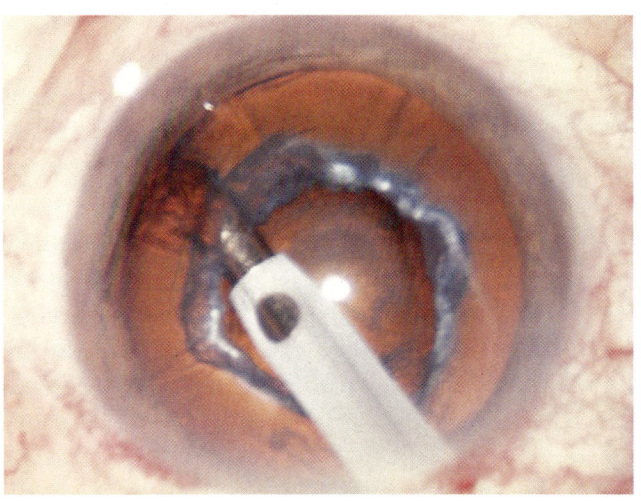

Figure 13.89 *The initial plug of peripheral nuclear rim has been withdrawn by the phacoemulsification tip suction.*

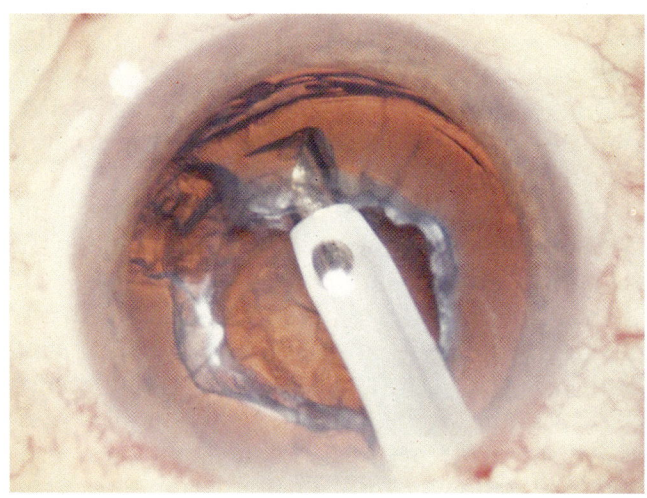

Figure 13.90 *A third wedge of peripheral nucleus is removed.*

Figure 13.91 *The peripheral anterior nucleus is drawn into the phaco tip when it is in suction mode.*

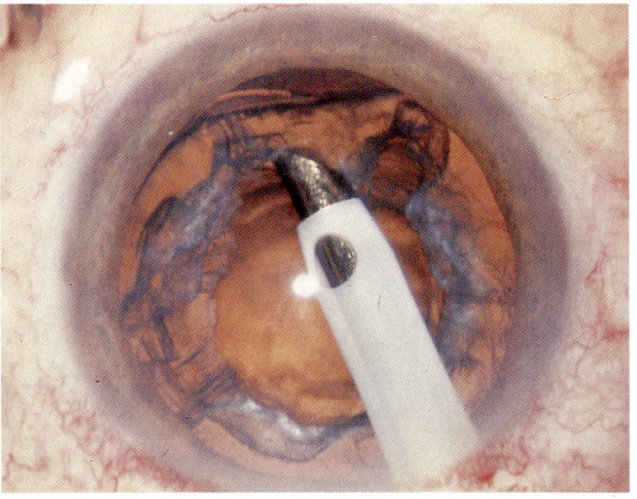

It is much safer and easier to turn the tip on its side and "sweep" the peripheral posterior nuclear surface (Fig. 13.87). This sweeping motion is effective for several reasons. First, the concavity of the posterior lens surface can be more easily paralleled by the sweeping tip when pivoted at the wound than during the usual superior to inferior driving motion, the thrust of which can cause the surgeon to overshoot the end point, giving the deeper nuclear drive a relatively high occlusion risk. Second, tip occlusion is virtually impossible since the tip's aperture is always pointed toward the more open cavity of the nuclear bowl. Third, visualization of the tip's action is excellent; that is, the depth of the remaining nucleus is visible immediately ahead of and behind the tip, enabling the surgeon to see how much material is being shaved. Instantaneous adjustments in depth can be made; thus, the posterior peripheral nucleus can be shaved quite thin. Fourth, the nuclear material immediately under the anterior capsular remnant can be emulsified without danger of aspiration. This enables the surgeon to see the deeper, more peripheral material and carve further peripherally and posteriorly.

Debulking the Inferior Equatorial Nucleus. The surgeon's mode of attack changes significantly at this stage. This is a transitional phase that occurs primarily between the cutting and suction modes. It actually involves both, but in very brief, low-power bursts.

As a safety measure in these soft nucleus cases, the maxium attainable power during linear control phacoemulsification is reduced to 50% from the usual starting point of 80%. This gives finer control and a greater measure of safety because the standard full pedal excursion distance is used for a shorter range of phacoemulsification energy. The actual observed phaco energy used through linear control is usually only 10% to 20% of maximum. My usual vacuum level of 101 mm Hg and aspiration flow rate of 17 cc/min remain unchanged when using the Alcon Series Ten Thousand. In the Alcon 9001 Series, the phaco vacuum is increased to its maximum adjustment of 35 inches of water. There are considerable differences in machines. The Storz Premier model, for instance, requires only about a 30% maximum power setting to be equivalent to the 9001's 80%.

To occlude the tip, the tip's aperture is engaged in a shallow fashion into the anterior peripheral nuclear remnant at the 3:30 clock-hour position. Very brief taps of the foot pedal while the phaco machine is set at the lowest energy level are used to remove a small section of peripheral nucleus (Figs. 13.88 and 13.89). This section does not have to be deep or large because each successive section will be a little deeper and larger. In this way, the tip does not become completely occluded by material that is directly attached to both sides of the remaining peripheral nuclear bulk, except during the first small initiating section (Fig. 13.90). After three or four pieces have been removed, the tip can be positioned on its side and deeper, newly exposed nuclear material can be shaved away.

Posterior Nuclear Thinning, Inward Collapse, and Aspiration of the Peripheral Nucleus. Once the transitional phase is completed, the ultrasonic tip can be operated at extremely low power, alternating between the suction and cutting modes. First, the aperture of the tip is applied like a suction cup to the 8 o'clock position on the peripheral nuclear remnant. As suction is applied across the aperture, a one to two clock-hour section of peripheral nucleus folds in centrally as the deeper fibers fracture. The folding and fracturing actions usually occur just central to the posterior equatorial zone, where the posterior nucleus has been thinned the most during the cutting mode. Brief taps of very low ultrasonic energy can be applied to encourage suction, infolding, and aspiration. It is important not to pursue peripheral nuclear material that does not come easily. The idea is to debulk only the peripheral nucleus by aspirating the anterior and equatorial level material, while letting the posterior layer drop back after the fracture and separation.

The lens nucleus is then rotated counterclockwise approximately three clock-hour positions. This rotation can usually be accomplished with only the cyclodialysis spatula, although a bimanual technique using the emulsification tip may be required as well. This rotational maneuver exposes another three clock hours of peripheral anterior and equatorial nucleus for aspiration with the assistance of low-power ultrasonic energy. The tip is returned to a cutting-shaving position in order to thin the deeper nuclear layers. Again, only low power is used and great care is taken not to occlude the tip and burst through the nucleus. If the deeper peripheral nucleus is adequately thinned, the remaining deeper fibers will fracture and the peripheral anterior nucleus will fold in and aspirate well. This deeper nuclear layer will fold and ultimately fracture as the anterior and equatorial layers are aspirated with suction and brief taps of low-power phacoemulsification energy (Fig. 13.91). Approximately half the peripheral nucleus has been debulked after this second three-clock-hour section has been brought into postion by the cyclodialysis spatula and emulsified.

After a third rotation is accomplished, the posterior nucleus is thinned using the cutting mode of the ultrasonic tip. Again, the tip is rotated 180 degrees, and the desired removal of the anterior and equatorial nuclear remnant is accomplished using suction (13.92).

The posterior thinning, infolding, and peripheral aspiration become easier with each rotation because the tip can be drawn more centrally while emulsifying and aspirating peripheral nucleus in the suction mode. This more central location is possible because of the diminished nuclear bulk and the resultant smaller nuclear diameter. Longer duration (but still low power) taps of emulsification energy can be used to emulsify and aspirate the infolded peripheral nucleus as it fractures. If too much material is drawn into the tip, or if the nuclear shell is pulled forward and endangers the perfection of the anterior capsular remnant, it can be pushed back by the spatula.

Removal of the Posterior Nuclear Disc. The superior pole of the posterior nuclear disc can be elevated slightly away from the posterior capsule by the cyclodialysis spatula and guided into position for safe ultrasonic tip exposure. Ultrasonic energy and suction can then be safely applied while the spatula continuously supports the nuclear material to protect the posterior capsule (Fig. 13.93). The shallow functional angle of attack of the 45-degree ultrasonic tip helps prevent posterior capsule aspiration. The spatula supports the nuclear fragments well away from the posterior capsule, which, if flaccid, can be easily aspirated if the tip is positioned deeply (Fig. 13.94). Remember, in most machines, the vacuum and flow rate parameters are not varied by foot position and are the same as at the start of emulsification. After the last fragments are drawn to the tip aperture by suction, ultrasonic energy has to be very low or the fragments will merely bounce off the tip and never be aspirated. The cyclodialysis spatula helps hold the material in place while protecting the posterior capsule (Fig. 13.95).

MEDIUM SOFT NUCLEI: MULTIPLE WEDGE TECHNIQUE

This technique works well for soft or even slightly firm lenses and is a variation of the suction-cutting method. It is a good technique to use if the nucleus seems too hard for the suction-cutting technique and the surgeon is uncomfortable with Gimbel and Shepherd's posterior cracking maneuver or if the surgeon finds that nuclear fracture is not possible. Thus, the multiple wedge technique is a valuable adjunctive strategy to the cutting-

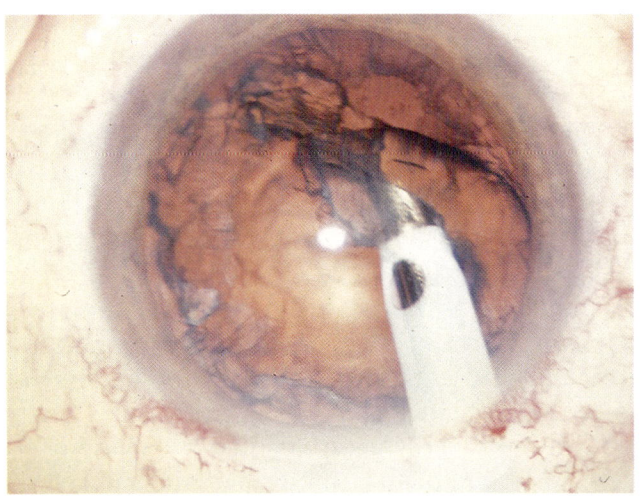

Figure 13.92 *Portions of the rim are nibbled away while the tip is positioned centrally.*

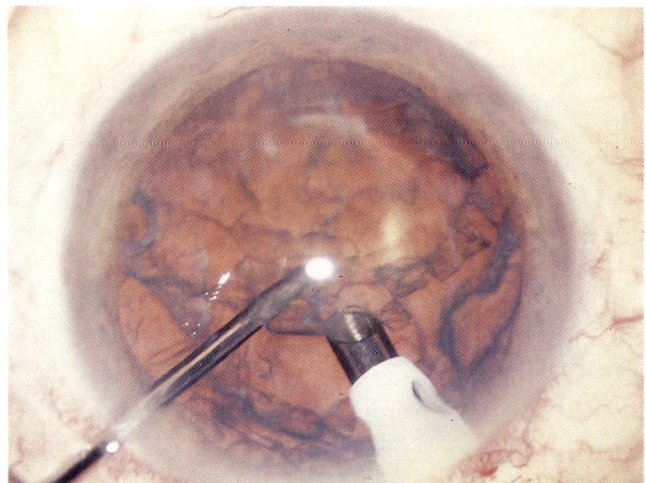

Figure 13.93 *As the posterior disc becomes smaller, the nuclear fragment can be held in a more central position away from the posterior capsule, improving visualization and enabling more aggressive use of the phacoemulsification tip.*

suction method or the fracture-quartering technique if the nucleus is too soft to crack.

In a very soft lens, hydrodissection is performed and the central nucleus is sculpted deeply, as with the cutting-suction technique. Deep and peripheral sculpting should be accomplished if nuclear cracking has been ineffective and unsuccessful in a firm lens. The first inferior three-clock-hour sections of the nucleus are cut away with the combined suction and tearing motion as in the soft nucleus strategy (Figure 13.96). This initial debulking will usually permit the nucleus to be loosened and rotated. The next three-clock-hour segment is rotated into an inferior position and its deeper peripheral nuclear layer thinned by the phaco tip in its cutting mode (Fig. 13.97). Three or four more wedges of nuclear rim are drawn in and torn away by aspiration.

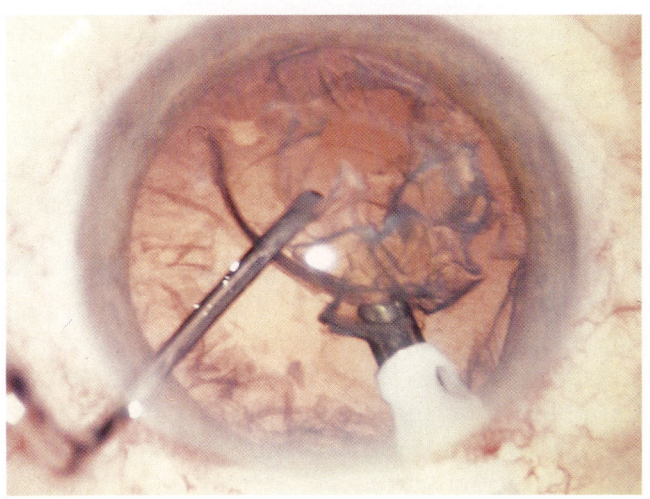

Figure 13.94 *The spatula continues to support nuclear fragments in a position away from the posterior capsule.*

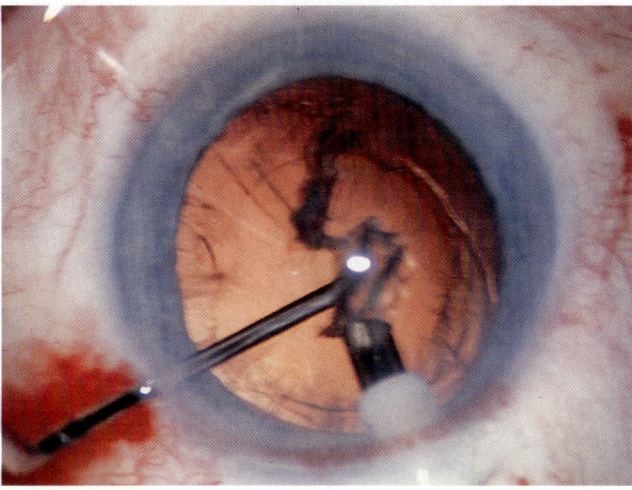

Figure 13.95 *The surgeon should be aware that a flaccid posterior capsule may be impaled easily just after the last fragment has been aspirated. It is important to keep the fragment away from the posterior capsule.*

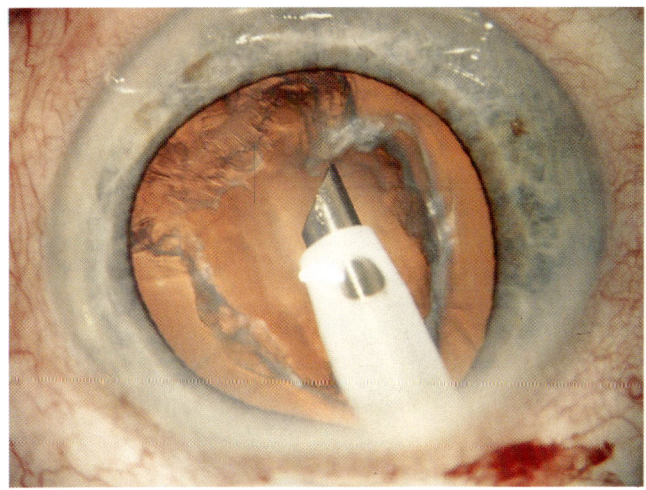

Figure 13.96 *Four small wedges of peripheral nucleus have been torn away by the occluded phaco tip in the aspiration mode without phacoemulsification. The nucleus is ready to be rotated three clock hours to expose a new quadrant for wedge removal.*

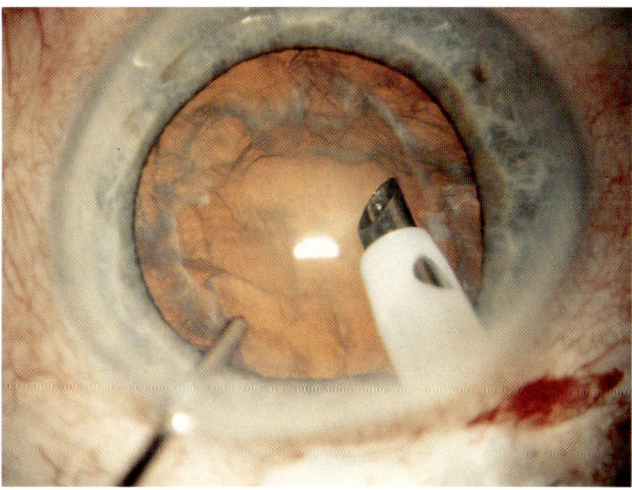

Figure 13.97 *A new quadrant has been rotated into position so the tip can be occluded with peripheral anterior material. First, however, the deeper peripheral nucleus must be thinned by the phaco tip in its cutting mode so the fibers just deep to the thinned portion will tear away as the overlying anterior peripheral wedge is pulled centrally.*

(Figs. 13.98 to 13.100). After additional rotations, the entire nuclear periphery is gone and the posterior nuclear disc can be removed just as with the cutting-suction strategy.

FIRM NUCLEI: POSTERIOR NUCLEAR FRACTURE AND QUARTERING HYBRID

This method is used in over 95% of cases in which the nucleus is firm enough to be efficiently manipulated by the phaco tip and the cyclodialysis spatula.

The first two strategies (cutting-suction and multiple wedge) depend on aspiration to remove relatively soft peripheral nucleus and tear away deeper peripheral segments. The tearing occurs across the peripherally thinned posterior nuclear shell. The peripheral posterior layer of firmer nuclei may be so hard that its fibers will not tear when the surgeon attempts to draw in the peripheral segment. The nuclear material may be so hard that it cannot effectively occlude the phaco tip and inadequate aspiration and poor followability result.

In these cases, fracturing the posterior nuclear plate into four pieces with a bimanual spreading motion (i.e., quartering the nucleus) makes each fragment manageable. Gimbel and Shepherd were the first to promote the bimanual spreading fracture of nuclear layers and separating the resulting nuclear segments for more convenient emulsification. As with soft or medium firm nucleus removal techniques, nuclear bowl segmentation has many variations. For example, Gimbel, Shepherd, and Dillman all prefer the 30-degree tip for this procedure while I like the 45-degree tip. The same principles of isolated cutting, suction, and manipulation apply to these fracture-quartering removal methods as well as to the removal methods for softer lenses.

After hydodissection, just enough anterior nuclear fibers are removed to maximize the red reflex and make the anterior capsulotomy plainly visible (Fig. 13.101). This first step, along with the initial groove in the nucleus, is performed with very low phaco power. Too much energy during this anterior dissection can cause substantial turbulence and fluttering of the iris, resulting in reduction in pupil size. The initial groove is about one and one-half phaco tip diameters wide. Again, it is safest to use as low a power as possible, especially while working deep and in the periphery of the nucleus (Figs. 13.102 and 13.103). Enough power must be used to keep the surgeon from pushing on the tip. If it is deliberately pushed, larger chunks of posterior plate will break away, suddenly exposing the posterior capsule to potential phaco tip trauma. Complete occlusion of the tip may be avoided by rotating the tip slightly to the side as the peripheral groove is created. Occlusion permits the establishment of vacuum and possible sudden aspiration with capsular damage.

After the first groove is completed, the nucleus is loosened and turned 90 degrees. The second groove is created in the superior hemisphere first in order to allow efficient access to the inferior hemisphere (Figs. 13.104 to 13.106). The cyclodialysis spatula and phaco tip then push on opposing nuclear walls to create a spreading and tearing

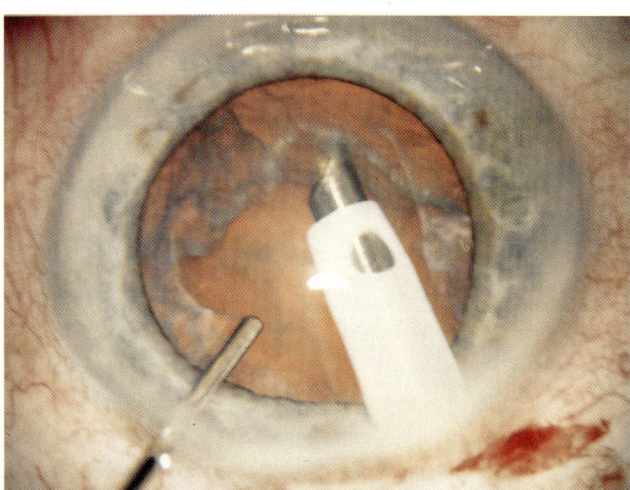

Figure 13.98 *The phacoemulsification tip is prepared to sink into the remaining anterior peripheral nucleus and pull a wedge of it over the thinner deep section. The deeper component is fractured passively so the middle and anterior portions can be freed and aspirated.*

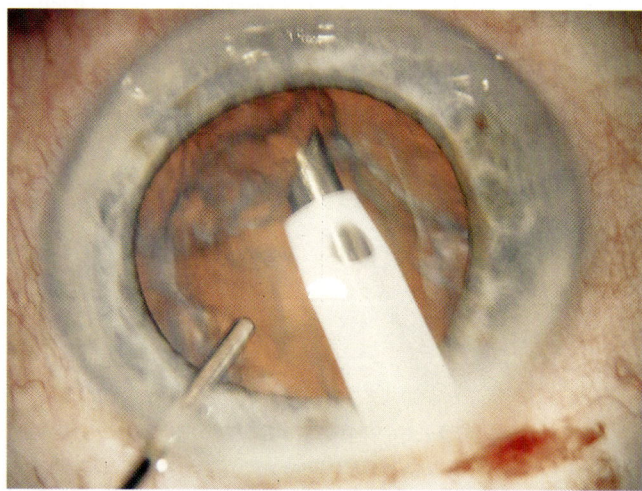

Figure 13.99 *The tip has been driven into the peripheral nucleus and the wedge of material is being drawn into the tip as it pulls centrally.*

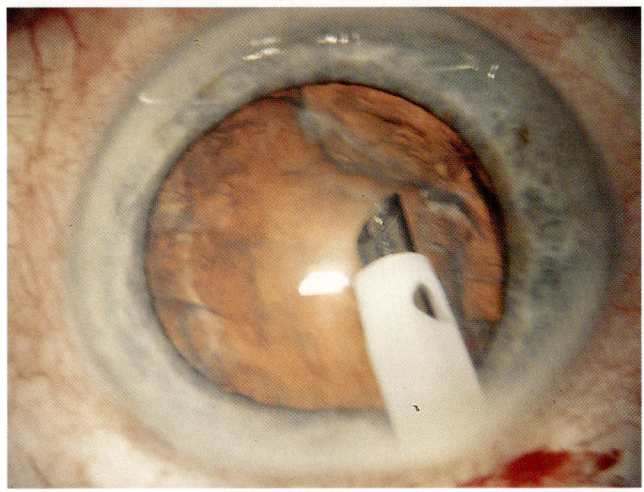

Figure 13.100 *A new section of nucleus is rotated into position while its deeper peripheral level is simultaneously thinned.*

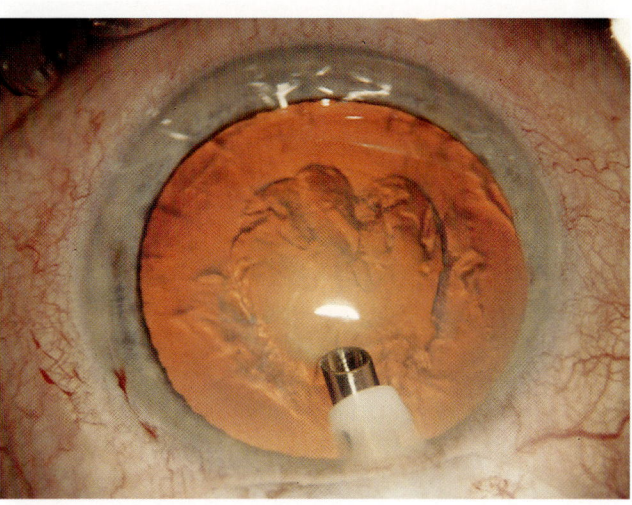

Figure 13.101 *The superficial optical irregularity of the lens is removed by sculpting the nucleus with very low phaco power to improve the red reflex and visualization of the capsulorhexis border.*

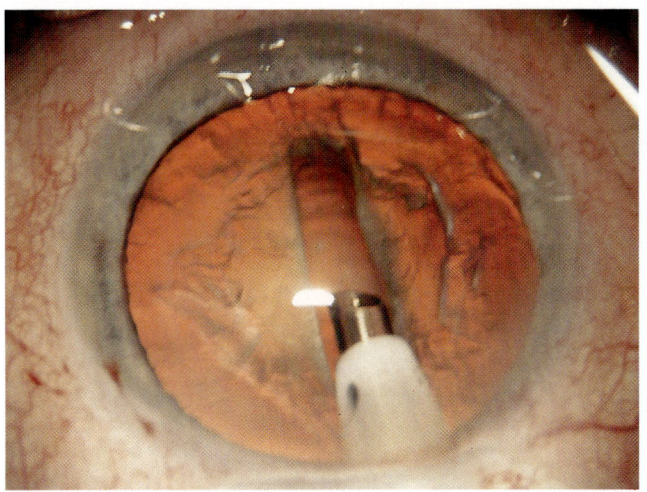

Figure 13.102 *A deep groove in the nucleus is cut with the 45-degree tip. Note the good visualization of the tip's cutting edge even at this extreme depth.*

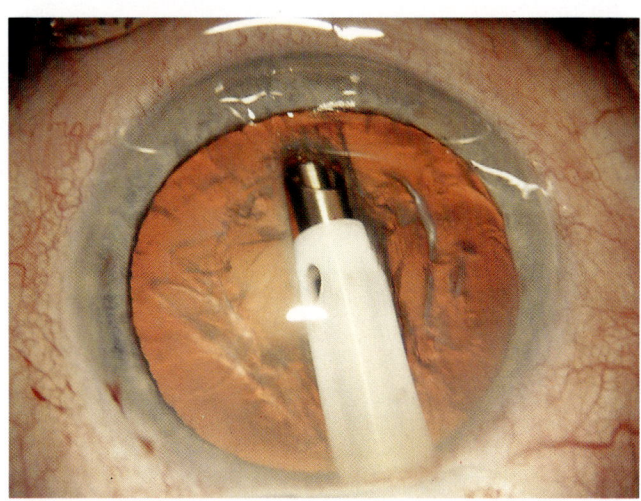

Figure 13.103 *In the far periphery, the tip may be rotated slightly so that it is not inadvertently occluded by capsule.*

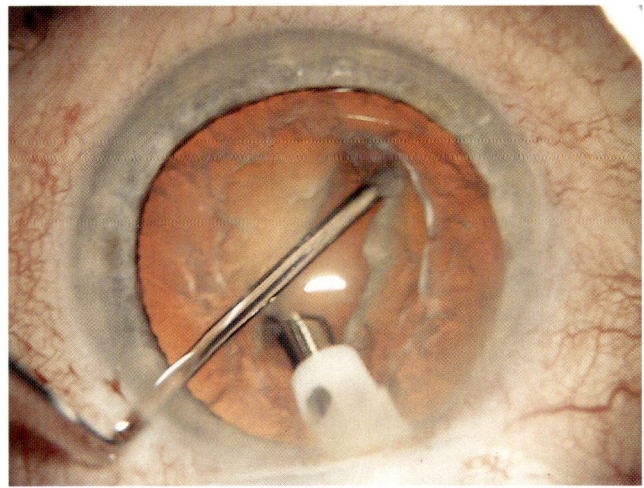

Figure 13.104 *The loosened nucleus is rotated carefully in a bimanual fashion.*

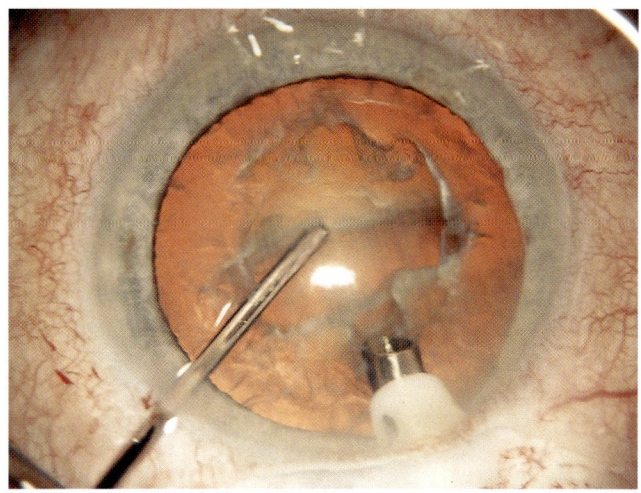

Figure 13.105 *The cyclodialysis spatula pushes the nucleus slightly inferiorly to improve exposure of the phaco tip to the superior hemisphere while creating its groove.*

of the deep fibers of the inferior posterior nuclear disc (Figs. 13.107 to 13.108). A similar spreading often can be accomplished in the superior hemisphere, causing the posterior nuclear plate to have a crack that extends from top to bottom. The nucleus is rotated 90 degrees and another cleft created in similar fashion. If superior fractures cannot be made easily, the hemisphere should be cracked after it is rotated to the inferior position. The nucleus has then been divided into four separate quadrants (Fig. 13.109).

The quadrants can be aspirated at this point if the lens is quite soft, but I usually prefer to remove much of the deep central nuclear material with the phaco tip in its cutting mode while the nuclear fragments are still in situ. (Figs. 13.110 and 13.111). The knife-like configuration of the 45-degree phaco tip can be applied to the nuclear plate very close to the posterior capsule. The aperture design prohibits complete inadvertent tip occlusion and inadvertent aspiration of the posterior capsule. Removal of the deep inner nuclear

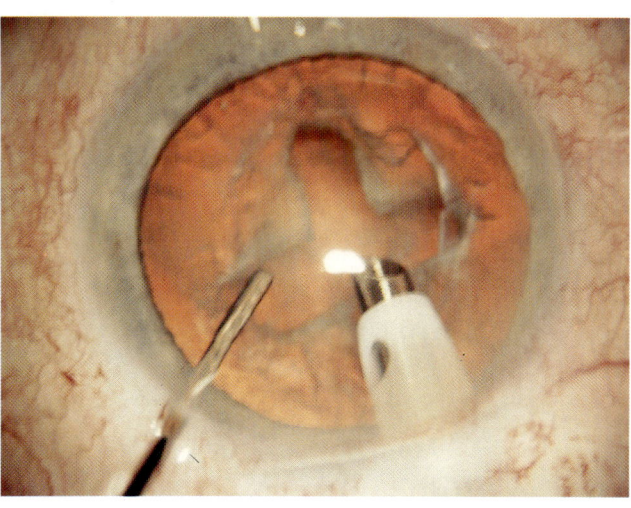

Figure 13.106 *The inferior groove is cut after the superior groove has been made. The nucleus is now ready for posterior fracture.*

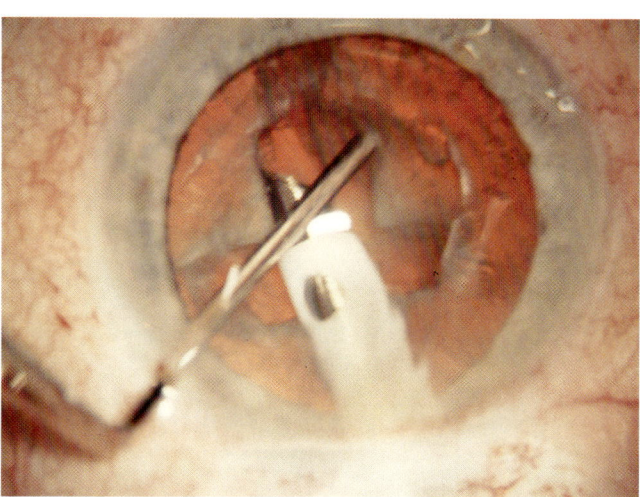

Figure 13.107 *A cross action pattern is seen with the two instruments pushing lightly on the deep aspect of the vertical walls of the cut nuclear grooves. This action is essential if the superior hemisphere is to be cracked in situ.*

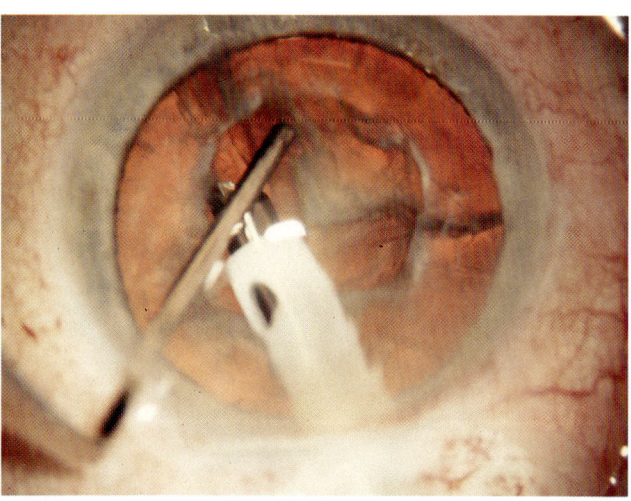

Figure 13.108 *The nucleus has been rotated 90 degrees and the second posterior nuclear fracture created.*

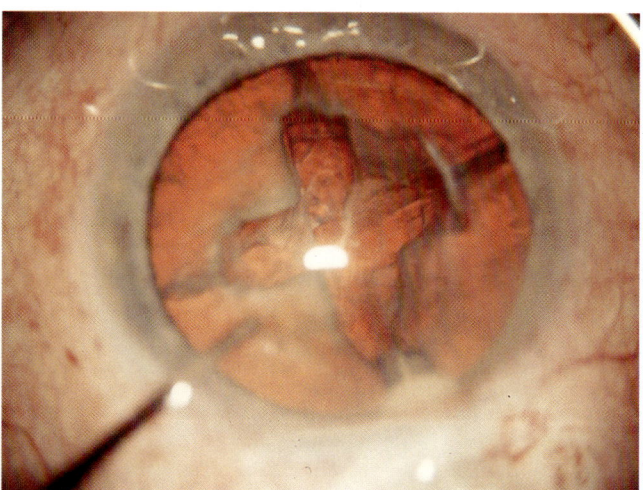

Figure 13.109 *The nucleus is ready for the inner nuclear debulking process.*

corners is more important in firmer nuclei; otherwise, large three-dimensional nuclear chunks may protrude into the anterior chamber or push on the posterior capsule or anterior capsular remnant. Shaving the corners away converts the chunks into relatively two-dimensional sheets awaiting aspiration. These sheets are less threatening to important adjacent features.

When all of the corners have been shaved and the deep nucleus thinned as much as practical, the phacoemulsification tip function is changed from the cutting mode to the suction mode (Figs. 13.112 and 13.113). This very deliberate change in attack mode permits the phaco tip aperture to be completely occluded by peripheral anterior nuclear material. It is burrowed into the sheet with brief taps of very low-power phaco energy so vacuum can be established. Because of adhesion between the phaco tip and the nuclear material, the sheet of nucleus can actually be moved to a slightly more central location within the capsular bag for safer, simultaneous application of pha-

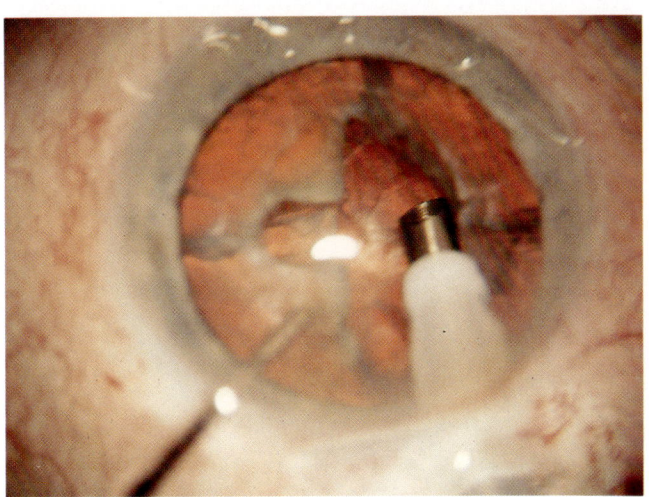

Figure 13.110 *The 45-degree tip is used at low power in the cutting mode to shave the corners off the nuclear quarters. Tip occlusion is not possible, thereby increasing safety.*

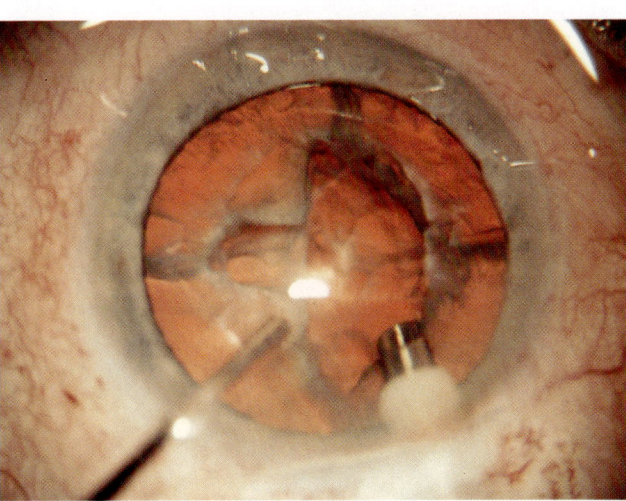

Figure 13.111 *Half of the nucleus has been debulked. This process will facilitate infolding and in situ emulsification of the subsequent smaller fragments.*

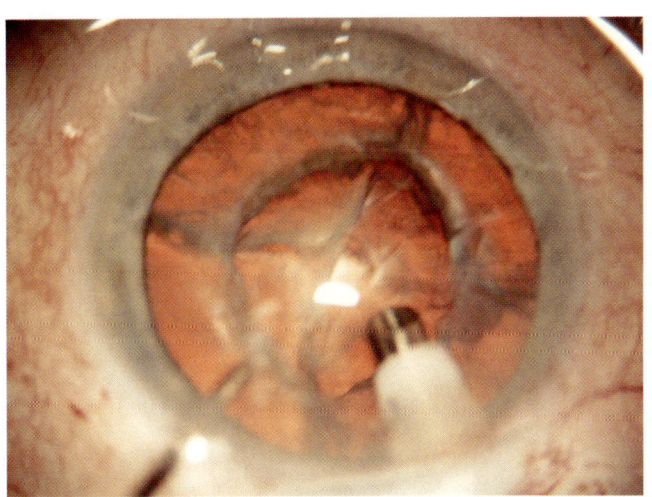

Figure 13.112 *The four corners have been shaved, the deeper nucleus debulked, and the deeper periphery thinned.*

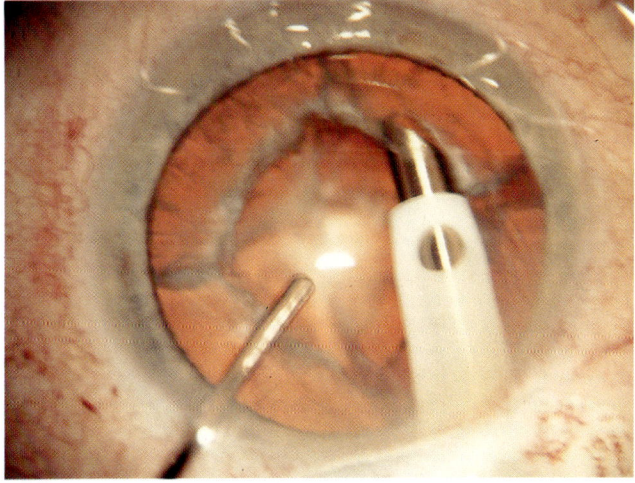

Figure 13.113 *Brief taps of the pedal provide low-power phaco energy and vacuum that are used to engage the peripheral anterior nuclear pillow at its thickest (safest) point.*

coemulsification energy and aspiration of formed nuclear material (Figs. 13.114 and 13.115).

Each quadrant is rotated into the inferior position for attack by the phaco tip in its suction mode. The last quadrant may present a special challenge, especially if it is firm. The surrounding capsule is relatively unprotected during removal of this quadrant so extra effort must be made to position it well away from important capsular structures before aspiration and phacoemulsification energy is engaged. This capsule can be supported with the cyclodialysis spatula during phacoemulsification at the iris plane (Fig. 13.116). The spatula acts as a physical barrier between the phaco tip and the posterior capsule, with the lens substance in between. This offers the best protection to the posterior capsule until the very last fragment has been removed (Fig. 13.117).

Aspiration of Cortex

There is a tendency to relax during cortical aspiration, a relatively easy post-phacoemulsification step. Unfortunately, it is still easy to tear the posterior capsule. Often, the first step in I/A is to remove small nuclear fragments (Fig. 13.118). The superior cortex should be removed before the rest as the handpiece is held almost vertically in order to effectively apply the 0.30 mm aperture to the cortical fibers, which are adherent to the anterior capsular remnant at the 11 o'clock position (Fig. 13.119).

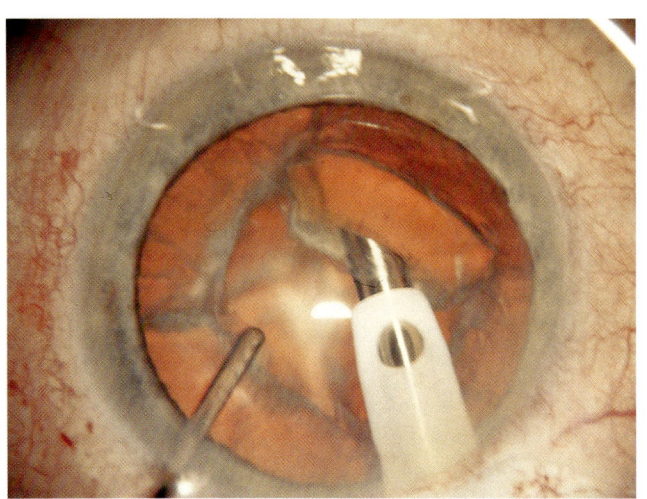

Figure 13.114 *As the nuclear quarter is engaged, it is drawn into a more central location within the capsular bag. While not exactly in situ, it is still within the capsular bag, which is a safer location for aspiration and phacoemulsification.*

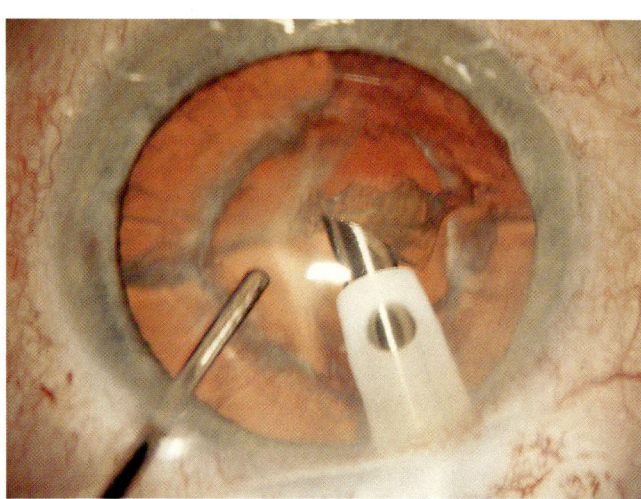

Figure 13.115 *Capsular aspiration is virtually impossible even when removing the last fragment.*

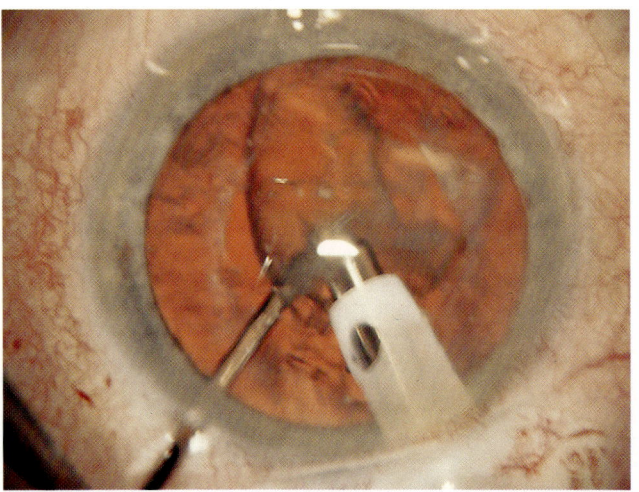

Figure 13.116 *The last nuclear quarter is held very carefully at about the iris plane by the cyclodialysis spatula.*

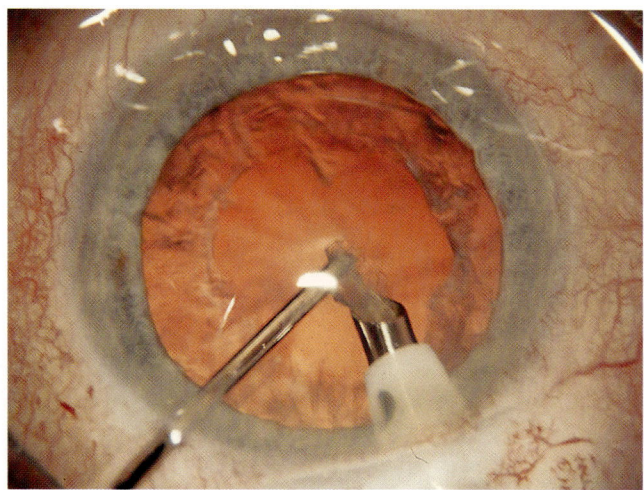

Figure 13.117 *The spatula stays in place, protecting the posterior capsule as the last fragment is aspirated.*

Some of the protruding fibers under the anterior capsular edge will be caught at either the 11 o'clock position or on either side of it. Anterior and equatorial cortex will strip away without difficulty when starting above and moving peripherally (Figs. 13.120 to 13.122). If the cortex is removed while progressing from inferior to superior, support and presentation is eventually lost adjacent to the 11 o'clock position. The cortical fibers protruding adjacent to the 11 o'clock position should be engaged early by the I/A tip so they can then help pull out the progressively larger triangular strips of

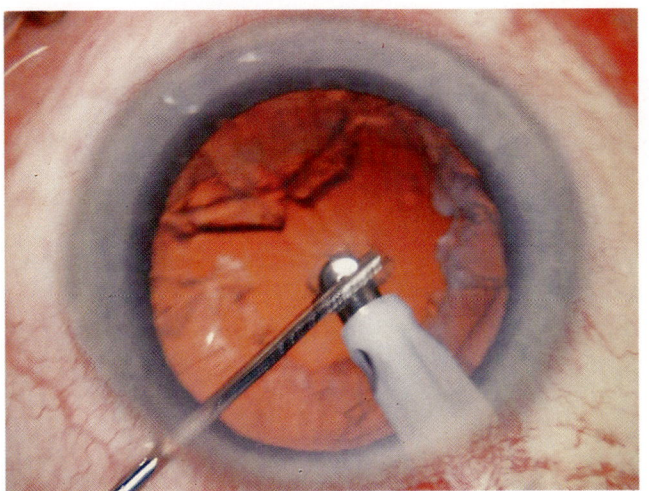

Figure 13.118 *Aspiration often starts by removing one or two small nuclear fragments and crushing them into the aspiration tip with the cyclodialysis spatula.*

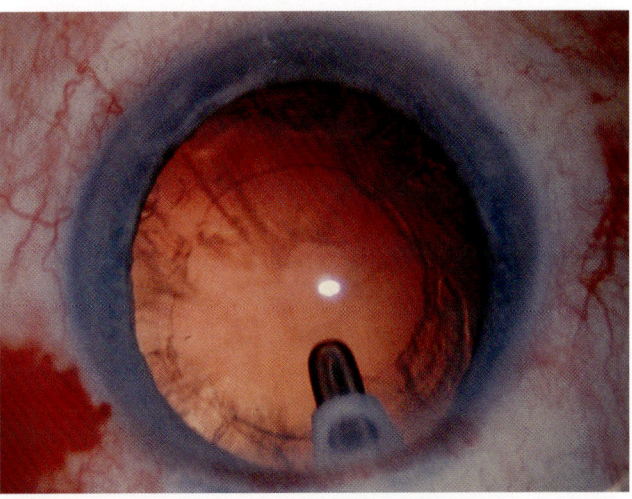

Figure 13.119 *The edge of the cortex is grasped at the 11 o'clock position just under the anterior capsular remnant.*

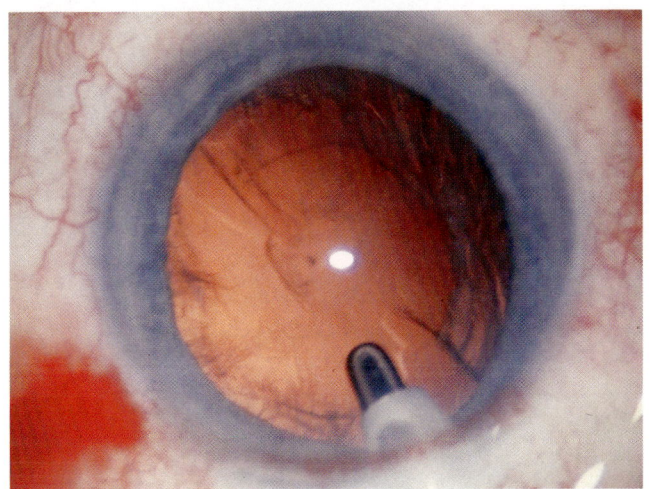

Figure 13.120 *This initial piece of cortex has been pulled away.*

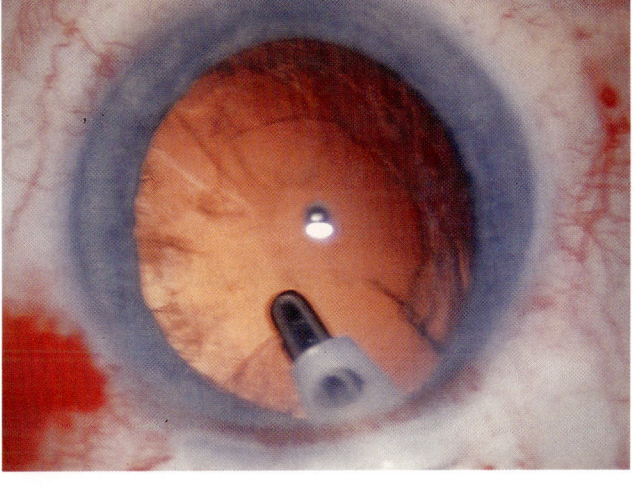

Figure 13.121 *Another small adjacent strip is grasped and withdrawn.*

Figure 13.122 *Superior cortex removal has been accomplished on the left side.*

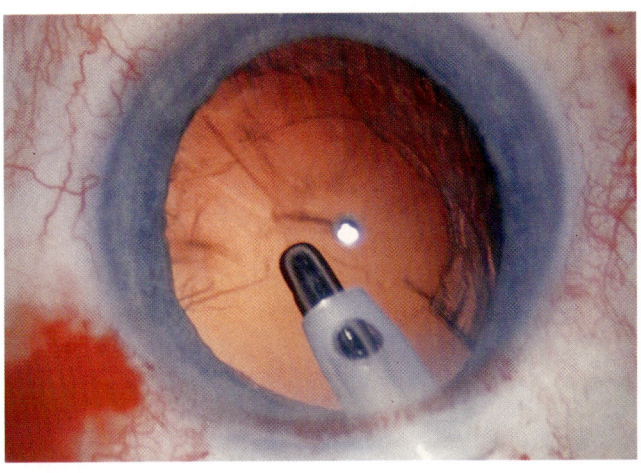

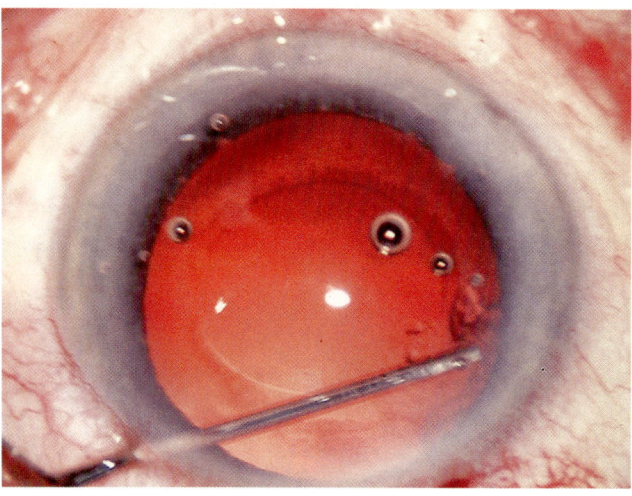

Figure 13.123 *After some viscoelastic is placed, the cortex is roughed up with a cyclodialysis spatula in an attempt to form an edge that can be grasped.*

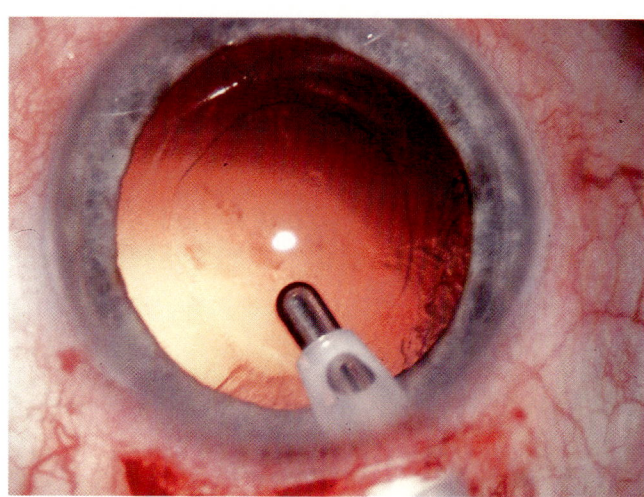

Figure 13.124 *The problem of superior cortex removal can be more troublesome in filmy posterior capsular cataracts than in other types. Sometimes it has to be left as it is.*

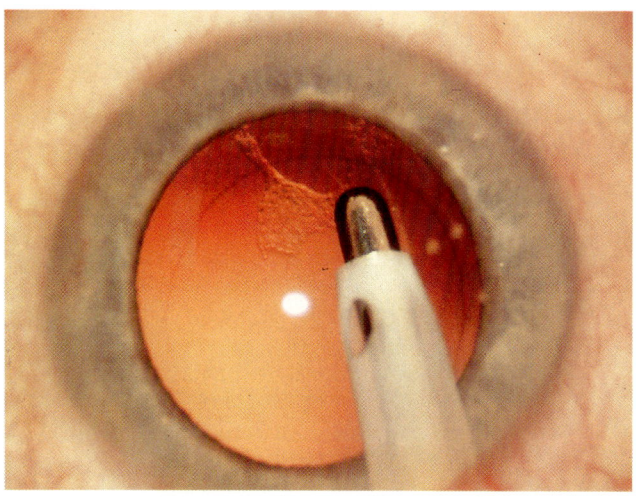

Figure 13.125 *Most of the capsule has been vacuumed.*

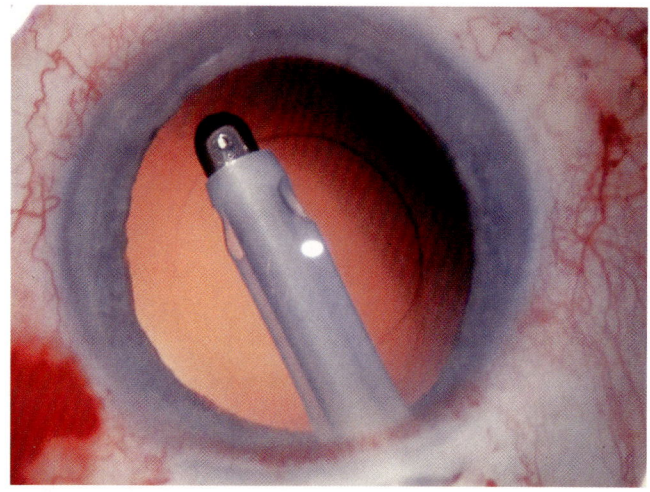

Figure 13.126 *Anterior capsule vacuuming may decrease epithelial cell complications.*

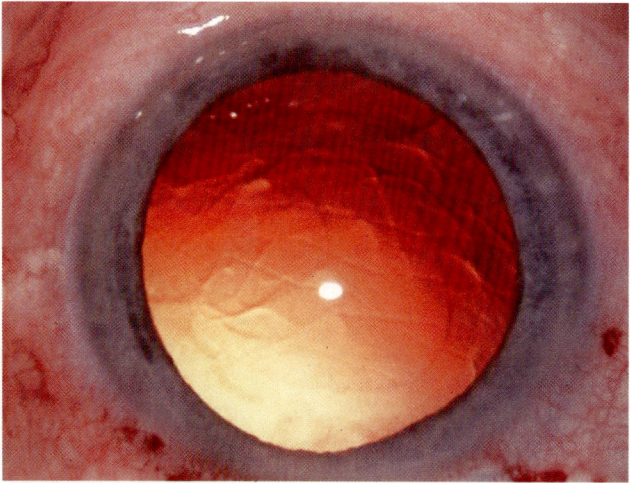

Figure 13.127 *The capsular bag has been filled with viscoelastic and the wound extended. Indivdual ribbons of viscoelastic can be seen. The posterior capsule is minimally concave, and the bag has not been overfilled.*

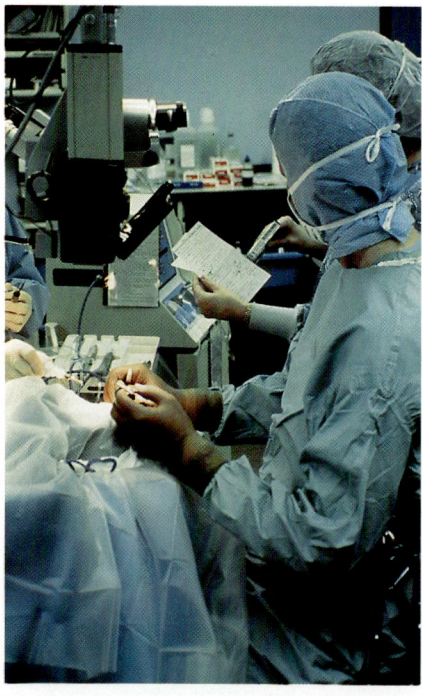

Figure 13.128 *A final last-minute check of the original IOL calculation sheet, the patient's name, the operative eye, and the IOL model and power.*

the surrounding cortex. Isolated wedges of peripheral cortex left within the capsular bag are often difficult to remove, since the peripheral component of the cortex may be stranded if the protruding fibers pull away during I/A tip engagement.

If a peripheral piece of cortex is left behind, the haptic knee of the IOL can be used as a "scratcher" to loosen it from the capsule. The I/A tip can then engage and remove the residual cortex later during viscoelastic aspiration. An angled I/A tip may be used, but even then, in some circumstances, some cortex may have to be left behind (Figs. 13.123 and 13.124).

The irrigation bottle is lowered to 40 cm above the eye, and the machine placed in a capsular vacuum mode. A 0.20-mm tip is used to vacuum the posterior capsule as well as any conveniently available anterior capsular remnants (Figs. 13.125 and 13.126).

Intraocular Lens Implantation

After capsular vacuuming, the anterior chamber is filled with enough viscoelastic to push back the posterior capsule so it is concave (Fig. 13.127). The wound incision is extended to 5.50 mm with lateral movement of the keratome. Of course, a smaller extension to only 4.00 mm may be necessary if a foldable IOL is to be used. I perform a last minute check of the IOL power calculation sheet (prepared in my script), match the desired IOL power to that on the IOL container, and verify the patient's name and operative eye (Fig. 13.128). I usually use a one-piece all-PMMA biconvex 6.00-mm UV filtering optic with a soft C-loop, a 12.00-mm overall length, and a six-degree posterior angulation (Fig. 13.129) or a three-piece folded silicone IOL. The haptics are very pliable and easily placed within the capsular bag using a Lester hook (Figs. 13.130 and 13.131). No manipulation of the superior haptic is required for insertion. This haptic configuration consistently centers the IOL in large or small eyes. During surgery, there is no distortion of the anterior capsular remnant, capsular equatorial zone, or posterior capsule. There is no tendency to generate ciliary body irritation secondary to

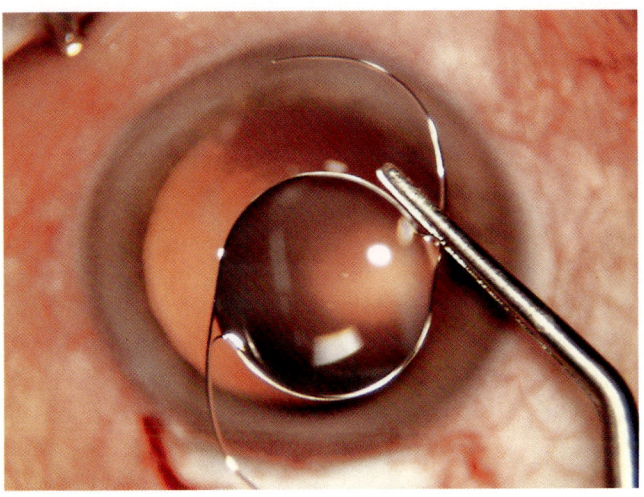

Figure 13.129 *For 6.00-mm optic IOLs, my preference is a one-piece all-PMMA IOL with biconvex UV filtered optic and a 12.00-mm haptic diameter with 6-degree haptic tilt and soft C-loop haptic design.*

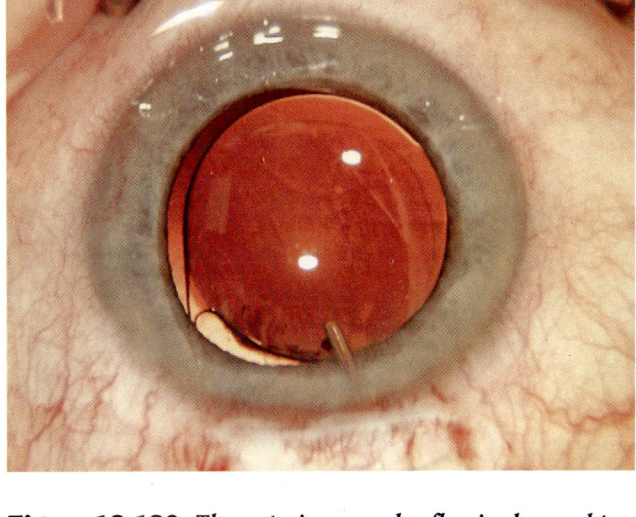

Figure 13.130 *The anterior capsular flap is observed to be anterior to the optic for 360 degrees. Only the superior haptic remains anterior to the anterior capsular remnant.*

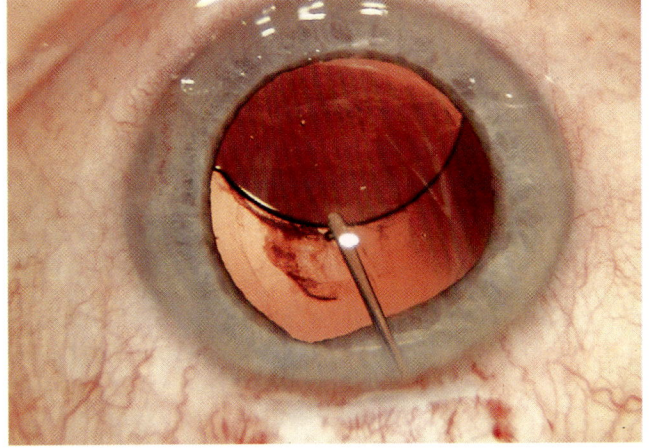

Figure 13.131 *The superior haptic is dialed into place through compression of the soft short inferior haptic. Compression is accomplished with the Lester hook on the superior optic edge. The one-piece all-PMMA construction provides good haptic memory and perfect centration, even after this vigorous compression.*

capsular bag overstretch, which can be seen with capsular bag implantation of longer, stiffer lenses better suited to ciliary sulcus implantation (Fig. 13.132). Long-term, a 12-mm, soft C-design seems to help balance the forces of capsular contracture and results in stable long-term optic centration.

A C-loop, 12.00-mm haptic configuration makes IOLs easy to implant when operative conditions are good. More importantly though, these lenses are safer to implant than longer, stiffer designs in less favorable situations. A moderately soft, shorter haptic IOL configuration allows easier management of conditions such as short eye, tight eye, small pupil, imperfect capsulorhexis, imperfect zonular support, very steep brow, or merely the restless patient.

Wound Closure

After suturing the wound with 10-0 nylon, sector iridectomies are repaired using a straight needle and 10-0 Prolene in a fashion described by Worst (Fig. 13.133). Viscoelastic is removed with the 0.30-mm I/A tip after the BSS bottle is lowered to 40 cm above the eye.

Wounds can be closed by a variety of suture techniques, depending on personal preference. As emphasized in the section on wound construction, if the wound has been perfectly created, wound closure is not a critical step. The objectives of any closure technique should include the creation of a secure leak-free wound, minimization of bleeding and postoperative hyphema, virtually immediate return of the wound to normal configuration without excessive induced with-the-rule astigmatism short-term or against-the-rule astigmatism long-term, and reasonable patient comfort with minimal postoperative irritation.

If a traditional running suture pattern is employed, final suture tightness should be obtained with keratoscopic control. The sutures are first tightened empirically and a triple throw knot made. The eye is inflated to a fairly firm level with a 30-gauge cannula through the side-port incision (Fig. 13.134). A surgical sponge is used to tamp down the wound while small amounts of BSS are expressed through the wound edge in order to check alignment and tightness (Fig. 13.135).

When the eye is at a "normal" firm pressure, a Maloney keratoscope can be used to check the keratoscopic reflex (Fig. 13.136). Figure 13.136 shows sutures pulled too tightly, and it appears that about 3.00 D of with-the-rule keratoscopic astigmatism has been induced. In these cases the suture is loosened slightly. Inflation, tamping, and keratoscopic checks are then repeated, yielding a more circular image. If any amount of against-the-rule astigmatism (vertically ovoid reflex) is noted, the sutures must be tightened. Finally, the position of the IOL should once again be confirmed to make sure that its position in the capsular bag has not changed during anterior chamber re-formation and suture tying (Fig. 13.137).

One of the problems with a running 10-0 nylon suture is its 25% elasticity. If wound construction technique is not good, then sutures must be extra tight to prevent leaks. Three diopters of with-the-rule astigmatism might not be a surprise the day after surgery. Moreover, faulty wound construction can cause such leaks and sometimes extra sutures must be placed, especially in high myopes (Figs. 13.138 and 13.139). Temporarily induced with-the-rule astigmatism can be increased substantially by wound compression from extra

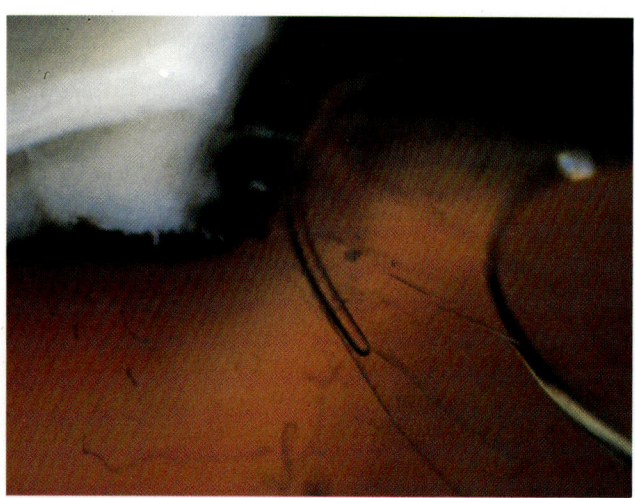

Figure 13.132 *A highly magnified view shows a 12.00-mm diameter haptic contained within the capsular bag but not pushed against the ciliary processes by capsular bag overstretch.*

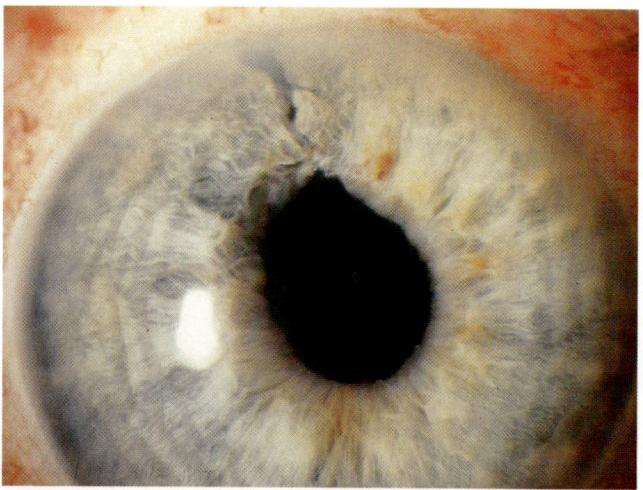

Figure 13.133 *Sector iridectomy has been repaired with two 10-0 Prolene sutures on straight needles, as described by Worst.*

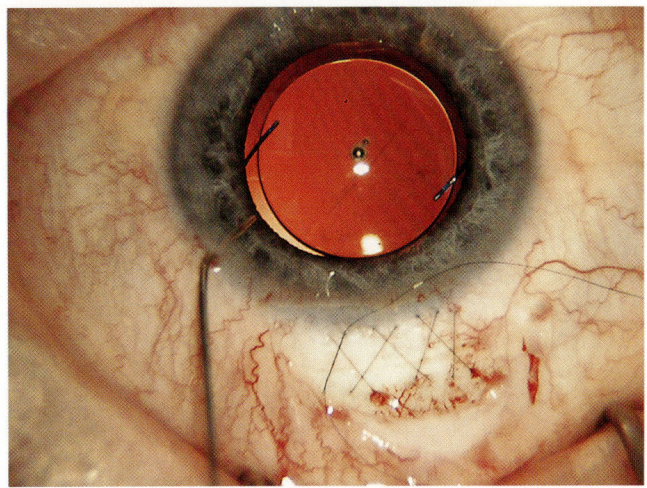

Figure 13.134 *The sutures have been brought up and secured by a triple thow knot. The anterior chamber is inflated with BSS through the stab incision with a 30-gauge cannula.*

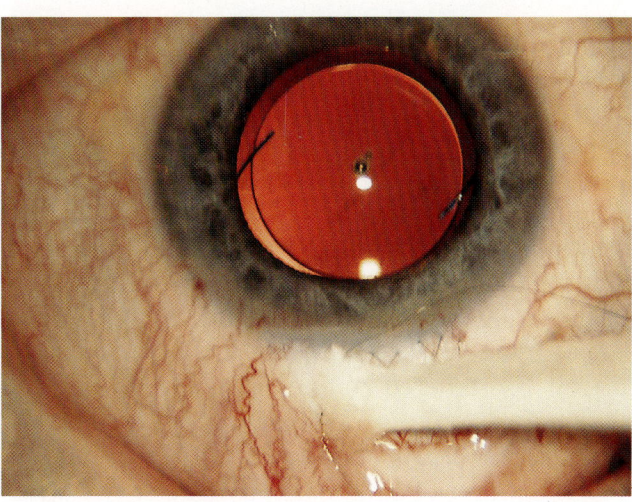

Figure 13.135 *The wound is tamped and checked for leakage and the eye is checked for firmness (for practical purposes, this is usually estimated by touch). It should be at a "normal" pressure of about 20 mm Hg to 25 mm Hg.*

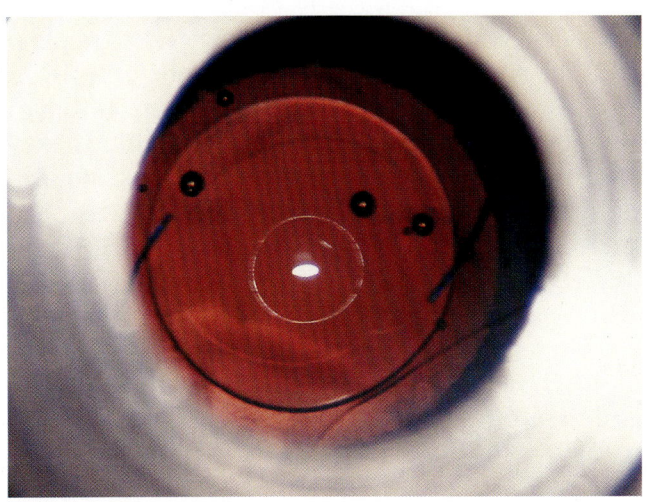

Figure 13.136 *The Maloney keratoscope is used; a horizontal ovoid reflection indicates about 3.00 D of induced with-the-rule astigmatism.*

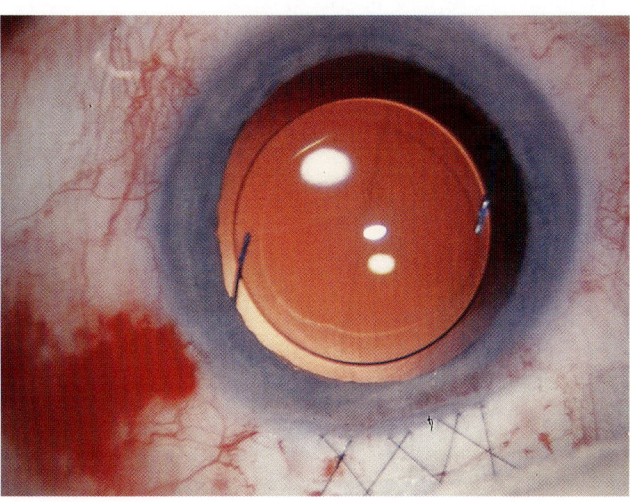

Figure 13.137 *A three-piece IOL is in good position within the capsular bag. No excessive viscoelastic remains. Surgical progress has been excellent up to this point.*

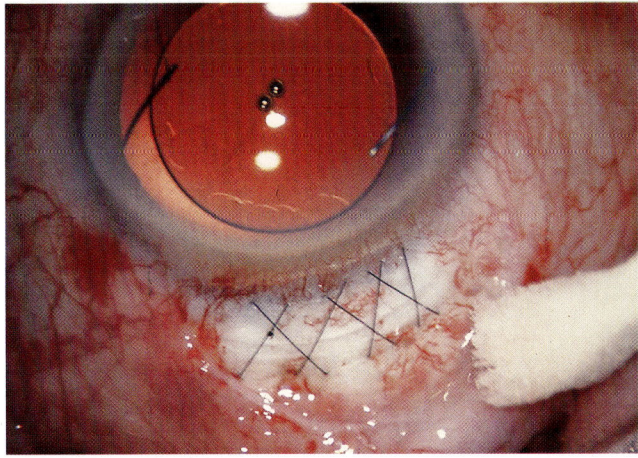

Figure 13.138 *The wound is checked, and a slight leak is identified at the right-hand extreme of the wound.*

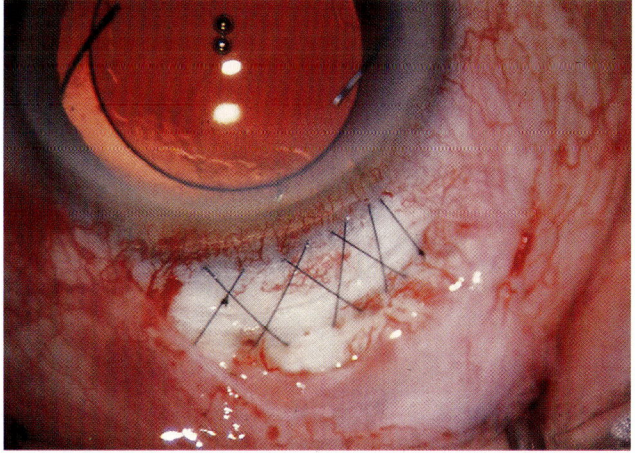

Figure 13.139 *The leak has been closed by an extra single radial suture.*

sutures and low intraocular pressure secondary to wound leakage.

John Shepherd, M.D., revolutionized small incision closure with his transverse suture concept (Fig. 13.140). Very little early with-the-rule astigmatism is induced with this method, and attainment of very impressive levels of vision is virtually immediate. Hybrids of this technique have been applied to larger wounds (Fig. 13.141). Any of these closures are fine if they are applied to well constructed competent wounds. The key to superior wound performance is in the entry to the anterior chamber. Normal intraocular pressure must press the internal lip against the outer flap for good tissue approximation. A balance between too central and too peripheral an entry must be sought. If anterior chamber entry is too peripheral, a fragile closure will result with occasional leaks or hyphemas (Figs. 13.142 to 13.144). If Descemet's entry is too central, increased endothelial trauma will occur but, even more important, anterior capsulotomy, phacoemulsification, cortex aspiration, and IOL implantation will all be more difficult because of poor visualization created by excessive corneal distortion (Fig. 13.145). Early on, my triplanar scleral pocket incisions were not consistently good, so I had more hyphemas, intercapsular-IOL blood, and anterior vitreous hemorrhages. Most important, some long-term against-the-rule astigmatism is being seen late in my tranverse closures of both 4.00 mm and 5.50 mm wounds.

My wound constuction technique is gradually improving. I usually use a simple double-X closure for 5.50 mm wounds (Figs. 13.146 to 13.149). I rarely see induced with-the-rule astigmatism of more than 1.50 D on the first postoperative day. Most patients have just less than 1.00 D of induced with-the-rule astigmatism. For 4.00 mm incisions, I usually use the same pattern. Results for these smaller incisions with this suture pattern are similar and the patients are delighted.

Long-term follow-up should demonstrate that improved construction of wounds 4.00 mm and 5.50 mm in length results in improved stability. The slight amount of with-the-rule astigmatism from the double-x closure may prevent some of the later against-the-rule astigmatism seen with transverse techniques.

Conclusion

Small incisions and increased biomechanical sophistication have made phacoemulsification the safest, most controlled, conservative modern cataract surgical technique available. Improved wound construction, which yields more uniform immediate and long-term visual results, makes the concept of concurrent transverse astigmatic keratotomy with phacoemulsification even more scientifically valid and reliable (Figs. 13.150 and 13.151). Concurrent transverse astigmatic keratotomy can help reduce preoperative keratometric astigmatism and may be valuable for about 5% of cataract surgery patients. Reduction of significant preoperative astigmatism will be of great importance to our patients with multifocal IOLs.

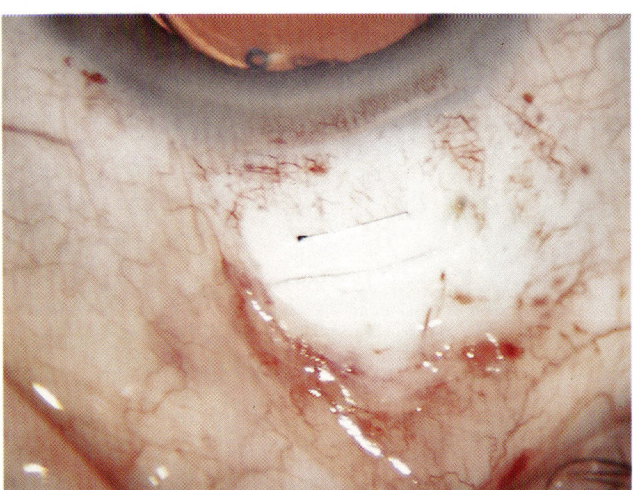

Figure 13.140 *Transverse suture of John Shepherd, M.D., for closure of 4.00 mm wounds.*

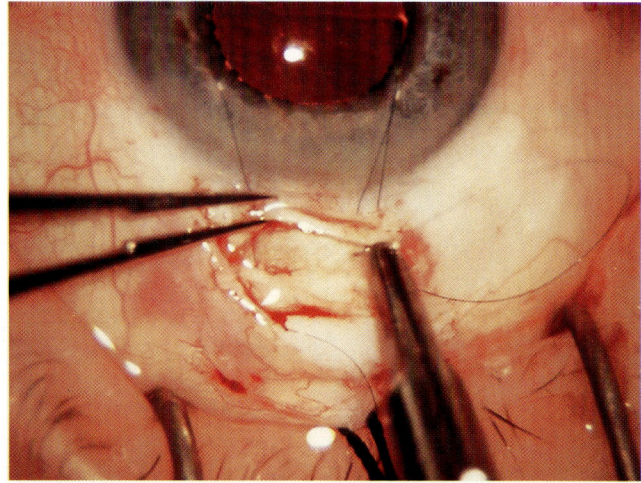

Figure 13.141 *One radial suture is on each side of the transverse suture. The deeper transverse bite is placed under direct visualization to insure adequate tissue bite while not completely penetrating the deeper layer.*

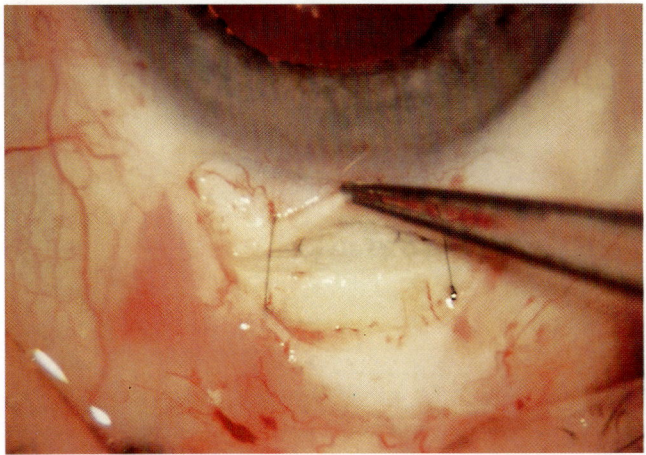

Figure 13.142 *The relatively fragile nature of the closure is identified by lifting the superficial flap.*

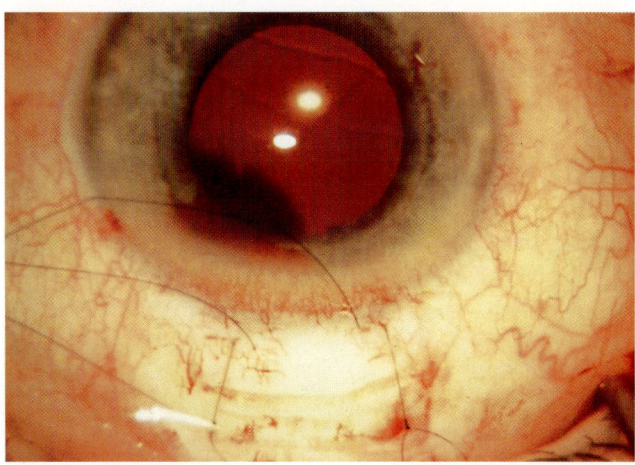

Figure 13.143 *Deep suturing can cause some fairly vigorous bleeding. If the wound is perfect, the blood can be removed by irrigation and the wound closed with less chance of a hyphema developing.*

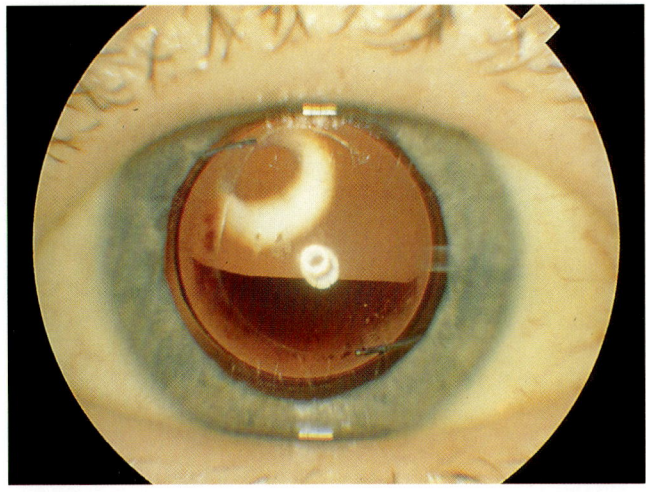

Figure 13.144 *Blood has migrated around the capsulorhexis and is trapped between the IOL and the posterior capsule. In this case, the patient's vision remained 20/20, but the blood was slow to resolve. An early YAG capsulotomy may release blood or disrupt a copper-stained capsule.*

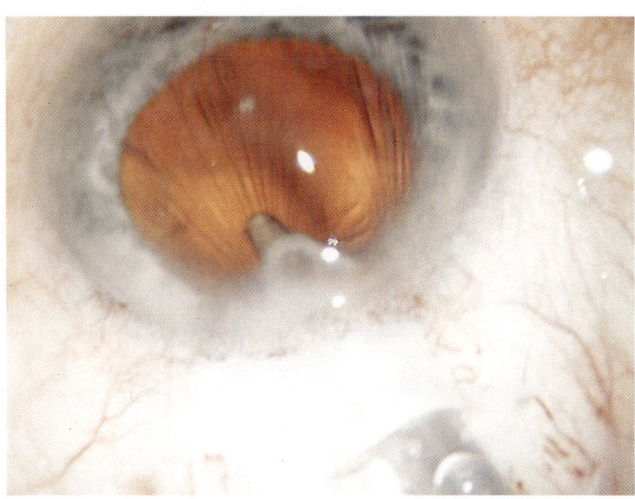

Figure 13.145 *Corneal distortion from too central an entry through Descemet's layer makes all stages of surgery difficult.*

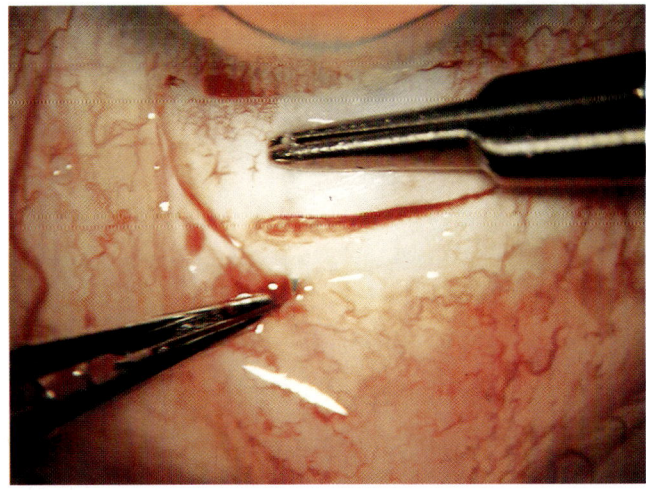

Figure 13.146 *Deep suture bites are used with 10-0 nylon.*

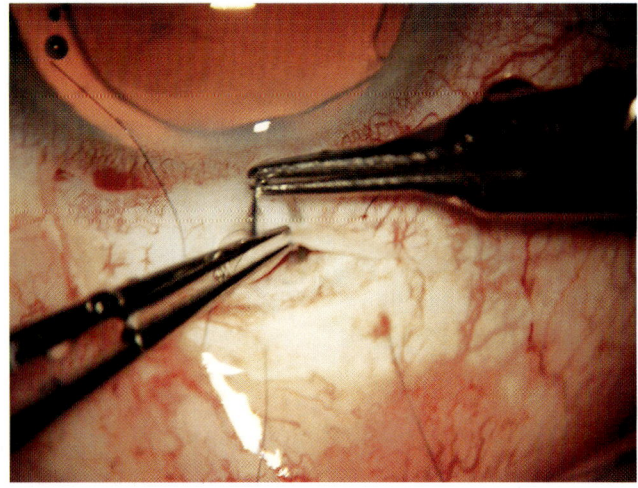

Figure 13.147 *The depth of each bite can be confirmed by elevating the superficial flap.*

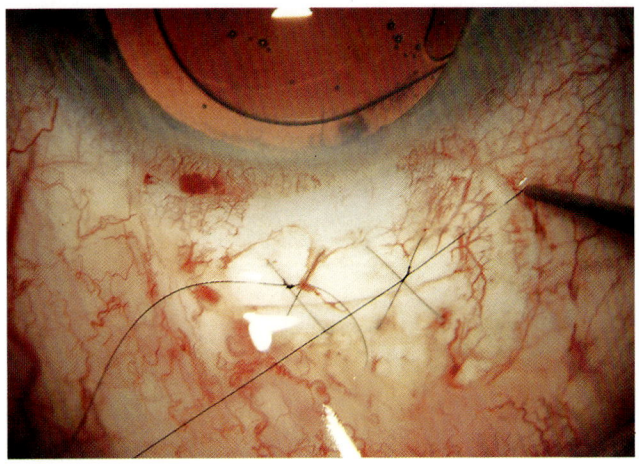

Figure 13.148 *A double-X wound closure with 10-0 nylon suture is complete. The suture is adjusted to the estimated correct degree of tightness and secured with a 3-1-1-1 knot. The suture will be cut at the knot. A keratoscope is not used. The knots are pulled to the scleral side.*

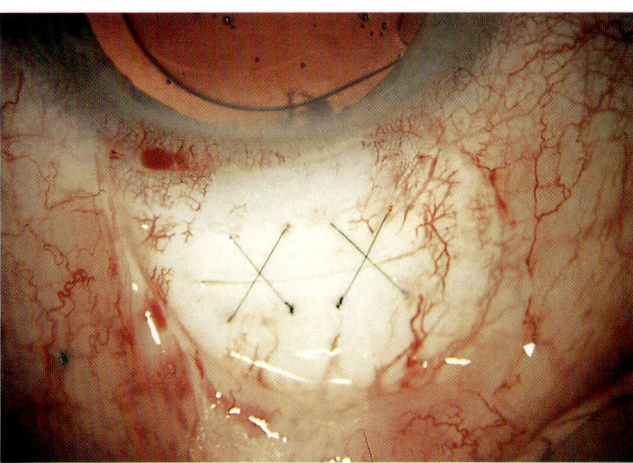

Figure 13.149 *The 5.50 mm wound has been closed and the knots pulled back. The double-X pattern closes a 5.50 mm wound adequately.*

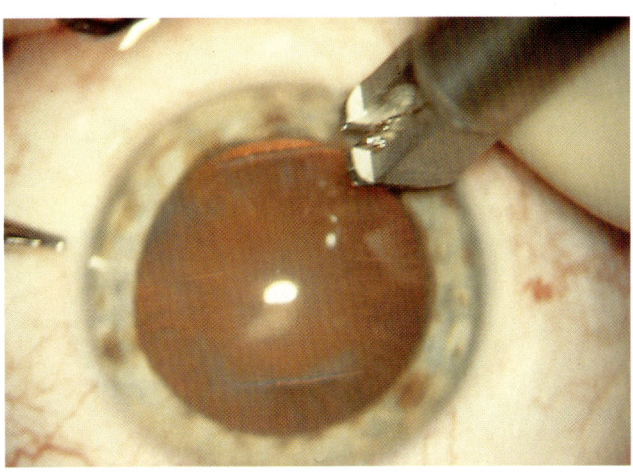

Figure 13.150 *Transverse astigmatic keratomy incisions with a 6.00 mm OZ have been made in the vertical corneal meridian, which greatly influence postoperative astigmatism.*

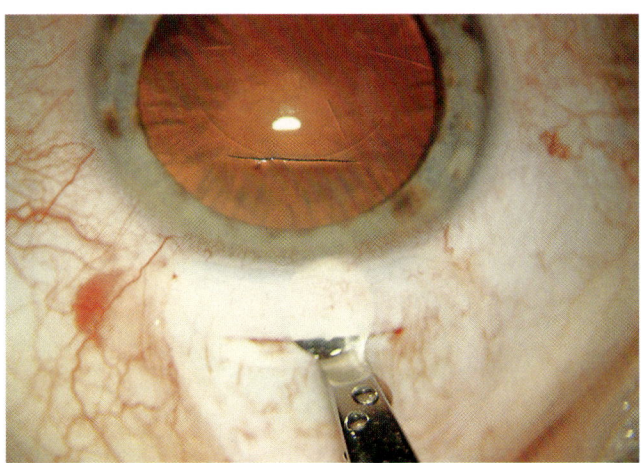

Figure 13.151 *In contrast to the TAK incisions, the beveled horizontal IOL wound starts 3.00 mm posterior to the limbus and has little influence on keratometric astigmatism.*

Clinical Points to Consider

☞ Currently, cataract extraction by phacoemulsification is the method that allows for the most rapid return of visual function.

☞ Phacoemulsification offers significant safety because the eye remains pressurized during the procedure.

☞ To perform excellent phacoemulsification, the surgeon must understand the functions of the machine and be able to troubleshoot problems effectively.

SMALL PUPIL PHACOEMULSIFICATION TECHNIQUES

I. HOWARD FINE, M.D.   SAMUEL MASKET, M.D.

Pupilloplasty Technique to Improve Cosmesis and Preserve Function After Cataract Surgery

I. Howard Fine, M.D

The pupil that dilates poorly (is fibrosed or hyalinized) is frequently the determining factor in the decision not to proceed with phacoemulsification. The small pupil is most commonly managed by performing a sector iridectomy, which requires suturing to prevent edge effects and other potential sources of glare caused by the implant. A sector iridectomy that has been sutured does not look natural and does not behave physiologically. The following procedure, however, creates a pupil of adequate size for either phacoemulsification or nuclear expression. Moreover, it will be cosmetically acceptable and physiologically functional postoperatively. This procedure can be used in all cases, no matter how small the pupil is preoperatively.

Surgical Procedure

The Rappasso scissors have an outer cylinder and a central rod, both with a blade at the end, which can be brought down against the blade attached to the cylinder, creating a shear force. The scissors are sufficiently small to fit through the smallest paracentesis incision used for capsulotomy (Fig. 14.1). The blades will shear when the spring-loaded hemicylinders on the instrument's handle are pressed (Fig. 14.2).

Multiple partial sphincterotomies are performed in the anterior chamber after the aqueous has been replaced by viscoelastic. After lysing any synechiae with a cyclodialysis spatula, eight tiny sphincterotomies (Fig. 14.3), measuring approximately 0.50 mm to 0.75 mm, are cut at equal intervals around the pupillary border. This results in a dramatic increase in the size of the pupil (Fig. 14.4).

It is important not to cut completely through the sphincter into the iris stroma. The sphincterotomies need not be exactly radial, but they must interrupt the continuity of the sphincter edge like a marginal myotomy in strabismus surgery. Almost all of the cuts appear radial following "healing."

After sphincterotomies have been cut in the inferior two thirds of the pupillary circumference, the blades of the scissors will have to be rotated in order to make sphincterotomies in the superior one third of the pupil. After completion of the sphincterotomies, the chamber is further deepened with viscoelastic, resulting in further dilation of the pupil, usually 5.50 mm to 6.00 mm in diameter. If the pupillary size is still inadequate, a Lester hook may be used to slowly stretch the pupil at each sphincterotomy site all the way to the root of the iris. I believe that this maneuver results in a rupturing of fibrous elements in the pupil while stretching only the muscular elements. This will almost always result in a pupil at least 7.00 mm in diameter through which cataract extraction can be easily performed.

Following completion of the cataract extraction and lens implantation, the Lester hook can be used gently to mechanically reduce the size of the pupil. Miochol (acetylcholine chloride, Iolab) is instilled into the anterior chamber. Pilogel oint-

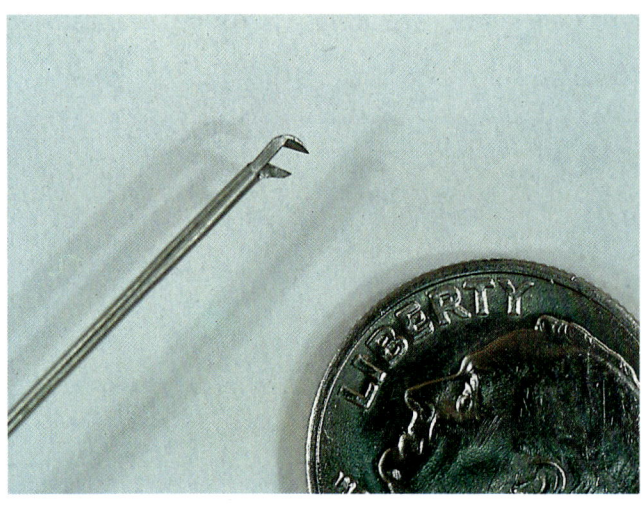

Figure 14.1 *The Rappasso scissors compared to a United States dime. The scissors are used to make multiple partial sphincterotomies. The angled tip allows the pupillary sphincter to be engaged for a full 360 degrees.*

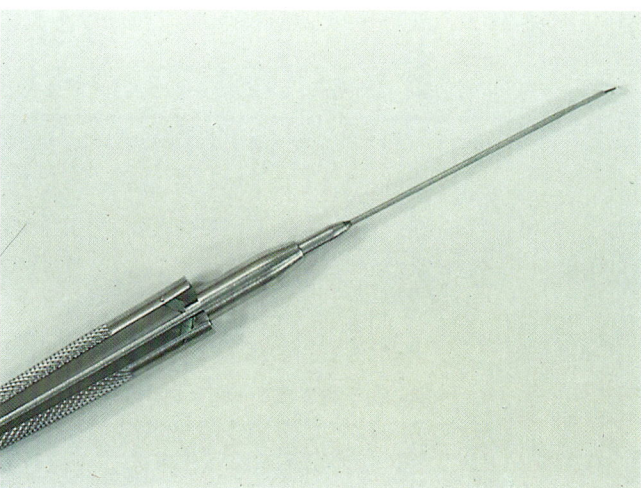

Figure 14.2 *The blades of the Rappasso scissors are activated by squeezing the long, narrow body of the scissors.*

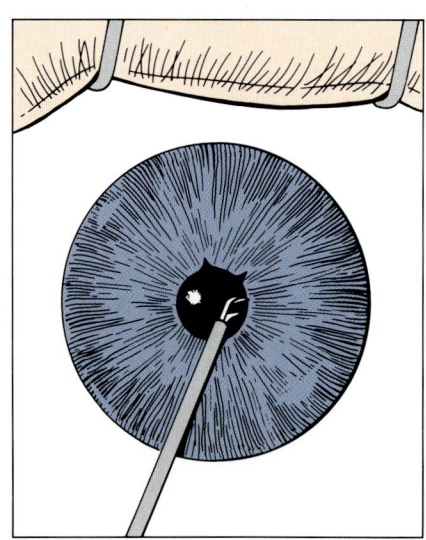

Figure 14.3 *Each sphincterotomy is about 0.50 mm to 0.75 mm in length. The width of the pupillary sphincter is about 1.00 mm.*

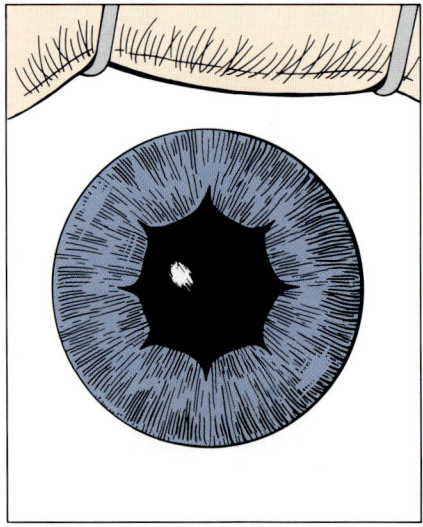

Figure 14.4 *A miotic pupil after eight partial microsphincterotomies.*

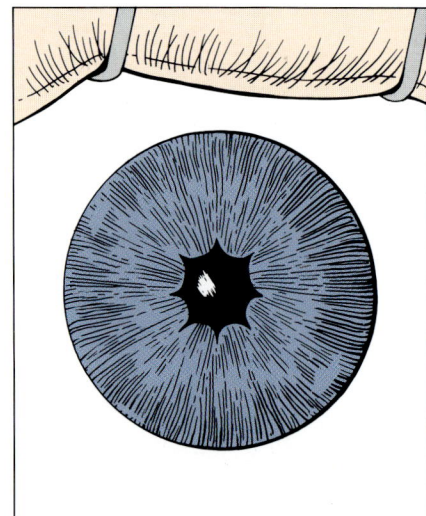

Figure 14.5 *The post-sphincterotomy pupil usually retains the ability to undergo physiologic constriction to light and maintain a relatively normal pupillary aperture.*

ment should be included in the medications instilled prior to patching. The pupil normally returns to a diameter very close to the preoperative diameter (Fig. 14.5), is more easily dilated, and reacts to light physiologically.

Clinical Results

Figure 14.6 shows the postoperative appearance of a pupil that was hyalinized after decades of miotic therapy and would not dilate to more than 3.00 mm preoperatively. Figure 14.7 shows the excellent postoperative appearance of an eye whose pupil was bound down over approximately two thirds of its circumference and would not dilate more than 3.00 mm preoperatively. The sphincterotomies appear healed.

Figure 14.8 is a postoperative photo of a patient who experienced multiple episodes of iritis over a period of years, resulting in synechiae and fibrosis of the pupil in all positions except superiorly from 11:30 to 1 o'clock. The synechiae were lysed. Six sphincterotomies were made in the hyalinized, fibrosed, and bound-down portion of the pupil; the pupil was stretched, and phacoemulsification was performed.

The same patient (Fig. 14.9) following five minutes of dark adaptation demonstrates physiologic dilation of the pupil. It is also of interest to note

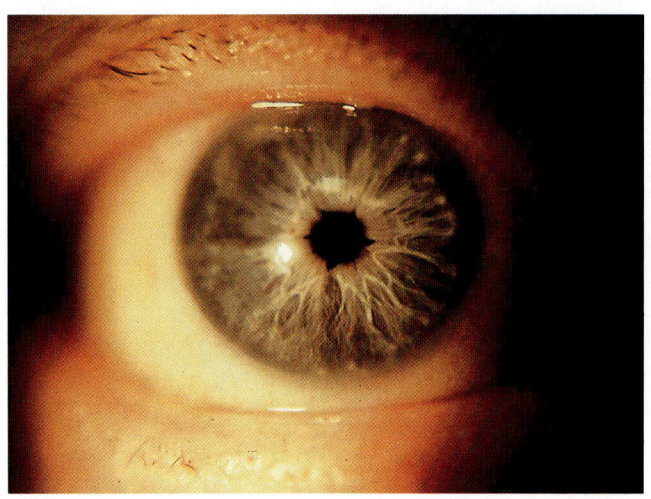

Figure 14.6 *The pupil, hyalinized after decades of miotic therapy, following pupilloplasty and phacoemulsification/ IOL surgery. Maximal preoperative dilation of the pupil was 3.00 mm.*

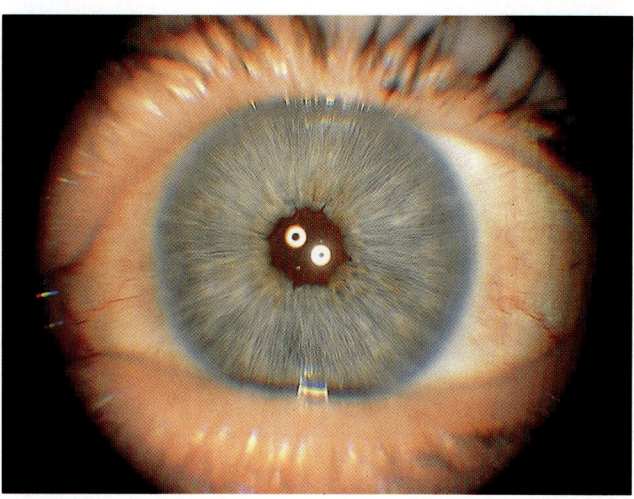

Figure 14.7 *The pupil, bound down over approximately two thirds of its circumference, after pupilloplasty and phacoemulsification/IOL surgery. Maximal preoperative dilation of the pupil was 3.00 mm.*

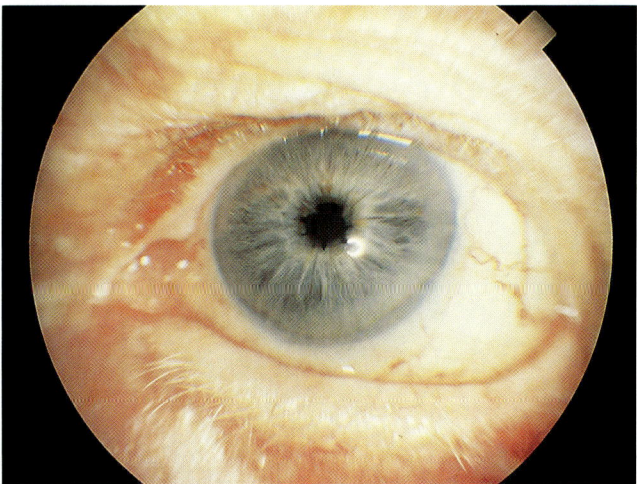

Figure 14.8 *The pupil after pupilloplasty and phacoemulsification/IOL surgery. Preoperatively, anterior synechiae had formed along the pupillary border everywhere except superiorly as a result of chronic iritis.*

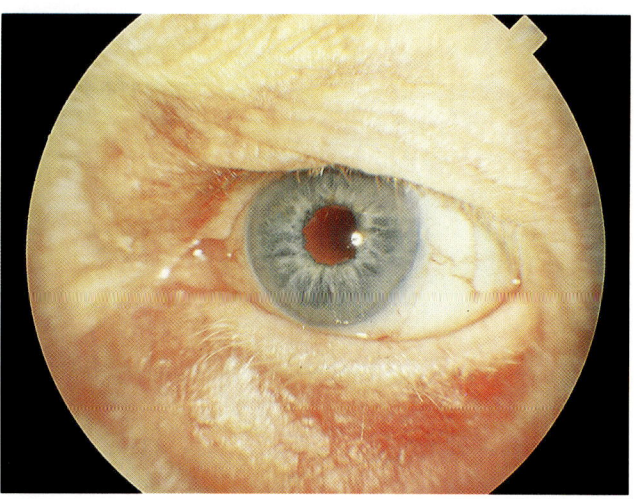

Figure 14.9 *The pupil of the patient in Figure 14.8 after five minutes of dark adaptation. Note the significant mydriasis.*

that, although we are frequently assured that the upper lid covers a sector iridectomy, this would certainly not have been the case for this patient.

Figure 14.10 shows apparent healing of a sphincterotomized and stretched pupil. Preoperatively, this pupil was hyalinized and fibrosed after years of miotic therapy and would not dilate more than 2.50 mm. Figure 14.11 shows that the same patient has excellent postoperative cosmesis; that is, the operated left eye and the unoperated right eye are symmetrical.

Conclusion

A miotic pupil that is not responsive to mydriatic agents can cause the phacoemulsification procedure to be significantly more difficult and risky. Pupilloplasty by multiple partial sphincterotomies usually allows enough mydriasis to permit reasonably safe phacoemulsification, yet obtain physiologic pupillary function postoperatively.

Preplaced Iris Suture Technique for Small Pupil Management in Phaco and Fracture Endolenticular Phacoemulsification

Samuel Masket, M.D.

The recent surgical advances in cataract rehabilitation have improved the risk/benefit ratio for the cataract patient. Moreover, the layperson's perception of the ease of cataract surgery combined with technical advances have altered both indications and patient demands for cataract removal. Frequently, patients request surgery for functional visual deficits, such as glare, rather than because of a major reduction in Snellen acuity. Therefore, it is imperative that cataract surgery relieve glare symptoms but not induce iatrogenic causes of glare disability. According to my study of best case cataract surgery in eyes free of pathology except for symptomatic cataracts, positive and statistically significant reduction of preoperative glare disability was measured and confirmed by the Miller–Nadler Glare Tester before and after surgery.

Maintaining a Functional Pupil

Surgical damage to the iris and pupil must be avoided; according to Brems and colleagues, irregular and unreactive pupils are likely to lead to postoperative glare symptoms if the optic edges are bared by the iris defects. This hypothesis was tested in a recent study that I designed to determine whether pupillary size has a significant bearing on measurable glare disability after surgery. Forty postoperative patients were selected because they demonstrated a clear cornea, normal iris architecture, normal pupillary shape, freedom from synechiae, and an intact, although not necessarily clean, posterior capsule. All surgery was performed by phaco and fracture endolenticular phacoemulsification (Fig. 14.12) with implantation of a one-piece PMMA IOL with a 6.50 mm optic within the capsular sac. Pupil diameter was measured with a template, and nonmasked Miller–Nadler glare testing was performed before pharmacologic pupillary dilation with 0.5% tropicamide. Following dilation the pupil size was remeasured and the glare testing repeated.

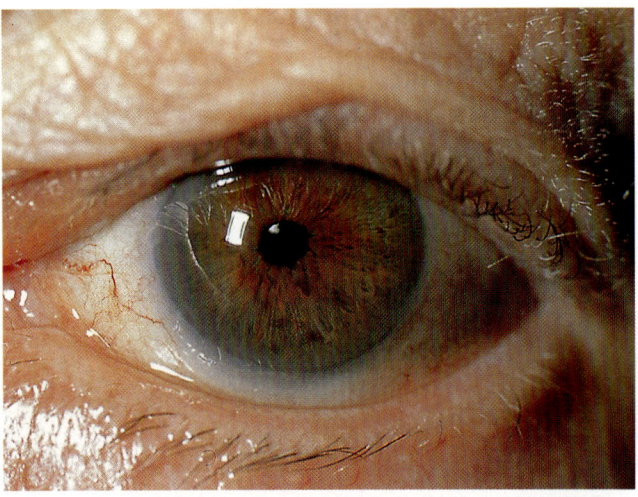

Figure 14.10 *A pupil following pupilloplasty and phacoemulsification/IOL surgery. Maximal preoperative dilation was 2.50 mm.*

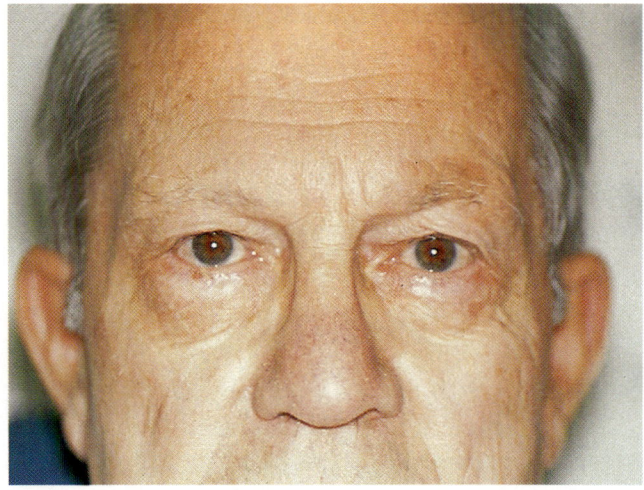

Figure 14.11 *The patient whose left pupil was presented in Figure 14.10. Note the symmetry of the pupillary apertures.*

The results of the study indicated that prior to dilation the mean pupil size was 2.80 mm and the Miller–Nadler glare score averaged 13.5%. After dilation the pupil averaged 5.50 mm and the glare score increased significantly to 28.1% (Table 14.13). The investigation clearly indicated that an enlarged pupil after surgery is associated with increased glare disability. Therefore, cataract surgery must not interfere with normal pupil size, shape, or function.

Modern cataract surgery is characterized by the reduced incision size of phacoemulsification and the use of foldable or reduced dimension implants as well as endolenticular emulsification with continuous tear capsulotomy. Unfortunately, pupils that dilate poorly may interfere with phacoemulsification. Some surgeons opt to perform manual nuclear removal in lieu of phacoemulsification when faced with a small pupil; as a result, the patient loses the advantages of small incision surgery, and the surgeon loses the exquisite control of the intraocular fluidic environment that phacoemulsification provides. Alternatively, a variety of surgical means for enlarging the pupil have been devised (Table 14.14).

Altering the pupil should be done only after the surgeon has exhausted nonsurgical methods of obtaining an adequately dilated pupil. Before surgery, miotic agents, if used for glaucoma, should be discontinued well in advance of the procedure; strong cycloplegics and mydriatics, unless contraindicated, should be applied; and a topical nonsteroidal anti-inflammatory should be employed as part of the preoperative regimen. Intraoperatively, synechiolysis as needed may enlarge the pupil, and the addition of nonpreserved, pure epinephrine to the irrigating solution may help prevent secondary surgical miosis. Secondary surgical miosis can be avoided by reducing iris trauma and maintaining a steady state of intraocular pressure during surgery.

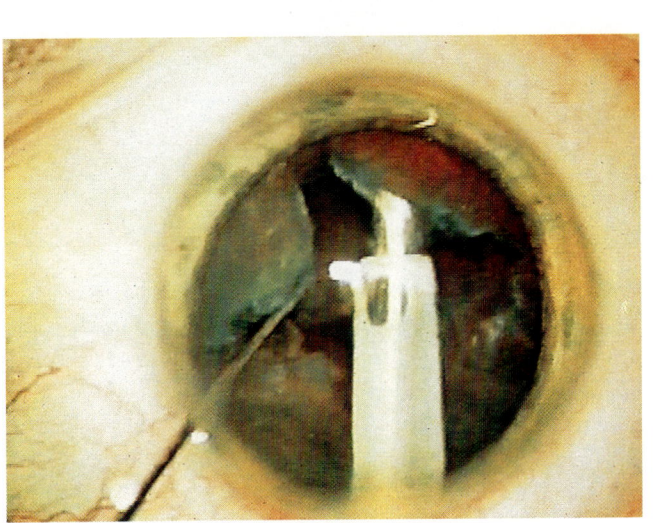

Figure 14.12 *Endolenticular phacoemulsification through capsulorhexis. Note the very adequate pupil dilation and nuclear dissection necessary for the phaco and fracture method.*

Table 14.13
Pupil Size and Postoperative Glare Disabiliy

	DILATION	
	Pre	Post
Diameter	2.80 mm	5.50 mm
Miller–Nadler	13.5%	28.1%
	$p < .05$	$p < .05$

Table 14.14
Surgical Methods For Pupil Enlargement

- Synechiolysis
- Sector iridectomy
- Inferior/radial sphincterotomies
- Multiple incomplete sphincterotomies
- Postplaced suture of iris defects

Nonetheless, certain cases, in particular those patients on long-standing topical miotic therapy or those with posterior synechiae, require surgical enlargement of the pupil for safe cataract removal. Figure 14.14 lists a variety of accepted means for operative pupillary manipulation. All of these methods, except synechiolysis, fail to leave the pupil physiologically reactive and/or cosmetically round after surgery (Fig. 14.15). Preplaced iris suture techniques, however, can allow for adequate working space intraoperatively and a normal pupil postoperatively. A method for a preplaced iris suture in conjunction with a superior radial iridotomy has been reported independently by Thomas Neuhann, M.D., and Harry Grabow, M.D. (Welch Cataract Congress, 1988). Preplaced iris suturing assures proper alignment of the iris pillars and prevents incorporation of the anterior lens capsule after lens implantation. The technique works well (Figs. 14.16 and 14.17) for phacoemulsification performed superiorly, in the standard two-handed manner. However, phaco and fracture endolenticular phaco methods, such as the *divide and conquer* or the nuclear cracking method, require greater visibility and space to work inferiorly rather than superiorly.

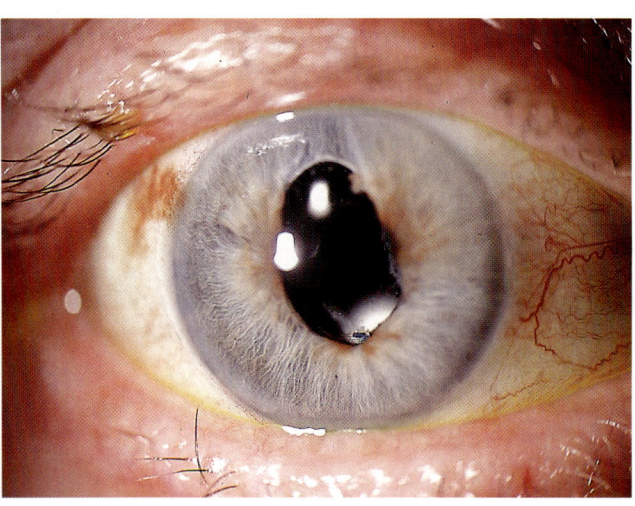

Figure 14.15 *Postoperative appearance of pupil after multiple sphincterotomies. The pupil is unacceptable aesthetically and functionally.*

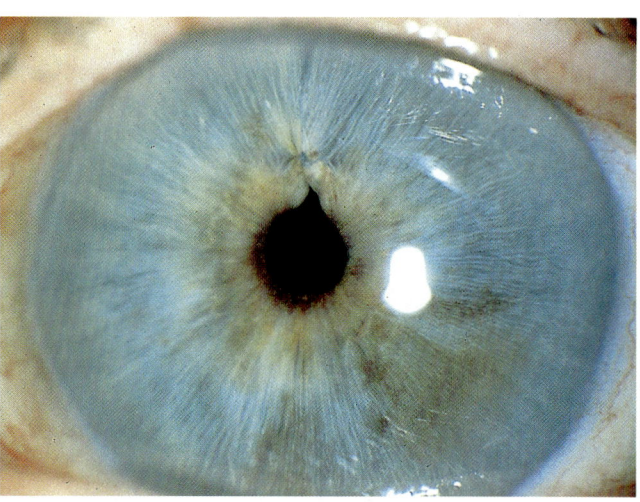

Figure 14.16 *Postoperative appearance of eye after superior preplaced iris suture method. Note the small, undilated, functionally normal pupil. The suture is visible adjacent to the superior pupil border.*

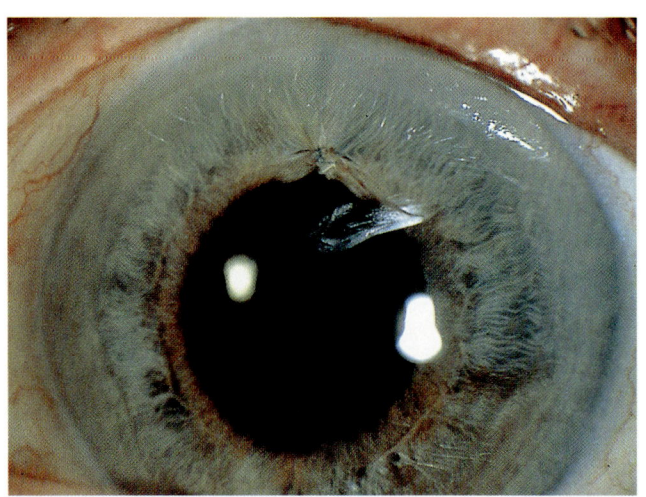

Figure 14.17 *The eye in Fig. 14.16 after pharmacologic pupillary dilation. The round shape affirms the benefit of preplacing the iris suture.*

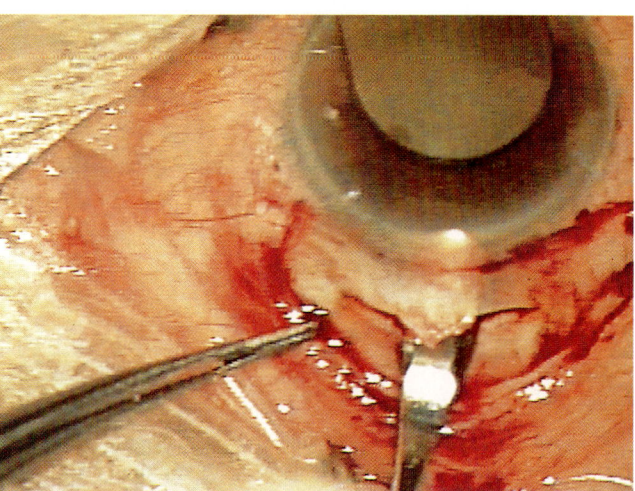

Figure 14.18 *A scleral pocket wound is created.*

Surgical Procedure

I have devised a system that incorporates a preplaced inferior iris suture with an inferior sphincterotomy to facilitate endolenticular phacoemulsification and also retain a physiologic pupil.

A superior scleral pocket is fashioned (Fig. 14.18). (In this case the flap is prepared for a combined trabeculectomy/glaucoma procedure.)

Synechiolysis is carried out bluntly with the aid of copious viscoelastic material (Fig. 14.19). After synechiolysis, however, the pupil is still too small for safe phacoemulsification.

A 10-0 polypropylene suture on a straight ultrasharp needle (Ethicon STC-6) penetrates the inferotemporal limbus (Fig. 14.20).

The needle is guided through full-thickness iris at the inferior sphincter. Ample viscoelastic is necessary to maintain deep anterior and posterior chambers in order to prevent damage to the lens capsule (Fig. 14.21).

The needle exits from the inferonasal limbus. The suture is noted to cross the chamber after the needle is withdrawn. A microhook is introduced through the superior incision, which has been opened with a keratome (Fig. 14.22).

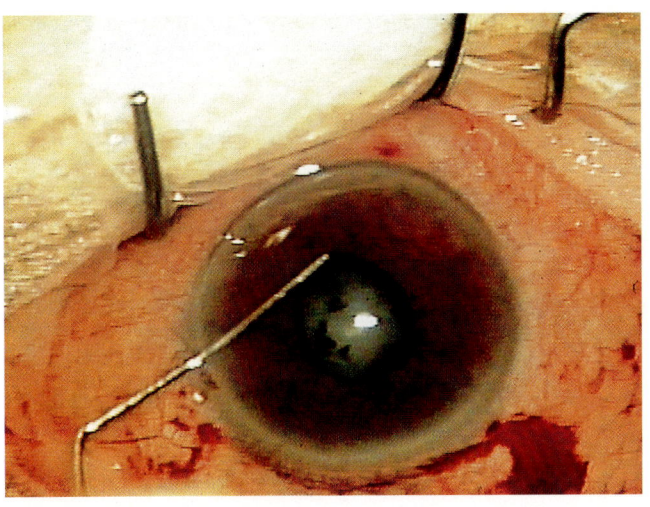

Figure 14.19 *Some posterior synechiae may be lysed by introducing viscoelastic into the anterior chamber. Further lysis may be accomplished using a spatula.*

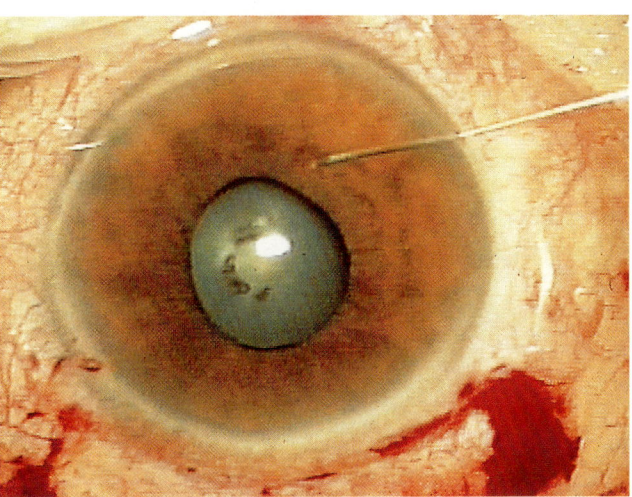

Figure 14.20 *A straight ultrasharp needle (Ethicon STC-6) swaged to 10-0 polypropylene (Prolene) suture is introduced into the anterior chamber through the inferotemporal limbus.*

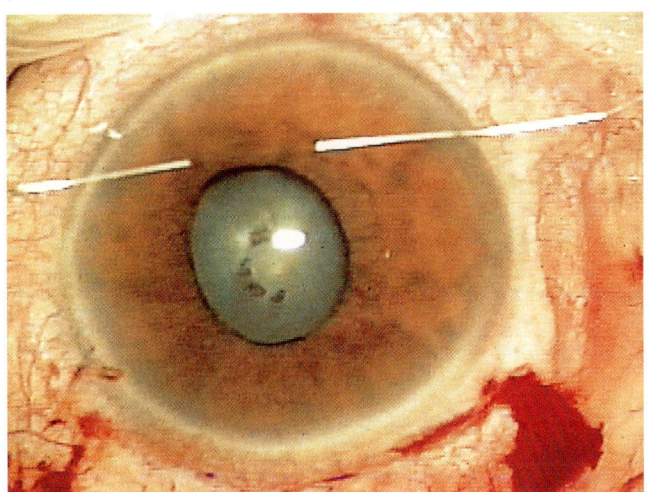

Figure 14.21 *The STC-6 needle proceeds through the inferior iris sphincter and exits from the anterior chamber through the inferonasal limbus.*

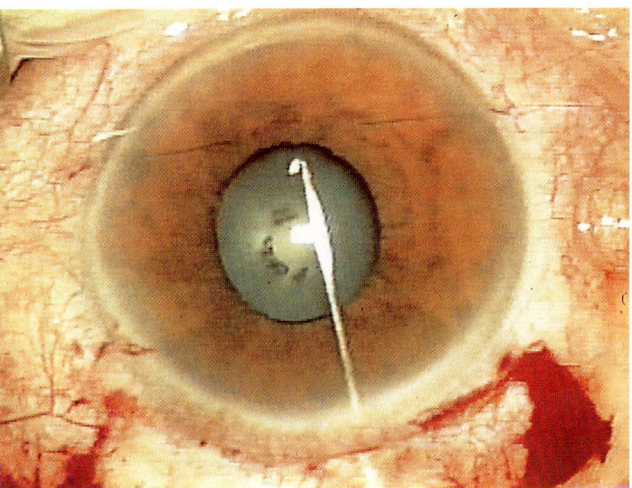

Figure 14.22 *A microhook is used to engage the 10-0 Prolene suture from beneath the iris at 6 o'clock.*

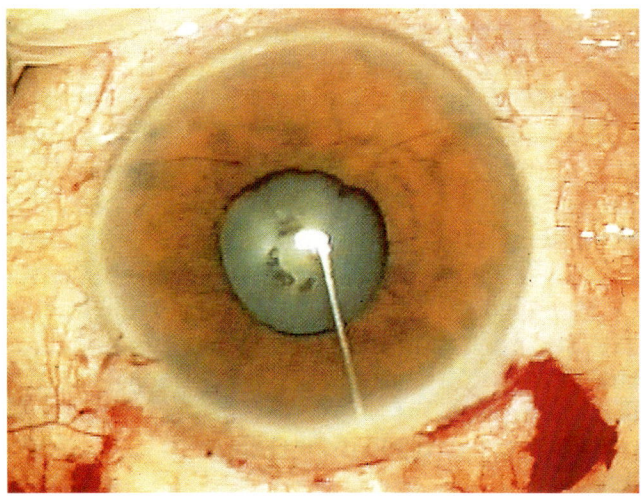

Figure 14.23 *The microhook is used to loop the 10-0 Prolene suture away from the inferior iris so that an inferior sphincterotomy can be performed.*

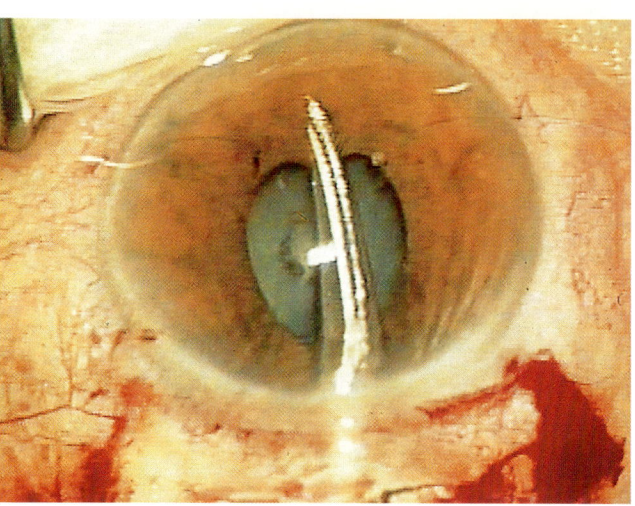

Figure 14.24 *An inferior sphincterotomy is performed.*

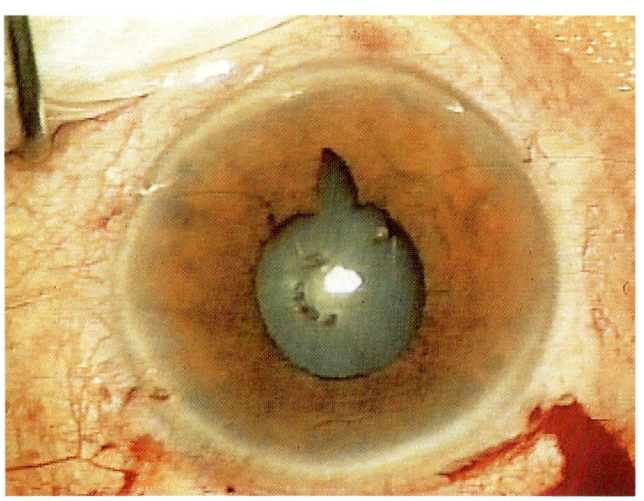

Figure 14.25 *A large inferior sphincterotomy enables pupil enlargement.*

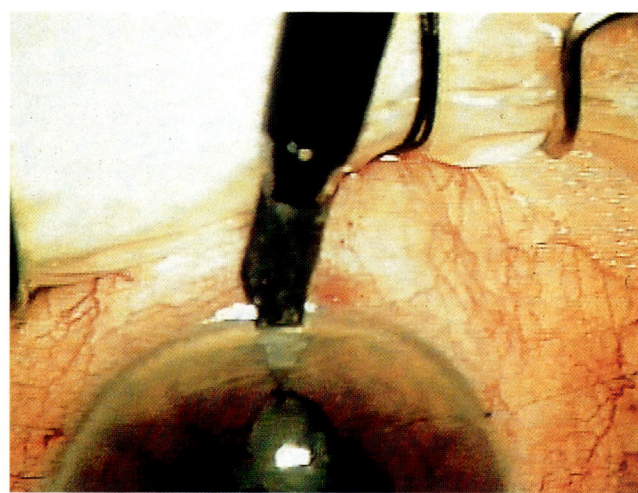

Figure 14.26 *An inferior limbal puncture into the anterior chamber is created.*

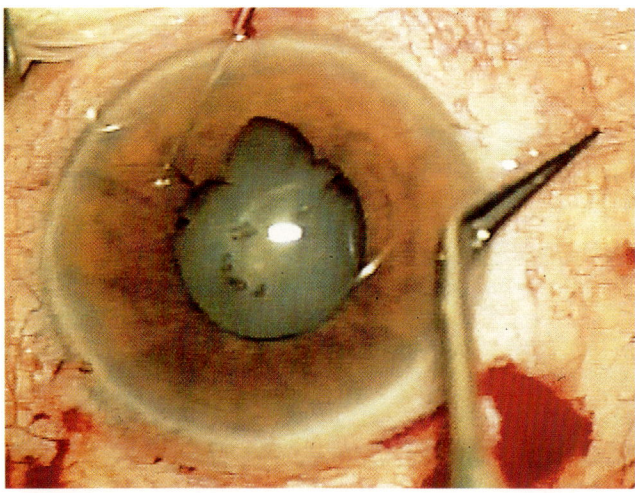

Figure 14.27 *The free end of the 10-0 Prolene suture is removed from the anterior chamber with a microhook.*

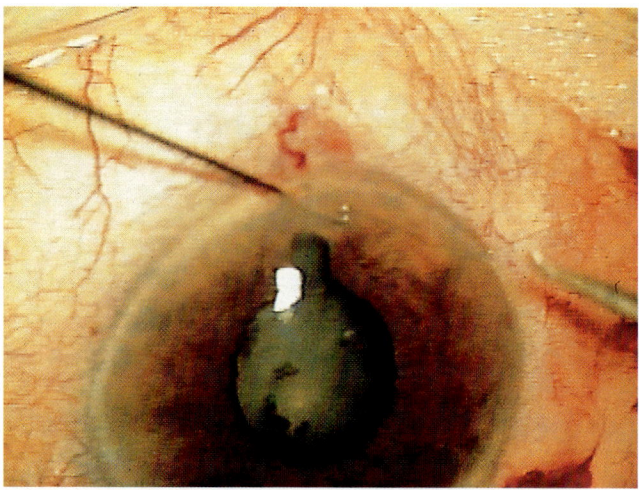

Figure 14.28 *The other end of the 10-0 Prolene suture is removed from the anterior chamber through the inferior puncture wound.*

The hook is used to loop the suture from under the inferior sphincter (Fig. 14.23).

With care taken to avoid the looped preplaced suture, a generous inferior sphincterotomy is performed (Fig. 14.24). The suture runs from one limbus to the other through the iris (Fig. 14.25).

An inferior limbal puncture is created (Fig. 14.26). In the fashion of a McCannell suture, the free end of the iris suture is brought out through the inferior puncture with a microhook while the other end is held with a tying forceps (Fig. 14.27).

The second end of the iris suture is brought through the inferior limbal puncture. Both suture ends are taped to the surgical drapes with a small Steri-strip (Fig. 14.28).

A tear capsulotomy is performed (Fig. 14.29). Endolenticular phacoemulsification is carried out (Fig. 14.31) using a nuclear *phaco and fracture* method. The cortex is removed with an angled (I/A) handpiece (Fig. 14.31).

After cortical cleanup the eye is ready for lens implantation. The iris suture is noted in the chamber (Fig. 14.32) and after the implant is placed into position, the iris suture is ready for tying (Fig. 14.33).

The suture is tied and cut at the inferior puncture and the iris is reposited. The inferior sphincter has been reapproximated. Surgery is completed after the trabeculectomy is carried out (Fig. 14.34).

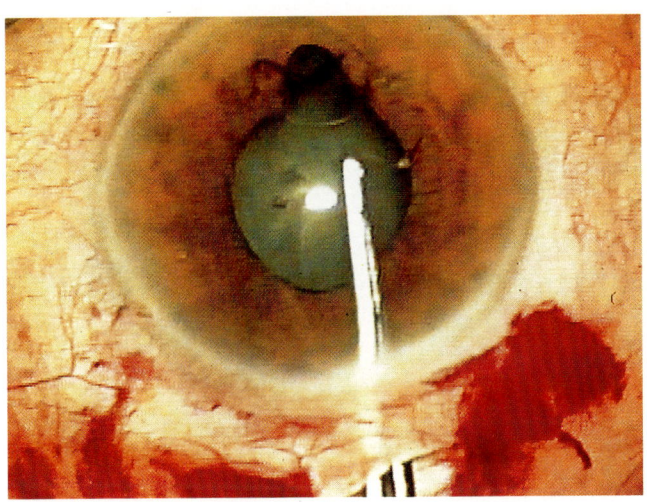

Figure 14.29 *Capsulorhexis is performed.*

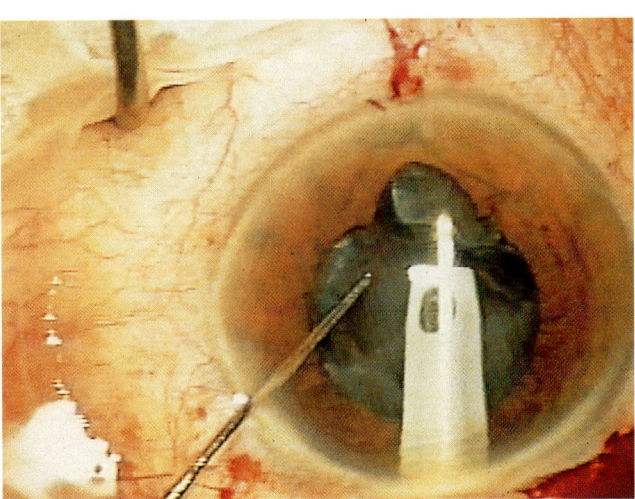

Figure 14.30 *Endolenticular phacoemulsification is performed.*

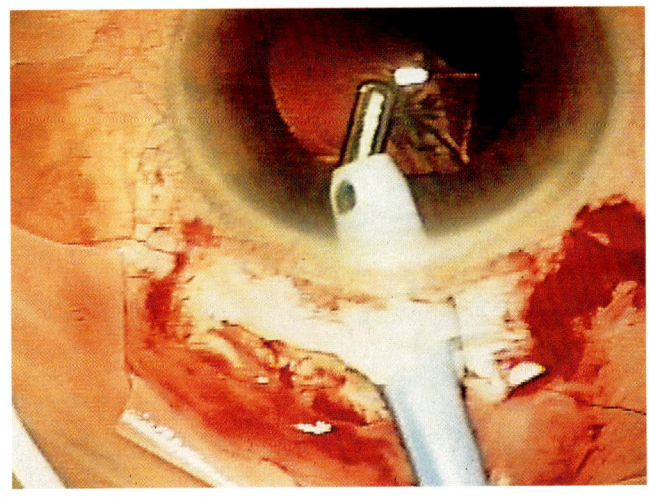

Figure 14.31 *The cortex is removed by automated I/A.*

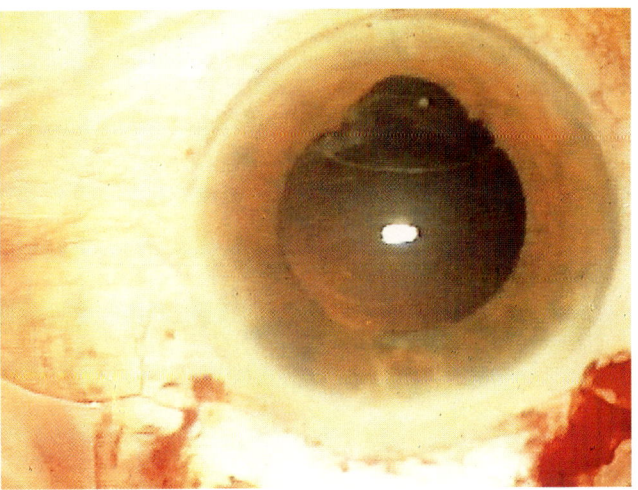

Figure 14.32 *After cortex removal, viscoelastic will be introduced into the anterior chamber and an IOL will be implanted. Note the 10-0 Prolene suture connecting the pillars of the inferior sphincterotomy.*

Conclusion

This procedure provides ample surgical exposure, and permits normal pupil shape and function after surgery. While the procedure adds time to the surgery, the reward, as noted in the postoperative photographs (Figs. 14.35 and 14.36), is a physiologically normal, aesthetically acceptable pupil.

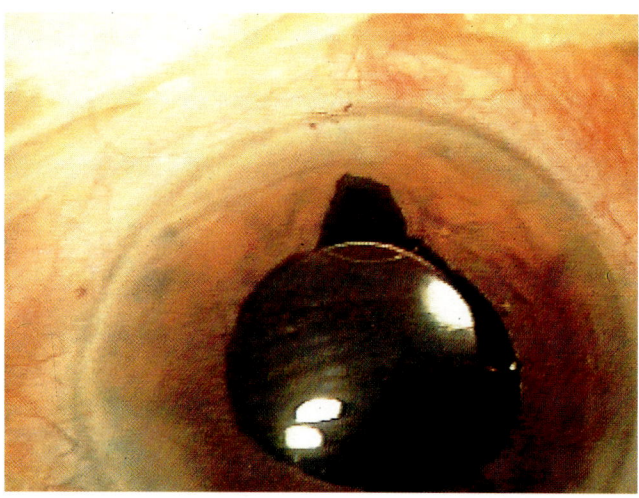

Figure 14.33 *After implantation of a posterior chamber IOL, the suture will be tied to close the inferior sphincterotomy.*

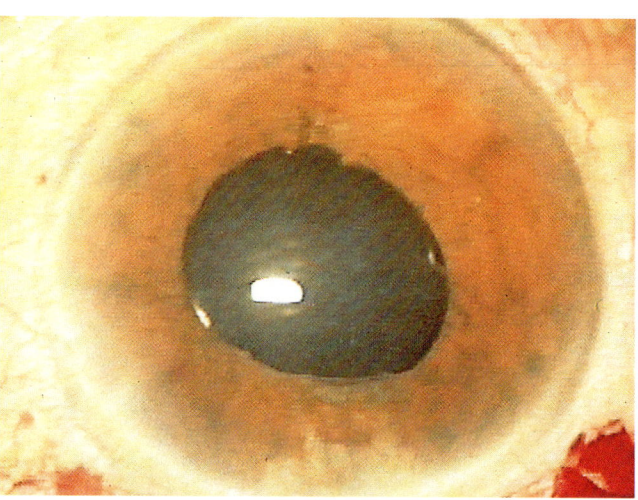

Figure 14.34 *The suture is tied through the inferior limbal incision and the knot cut short. The inferior sphincterotomy has been closed.*

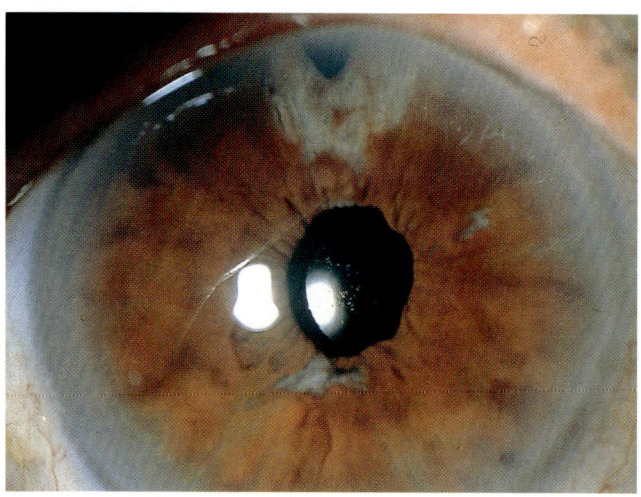

Figure 14.35 *Postoperative, undilated appearance of the eye. Note the essentially round, physiologic pupil. A superior peripheral iridectomy was performed as part of the combined glaucoma/cataract procedure.*

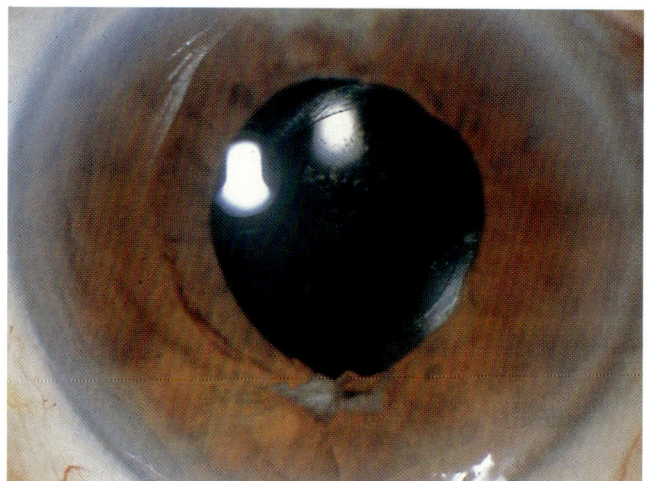

Figure 14.36 *The eye after pharmacologic pupillary dilation. Note the aesthetically normal pupil.*

Clinical Points to Consider

- A small pupil can make creation of an adequate capsulotomy difficult.

- The surgeon should have a specific plan for enlarging the miotic pupil prior to phacoemulsification.

- The surgeon must decide on an in-the-bag or iris plane phacoemulsification technique when a small pupil is present.

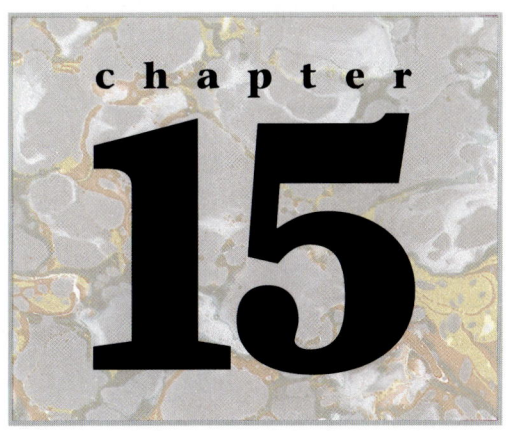

chapter 15

SMALL INCISION INTRAOCULAR LENS IMPLANTATION

STEPHEN F. BRINT, M.D.

The replacement of a cataractous lens with an artificial implant has been a recognized surgical procedure since 1949, when Ridley first used a polymethylmethacrylate (PMMA) lens as a pseudophakos.

By the mid 1970s, several surgeons around the world were beginning to consider the possibility of intraocular implants made of soft materials. It was hoped that these implants would be more compatible with the normal soft tissues of the eye than previous implants, matching their elasticity and plasticity. Epstein in South Africa began to investigate both silicone and hydrogel materials, Mehta performed human implantation of a hydrogel lens in 1978, and Fyodorov in Russia and Zhou in China pioneered the use of silicone intraocular lenses (IOLs). Early studies demonstrated less damage to the corneal endothelium upon touch with either silicone or hydrogel IOLs than that seen with PMMA IOLs.

The soft IOL implants currently available can be traced back to August 1983, when Graham Barrett, M.D., implanted the first IOGEL (HEMA) IOL (Alcon) in Australia and to April 1984, when Tom Mazzocco, M.D., implanted the first silicone IOL (Staar Surgical) in the United States. Early enthusiasm was fueled by the biocompatibility of the eye and the implant as well as the ability of the lens to be folded and implanted through a small incision. These factors lessened the trauma associated with the surgical procedure, thereby resulting in faster recovery and less induced astigmatism. Tremendous progress has been made since these implants were introduced. Initially there were unacceptably high complication rates due to either design flaws or faulty surgical technique, but in October 1989 the FDA approved the Allergan Medical Optics (AMO) SI-18NB silicone IOL as safe and effective.

The original Staar RMX-1 silicone IOL was one piece and had an overall length of 11.00 mm. It was opalescent and had very flimsy haptics. The visual acuity results with this early lens design compared favorably to those obtained with PMMA IOLs; however, the complication rate was remarkably high. The complications, which included subluxation, decentration, corneal edema, and elevated intraocular pressure, have since been attributed to the one-piece, one-size-fits-all IOL. When this IOL was implanted in the capsular bag, occasionally a serious problem—the *Z syndrome*—occurred; that is, the bending at the optic/haptics junction caused lens tilting. This lens tilt induced lenticular astigmatism or caused the IOL to vault forward, creating iris bulging, or backward, creating depression. These problems could be corrected by manipulating the IOL from the bag into the sulcus, which was technically easy because the IOL did not adhere to the capsular bag.

Traditionally, the ciliary sulcus has been an adequate location for haptic placement because polypropylene and PMMA loops are well tolerated by uveal tissue. Both silicone and hydrogel materials cause little tissue reaction; however, both of these materials in the one-size-fits-all design may not fixate well in the sulcus, causing pigment dispersion and possibly edge glare when placed in a large eye. The sulcus placement of the silicone IOL accounted for early posterior capsular opacification due to a lack of stretch on the posterior capsule.

It has been shown that the incidence of opacification requiring capsulotomy is significantly higher for sulcus-placed silicone IOLs than it is for capsular bag-placed silicone IOLs. Biomicroscopy reveals that sulcus-placed IOLs cause the posterior capsule to be heavily wrinkled while capsular bag-placed silicone IOLs and hydrogel IOLs result in an extremely smooth posterior capsule. These problems, as well as other problems associated with the bulky folding instrumentation required for implantation, have been well chronicled in the literature.

The present generation of soft IOLs, along with improvements in surgical technique, such as

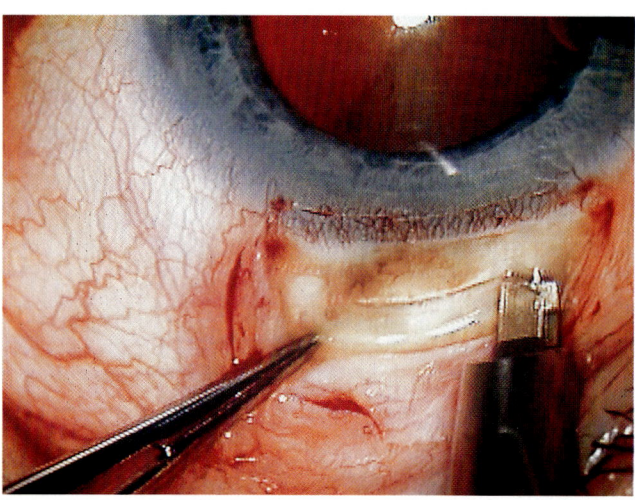

Figure 15.1 *A 4.00-mm groove is made with the diamond step knife 2.50 mm to 3.00 mm posterior and parallel to the limbus.*

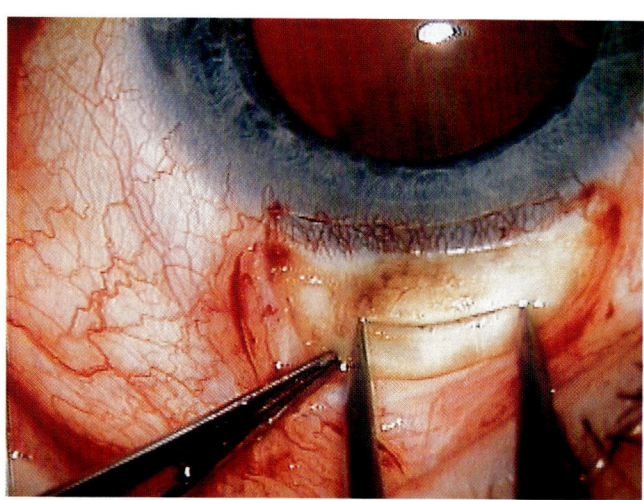

Figure 15.2 *The 4.00-mm length of the incision is verified.*

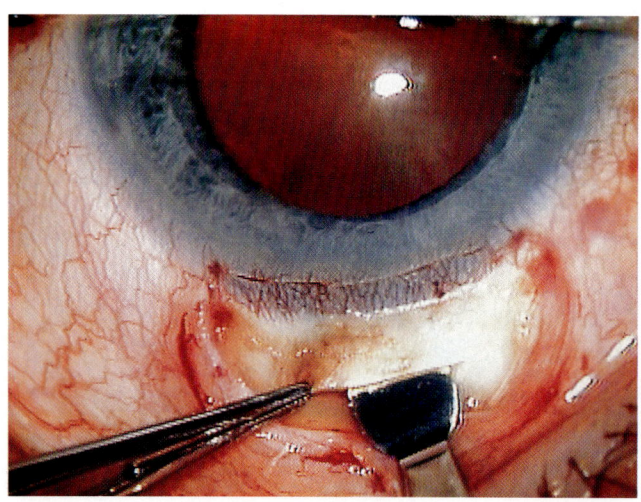

Figure 15.3 *A No. 21 Grieshaber blade is used to dissect a scleral pocket.*

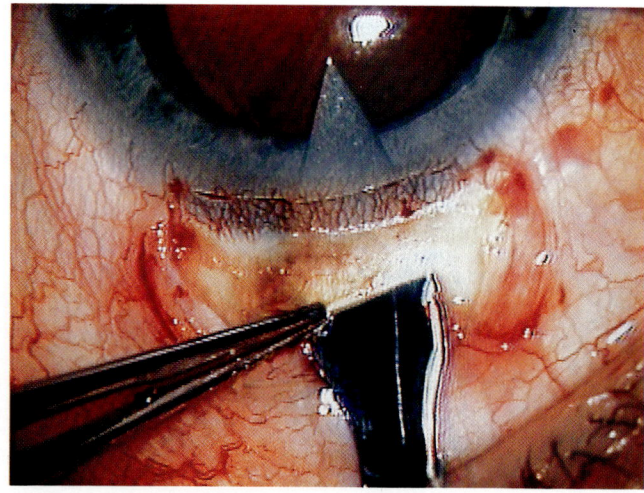

Figure 15.4 *The 3.00-mm metal keratome enters the anterior chamber well anterior to the iris root.*

continuous circular capsulorhexis and endolenticular phacoemulsification, have largely solved all of these early problems.

Surgical Procedure

My surgical technique is the same for all the currently available soft foldable IOLs until I reach the point of IOL implantation. After peribulbar anesthesia and softening of the orbital contents using a Honan balloon, the patient is brought to the surgical suite, where routine prepping and draping is done. Inferior and superior rectus bridle sutures obviate the need for a lid speculum. A 5.00-mm conjunctival peritomy is performed with relaxing incisions at either end. The perilimbal area is cleaned and lightly cauterized. A diamond knife is used to make a 4.00-mm groove that is 0.30 mm in depth and 2.50 mm to 3.00 mm posterior concentric to the limbus. A No. 21 Grieshaber blade is then used to dissect a scleral pocket, with the surgeon making certain not to enter the anterior chamber prematurely. Using a 3.00-mm keratome and a 2 o'clock side-port incision, the anterior chamber is entered and filled with viscoelastic (AmVisc Plus) (Figs. 15.1 to 15.4).

Capsulorhexis is performed by puncturing the center of the capsule with a bent 25-gauge cystotome and carrying it to the midperiphery toward the 9 o'clock position. The cystotome is then placed underneath the capsule and lifted, which causes a gentle tear to begin. The torn capsule is flipped over and engaged with the point of the cystotome and torn toward the 6 o'clock position. The Kraff-Utrata capsule forceps are used to grasp the margin of the torn capsule and continue the tear in a counterclockwise direction. The capsule should be regrasped approximately every 90 degrees in order to maintain control of the tear (Figs. 15.5 and 15.6).

Hydrodissection is performed with a 25-gauge, flat Visitech cannula, and the BSS is injected just under the margin of the anterior capsule in several locations (Fig. 15.7). Endolenticular phacoemulsfication is performed using a 45-degree phaco tip with a one-hand technique for soft

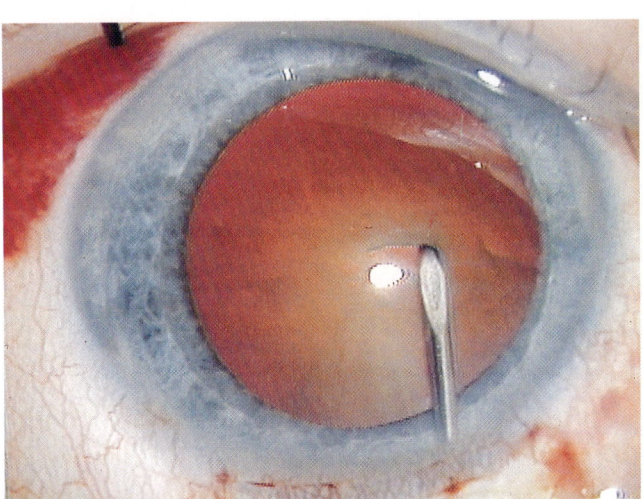

Figure 15.5 *A bent 25-gauge needle is used as a cystotome to begin the continuous circular capsulorhexis by puncturing the anterior capsule at the center of the pupil and tearing toward the 9 o'clock position.*

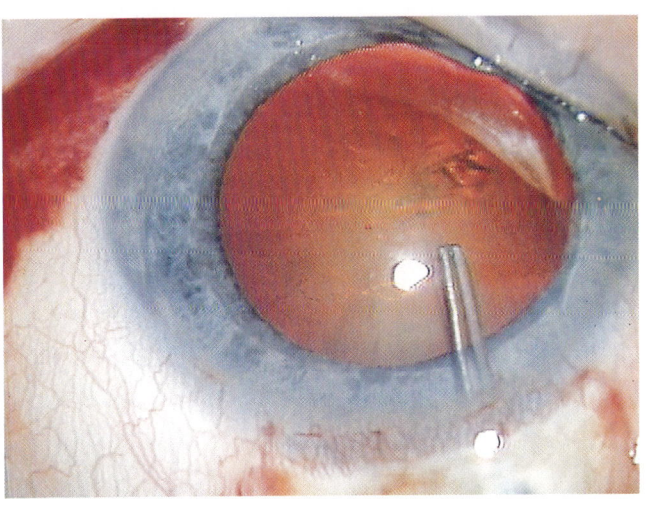

Figure 15.6 *The capsulorhexis is completed using the Kraff-Utrata forceps.*

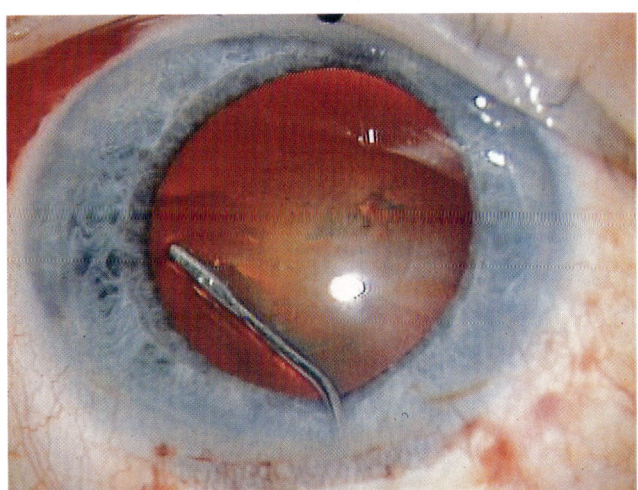

Figure 15.7 *Hydrodissection under the margin of the anterior capsule at several points releases the nucleus from its corticocapsular attachments.*

nuclei or the Shepherd modification of Gimbel's *divide and conquer* technique for medium to firm nuclei. After cortical aspiration, a perfect bag with a central opening of approximately 5.00 mm remains and houses either a one-piece hydrogel or silicone IOL or a three-piece silicone implant (Figs. 15.8 to 15.14).

Three-Piece Silicone Lens Implants

The presently available three-piece silicone IOLs include the AMO SI-18NB and SI-20NB, the IOLAB LI-3OU, which combines silicone optics with polypropylene haptics, and the Staar elastimide AQ-1000 IOL with polyamide haptics. Cross action Faulkner forceps are used to insert these composite IOLs. This system, originated by Gerald Faulkner, M.D., consists of holding the optic with forceps that have rounded jaws (similar to Kelman-McPherson forceps). Then, while the Faulkner forceps fold the IOL, the holding forceps are removed. I prefer stainless steel holding forceps (Katena) and titanium Faulkner forceps (Western Medical).

The method of folding can be either lengthwise or crosswise. If the IOL is folded and inserted lengthwise (Figs. 15.15 to 15.17), the forceps are first turned to the left so that the IOL is inserted sideways, and the inferior haptic is placed under the margin of the capsulorhexis. The forceps are then rotated upright and the IOL is released gently. The optic can then be nudged under the margins of the capsulorhexis, and the superior or trailing haptic placed with forceps in the tradi-

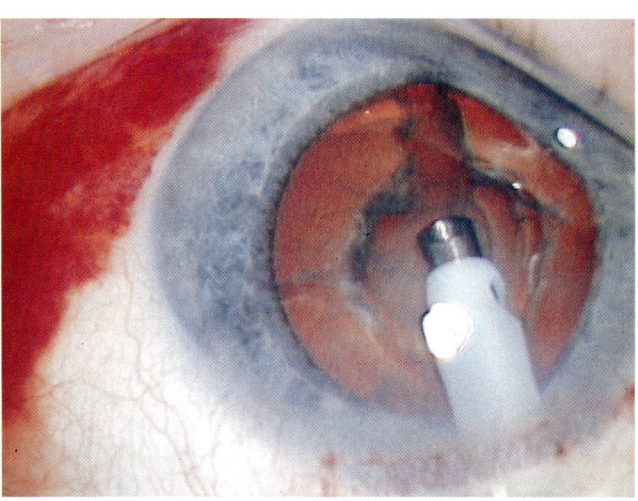

Figure 15.8 *Central sculpting with the 45-degree phaco tip has been accomplished. The first of four grooves is sculpted with the 45-degree phaco tip as deeply as is comfortable without going too far peripherally.*

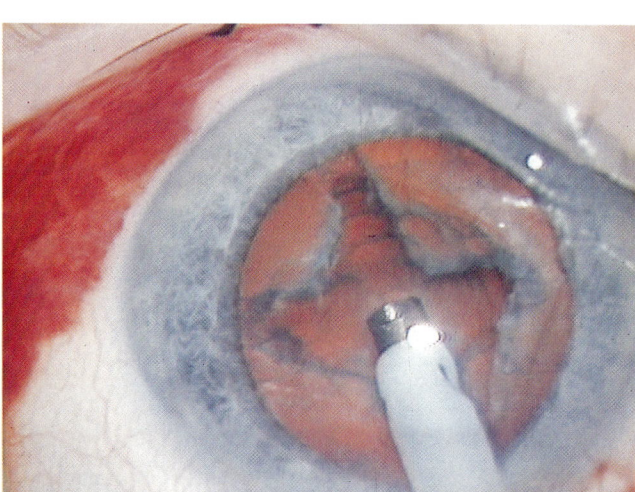

Figure 15.9 *By rotating the nucleus one quadrant at a time, the last of the four grooves is created.*

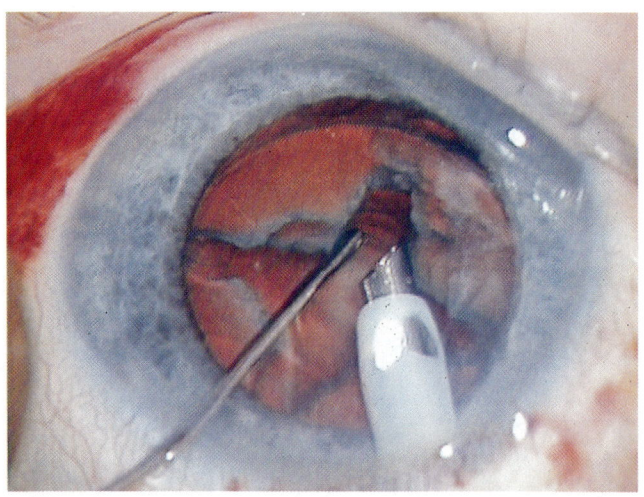
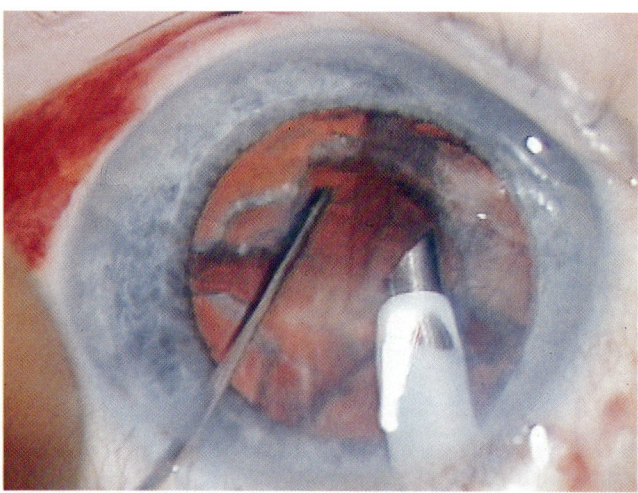

Figure 15.10 (left and right) *The Knolle spatula and back of the 45-degree tip are used to fracture the nucleus into quadrants, usually using* foot-position 0.

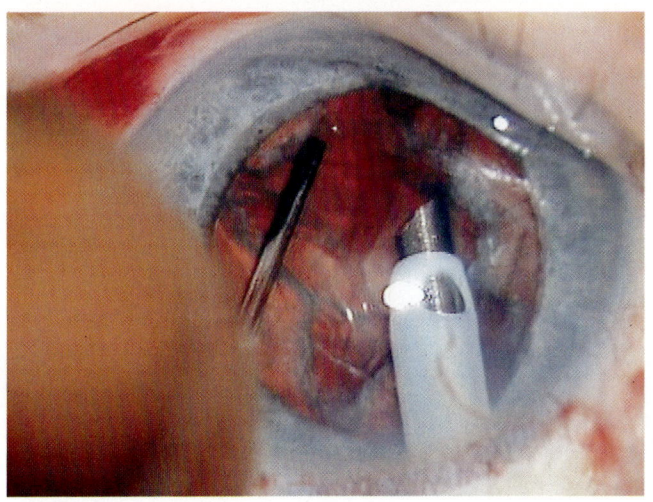

Figure 15.11 *The last fracture is accomplished, thus the nucleus is seperated into four mobile quadrants.*

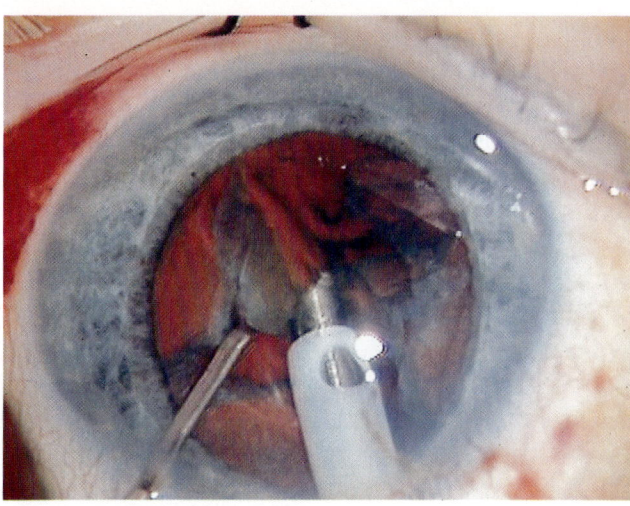

Figure 15.12 *The first of the four quadrants is brought to the center of the pupil and emulsified.*

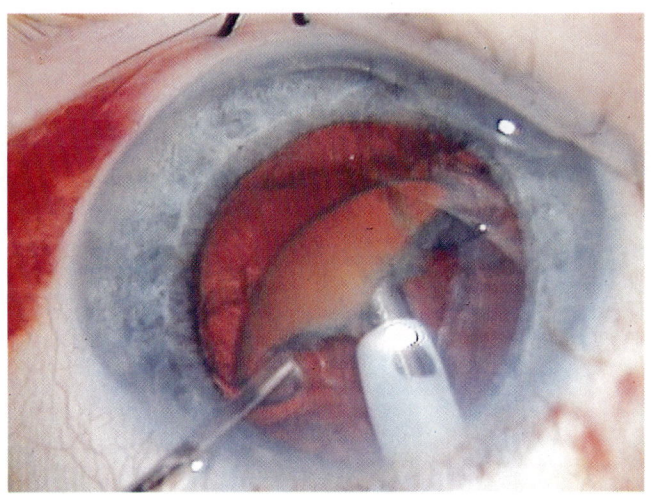

Figure 15.13 *The last of the four quadrants is emulsified.*

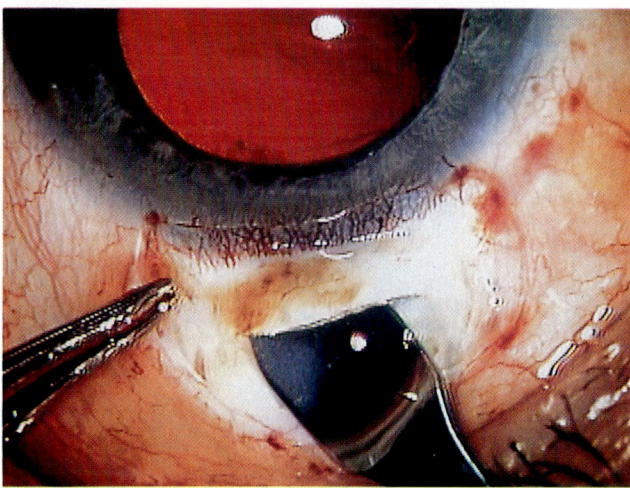

Figure 15.14 *After completing cortical aspiration and refilling the anterior chamber and capsular bag with viscoelastic, the cutting edge of the keratome is used to enlarge the incision in the same plane up to the limits of the 4.00-mm groove.*

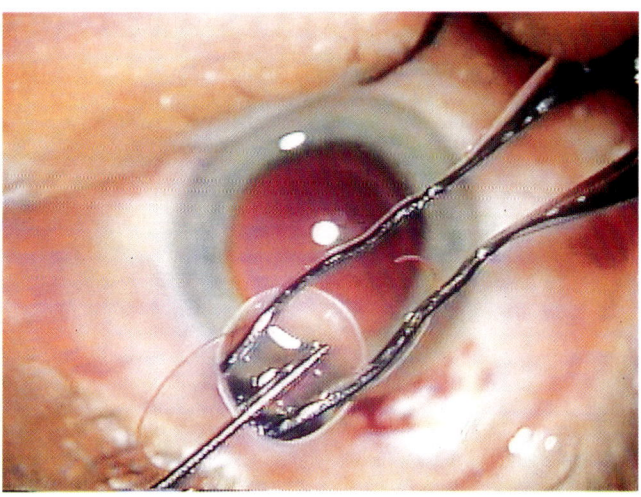
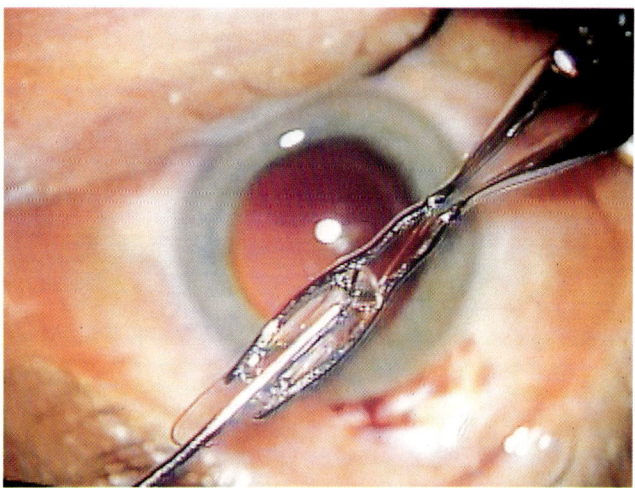

Figure 15.15 *The IOL is bisected with the holding forceps in a longitudinal manner* **(left)**, *and the IOL is folded with the Faulkner forceps* **(right)**.

tional manner. When the crosswise technique is used (Figs. 15.18 to 15.22), both of the haptics as well as the optic should enter the capsular bag in one continuous motion. Occasionally the optic will need to be nudged in or one of the haptics will enter the sulcus rather than the bag and have to be retrieved and placed manually in a conventional manner.

The most common problem I have found when using the Faulkner forceps is that when the wound is open, there is a tendency to have a mini-iris prolapse; that is, the iris engages on the lower jaw of the Faulkner forceps. When this is anticipated because the eye has a shallow chamber, or when this actually occurs, a lens glide should be used. It will have to be trimmed slightly, as it is wider than the 4.00-mm incision, but when placed over the iris, it greatly facilitates the entrance of the Faulkner forceps into the eye. When the IOL is centered over the capsulorhexis, the glide can be gently removed by the assistant.

When the Faulkner forceps are removed from the eye, it is helpful to stabilize the globe with toothed forceps. Also, gently closing and releasing the jaws of the forceps helps prevent the forceps from adhering too much to the underlying IOL.

A new injection instrument, the Prodigy (AMO), may be packaged with the AMO SI-18NB IOL. The

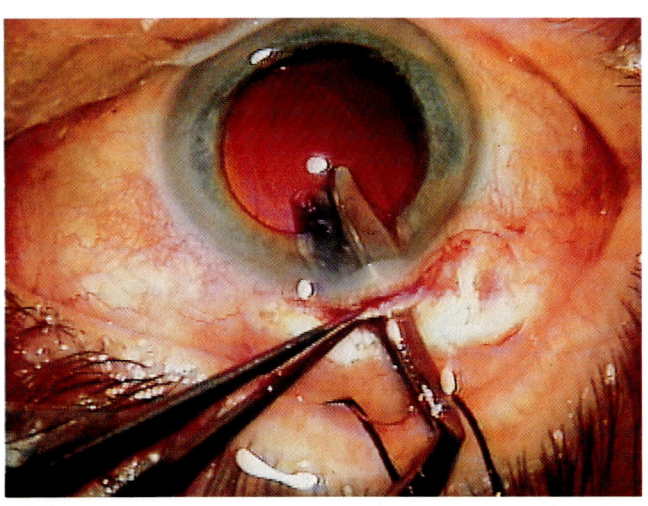
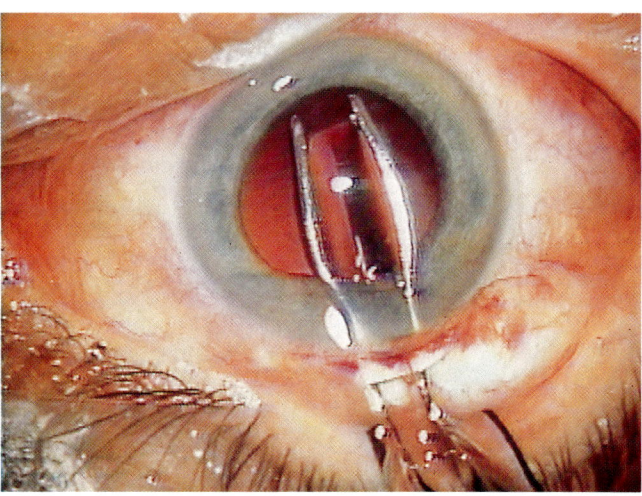

Figure 15.16 *The Faulkner forceps are rotated to the side, and the inferior haptic is tucked under the margin of the capsulorhexis* **(left)**. *The forceps rotate the lens upright* **(right)** *and gently release it into the capsular bag.*

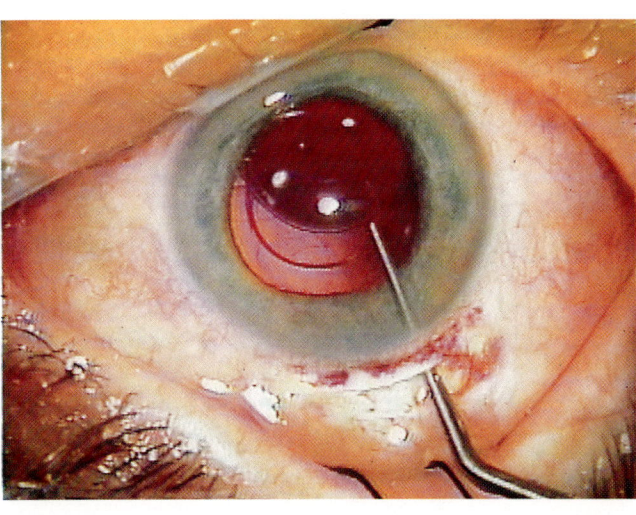

Figure 15.17 *The superior haptic is placed in the capsular bag in a routine manner.*

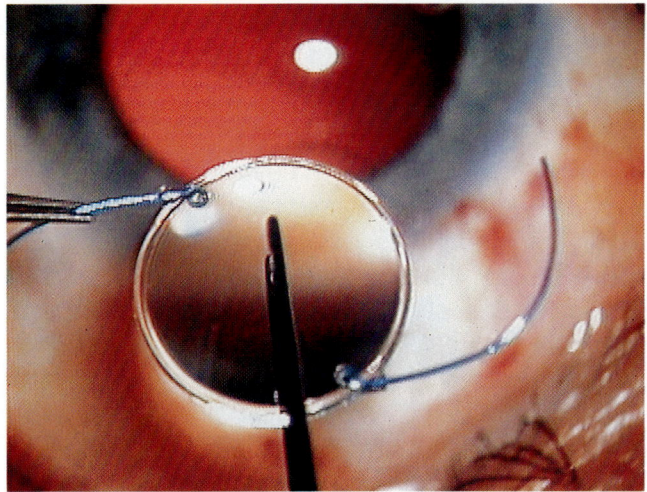

Figure 15.18 *The SI-20NB is grasped crosswise and bisected with the holding forceps.*

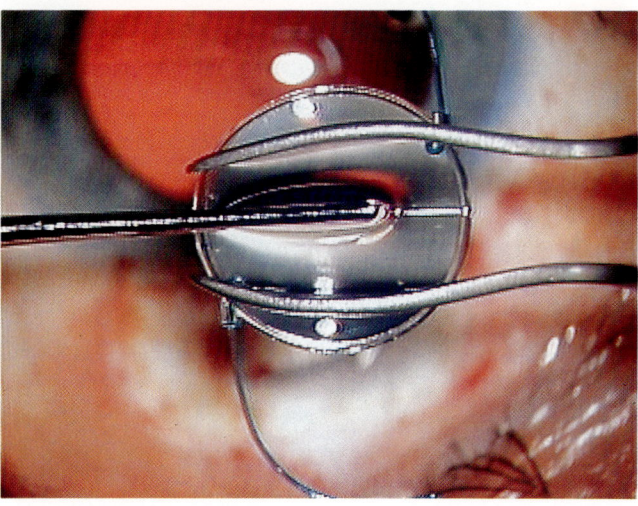

Figure 15.19 *The Faulkner forceps fold the lens and the accessory forceps are removed.*

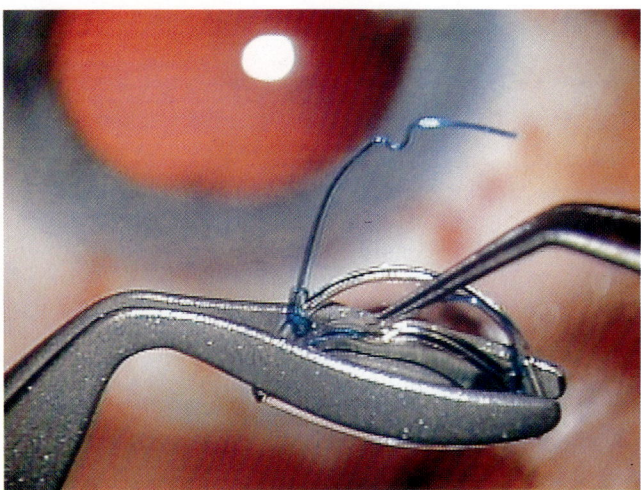
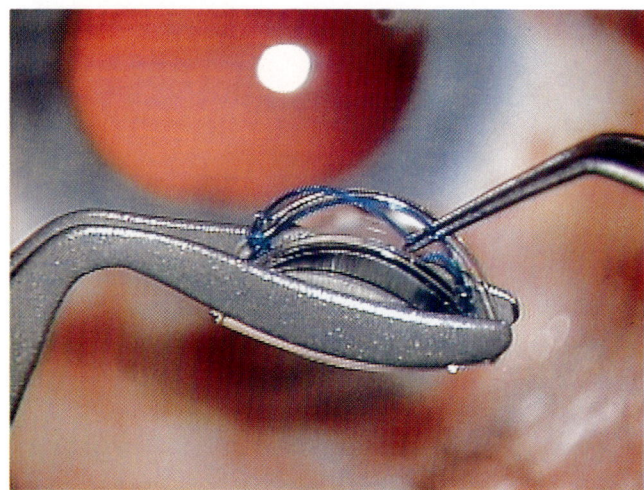

Figure 15.20 (Left and right) *The Prolene loops are tucked into the folded IOL.*

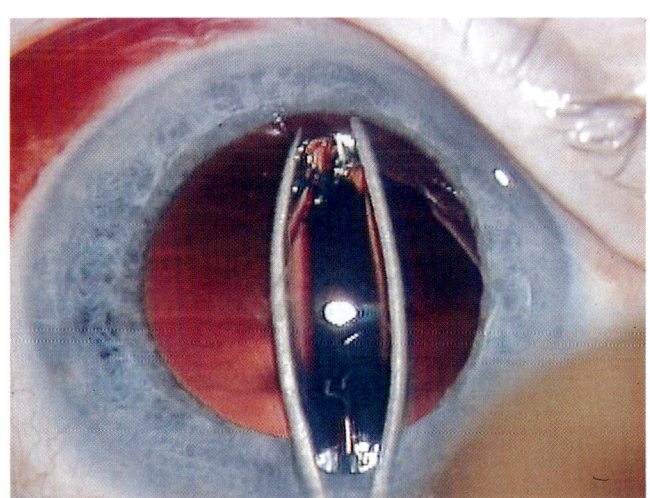

Figure 15.21 *The folded IOL may be inserted with the Faulkner forceps either upright or rotated horizontally to the left. The lens is centered over the capsulorhexis and then gently released. Both haptics and optic enter the bag in one continuous motion.*

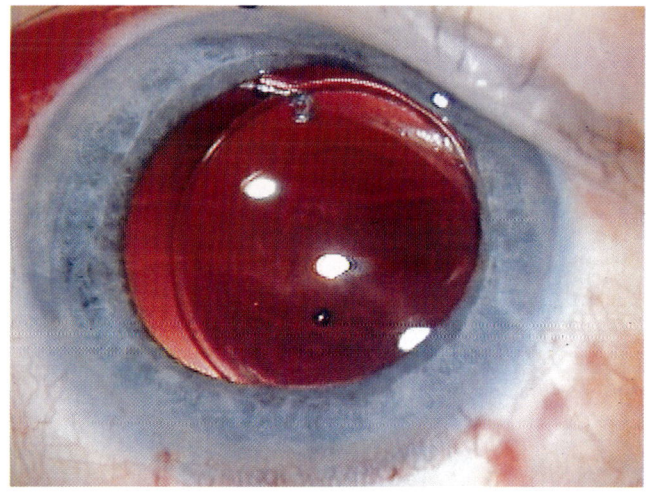

Figure 15.22 *The centered silicone lens requires no additional manipulation.*

SURGICAL REHABILITATION OF VISION

Prodigy is designed to gently release the SI-18 IOL into the bag in one continuous motion (Figs. 15.23 to 15.28)

It is important that any instrument making contact with the silicone IOL be carefully cleaned and all debris and rust removed because of the high propensity for particulate matter to adhere to silicone material. Also, for the Faulkner forceps to maintain a firm hold on the outer lens surface, the surface must be dry and free of BSS or viscoelastic.

Small incision IOLs have also been developed using traditional PMMA materials. Initial clinical experience has shown that the AMO Kelman Phacofit PC-28LB collapsible IOL (Fig. 15.29) can be easily placed in the capsular bag through a 3.50-mm incision (Figs. 15.30 and 15.31) and that visual rehabilitation is rapid due to reduced astigmatism. The Phacofit IOL has a distinct advantage: The long-term effects of PMMA in the eye are well known while those of the silicone and HEMA IOLs are undetermined. The PC-28LB has expanded opacified wings that can be flexed posteriorly to allow insertion through an incision only slightly larger than the 3.00-mm-wide optic (see Figs. 15.18 to 15.20). Some surgeons remain wary of this IOL because they fear that decentration might compromise vision by offsetting the clear portion of the optic from the visual axis.

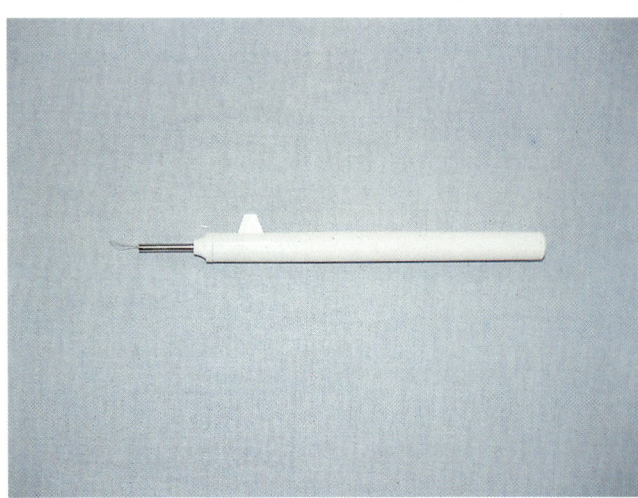

Figure 15.23 *The Prodigy system is two-part: a special lens-holding forceps, and an injector with a silicone sleeve that is retracted into a metal nose cone by a sliding thumb control.*

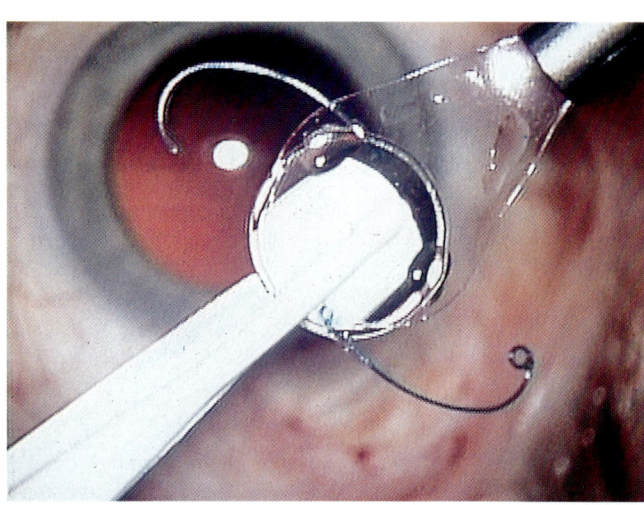

Figure 15.24 *The AMO SI-18NB is placed perpendicular to the long axis of the holding forceps on the platform, allowing 1.00 mm of the lens to overhang the platform. The paddle is then placed over the lens, also allowing a 1.00-mm lens overhang from the paddle.*

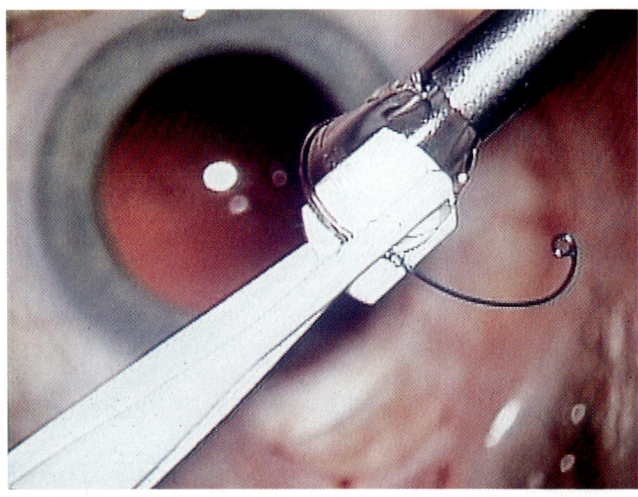

Figure 15.25 *The lens is retracted into the metal nose cone. The forceps are released when retraction is secure.*

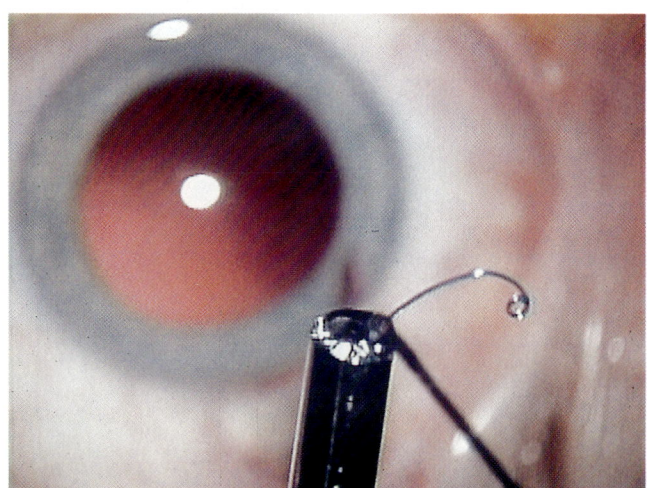

Figure 15.26 *After the lens is retracted into the nose cone, viscoelastic may be instilled to prevent any trapped air bubbles.*

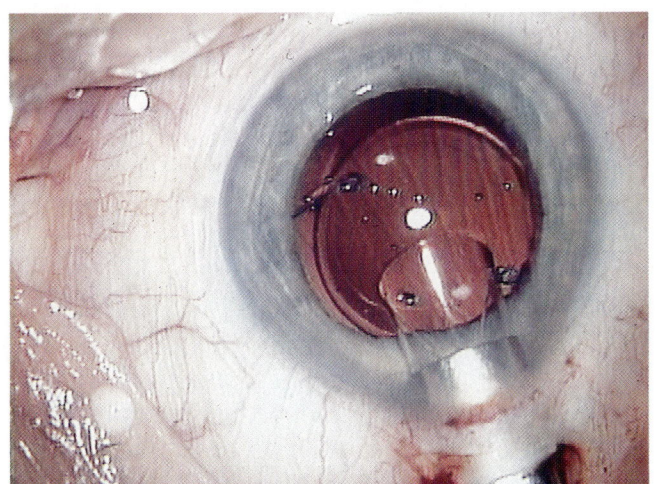

Figure 15.27 *The nose cone is placed in the 4.00-mm scleral pocket. The slide control is pressed forward with the thumb of the right hand until the haptics and optic are gently released into the capsular bag. The paddle is retracted back into the nose cone prior to removing the metal nose cone from the eye.*

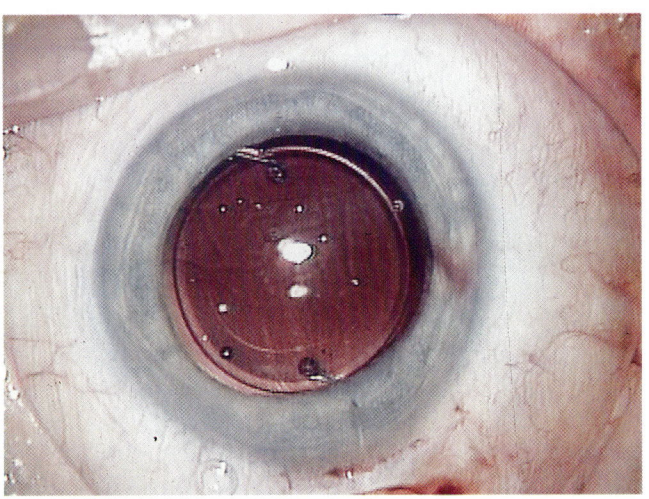

Figure 15.28 *The IOL spontaneously centers itself in the capsular bag.*

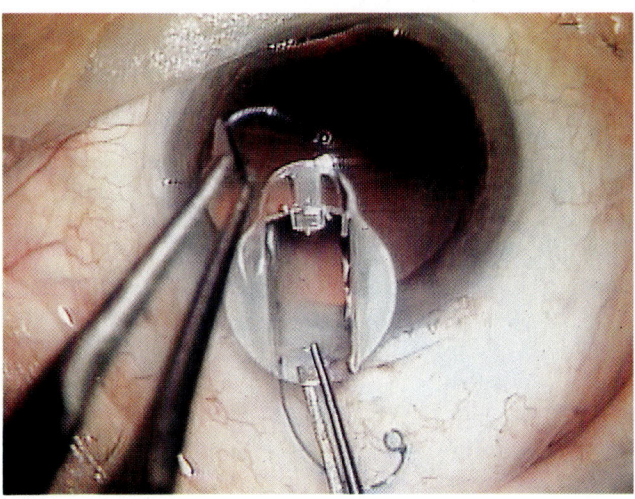

Figure 15.29 *The AMO Kelman Phacofit PC-28LB IOL.*

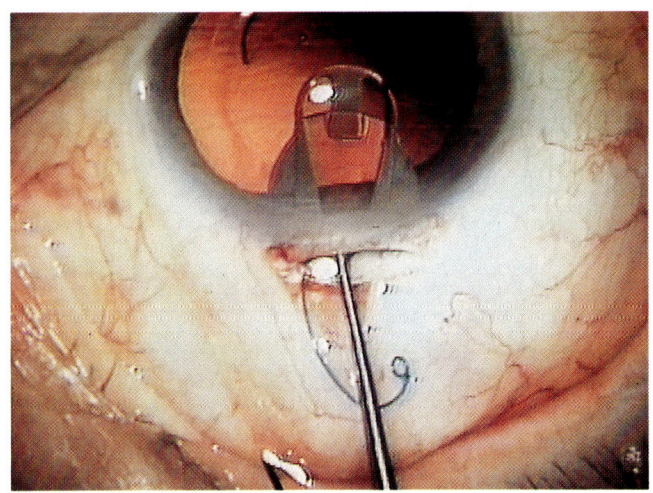

Figure 15.30 *The IOL is grasped at the clear optic and gently nudged through the 4.00-mm incision, allowing the "wings" to fold posterior to the optic.*

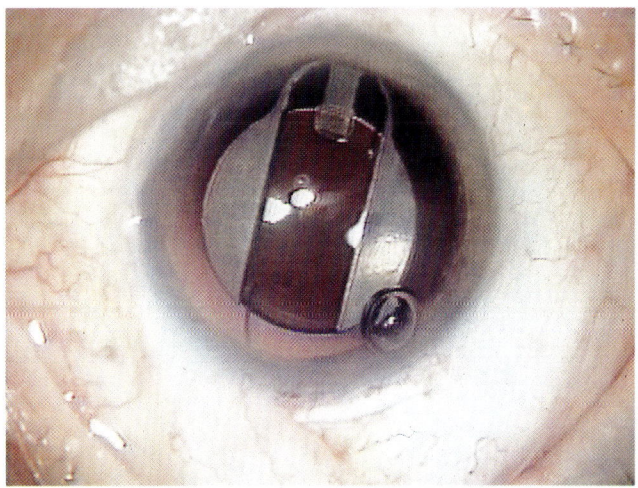

Figure 15.31 *The "wings" spontaneously unfold and the trailing prolene loop is placed in the bag in a conventional manner. The lens centers well.*

One-Piece Implants

Presently available one-piece designs include the Alcon IOGEL 38% water content poly-HEMA IOL and the Staar plated haptic AA-4203C silicone IOL.

IOGEL IOLs with a 12.00-mm overall length (PC-12) and an 11.30-mm overall length (PC-1103) are now available. The posterior surface of the optic and the flanges of the IOL have a single continuous arc of curvature that is designed to maximize contact with the posterior capsule. With symmetrical compression—the result of capsular bag contraction—the lens is designed to vault minimally posteriorly, not buckle or decenter.

The Staar AA-4203C is a uniplanar biconvex one-piece design, with an overall length of 10.50 mm. It also maintains even distention of the posterior capsule.

The IOGEL IOL is easily implanted using the Faulkner forceps (Figs. 15.32 to 15.34). The IOL is grasped lengthwise with the accessory rounded forceps and then folded lengthwise with the cross action Faulkner forceps. The accessory forceps are then removed. Once folded, a few drops of BSS are applied to maintain hydration of the hydrogel lens. It can then be implanted through the 4.00-mm scleral pocket incision without rotating the Faulkner forceps to the side. With

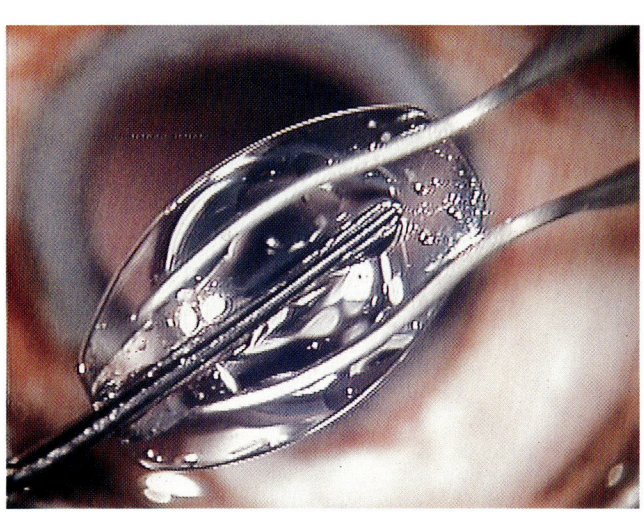

Figure 15.32 *The IOGEL IOL is held lengthwise, bisected with the holding forceps, and then folded with the Faulkner forceps.*

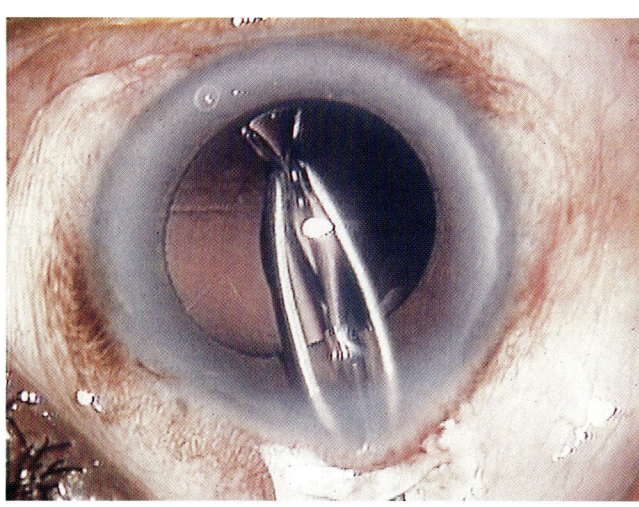

Figure 15.33 *The IOL is gently placed into the eye, tucking the inferior haptic under the margin of the capsulorhexis, which acts as its own lens glide.*

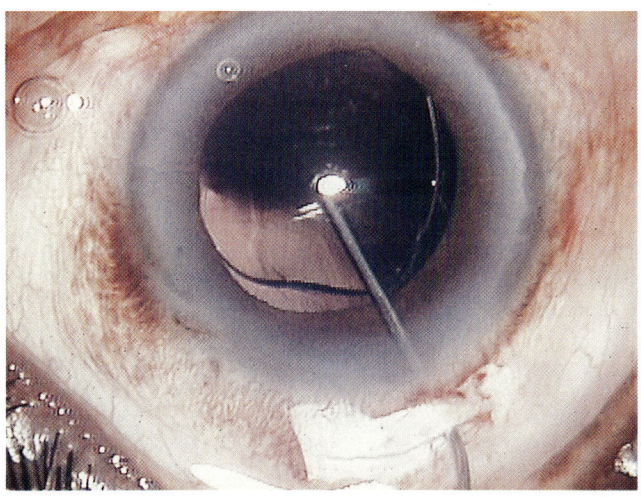

Figure 15.34 *After release of the IOL, the superior haptic is tucked into the bag by gentle pressure at the optic/haptics junction, using a viscoelastic cannula.*

the IOL itself acting as a lens glide, the inferior haptic is tucked into the capsular bag. The Faulkner forceps are then released. The IOL gently unfolds and the Faulkner forceps are removed from the eye. The superior haptic can be tucked under the margin of the capsulorhexis, using either the viscoelastic cannula, which is placed at the optic/haptic junction, or a special mushroom-shaped lens manipulator (Alcon). Once in the bag, the IOL spontaneously centers itself quite nicely.

Using a similar technique, the Staar AA-4203C IOL can also be inserted with the Faulkner forceps. It is preferable, however, to turn the Faulkner forceps to the side for insertion of the IOL before turning the forceps upright to release the IOL. Normal procedure for placing the superior haptic of the Staar IOL uses a Lester lens manipulator to engage the superior positioning hole and depress slightly posteriorly and toward 6 o'clock, allowing the superior haptic to buckle underneath the margin of the capsulorhexis into the bag. If this appears to cause excessive stress to the zonules, the superior margin of the capsular bag can be retracted using a blunt iris hook to facilitate the placement of the haptic.

An alternate method for insertion of the Staar one-piece IOL is the Softrans injector instrument (Figs. 15.35 to 15.41). This technique is generally preferred by most surgeons as it allows a 3.50-

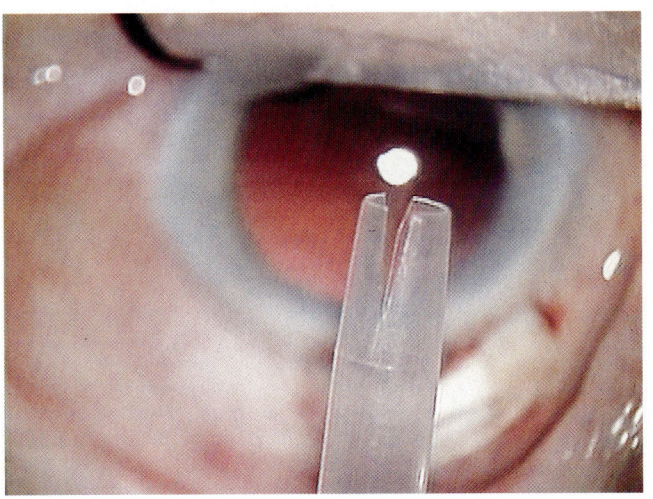

Figure 15.35 *Slits in the silicone nose piece are made by the surgeon to allow for a more gentle lens release.*

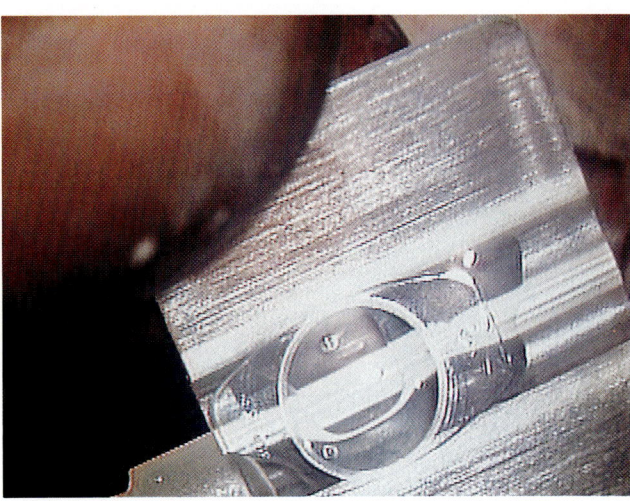

Figure 15.36 *The wings of the injector cartridge are opened. Viscoelastic is placed in the proximal end of the nose cone and the bed of the cartridge. The margins of the Staar AA-4203C are tucked under the edges of the bed.*

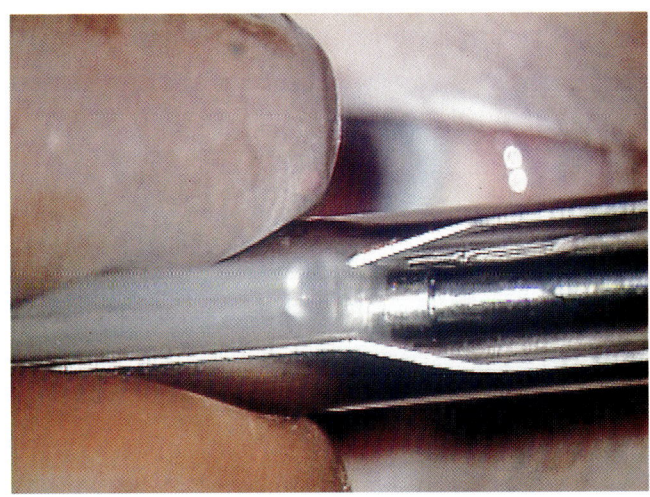

Figure 15.37 *Having folded the wings together, the nose cone is inserted in the metal sleeve with the push rod placed in the rear of the injector cartridge.*

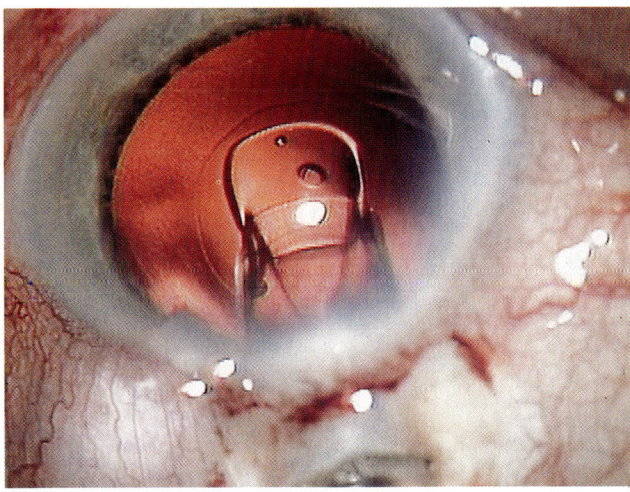

Figure 15.38 *The thumbscrew is rotated and the IOL begins to emerge into the capsular bag.*

mm incision, rather than the 4.00-mm incision required by the Faulkner forceps, and a more gentle release of the IOL into the eye. With this instrument, the superior haptic can sometimes be placed into the bag in one continuous motion. Alternatively, it may be placed manually, as previously described, with the Faulkner forceps method.

When using the one-piece hydrogel lens as well as the one-piece silicone lenses, it is important that both haptics are securely under the margins of the capsulorhexis. It is also important to remove viscoelastic as thoroughly as possible, making sure to massage out any viscoelastic retained behind the implant, so as not to induce excessive postoperative intraocular pressure. There has been one case reported in which the IOGEL lens, instead of vaulting posteriorly, vaulted anteriorly, occluding the opening of the capsulorhexis with retained viscoelastic material. This capsulorhexis block phenomenon can be corrected, using the YAG laser to make a small peripheral anterior capsule puncture so the lens spontaneously returns to its proper position.

Closure

My preferred method of closure is a single horizontal suture, as described by Shepherd (Figs. 15.42 to 15.44). With this technique, either a 10-0 or 11-0 nylon suture on a conventional needle is

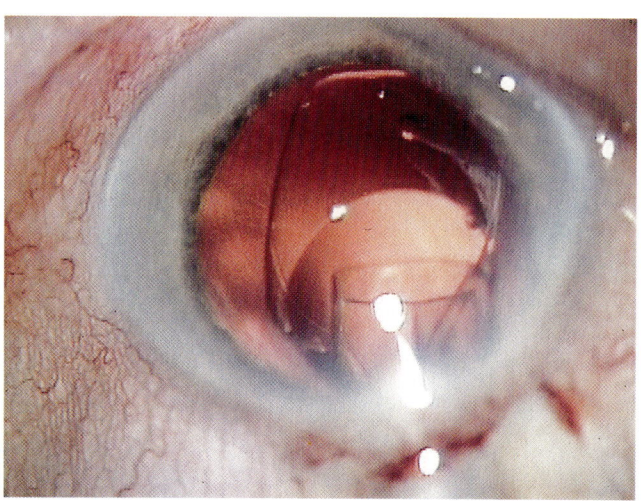

Figure 15.39 *A gentle release of the lens is accomplished because of the previously made slits.*

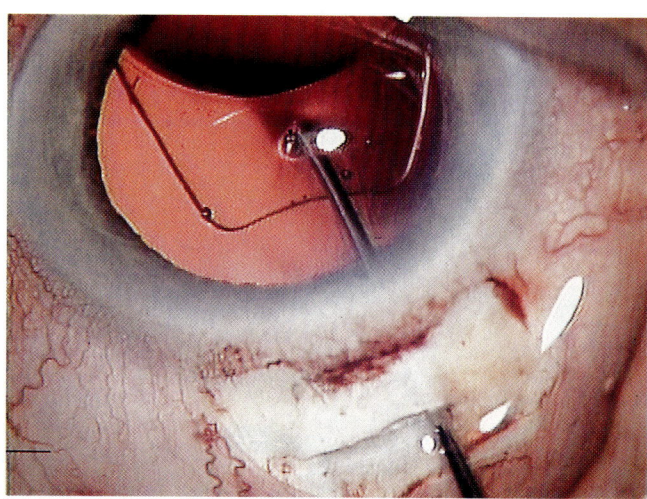

Figure 15.40 *A Lester lens manipulator engages the superior positioning hole, and the lens is tucked under the margin of the capsulorhexis.*

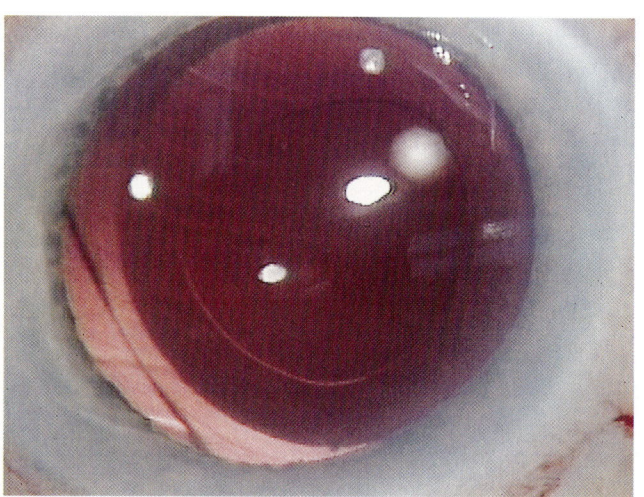

Figure 15.41 *The 10.50-mm lens centers well in the capsular bag.*

passed through the superficial sclera at a point that bisects the limbus and the scleral groove and is approximately 1.00 mm central to the lateral margin of the groove. The needle is driven perpendicularly and one can feel it pass through the superficial sclera and the deep sclera. When the deep sclera is entered, the needle is passed transversely and then brought up through the corresponding symmetrical point on the opposite side. The superficial scleral lip is lifted and a Weck-cel is used to clean the scleral bed so that one can see that the suture has indeed passed through both layers of the sclera. Prior to tying the suture, the irrigation/aspiration (I/A) instrument is used to meticulously remove as much of the viscoelastic as possible, especially massaging the one-piece IOL. The suture is tied snugly, but not too tightly, with a 3-1-1 throw knot, which is cut and rotated. The conjunctival flap is pulled down, and appropriate subconjunctival injections are given.

The principal advantage of soft foldable IOLs is their ability to be placed through a 3.50-mm to 4.00-mm wide scleral pocket incision that can be closed with a single horizontal suture. Shepherd demonstrated that this type of closure induced 0.13 D (±0.67 D) with-the-rule astigmatism at one week, which stabilized at 0.22 D (±0.47 D) against-the-rule at twelve weeks. The postoperative mean change from one week to twelve weeks was 0.36 D.

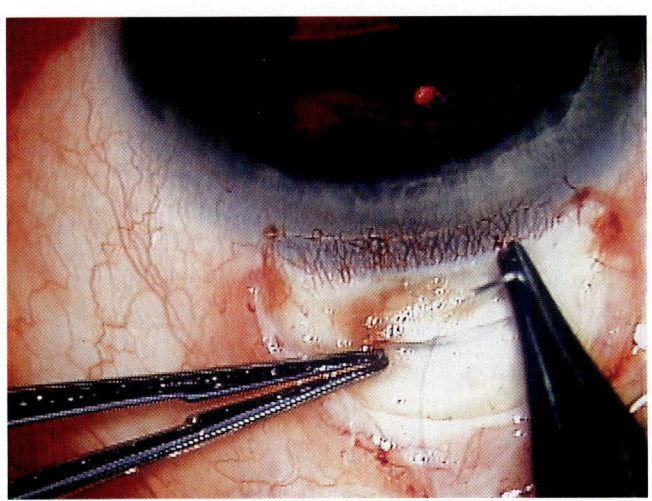 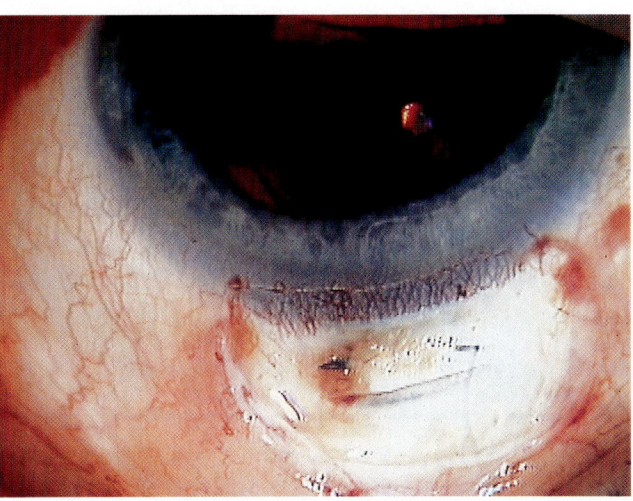

Figure 15.42 (Left and right) *After having completed lens implantation, the wound is closed with a single horizontal suture of 10-0 or 11-0 nylon. The entry point is halfway between the limbus and the groove and 1.00 mm central to the lateral margin of the groove. The needle is driven perpendicular to the sclera and then, as it passes into the deeper layer, tangentially. It is removed at the symmetrical point on the other side.*

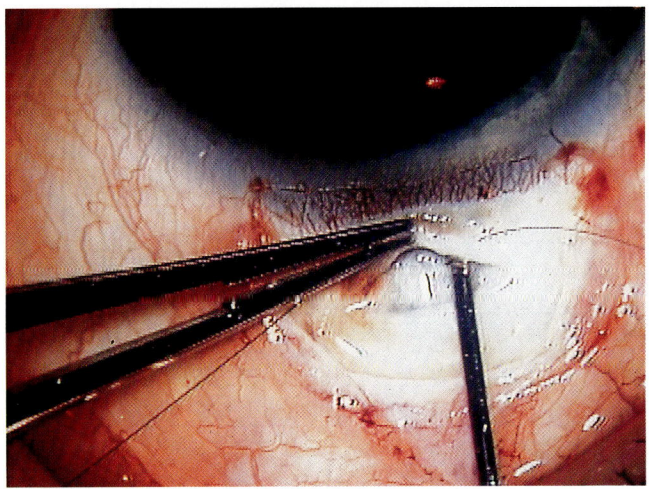 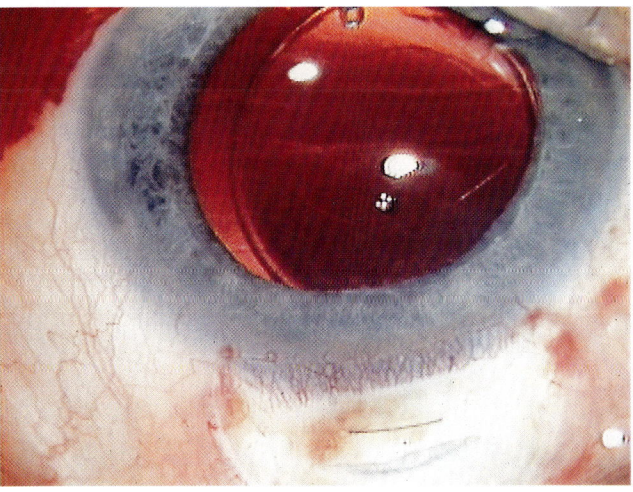

Figure 15.43 *The superficial scleral layer is lifted and it is confirmed that a deep, as well as superficial, scleral bite has been obtained.*

Figure 15.44 *The folded silicone lens is well centered in the capsular bag, and the wound is closed with the horizontal suture. The slight wound gape creates no problem with maintaining a water tight wound.*

The two-year follow-up of Shepherd's series demonstrates that this minimal, surgically induced astigmatism has remained stable during this period. My own study supports this finding—90% of my patients who had this type of incision achieved 20/40 or better uncorrected vision two weeks postoperatively compared to 31.6% of a similar group of patients who underwent phacoemulsification with implantation of a 7.00-mm PMMA IOL. This remarkably quick visual rehabilitation and stabilization has greatly increased patient satisfaction with cataract surgery. With this small incision technique, the eye remains a stable platform on which other procedures for correcting pre-existing astigmatism can be performed, further enhancing refractive results.

An additional benefit of the relatively low index of refraction, thick IOLs, and in-the-bag fixation and capsulorhexis, is a remarkably low instance of posterior capsular opacificaton. In my own hands, the YAG rate at one year for hydrogel implants is 1.5% and 3% after silicone implants. This mirrors other previously reported capsulotomy rates by investigators who used hydrogel and silicone materials.

Complications

Once the technique of inserting three-piece silicone lenses has been mastered, there is no reason to expect that the incidence of complications would be any different than with a similar group of PMMA lenses with polypropylene haptics. Because these three-piece foldable IOLs may be implanted without a perfect capsulorhexis, the AMO SI-18NB is the small incision IOL of choice as of 1990.

When using one-piece hydrogel and silicone IOLs, it is incumbent on the surgeon to perfect his or her surgical technique. The surgeon should be able to reliably produce an intact margin of the capsulorhexis with no radial tears and an intact posterior capsule in order to implant these types of lenses with optimum results. Any radial extension of the capsulorhexis or tear of the posterior capsule predisposes these IOLs to decenter or dislocate, either anteriorly or into the vitreous.

Recently reported were five cases of capsular bag-placed IOGEL lenses that were lost in the vitreous when a YAG posterior capsulotomy was performed prior to three months following surgery. Surgeons implanting the Staar one-piece IOL also had similar problems, i.e., IOLs dislocating into the vitreous following premature YAG. Thus, it is recommended that the surgeon wait at least six months after placing a one-piece IOL before performing a YAG posterior capsulotomy or a small circular posterior capsulotomy.

Future Developments

With the superior results being obtained using the surgical procedure described in this chapter and foldable IOLs, the future of small incision surgery is bright. Just around the corner are acrylic IOLs with a higher index of refraction, which will be available from IOPTEX and Alcon–Cilco. Also available will be the memory IOL, a thermal labile IOL with a 25% water content that can be placed through a 3.20-mm incision in its rolled state, inserted with no special instrumentation, and unfolded according to the temperature of the aqueous.

Exciting work continues in the area of injectable, pliable IOL materials, capable of accommodation and usage following intercapsular phacoemulsification. These developments may help redefine our concept of small incision cataract surgery.

Clinical Points to Consider

☞ Small incision cataract/IOL surgery can significantly improve the percentage of patients who obtain the best possible uncorrected visual acuity.

☞ A three piece Sinskey-style foldable IOL with a 6.00-mm optic allows implantation through a 4.00-mm incision with the least number of complications.

☞ The Faulkner forceps may provide more controlled delivery of a folded IOL into the anterior chamber than the current generation of injectors.

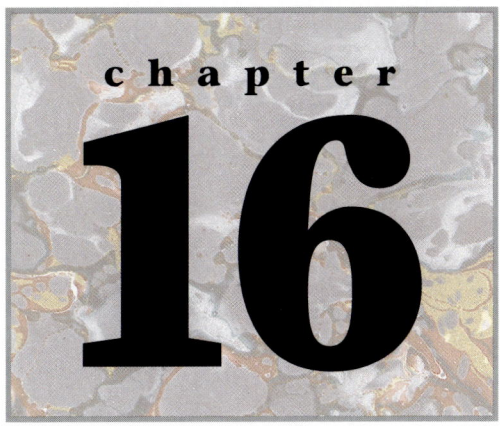

COMPARISION OF CATARACT WOUND SIZES

PAUL S. KOCH, M.D.

Ideas concerning cataract surgery incisions have changed in the past decade. Knowledge of how incision location, suture placement and orientation, and vector forces affect the cornea has prompted surgeons to investigate and create more sophisticated cataract surgery incisions. Formerly, surgeons selected the incision that provided the easiest access into the anterior chamber; now they choose the incision that permits the best postoperative healing. Thus, for many surgeons, the longer midlimbal incision demanded by classic extracapsular cataract extraction (ECCE) has been replaced by phacoemulsification's shorter incisions (the *posterior limbal*, the *pocket*, and the *scleral flap* (*shelf*) incisions). These incisions allow the patient quicker visual rehabilitation and less chance of surgically-induced astigmatism than is likely with other types of cataract surgery. This chapter will focus on the 6.00-mm phacoemulsification flap incision; however, the concepts involved should be valuable to cataract surgeons who want to minimize postoperative recovery time and increase the chances of best uncorrected visual acuity following cataract/intraocular lens (IOL) surgery.

The Scleral Flap Incision

The scleral flap incision has three dimensions (Fig. 16.1):

1. Depth: the thickness of the flap
2. Width: the perpendicular distance from the scleral groove to the line of entry into the anterior chamber
3. Length: the distance between the ends of the incision measured along the contour of the incision

This chapter will confine itself to the traditional tangential incision (when the incision and the limbus are concentric). Steven Siepser, M.D., (American Society of Cataract and Refractive Surgery meeting, 1990) has presented an innovative partial scleral incision that is placed perpendicular (radially) to the limbus with a tangential entry into the anterior chamber by lateral dissection of the sclera at a deeper layer (see Chapter 19). In theory, this incision can be used for phacoemulsification and implantation of a foldable IOL with absolutely no vertical tension forces placed on the cornea. As of this writing, however, experience is too limited to comment further on the advantage of this incision compared to a 4.00-mm tangential incision, which is more easily produced and also causes minimal change in corneal topography.

Depth

Scleral flap incisions can be dissected to virtually any predetermined depth. The sclera at 2.00 mm posterior to the limbus is roughly 0.60 mm thick, so the incision depth's practical range is from 0.10 mm to 0.50 mm. Flap depth can be determined accurately using a guarded, calibrated diamond knife held perpendicular to the scleral surface for the initial groove.

There are two problems with a very thin flap. First, it has a tendency to tear with manipulation, sometimes shredding because of the toothed forceps. Second, a thin flap can stretch, allowing an otherwise adequate closure to develop against-the-rule astigmatism.

Thick flaps are usually not a problem, provided one does not dissect so deeply that a suture bite cannot be adequately anchored in the underlying scleral bed. There is a trend toward using closure techniques that require suture placement parallel to the limbus. This closure demands that the suture be anchored well in the underlying scleral bed where a deep suture bite by a curved needle will often nick the underlying choroid, causing end-of-case bleeding. Straighter needles have been designed to prevent this problem. Nevertheless, in order to avoid the choroid and still have a good bite of tissue underneath the flap, a fairly thick scleral bed is required. This, naturally, necessitates a thinner scleral flap. It appears that the optimal incision depth is about 0.20 mm, or about one-third the thickness of the sclera.

Width

The distance between the external groove and the internal entry into the anterior chamber is the width of the incision. For production of an "astigmatism neutral" incision (i.e., one that creates no corneal astigmatism when closed watertight), the external incision should be as posterior as possible to minimize the effect of the sutures. The maximum permanent against-the-rule astigmatism that may develop as a result of a sceral flap incision of a given length and location is indirectly proportional to the surface area of the flap. In other words, the wider the flap, the less astigmatic effect because the lateral "pillars" of the wound help support the existing shape. Because the eye is a round structure, however, there is a practical limit as to how far back one can go before working around a curve (the limit is about 4.00 mm).

The anterior limit of a scleral pocket incision is about 1.00 mm back from the posterior aspect of the limbus. This is the shortest distance one can use and assure that the anterior aspect of the closure suture bites will be placed in white scleral tissue. A width less than 1.00 mm means that the sutures will be too close to the cornea and cause astigmatism postoperatively.

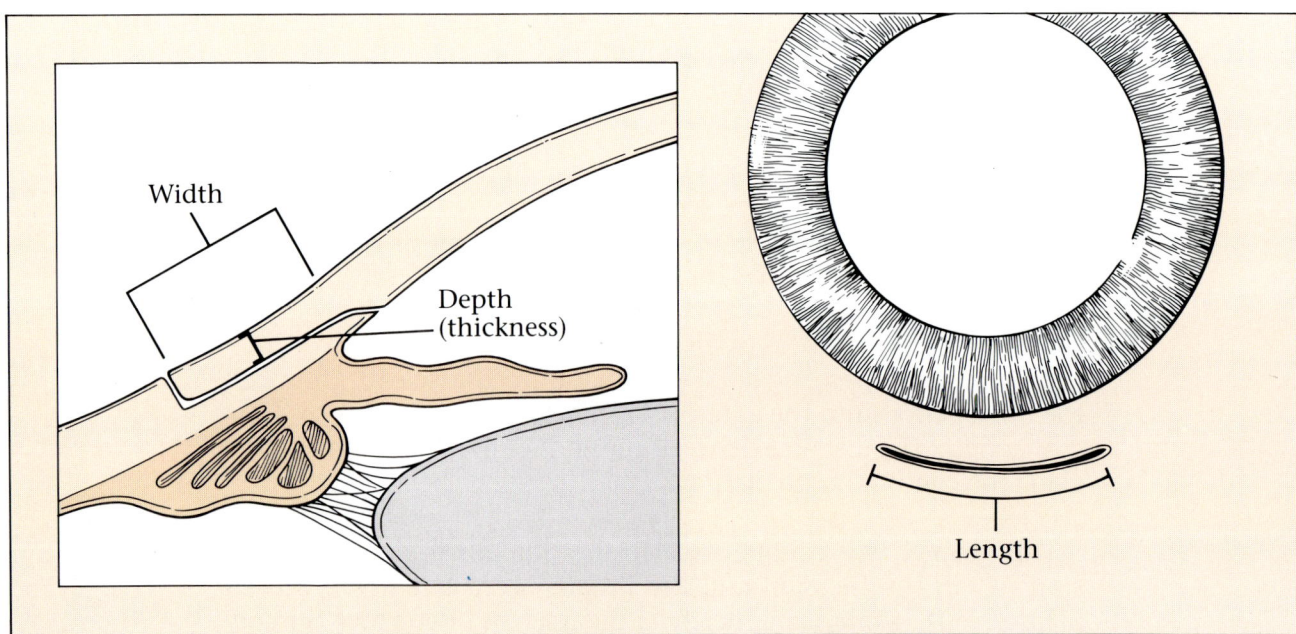

Figure 16.1 *The scleral flap incision has three dimensions: depth, width, and length.*

The surgeon must be aware of the location of the surgical limbus. The limbal area is really a zone about 1.00 mm wide (Fig. 16.2). Many patients have significant pannus formation in the 12 o'clock area that obscures the limbus. Often a surgeon will be fooled into using the insertion of the conjunctiva on the cornea as a reference mark. The change in shape between the cornea and the sclera, as well as the darker gray-blue appearance of the corneal transition tissue, helps to properly determine the posterior aspect of the limbus (Fig. 16.3).

The desire to move posteriorly has to be tempered with an understanding of the amount of bleeding that may be encountered during dissection of the flap. Simply put, the more posteriorly one proceeds, the more bleeding one will encounter. Staying away from the cornea while trying to avoid unnecessary bleeding means that most incisions will have a width of about 1.50 mm to 2.00 mm.

Length

Douglas Koch, M.D. (no relation) and others have shown that no incision length can be free of astigmatism considerations. An incision of 3.00 mm or less however, disturbs so little of the circumferential corneal ring that wound sag does not occur and no against-the-rule astigmatism is produced. Therefore, there is no advantage to making an incision smaller than 3.00 mm, assuming the incision is closed in a watertight, astigmatism-neutral fashion, in the patient with low preoperative astigmatism.

John Shepard, M.D., reasoned that if a 3.50-mm to 4.00-mm incision does not cause astigmatism by wound sag, then closing the wound in a watertight fashion without inducing with-the-rule astigmatism would allow for extremely rapid visual recovery following phacoemulsification/foldable IOL surgery. He achieved his goal by eliminating radial sutures and substituting horizontal

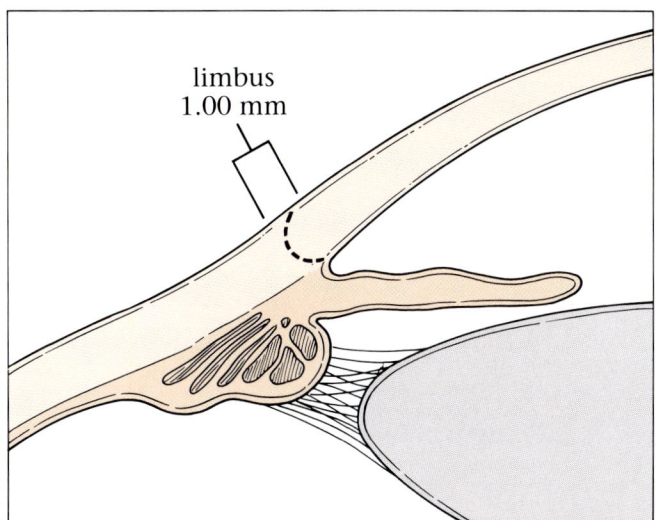

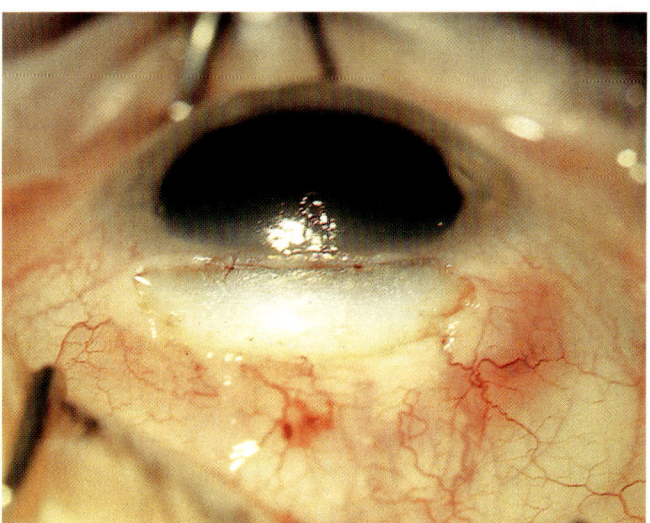

Figure 16.2 *The surgical limbus, an area about 1.00 mm wide, looks blue-gray to the surgeon. The change in shape between the cornea and the sclera and the color of the corneal transition tissue enables the surgeon to identify the posterior aspect of the limbus. An incision commencing at the posterior aspect of the surgical limbus must be beveled when entering the anterior chamber to avoid the iris root and ciliary body.*

Figure 16.3 *The surgeon's view of the surgical limbus just prior to performing a scleral flap incision for phacoemulsification.*

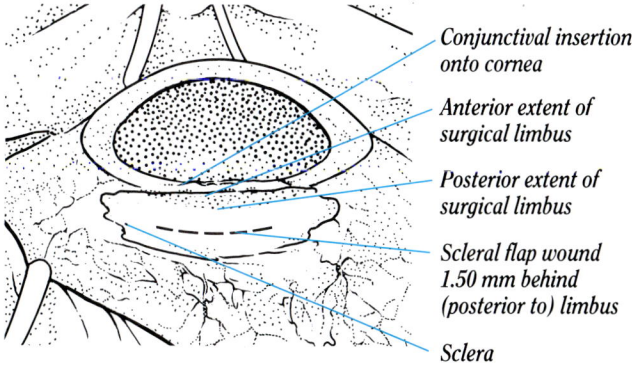

sutures. This breakthrough in cataract surgery is one of the greatest single advances to occur during the past five years. Howard Fine, M.D., has popularized the *infinity suture* for 6.00-mm wounds as well (see Chapter 20), which works on the same principle, i.e., not creating transient surgically induced astigmatism.

However, IOLs that can be inserted through a 3.00-mm incision do not exist at this time, although they certainly are desirable. A foldable silicone IOL can be inserted gently through a 4.00-mm wound, but most surgeons who perform phacoemulsification use a 6.00-mm incision to accommodate the PMMA IOL optic of the same diameter. Those surgeons who perform nucleus expression use 10.00-mm to 12.00-mm incisions.

Our search for astigmatism-neutral cataract surgery compels evaluation of the radial vector forces on the cornea when the circumferential corneal ring is opened by varying amounts.

Vertical Corneal Instability

It is possible to construct a mathematical model of the cornea using vector analysis to evaluate the vertical integrity of the cornea following circumferential incisions of different lengths. Calculations in this model were made with a flap incision width of only 1.00 mm, essentially making these calculations reflect a worst-case scenario. The classic ECCE 10.00-mm to 12.00-mm beveled corneoscleral incision is not easily com-

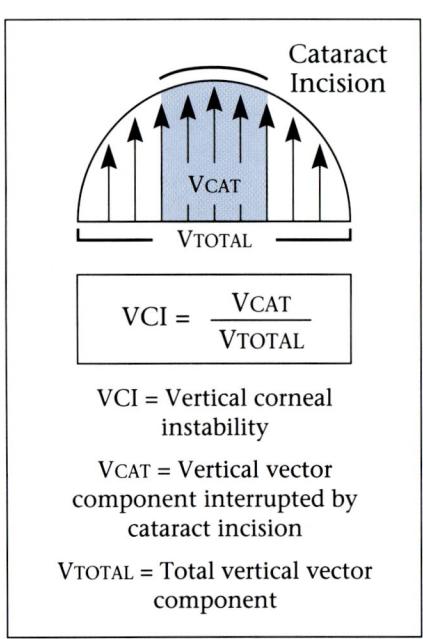
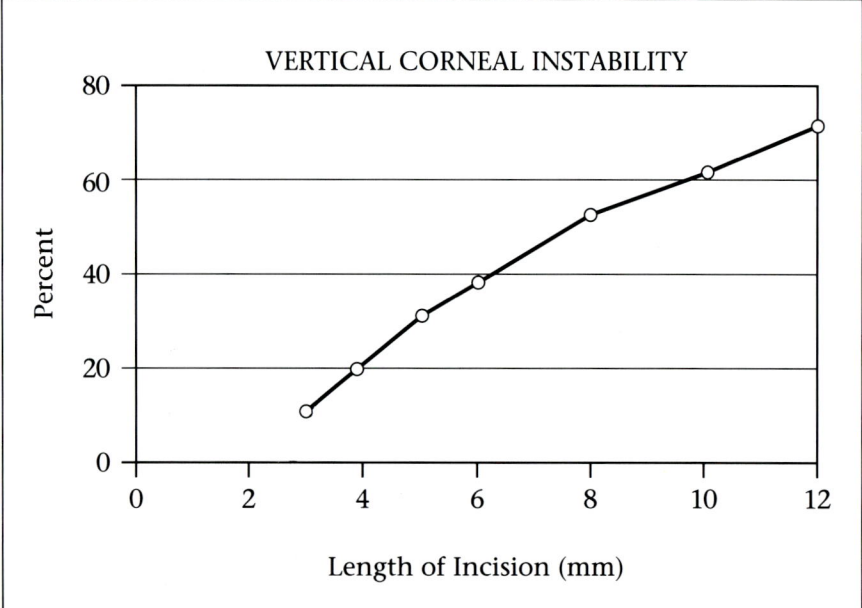

Figure 16.4 (Left) *Vertical corneal instability (VCI) is the percentage of vertical vector forces that are disrupted by a corneoscleral incision.* **(Right)** *Graphic representation of VCI correlated to cataract wound length.*

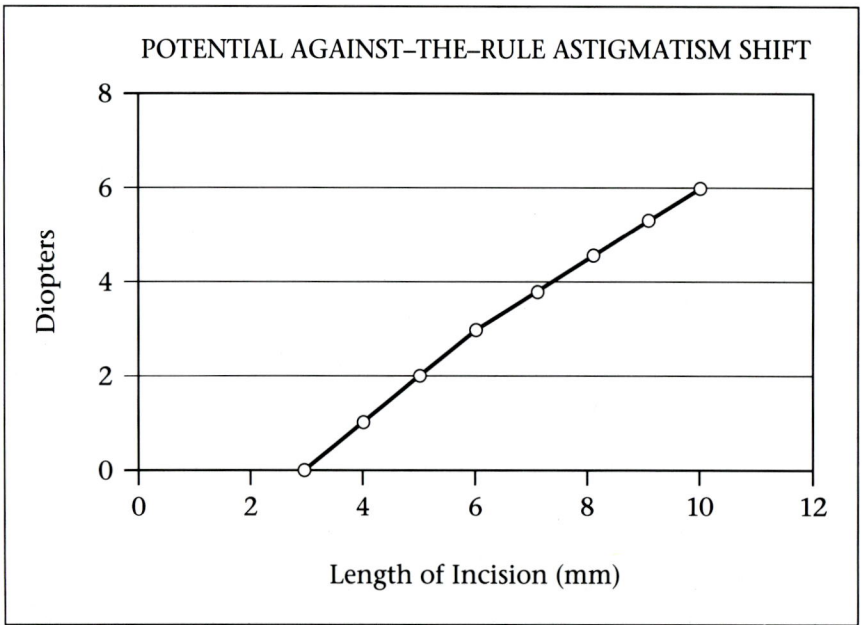

Figure 16.5 *This graph depicts the potential increase in against-the-rule astigmatism resulting from limbal corneoscleral incisions of various lengths.*

patible with a 1.00-mm scleral flap component. Therefore, wounds of this length usually employ only beveled incisions for entrance into the anterior chamber. Theoretically, a scleral incision would induce the least astigmatism when entering the anterior chamber as posteriorly as possible since it comprises less of the circumference of the corneal ring and, therefore, creates less wound sag.

Actually, a 6.00-mm long, 1.00-mm wide scleral flap incision enters the anterior chamber rather centrally, and its effect on astigmatism is essentially the same as a nonflap 6.00-mm incision. This flap incision is desirable, however, because the large amount of scleral contact creates a watertight wound during surgery, which heals in the preoperative position, and the sutures peripheral to the limbus affect the cornea less than a narrower incision would.

Vertical corneal instability is defined as the sum of the vertical vector components that are interrupted by the cataract wound. Therefore, the vertical corneal instability is 0% if no incision has been made and 100% if a 180-degree incision has been made. All calculations are relative to these two standards. Remember that the corneal meridian involved by a wound concentric with the limbus becomes flatter (longer radius of curvature, less refractive power), thereby creating against-the-rule astigmatism.

Tight radial sutures can cause with-the-rule astigmatism by steepening the involved meridian but *only transiently*. Nonabsorbable sutures, even though they do not readily biodegrade, have less effect on corneal curvature with time. The scleral tissue 2.00 mm behind the limbus is less dense than limbal tissue, so cheesewiring, scleral stretch, and preoperative curvature of the eye cause preoperative astigmatism to return six to 12 months postoperatively, despite the continued presence of these sutures.

Figure 16.4 is a graph showing the relationship between length of incision and vertical corneal instability as measured by the reduction in the 90-degree meridian force vector that maintains the domed shape of the cornea. The relationship is not a straight line correlation but rather a mild hyperbolic curve.

A 3.00-mm incision causes vertical corneal instability of 15% but is clinically irrelevant since virtually no astigmatism is induced. The surgeon must ask: What degree of vertical corneal instability is clinically relevant?

An incision will seek to return to its original orientation unless acted upon by some force that, unfortunately for cataract surgeons, includes suture tension, wound healing, incision sag, intraocular pressure, and preoperative shape. Attempts to orient the incision to correct pre-existing astigmatism are valuable but, of course, have limits in affecting permanent wound position. Figure 16.5 shows the maximum potential change possible in astigmatism after recessing limbal wounds of varying lengths when all the sutures have been removed. Table 16.6 correlates vertical corneal instability to astigmatism change.

It is important to note that no increase in vertical corneal refractive power has been calculated for a tight wound. Clinical experience has shown that tight sutures have only a transient effect on corneal curvature. Therefore, *tight sutures, even combined with wound resection (wedge resection), cannot be used to make a flatter meridian become steeper permanently.* Wound recession is

Table 16.6
Astigmatism Versus Incision Length

VERTICAL CORNEAL INSTABILITY	Incision Length (mm)	Vertical Corneal Instability (percent)	Potential Against-The-Rule Astigmatism (diopters)
Assumptions:	3.00	15	0.00
1. Corneal wound centered at 12 o'clock	4.00	20	1.00
2. Anterior chamber entered just posterior to	5.00	29	2.00
Schwalbe's ring	6.00	38	3.00
3. 3.00-mm to 7.00-mm wounds, scleral flap incision	7.00	45	3.75
4. 8.00-mm to 12.00-mm wounds, midlimbal incision	8.00	52	4.50
5. Intraocular pressure: 16 mm Hg	9.00	57	5.25
	10.00	61	6.00
	12.00	70	6.70

a stable method of astigmatism correction. With-the-rule astigmatism can be corrected by recessing a wound of the proper length, but *correction of against-the-rule astigmatism must employ either a lateral wound oriented on the steeper meridian or an astigmatic keratotomy combined with a wound oriented above on the flatter meridian.*

Conclusion

The use of a small incision depends not only on the goal of the operation, but on the surgeon's preference and surgical technique. A small incision is of no value if the goal of the procedure is to make a permanent change in the patient's preoperative astigmatism. On the other hand, a large incision is troublesome if the surgeon wants to preserve a preoperative corneal curvature or provide the patient with rapid postoperative stability of refraction.

Incision length considerations do not exist in a vacuum. The method of incision closure may allow significant against-the-rule astigmatism to develop if the wound is of sufficient length. Single horizontal suture techniques are rapidly gaining acceptance for small incisions, while multiple, running, and hybrid horizontal suture techniques are being used for larger incisions. The surgical result depends on incision length and closure; incision length must be considered in relation to the closure method employed in order to achieve best uncorrected visual acuity in the shortest possible time—the goal of cataract/IOL surgery.

Clinical Points to Consider

☞ Astigmatism is usually the limiting factor to good vision following cataract/IOL surgery.

☞ The ideal cataract/IOL wound induces no astigmatism but allows excellent access to the anterior chamber.

ANTERIOR VITRECTOMY

PAUL S. KOCH, M.D.

Vitreous loss is the unintentional movement of vitreous outside the globe through the surgical wound. When vitreous loss occurs during surgery, an emmetropic result may be undermined for the following reasons:

1. Typically, the surgeon disregards the surgical plan and instead concentrates on correcting the miserable immediate situation.
2. Cases involving vitreous loss have a cystoid macular edema rate of 30% to 50%.
3. Once the vitrectomy is complete, the lens usually has to be placed in the ciliary sulcus, which requires a change in the lens power from the predicted in-the-bag value. Usually the lens power has to be reduced 0.50 D.

The third problem is not serious and can be solved by adhering to a standard policy of changing lens power whenever a vitrectomy is performed. Dealing with the first two problems is more complicated because both the surgeon's technique and ego are factors.

Vitreous loss does not have to be a disaster—the ultimate outcome can be positive. The better the vitrectomy technique, the better the results will be and the less the surgeon's confidence will be damaged. In this chapter I will discuss the vitreous in relation to phacoemulsification, how it reacts when the posterior capsule opens, how vitreous loss can be limited, and how a relatively atraumatic vitrectomy can be performed with excellent results.

Characteristics of the Vitreous

It is helpful to study vitreous dynamics by using the image of a spring (a Slinky toy) with one end attached to the vitreous base and the other attached to the vitreomacular interface. The Slinky varies in size and color, just as the vitreous varies. When there is mild tension on a Slinky, the force is absorbed by the first few coils and not much else happens (Fig. 17.1). With greater tension, however, the entire coil stretches out and exerts tension at its base (Fig. 17.2). If the Slinky were the vitreous, this type of tension could cause a detached retina and cystoid macular edema at the vitreomacular interface.

In the vitreous wick syndrome, a small, narrow band of vitreous is stretched to the incision, and the resultant vitreous contraction may disturb the retina and cause cystoid macular edema. Severing the vitreous band near the incision causes it to retract quickly as would a spring. Often the cystoid macular edema will resolve.

The spring-like nature of the vitreous is also evident when performing a vitrectomy with small surgical sponges (e.g., Weck-Cel) and scissors. During this procedure small amounts of vitreous are pulled from the eye and excised. The remaining vitreous retracts quickly into the eye.

The Vitreous in Phacoemulsification

Vitreous loss is directly related to the size of the incision and to the liquidity of the vitreous gel. Thus the vitreous acts differently during phacoemulsification than it does during nucleus ex-

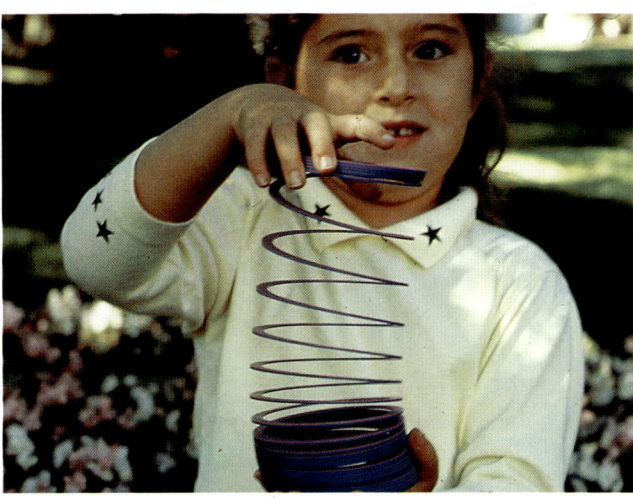

Figure 17.1 *Gentle stretching of a spring disturbs only the first few coils. The main body is undisturbed.*

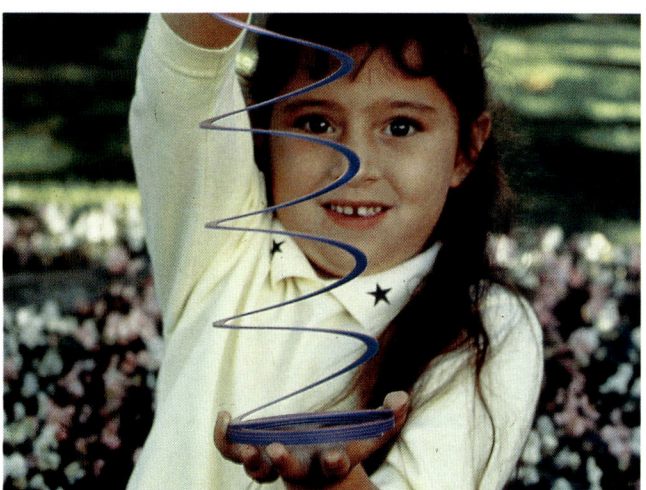

Figure 17.2 *If there is a lot of tension on a spring, all of the coils are disturbed and the tension is reflected right down to its base.*

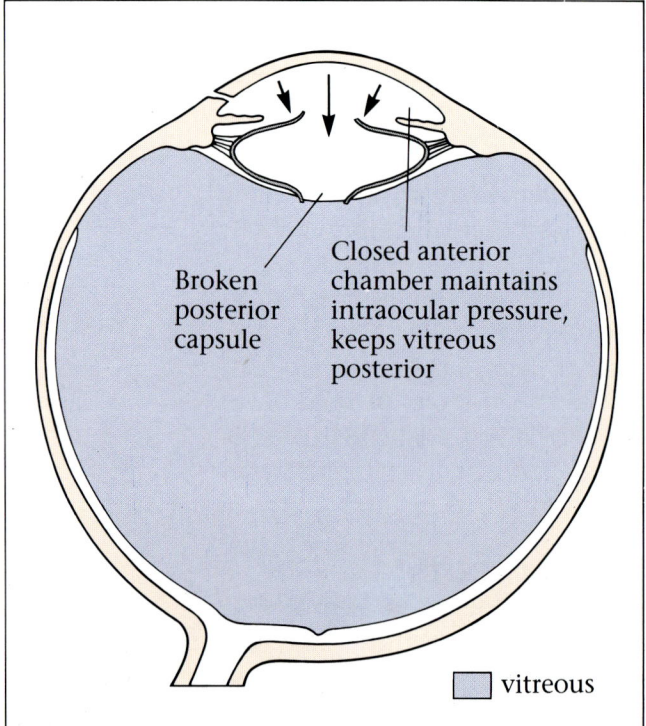

Figure 17.3 *Phacoemulsification's closed system helps limit vitreous loss. Pressure in the anterior chamber will press against the vitreous, preventing it from moving forward.*

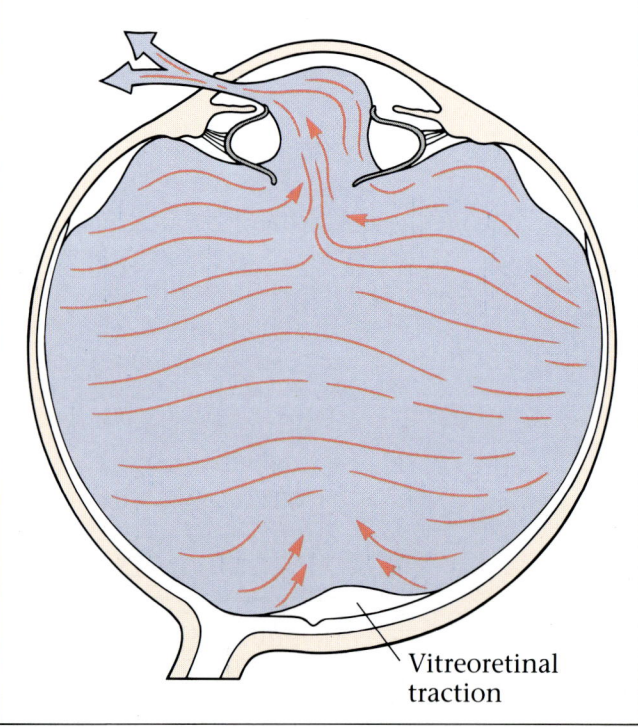

Figure 17.4 *In procedures without a closed system, such as ECCE with nucleus expression or ICCE, vitreous loss can be significant and may cause traction to be exerted at the vitreomacular interface and the vitreous base.*

pression procedures. If vitreous loss occurs during a nucleus expression procedure, there are no natural forces to limit the flow of vitreous out of the eye. In phacoemulsification, the constant pressure in the anterior chamber helps to hold the vitreous back, and the small incision limits how much vitreous will be extruded from the eye. Phacoemulsification's closed system limits the damage caused by vitreous loss and enhances the surgeon's ability to perform an appropriate vitrectomy.

If the posterior capsule is opened during the operation but the vitreous face remains intact, anterior chamber pressure can hold the vitreous back and prevent vitreous loss. Even if the vitreous face is disturbed and vitreous movement toward the wound is imminent, the pressure in the anterior chamber may prevent vitreous loss or at least limit vitreous movement to a mild prolapse into the anterior chamber (Fig. 17.3).

If the posterior capsule opens suddenly or in such a way that the surgeon does not immediately recognize it (e.g., if it occurs behind the nucleus), extensive vitreous loss may occur. The aspiration port of the phacoemulsification handpiece will remove fluid from the anterior chamber, and the fluid will be replaced partially by solution from the irrigation bottle and partially by vitreous. Further aspiration may cause vitreous to be aspirated into the phaco tip, resulting in additional vitreous loss. The amount of vitreous loss is directly related to the amount of time that passes from the opening of the posterior capsule to the surgeon's recognition of the problem (Fig. 17.4).

Vitrectomy Principles

The first principle of vitrectomy is *do not stretch the vitreous*. The best way to prevent stretching is to maintain an intact posterior capsule. When this is not possible, the integrity of the vitreous must be maintained; that is, the tear must be recognized as quickly as possible so that aspiration can be stopped. If vitreous moves into the anterior chamber, however, a vitrectomy will have to be performed in a way that does not disturb the posterior vitreous (i.e., the deeper vitreous body must not be violated by infusion or aspiration). If the vitrectomy is performed with a coaxial infusion cannula slipped over the vitrectomy tip, a one-handed vitrectomy can be performed, but this disturbs the vitreous three ways (Fig. 17.5):

Extension of the posterior capsular tear
Hydration of the vitreous
Flushing the vitreous

Extension of the Posterior Capsule Tear. Because the force of infusion is aimed in the same direction as the tip, the infusion is directed downward into the deep areas of the eye. As the tip passes down toward the opening in the posterior capsule, the infusion flow will strike the capsular flaps, forcing them apart. This separation causes the capsular tear to extend and the opening to enlarge, enabling more vitreous to prolapse forward and stretch (Fig. 17.6).

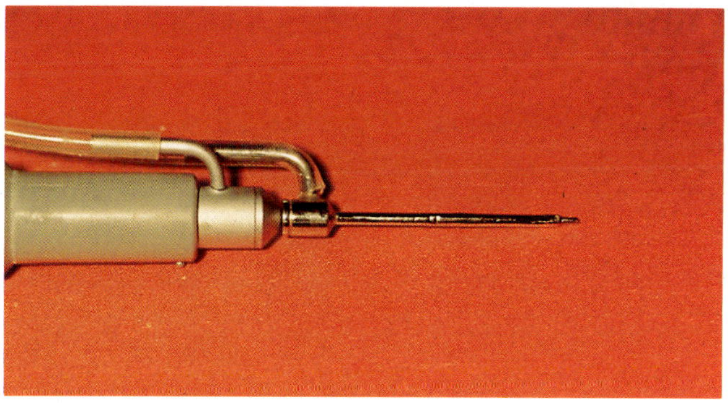

Figure 17.5 *Vitrectomy tip with a coaxial cannula. This combination should not be used.*

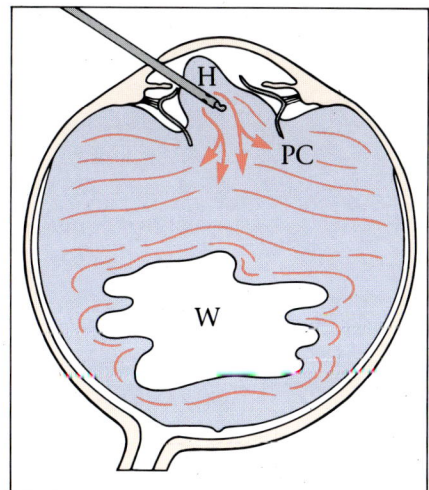

Figure 17.6 *Coaxial infusion rips open the posterior capsule (PC), permitting more vitreous to prolapse and stretch; hydrates (H) the vitreous, forcing more of the vitreous into the anterior chamber as it becomes stretched; and flushes vitreous toward the anterior chamber, stretching and wiggling (W) the vitreous.*

A small capsular tear limits the forward prolapse of vitreous because the rest of the posterior capsule serves as a barrier. Enlarging the tear reduces the size of the barrier and permits more vitreous prolapse. Traditionally, the posterior capsule has been considered the only structural barrier to vitreous movement, but the anterior capsule is also a barrier. If the anterior capsule has a large capsulotomy, the barrier is weak, but if it has a small capsulorhexis, there is a very strong barrier. The small opening in the anterior capsule will not rip open when the vitrectomy tip is inserted because the barrier integrity is maintained.

Trying to get vitreous to prolapse through a 4.50-mm capsulorhexis is like trying to squeeze toothpaste through the top of the tube. The small, rigid opening restricts movement and limits vitreous prolapse. This limits the extent of vitreous stretch and may turn out to be one of the most significant benefits of the capsulorhexis capsulotomy.

Hydration of the Vitreous. The infusion fluid hydrates the vitreous, causing it to increase in volume and expand. The vitreous is able to expand only through the opening in the posterior capsule toward the anterior chamber. This forward motion stretches the vitreous (Fig. 17.7).

Flushing the Vitreous. The force of the infusion acts like a hydraulic hose, pushing the vitreous around, shaking, wiggling, and forcing it every which way. The force causes trauma to the vitreous, the vitreous base, and the vitreomacular interface. Even with low flow systems the vitreous moves, creating microtraumas (Fig. 17.8).

The end result of this movement is the flushing of the vitreous out of the back of the eye toward the anterior chamber. This flush pulls the vitreous base toward the anterior chamber, increasing the amount of vitreous that needs to be removed. This is what occurs when a small vitrectomy turns into a large one as the anterior chamber is constantly refilled with new, previously untouched vitreous. Ultimately, little additional vitreous moves forward because most of it has already been removed (Fig. 17.9).

These three factors have an adverse effect on the integrity of the vitreous because they cause the vitreous to stretch, which exerts force at its base. It is not surprising that vitrectomy following vitreous loss in cataract surgery has a postoperative complication rate of 30% to 50%.

Bimanual Vitrectomy

When performing a vitrectomy, *touch the vitreous as little as possible.* Remember that phacoemulsification, performed in a closed system with a small wound, inherently limits vitreous movement. The primary goal is to avoid violating the vitreous more than is necessary. If vitreous in the anterior chamber can be removed without disturbing the remaining vitreous (which overlies the vitreous base or the vitreomacular interface), there should be very few postoperative problems.

To avoid the problems caused by coaxial infusion, remove the coaxial sleeve and replace it with

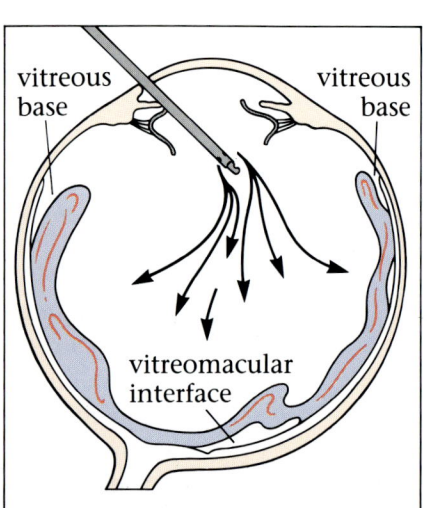

Figure 17.7 *After removal of the vitreous that was washed into the anterior chamber, much of the vitreous cavity has been disturbed, including the vitreomacular interface and the vitreous base.*

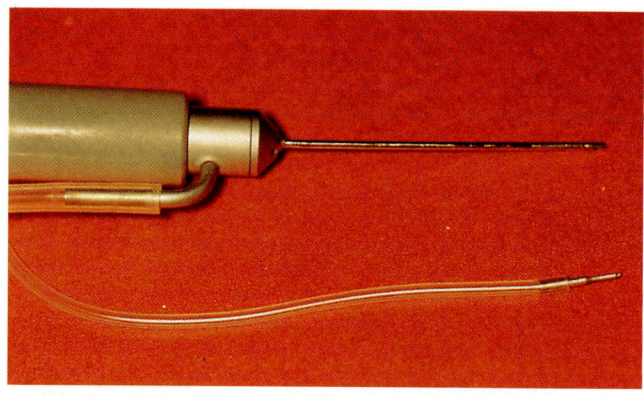

Figure 17.8 *Bimanual vitrectomy is performed after separating the infusion from the cutting tip. The separate infusion line is attached to the infusion line of the vitrectomy unit. The aspiration line is still attached to the cutting tip.*

a separate infusion line. A chamber maintainer is a short piece of silicone tubing, with a female Luer-Lok connector on one end and a short hub on the other. Attach the female Luer-Lok connector to the infusion line from the vitrectomy infusion bottle. The tubing can be held in the left hand and the hub placed into the side-port incision when needed (Fig. 17.10).

The vitrectomy unit should be held in the right hand and passed into the eye, down through the vitreous in the anterior chamber, through the opening in the posterior capsule, and held a millimeter or two behind the posterior capsule. Direct the aspiration post upward toward the cornea.

The vitreous in the anterior chamber should be drawn down to the vitrectomy tip until the anterior chamber is free of vitreous. No more vitreous should be removed from the vitreous cavity than is necessary to clean around the posterior capsule. The body of the vitreous should not be disturbed (i.e., the base should not be disturbed).

After the vitrectomy tip is in position just behind the posterior capsule, gentle cutting and aspiration can be activated in order to draw the vitreous from the anterior chamber down to the vitrectomy tip. This does not disturb the rest of the vitreous, but it does soften the eye. After a second or two of vitrectomy, the eye needs to be firmed up again using irrigation.

The irrigation line is placed in the side-port incision, and the fluid is directed across the anterior chamber in the plane of the iris. Refill the anterior chamber without pushing any of the irrigation fluid behind the posterior capsule. There may be some admixing of the fluid and the vitreous in the anterior chamber, but this is of no consequence because it will be removed anyway. Irrigation fluid and vitreous should not be mixed behind the posterior capsule because the hydration will lead to new vitreous prolapse.

The vitrectomy should proceed until the vitreous is posterior to the postcapsular remnants so that any traction or adhesions can be eliminated before the procedure is finished. The posterior capsule is usually unaffected by the vitrectomy. Insertion of a posterior chamber intraocular lens (IOL) can be performed without difficulty, though usually in the ciliary sulcus rather than in the capsular bag; however, this depends on the size of the opening in the posterior capsule.

Cortical Aspiration

If there is residual cortex in the capsular bag, it can be removed with the vitrectomy tip using a combination of aspiration and cutting. Aspiration of the cortex sometimes leads to new vitreous prolapse, so at the first sign of aspiration block-

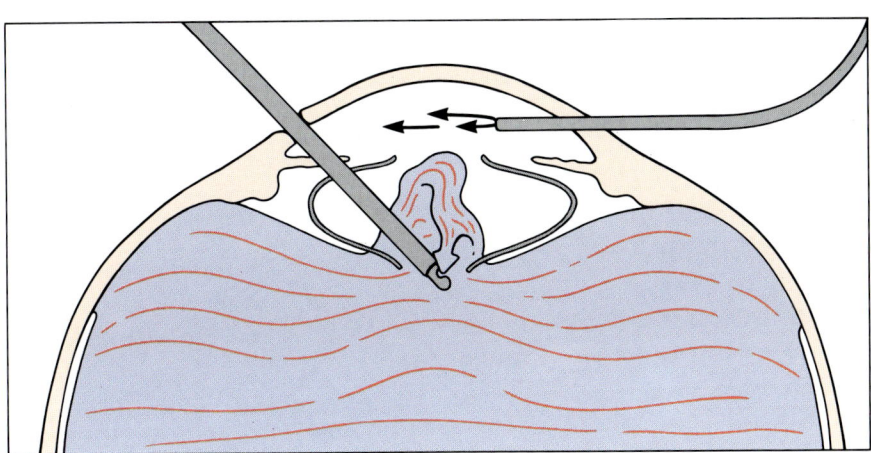

Figure 17.9 *Infusion is directed parallel to the iris. The cutting tip is placed behind the posterior capsule, and the vitreous in the anterior chamber is aspirated downward. The body of the vitreous is not disturbed.*

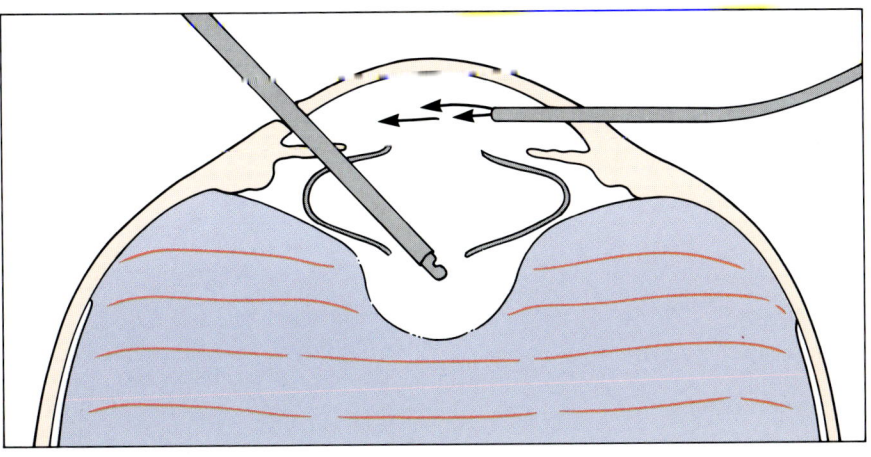

Figure 17.10 *At the end of the vitrectomy, the vitreous has been removed from the anterior chamber, the capsular bag, and the region just behind the posterior capsule. The rest of the vitreous has not been touched.*

age, the cutter should be activated in order to sever the vitreous before any tension is exerted.

Another method of cortical aspiration that may work well in the presence of only a small defect in the posterior capsule is to hold the vitreous back with viscoelastic and remove the cortex with a manual aspirator (e.g., a cortex cannula on a syringe). If the anterior chamber shallows during cortical aspiration, it will have to be refilled with viscoelastic to maintain positive pressure against the vitreous.

Results

A review of 2,000 consecutive cases of phacoemulsification with lens implantation that I have performed reveals that the posterior capsule was inadvertently opened in 60 cases (3%), but there was vitreous loss in only 16 cases (0.8%). I attribute the low rate of vitreous loss in these open posterior capsule cases (26.6%) to the unique advantages of the closed system in phacoemulsification and to the fact that aspiration was terminated before the vitreous was aspirated.

The 16 cases of vitreous loss were treated exactly as described in this chapter, and all of the patients had a normal postoperative course. Each patient had a corrected visual acuity of 20/20 by the third postoperative week and was followed for over a year, during which time the 20/20 vision has been maintained (Table 17.11).

This does not mean that decreased visual function after vitreous loss during phacoemulsification will not occur, but that the incidence of visual loss due to cystoid macular edema is certainly reduced from the usually reported 30% to 50%.

Conclusion

Vitreous loss during phacoemulsification can be limited because the operation is performed in a closed system. If the vitrectomy is also performed in a closed system and the integrity of the vitreous body is respected, visual complications can be reduced.

The vitrectomy should be performed using a bimanual technique. The main body of the vitreous should not be disturbed, and the vitreous in the anterior chamber should be aspirated downward below the plane of the posterior capsule. Irrigation should be gentle and limited to the anterior chamber.

Using the Slinky toy for visualization of these principles helps us understand that coaxial infusion vitrectomy leads to additional retinal problems because of extension of the capsular tear, hydration of the vitreous, and flushing of the vitreous.

Bimanual vitrectomy is a gentler and safer way to perform vitrectomy after vitreous loss during phacoemulsification because it does not "stretch the Slinky." By following the principles presented, it is possible to have similar morbidity and visual acuity in eyes with vitreous loss as in those without vitreous loss.

Table 17.11
Vitreous Loss During Phacoemulsification

VITREOUS LOSS			TIMING OF VITREOUS LOSS		
Number of Cases	2,000	100%	Number of Cases	16	100%
Posterior capsule openings	60	3%	During emulsification	2	12.5%
Vitreous loss	16	0.8%	At end of emulsification	10	62.5%
			At end of cortical aspiration	4	25%
Posterior capsule openings resulting in vitreous loss		26.6%			

Clinical Points to Consider

☛ Anterior vitrectomy technique during a cataract/IOL procedure should minimize trauma to the vitreous and vitreous base, remaining posterior capsule, and corneal endothelium.

☛ After vitreous loss, the remaining anterior capsular flap following capsulorhexis can provide support for a posterior chamber IOL, if necessary.

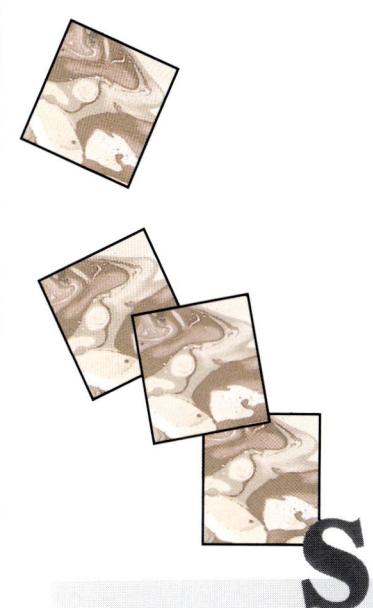

SECTION FOUR
INNOVATIVE CATARACT SURGERY

CHIP-AND-FLIP PHACOEMULSIFICATION

I. HOWARD FINE, M.D.

As Thomas Neuhann, M.D., and Howard Gimbel, M.D., predicted, it has become apparent that the continuous tear circular capsulorhexis with a wide anterior capsular flap has definite advantages over a can-opener type anterior capsulotomy. The advantages include avoiding extensions of anterior capsule tears to the posterior capsule and insuring in-the-bag placement and centration of posterior chamber implants. However, there are also disadvantages, the most important of which is the inability to easily dislocate the superior pole of the nucleus for pupillary plane phacoemulsification. Because of this, many surgeons have returned to the one-handed phaco techniques (which they had abandoned for the two-handed techniques they felt offered more control and safety).

Chip-and-flip phacoemulsification, a two-handed technique using a small circular capsulorhexis, increases safety and control when doing phacoemulsification within the capsular bag. With this technique, the surgeon need never sculpt deeply near the posterior capsule, nor work in the capsular fornix or under the iris. The surgeon is always working near the center of the pupil in the deepest part of the capsular bag, which for endolenticular phaco is considered the "safety zone." In all cases, an easily identifiable anatomic landmark, the hydrodelineation circle, is present.

Surgical Procedure

Using a blunt dissection technique, a Beaver blade is used to make a groove and dissect a scleral tunnel. The side-port incision is made to the left with a super-sharp instrument, and viscoelastic is used to replace aqueous humor. The keratome is then used to enter the anterior chamber through the scleral tunnel. Using a bent needle, the circular capsulorhexis is started by making a small cut at the center of the lens, pulling directly toward the incision, and curving toward the left. This creates a central flap that tears in a circular pattern to the right (Fig. 18.1). The flap is folded over, purchased with Utrata-Kraff forceps, and pulled by the forceps in a circular motion so the force at the point of tear is tangential to the circumference of the circle (Fig. 18.2). It is necessary to repurchase the capsular flap closer to the tear point during the course of the capsulotomy (Fig. 18.3). To prevent a nick in the capsular ring, the completion of the tear comes from slightly outside toward the inside (Fig. 18.4).

Hydrodelineation is performed using the technique taught me by Neuhann. A 26-gauge cannula is directed toward the center of the nucleus as deeply as one can go, and then balanced salt solution is injected tangentially, resulting in hydrodelineation of the hard central and the soft outer nuclear zones (Fig. 18.5). A second hydrodissecting fluid wave may be placed just under the anterior capsule to facilitate rotation of the lens within the capsule.

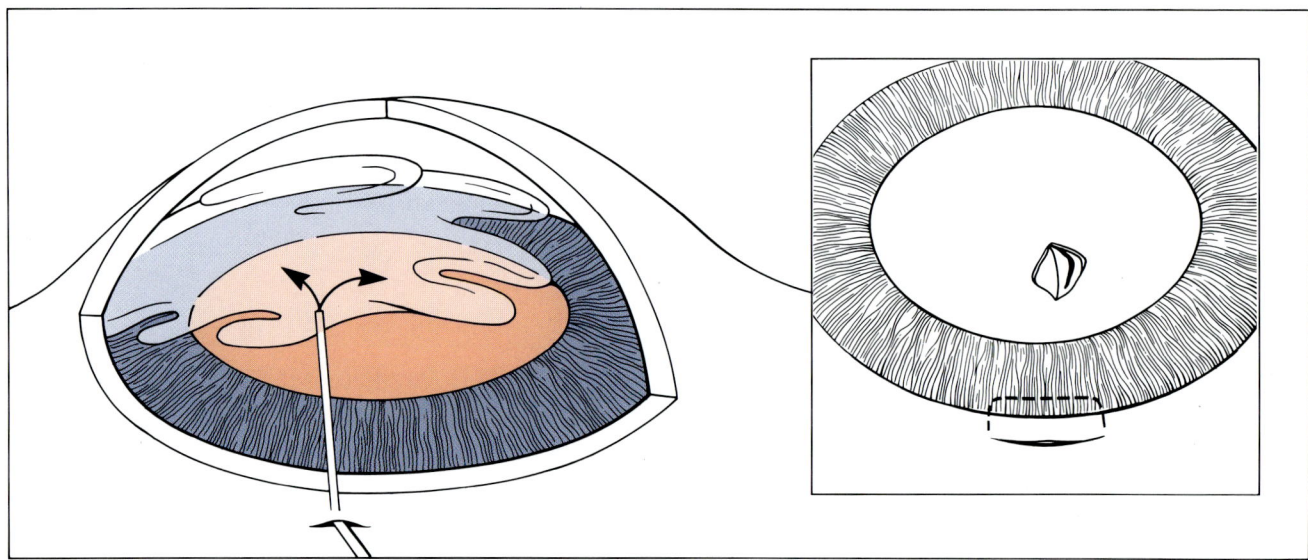

Figure 18.1 *Viscoelastic is injected into the anterior chamber. A bent needle is used to create a central, circular tear in the anterior capsule* **(inset)**.

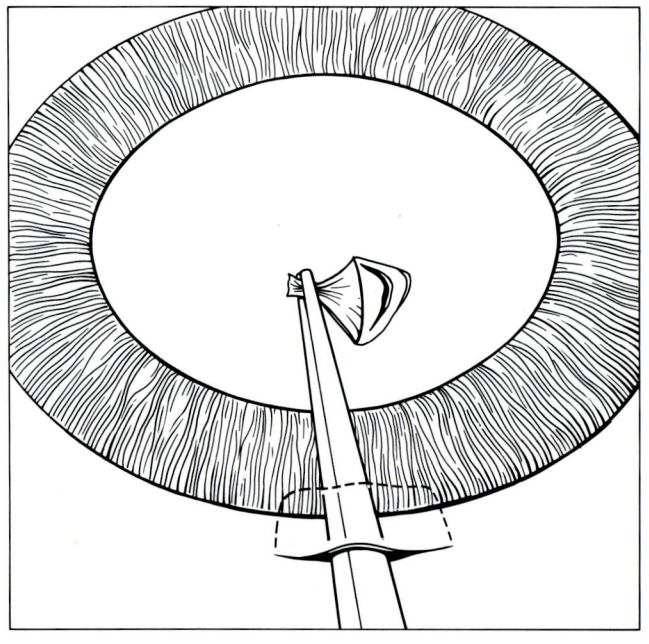

Figure 18.2 *The central tear is enlarged using Utrata-Kraff capsular forceps. The capsule is folded over before it is grasped by the capsular forceps.*

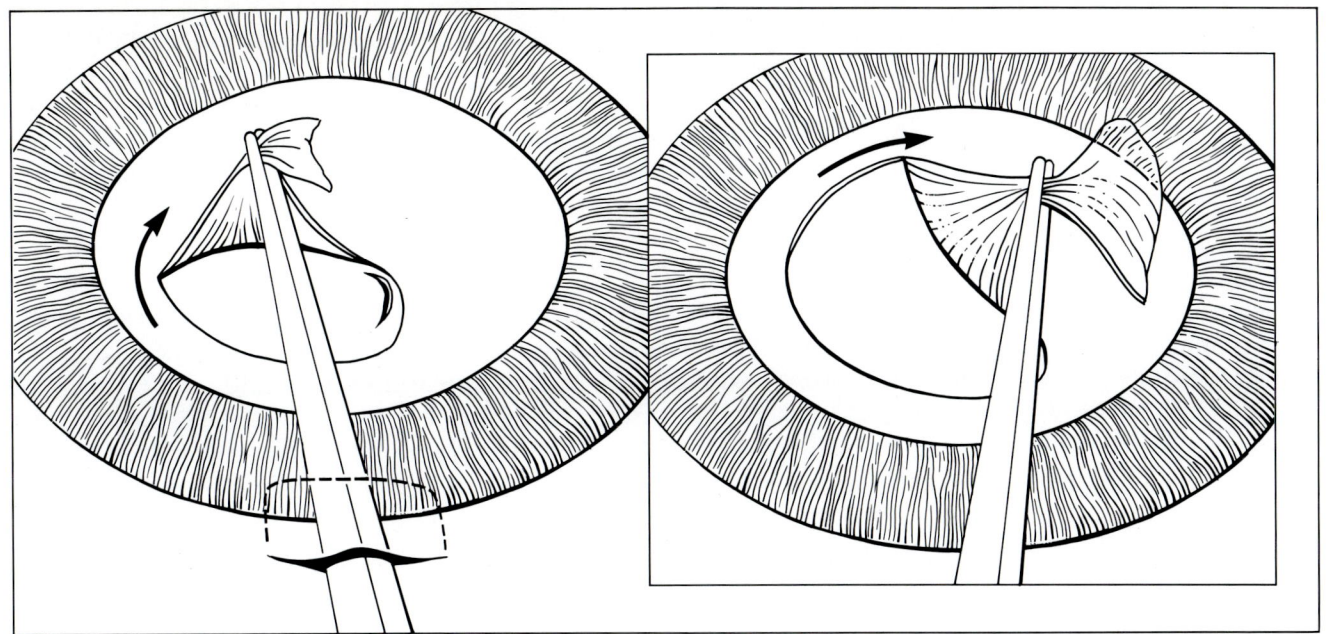

Figure 18.3 *The capsular flap is regrasped closer to the tear point as the capsulotomy is enlarged* **(inset)**.

Figure 18.4 *Completion of the tear proceeds from the outside toward the inside to prevent a nick in the capsular ring.*

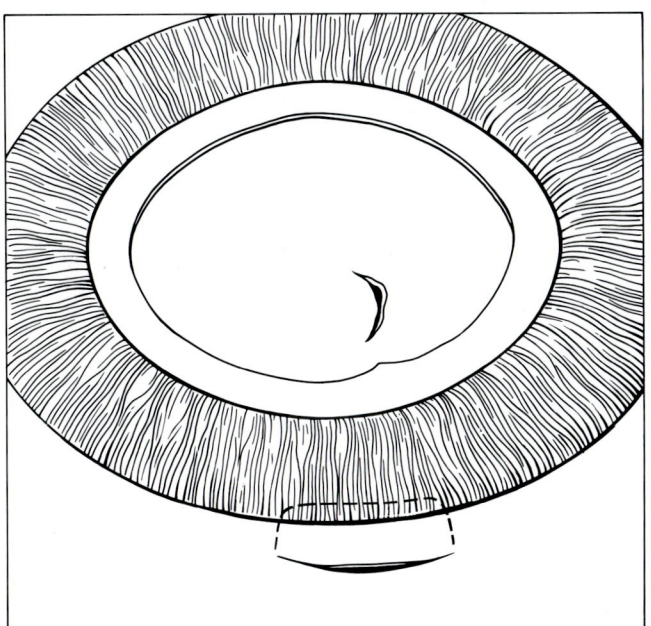

Figure 18.5 *Hydrodelineation is achieved with a 26-gauge cannula, which is directed toward the center of the nucleus. Hydrodelineation separates the hard, central nucleus from the soft, outer nucleus.*

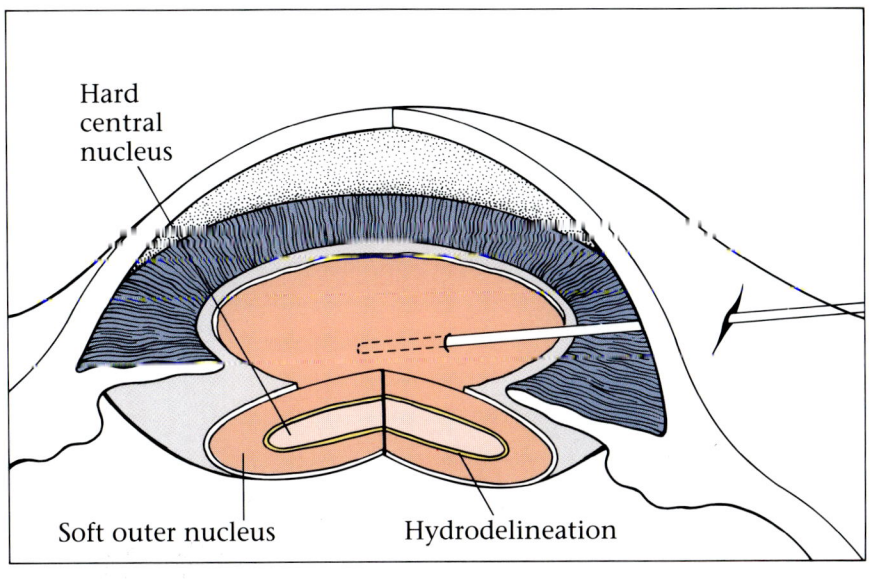

Phacoemulsification takes place through the small circular capsulorhexis. Central sculpting to 50% of the nuclear thickness is accomplished in the usual manner (Fig. 18.6). The Bechert nucleus rotator is brought into the anterior chamber and the nucleus is pushed *toward 12 o'clock* with the Bechert nucleus rotator under the tip of the phaco handpiece. The rim of the inner nuclear bowl is removed at the 5 o'clock to 6 o'clock positions (Fig. 18.7), the nucleus is rotated clockwise, and another hour of rim is removed at 5 o'clock to 6 o'clock. Pulsed phacoemulsification adds additional control; it helps prevent breaking through to the outer nuclear rim while segmentally removing the entire rim of the inner nuclear bowl (Fig. 18.8).

There is usually a clear-cut demarcation line between the hard inner nuclear bowl and the soft outer nuclear bowl. *The displacement of the nucleus toward 12 o'clock with the emulsification taking place in the 5 o'clock to 6 o'clock area protects the capsule* because the part of the nucleus being emulsified is brought away from the capsular fornix and out from under the iris, even in the presence of a small pupil. Emulsification takes place just under the anterior capsular flap and close to the center of the deepest part of the anterior chamber.

Once the rim of the inner nuclear bowl has been removed, the side-port instrument can be brought into the cleavage plane between the inner nuclear chip and the outer nuclear bowl (the hydrodelineation circle) and swept under the chip, elevating it into the center of the capsular bag (Fig. 18.9). Using the side-port instrument to control the nuclear chip, the chip can be quickly and safely removed (Fig. 18.10). Pulsed phacoemulsification dramatically reduces "chattering" of the chip.

The soft outer nuclear bowl, which has cushioned all previous phacoemulsification, is now displaced from the capsular fornix at 5 o'clock to 6 o'clock. This is done by either pushing the 12 o'clock rim *toward* 12 o'clock, thus bringing the

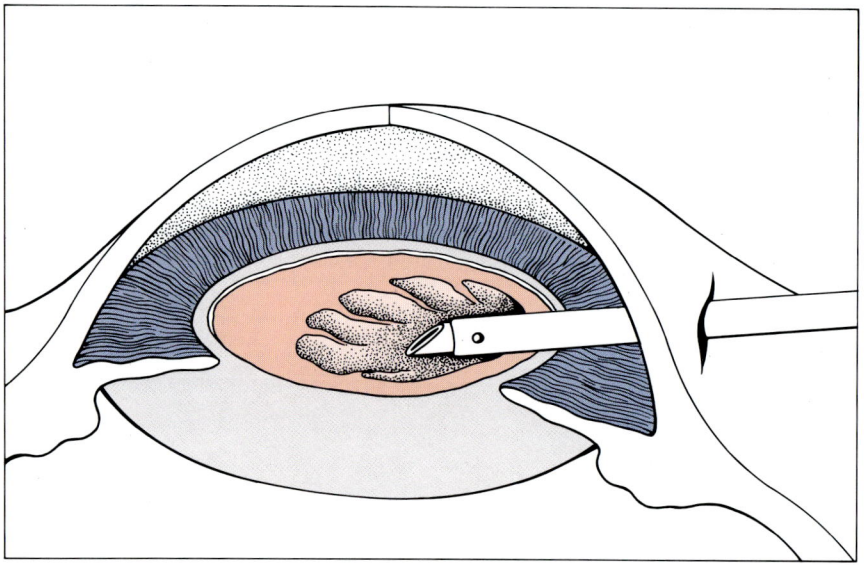

Figure 18.6 *The nucleus is sculpted using the tip of the phacoemulsification handpiece.*

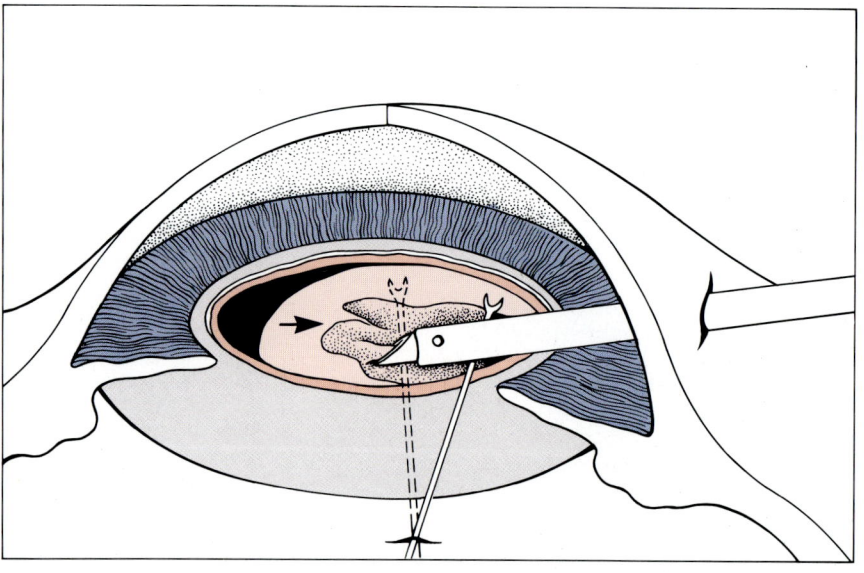

Figure 18.7 *The nucleus is pushed toward 12 o'clock by the lens manipulator as the tip of the phacoemulsification handpiece removes the rim of the inner nuclear bowl at the 6 o'clock position.*

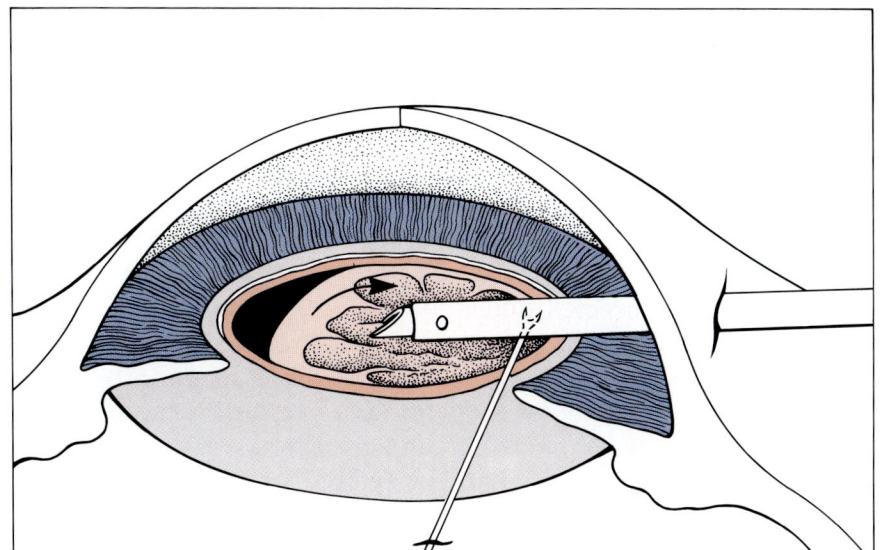

Figure 18.8 *The entire nuclear rim has been removed.*

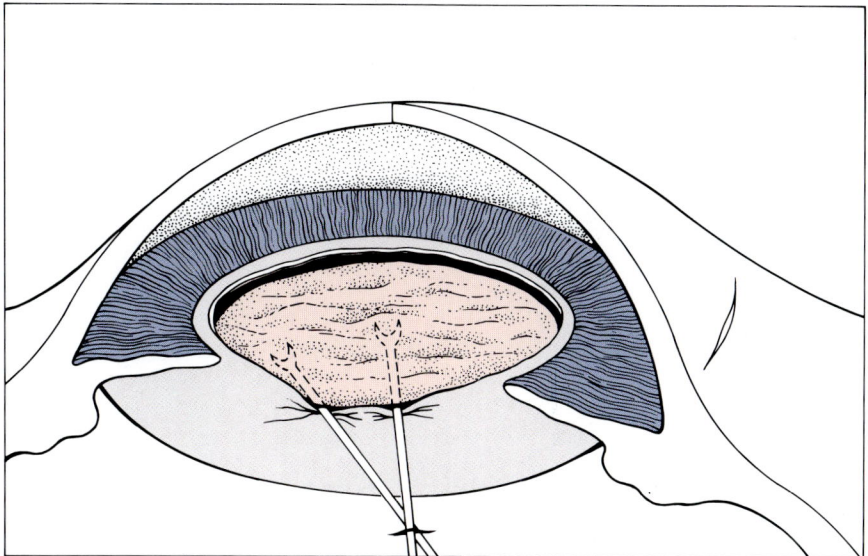

Figure 18.9 *The inner nuclear chip is elevated into the center of the capsular bag by placing the lens manipulator into the cleavage plane between the inner and outer nuclear portions.*

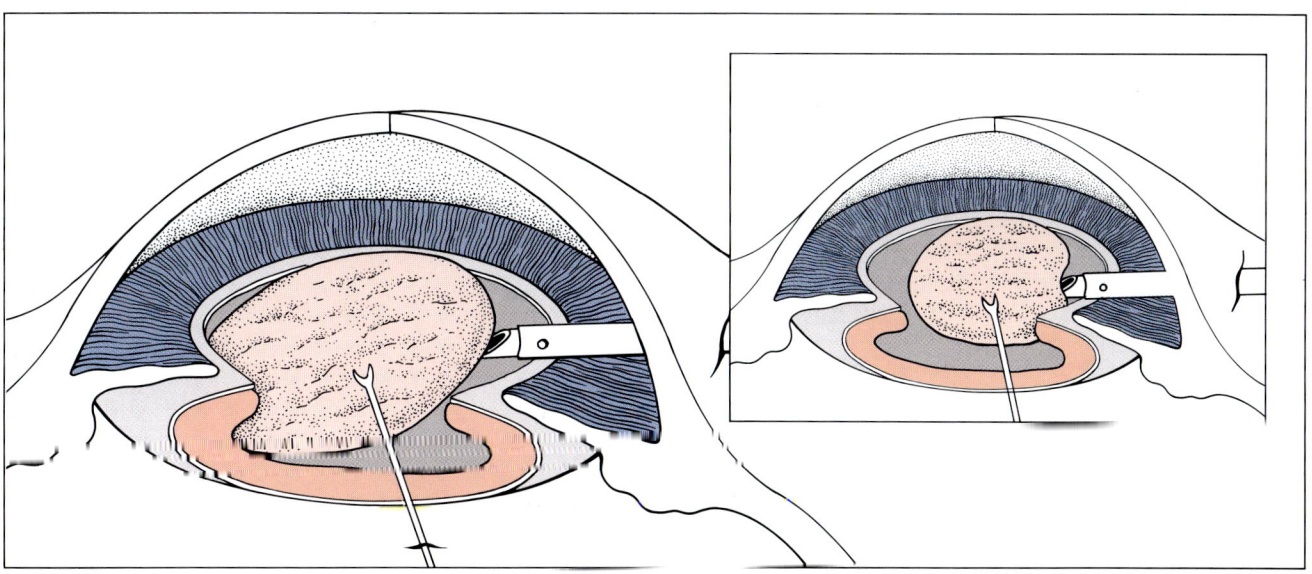

Figure 18.10 *The inner nuclear chip is removed by phacoemulsification* **(inset)** *in the center of the capsular bag.*

5 o'clock to 6 o'clock rim out of the fornix, or by pushing the center of the bowl *toward* 5 o'clock to 6 o'clock, causing the 5 o'clock to 6 o'clock rim to curl out of the fornix and under the anterior capsulotomy flap back toward the 12 o'clock position. Using the phaco tip, in the irrigation and aspiration mode (without phaco)—*foot-position 2*—the nuclear bowl is mobilized by pulling the rim at 5 o'clock to 6 o'clock toward 12 o'clock and pushing with the side-port instrument at the bottom of the nuclear bowl toward 5 o'clock to 6 o'clock to tumble or flip the soft outer nuclear bowl (Figs. 18.11 to 18.13). Several attempts at this maneuver, with rotation of the bowl following each attempt, may be necessary in order to achieve the tumbling. By flipping the bowl away from the capsule, it can be removed safely with either aspiration or low power emulsification without jeopardizing the capsule (Fig. 18.14).

The cortex strips easily and safely in the absence of capsular tags and the capsular bag is filled with viscoelastic (Fig. 18.15). The implant is directed under the anterior capsular flap and the optic is placed at least halfway through the anterior capsulorhexis. The trailing loop can be dialed in and the distortion in the anterior capsular ring at 3 o'clock is visible as it peaks toward the pupil and snaps back when the haptic goes under the

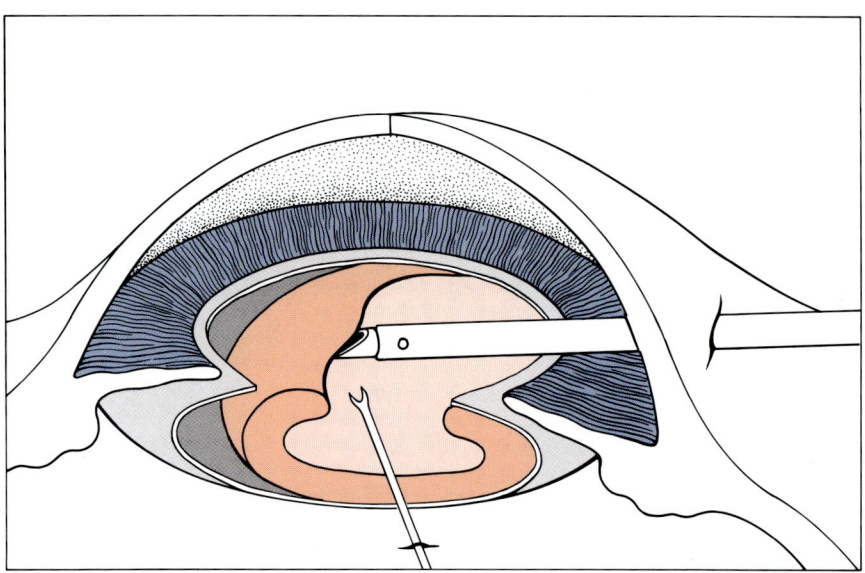

Figure 18.11 *The outer nuclear bowl is aspirated at 6 o'clock and pulled toward 12 o'clock.*

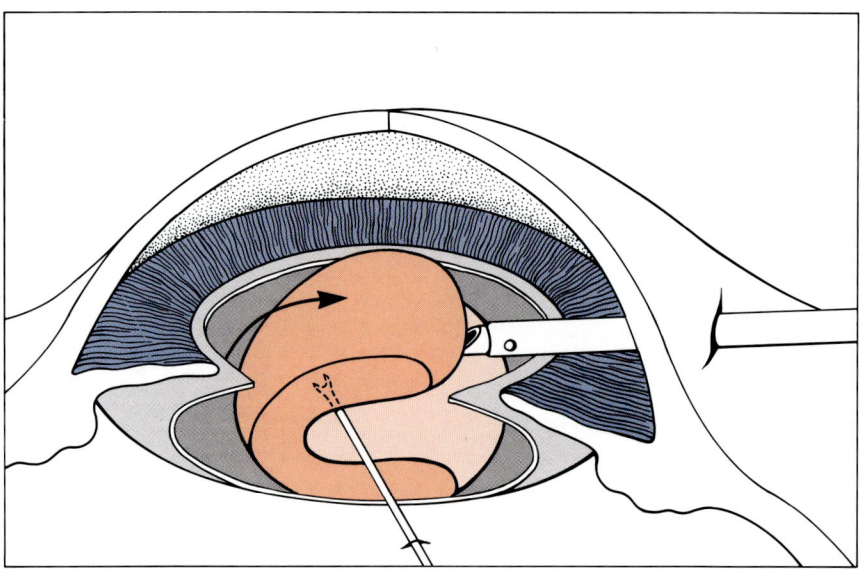

Figure 18.12 *The lens manipulator helps flip the outer nuclear bowl upside down by pushing the chip toward 6 o'clock as the phacoemulsification handpiece pulls it toward 12 o'clock.*

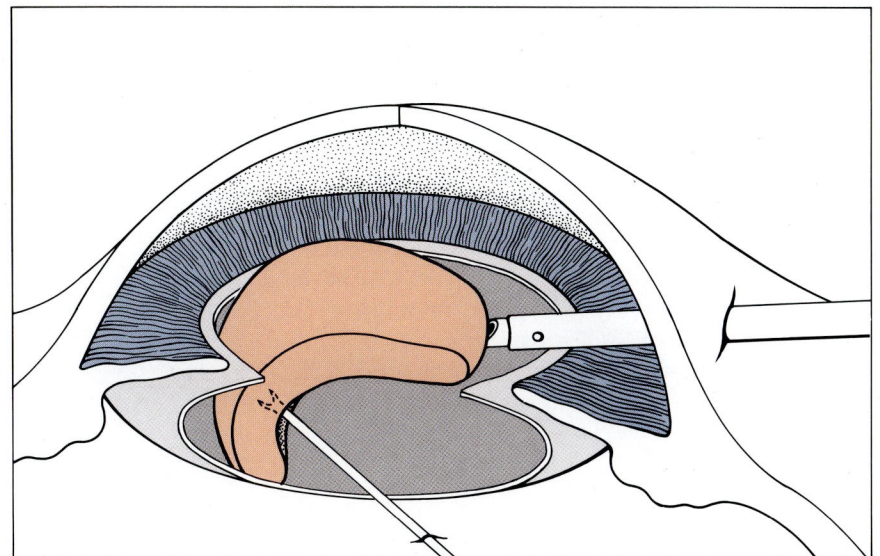

Figure 18.13 *The outer nuclear bowl has been completely flipped into the center of the capsular bag.*

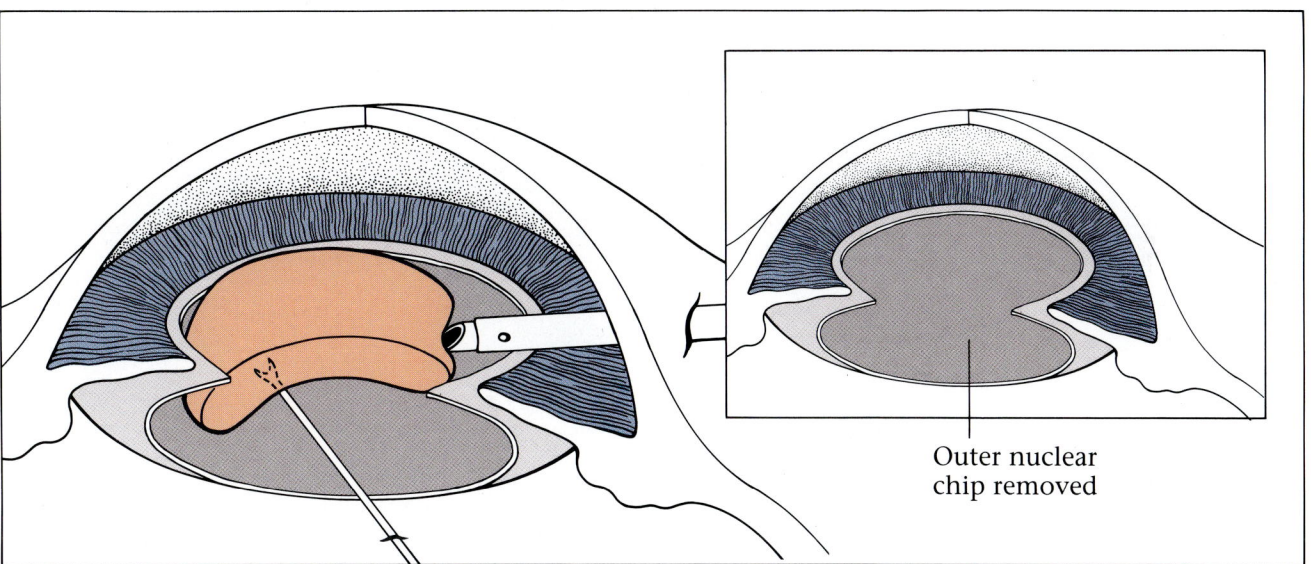

Figure 18.14 (Left and right) *The outer nuclear bowl is removed by either phacoemulsification or aspiration.*

Outer nuclear chip removed

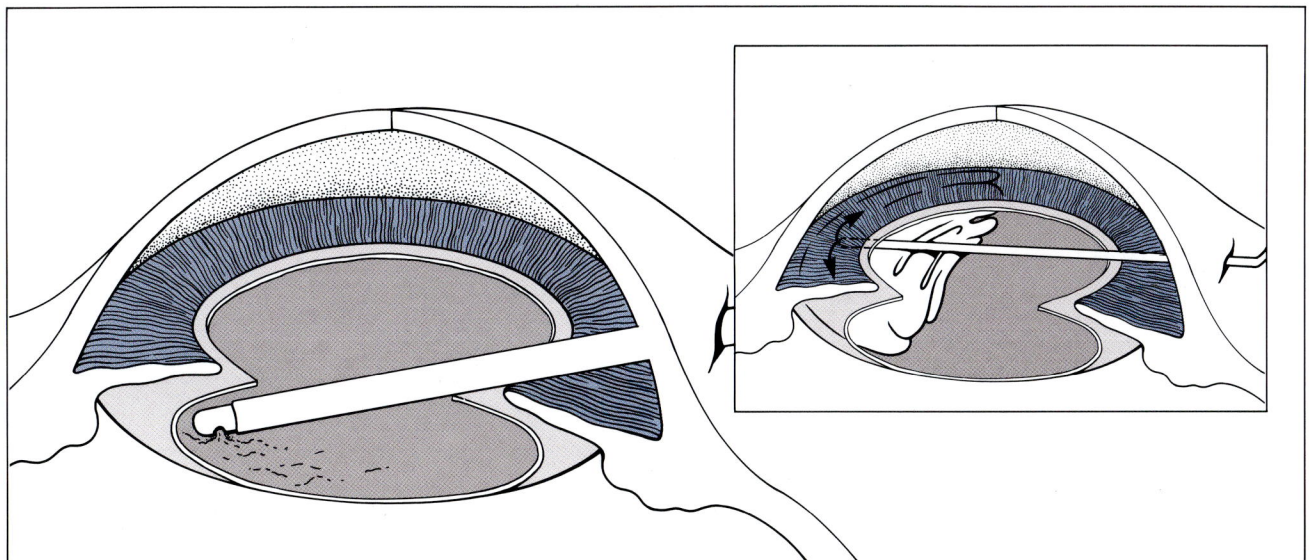

Figure 18.15 *The cortex is removed by aspiration. The capsular bag is filled with viscoelastic* **(inset)**.

anterior capsular flap. It can be visually confirmed that the implant is placed within the capsular bag and that centration is excellent (Fig. 18.16). Figure 18.17 is a photograph of a patient two months postoperatively, demonstrating implant position and centration.

Conclusion

Phacoemulsification by the chip-and-flip method provides the cataract surgeon with a safe way to achieve in-the-bag removal of the nucleus. In addition, capsulorhexis, hydrodelineation, which separates the hard central nucleus from the soft outer nucleus, and hydrodissection, which separates the nucleus from the cortex, should also be employed. At the conclusion of phacoemulsification by chip-and-flip, the IOL positioned in the capsular bag should remain well-centered, providing the patient with excellent function.

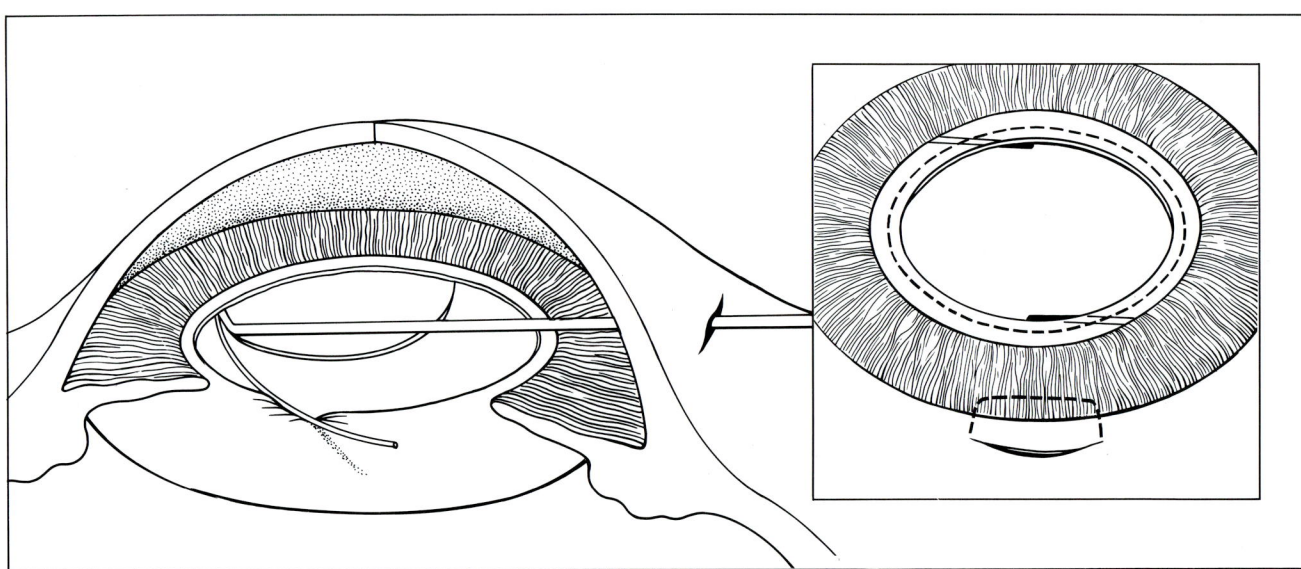

Figure 18.16 *The inferior haptic of the IOL is placed into the capsular bag interiorly and the superior haptic is dialed into the bag. The distortion of the anterior capsular ring at 3 o'clock disappears as the superior haptic goes under the anterior capsular flap.* **(Inset)** *The implant is totally within the capsular bag and well centered.*

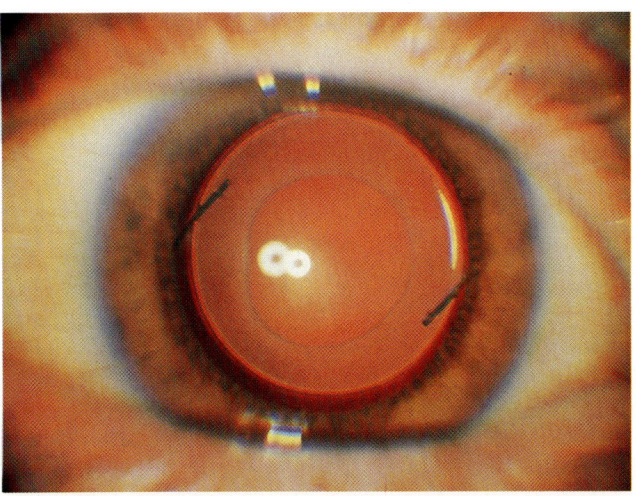

Figure 18.17 *A patient two months postoperatively following capsulorhexis, chip-and-flip phacoemulsification, and IOL implantation in the capsular bag.*

Clinical Point to Consider

☛ Chip-and-flip allows phacoemulsification in the central portion of the capsular bag, which is considered a safer location.

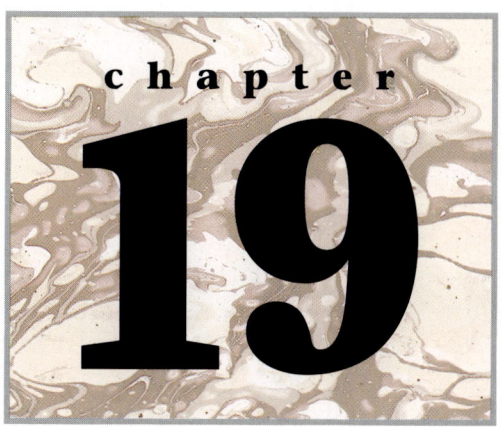

RADIAL-TRANSVERSE CATARACT INCISION

STEVEN B. SIEPSER, M.D.

The desirability of a self-sealing wound that allows for cataract extraction and intraocular lens (IOL) implantation without inducing any astigmatism is obvious. This chapter will discuss such a cataract wound, the radial-transverse (R-T) incision, which I developed in 1989 and have used successfully in more than 100 cases as of September 1990.

The History of Cataract Surgery

Before the 1700s, cataracts were removed by couching, a process in which an opaque lens was dislocated. The sclera was indented with a forklike instrument, which ruptured the zonules and caused the lens to fall into the vitreous. Vision improved, although subsequent inflammation and glaucoma often destroyed the eye.

In the 1700s, the French popularized a form of extracapsular cataract extraction (ECCE), in which the anterior capsule was broken and the central portion of the lens was scooped out. A German ophthalmologist, von Graefe, became famous for the Graefe knife incision. A Graefe knife is a thin, flat blade that creates a cataract incision by entering the anterior chamber through the limbus at a lateral position and exits the limbus directly across from the entry location. The Graefe knife is then advanced superiorly with a sawing motion to create a 180-degree beveled superior incision.

Everting the cornea after a Graefe knife incision enabled entry into the anterior chamber so that the lens could be manipulated by either forceps or an erisophake, an instrument that uses vacuum to adhere to the anterior capsule of the lens. In the 1960s, Kelman, in New York City, developed the cryoprobe for facilitating the removal of the lens by intracapsular cataract extraction (ICCE). Removal of the lens in an intracapsular fashion became the most common method of cataract extraction, and Barcelona's Joaquin Barraquer contributed the use of alpha-chymotripsin to dissolve zonules and greatly reduce the incidence of unplanned ECCE.

At first, Graefe knife incisions were closed by apposition and by keeping the patient as motionless as possible for several weeks at least. Early suture material included horsetail fibers and rat tail tendon. Such unsterile organic suture material and large needles often caused inflammation and infection. Silk, in one form or another, became the standard suture material for cataract surgery until the 1960s. Troutman, also in New York, was instrumental in introducing the operating microscope and nylon suture to anterior segment surgery.

In the early 1950s, Ridley, of Great Britain, pioneered the implantation of IOLs after realizing that intraocular plastic windshield fragments sustained by British Spitfire pilots during World War II were well tolerated. Ridley was prompted to investigate IOLs after a medical student asked why a cataract that had been removed was not replaced by another lens. The high incidence of complications associated with early IOLs limited their use until the 1960s, when Binkhorst, a Dutch eye surgeon, developed IOLs that were fixated within the capsular bag after ECCE by nucleus expression and manual irrigation and aspiration (I/A) of the cortex.

By the early 1970s, Kelman had developed ECCE by phacoemulsification, which used ultrasound to fragment the nucleus, thus enabling cataract removal through a 3.00-mm wound. Soon, phacoemulsification was combined with anterior chamber IOL implantation. Shearing introduced the posterior chamber IOL, and Mazzacco popularized the foldable silicone posterior chamber IOL, which could be implanted through a 4.00-mm incision. Recent developments in cataract surgery techniques include creating an anterior capsulotomy by capsulorhexis (Fercho and Neuhann), hydrodissection of the nucleus, and attempts to minimize postoperative astigmatism by wound manipulation or astigmatic keratotomy.

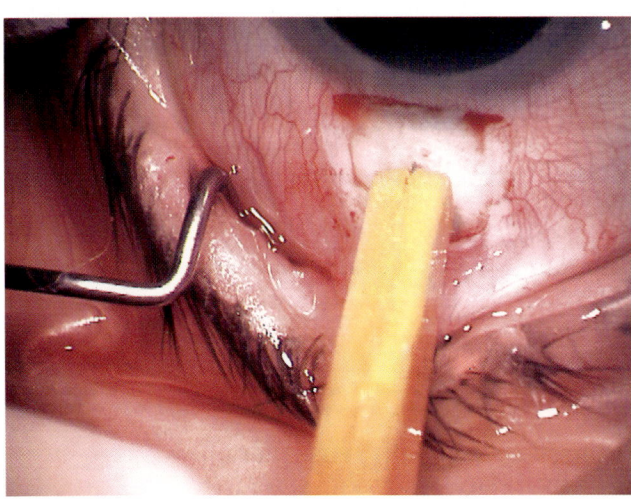

Figure 19.1 *The radial (R) portion of the R-T incision is made to a depth of midsclera using a microsclerotomy knife.*

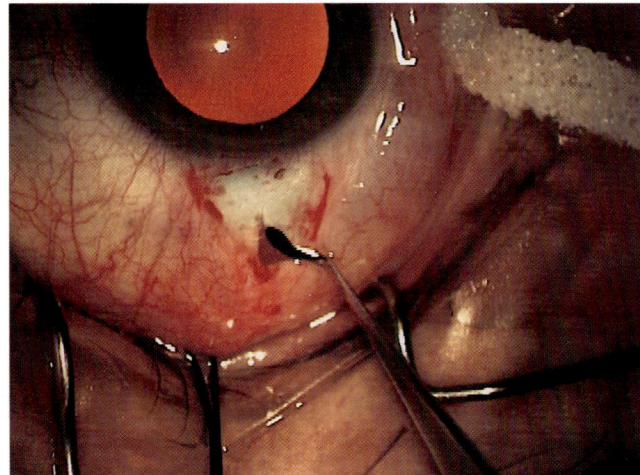

Figure 19.2 *The transverse (T) intrascleral pocket dissection of the R-T incision is performed with a microsclerotome.*

Figure 19.3 *The transverse (T) incision's location of entry into the anterior chamber is near Schwalbe's line.*

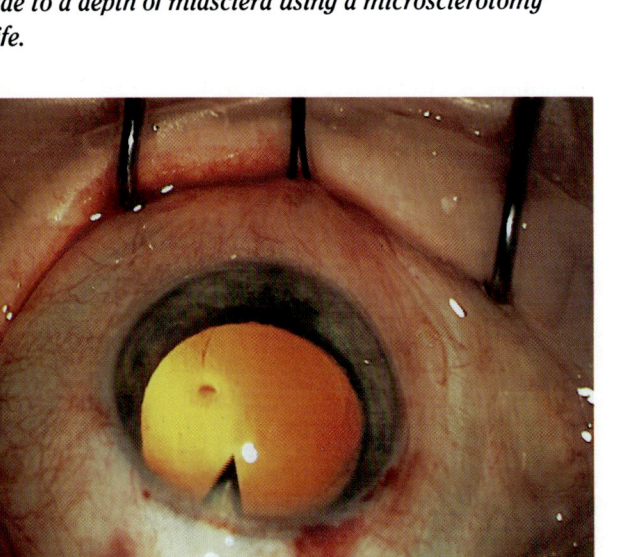

The goal of modern cataract extraction with IOL implantation is to provide the patient with best *uncorrected* visual acuity. Wound design for cataract/IOL surgery must enable efficient cataract removal and IOL implantation while inducing no astigmatism and allowing for rapid, stable recovery of visual acuity. The R-T incision fulfills these goals and requires that the surgeon be adept at phacoemulsification and foldable IOL implantation techniques. The R-T incision is inherently self-sealing because of its geometric configuration and requires no support from or involvement with the conjunctiva.

Surgical Procedure

The R-T incision is created by making a radial sclerotomy with a Medical Sterile Products (MSP) guarded 0.30-mm microsclerotomy knife just posterior and perpendicular to the limbus down to the depth of midsclera (Fig. 19.1). Dissection of the intrascleral pocket parallel to the front surface of the sclera is performed with an MSP microsclerotome specifically designed for this maneuver (Fig. 19.2). Entry into the anterior chamber is made with a 2.00-mm-wide keratome and widened to 3.00 mm to admit the phaco tip. This entrance incision into the anterior chamber is located well in front of the iris root (near Schwalbe's line), as it is with a scleral flap wound (Fig. 19.3).

The superficial radial (R) incision and the deeper transverse (T) incision allow the anterior chamber to be entered through one opening, but the two-layer wound allows closure with the incisions perpendicular to each other, thus creating a totally watertight seal (Fig. 19.4).

The radial incision is about 3.50 mm to 4.00 mm long and commences 1.00 mm posterior to the surgical limbus. After phacoemulsification

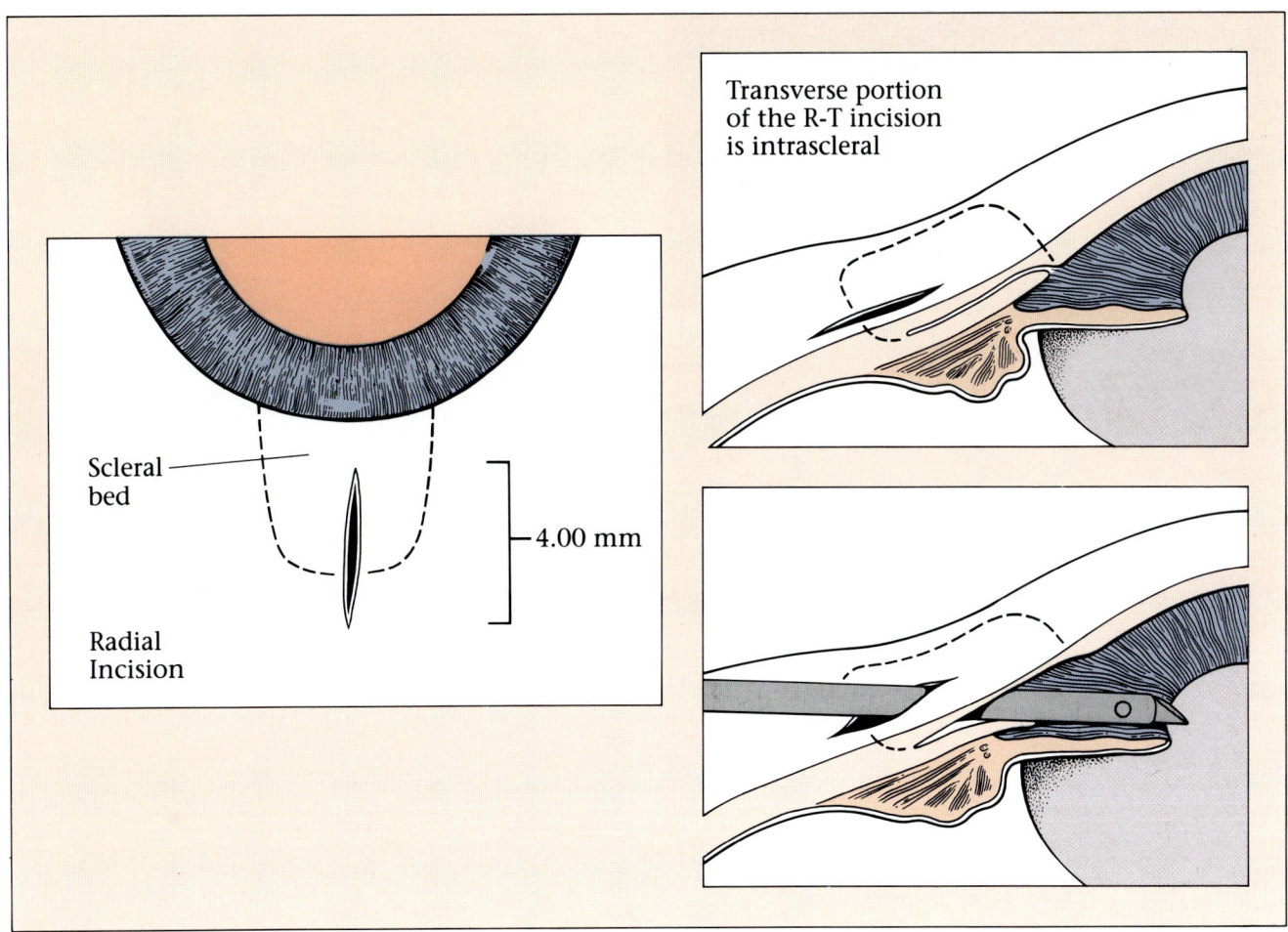

Figure 19.4 *The R-T incision. The anterior chamber is entered through one opening, which when sealed is watertight.*

(Fig. 19.5), the transverse dissection must be widened enough to accommodate implantation of the foldable IOL. A silicone foldable IOL such as the Allergan Medical Optics SI-18 requires a 3.60-mm- to 4.00-mm-wide entrance into the anterior chamber and an IOL injector device (e.g., the Prodigy) (Fig. 19.6). A Faulkner forceps delivery system for foldable IOL insertion has been tried but the wound configuration makes it rather difficult to use.

Clinical Considerations

The advantages of the R-T incision are quickly discernible. No suture, glue, or other means of closure is necessary, and the truly watertight wound does not violate any principles of wound construction. The radial incision leaves virtually all the superficial sclera intact in an antero-postero direction so that no wound gape and, therefore, no change in astigmatism, is possible.

When the R-T incision is compared to a 3.00-mm to 5.00-mm scleral flap incision that has vertical incisions at the inner extremes of the incision in order to admit an IOL, the mechanical advantages of the R-T incision are apparent. Furthermore, an undesirable scleral defect at the junction of the horizontal flap incision and its vertical enlargement increases the possibility of aqueous leakage. Also, with these wounds, the

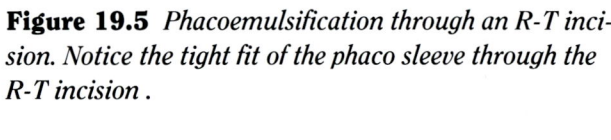

Figure 19.5 *Phacoemulsification through an R-T incision. Notice the tight fit of the phaco sleeve through the R-T incision.*

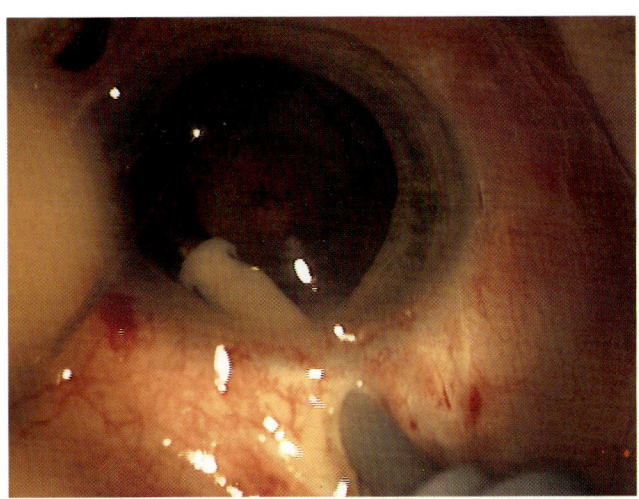

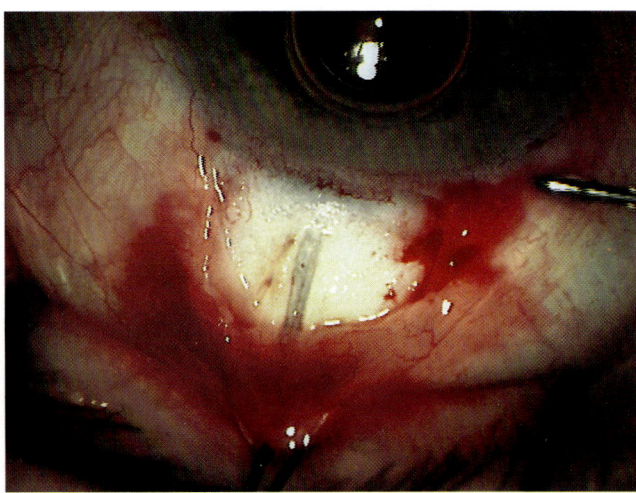

Figure 19.6 (Left) *Inserting an AMO SI-18 silicone IOL with the Prodigy injector through an R-T incision.* **(Right)** *The R-T incision after performing cataract extraction by phacoemulsification and posterior chamber IOL implantation.*

repositioned conjunctiva is used to secure the scleral flap, which is structurally unsound. A 4.00-mm scleral flap that is not unsecured can induce up to 1.00 D of unwanted against-the-rule astigmatism.

The main disadvantage of the R-T incision, besides the more involved wound dissection, is that it makes phacoemulsification and IOL implantation more difficult. The friction between the phaco tip sleeve and the scleral edges of the radial incision reduce the maneuverability of the phaco tip. More importantly, with soft irrigation sleeves, the flow of irrigating fluid may be slowed, causing anterior chamber collapse.

The R-T incision may be extended to allow for ECCE without undue difficulty by performing a vertical posterior limbal groove and joining it with the underlying horizontal scleral entrance wound. Then a blade, keratome, or corneal-scleral scissors may be used to lengthen the wound to the desired size.

Conclusion

The R-T incision can be used when the patient has low preoperative astigmatism, desires very rapid recovery, and the surgeon is skilled at both phacoemulsification and foldable IOL insertion. A 4.00-mm scleral flap wound with a single horizontal suture is certainly an excellent alternative to an R-T cataract incision. As of this writing, a nontoxic, inexpensive scleral tissue glue that is not derived from pooled blood products has not been developed. Such a substance would also facilitate small scleral flap wound closure.

The R-T cataract incision is specifically designed to provide a sutureless, watertight wound that induces no postoperative astigmatism. Under the appropriate conditions, the R-T cataract incision provides significant advantages for both the patient and surgeon.

Clinical Point to Consider

☛ The advantages of the R-T incision (no sutures, no induced astigmatism) must be balanced against the increased difficulty of the surgical technique.

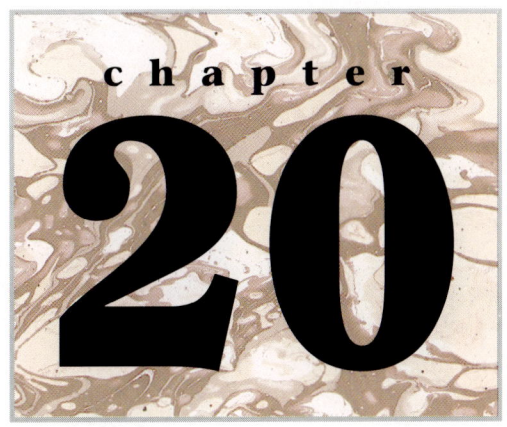

THE INFINITY SUTURE

I. HOWARD FINE, M.D.

The horizontal mattress suture, introduced by John Shepherd, M.D., has helped improve the already dramatically decreased rate of surgically induced astigmatism following small incision intraocular lens (IOL) implantation. The possibility that a similar principle could be used for conventional 6.50-mm phacoemulsification incisions is intriguing. Over the past year, I have used a variation of Shepherd's suture that requires the use of a scleral tunnel incision. It appears tremendousy promising.

Surgical Procedure

Following phacoemulsification and IOL implantation, the incision is closed by suturing the roof of the scleral tunnel to the floor of the scleral tunnel with a suture that in cross section resembles the mathematical symbol for infinity. For this reason, I have called this closure the *infinity suture*. The first loop covers approximately 40% of the tunnel width, with the needle entering at the right end of the incision and exiting at about the center (Fig. 20.1). The suture is then brought further left, with the needle entering at the left end of the incision and exiting at about the center. This second bite also incorporates approximately 40% of the tunnel width (Fig. 20.2). The two ends of the suture can then be pulled snug, closing the left side of the incision while the irrigation/aspiration (I/A) handpiece is used to remove residual viscoelastic (Fig. 20.3). Alternatively, the left half of the tunnel can be held closed using an instrument such as the Colibri forceps, while the right half of the incision is used for viscoelastic removal.

Following aspiration of the viscoelastic, the suture is pulled up tightly and tied without keratometric control, and the suture ends are cut flush with the knot (Fig. 20.4). The conjunctival flap is then draped back over the incision. An alternative suturing technique involves placing the second bite, with the second needle of a double-armed suture, just to the right of the exit point of the first bite and advancing the needle from right to left.

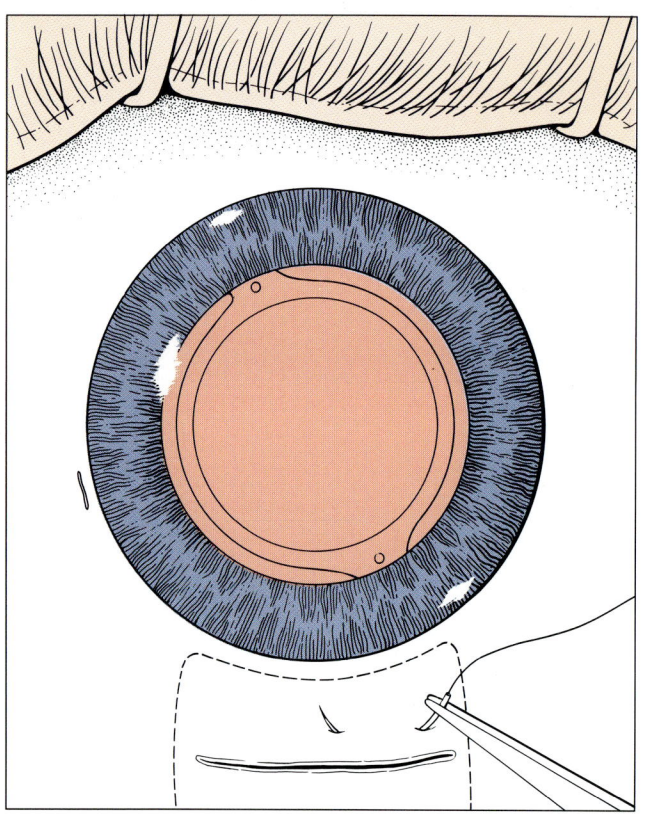

Figure 20.1 *The first bite of the infinity suture incorporates about 40% of a 6.00-mm scleral tunnel.*

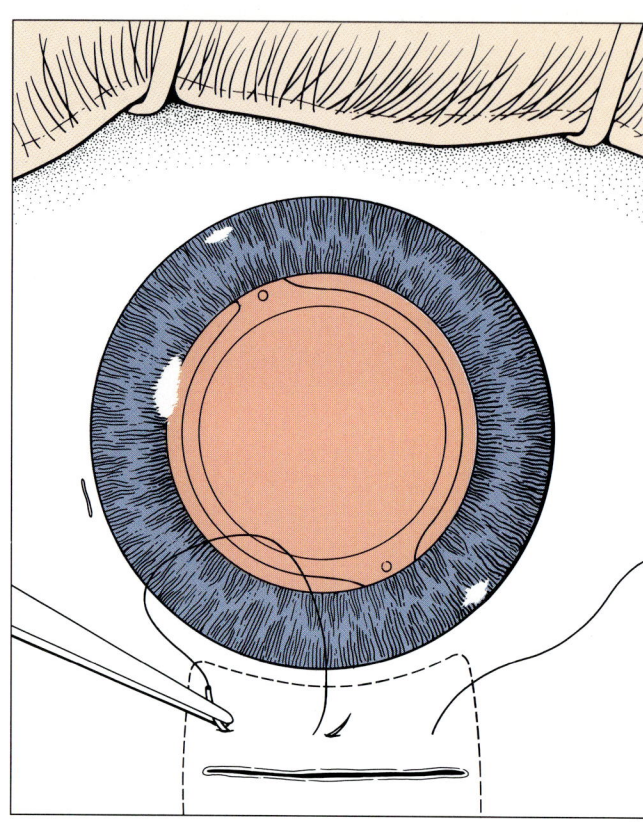

Figure 20.2 *The second bite of the infinity suture incorporates about 40% of a 6.00-mm scleral tunnel.*

Figure 20.3 *When viscoelastic is aspirated from the anterior chamber with the infinity suture in place, it is likely that a closed system will be maintained.*

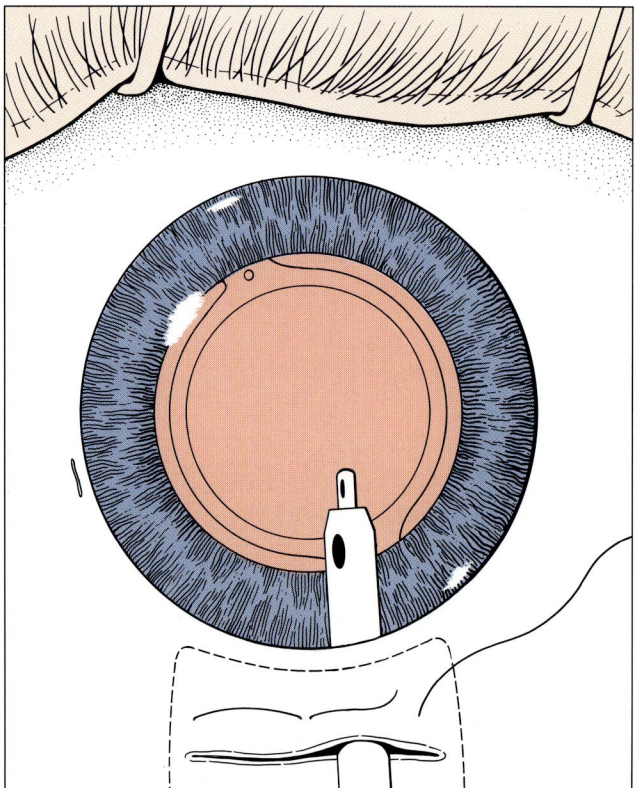

Conclusion

The great advantage of this type of closure is that there is no suture crossing the lips of the incision radially and, therefore, no force is exerted at the limbus in a manner that significantly alters corneal curvature. Alternatively, the compressive forces of the suture are tangential to the cornea and exhibit little or no effect on corneal curvature. The fact that the lips of the incision gape considerably after the suture is tied may intimidate some surgeons. One should bear in mind, however, that following the placement of a groove and the dissection of a scleral tunnel up to the point of entry into the anterior chamber, there is considerable gaping of the lips of the wound, yet the keratometry readings have not changed at all.

The preliminary results for this suture have been excellent. I have used it on approximately 100 patients and have not experienced any wound leaks, filtering blebs, anterior chamber depth shallowing, or hyphemas. In 65 patients using 11-0 Mersilene, the surgically induced cylinder by vector analysis was -0.75 D at two weeks and -0.70 D at two months. In 20 consecutive patients using 10-0 nylon, the surgically induced cylinder by vector analysis was -0.17 D at two weeks and -0.23 D at two months (Fig. 20.5). Both materials demonstrate enormous stability between two weeks and two months postopera-

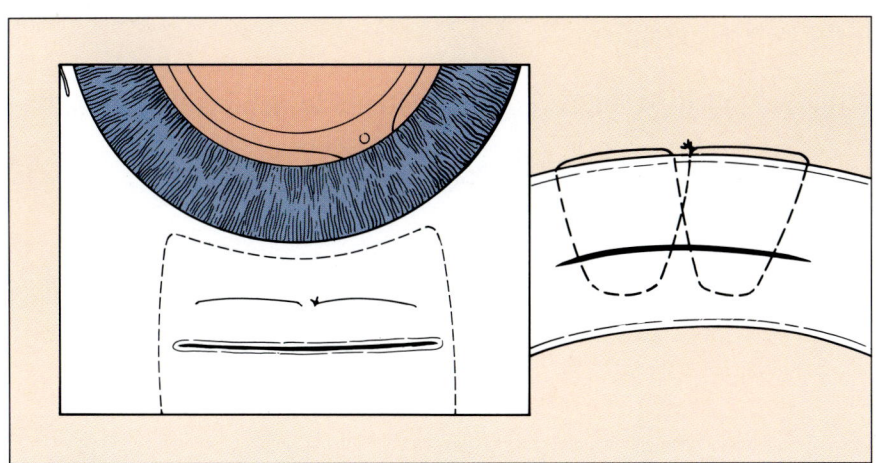

Figure 20.4 *The infinity suture is tied and the knot cut short without keratometric control.*

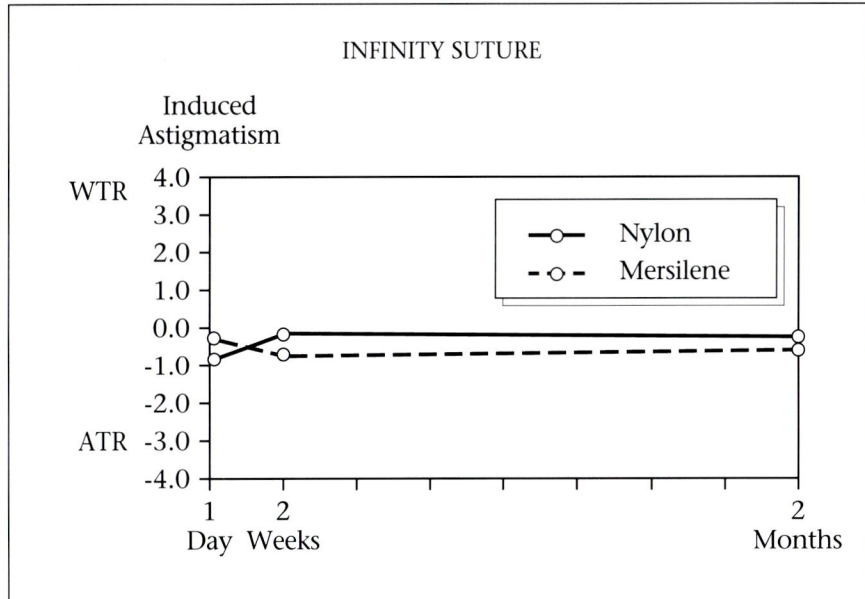

Figure 20.5 *In 20 consecutive phacoemulsification/IOL patients who had the infinity suture, only -0.17 D of astigmatism was induced two weeks postoperatively and only -0.23 D of astigmatism was induced two months postoperatively. All 20 patients had clinically stable refractions.*

tively, resulting in an ability to prescribe spectacles by two weeks postoperatively and in many cases prior to two weeks.

The difference between the two suture materials is speculative. At this time, my belief is that the 11-0 Mersilene suture is too strong and fine, causing it to "cheesewire" very early in the postoperative period. This would result in some recession of the roof of the tunnel, thereby inducing a small against-the-rule cylinder. Once the healing process begins, however, and the scleral tunnel is stable, there appears to be no further regression during the first two postoperative months.

What remains to be seen with this type of incision closure, is how much regression will occur over a period of several more months to several years. Its initial use, however, has been extremely gratifying and very promising because it does not result in the significant postoperative astigmatism that radial suturing techniques induce.

Clinical Points to Consider

☞ Radial suturing techniques can induce significant postoperative astigmatism.

☞ The infinity suture may significantly reduce the number of patients who require suture cutting to reduce postoperative with-the-rule astigmatism.

☞ Nonradial sutures may allow the wound to stabilize and the patient to achieve functional vision more quickly.

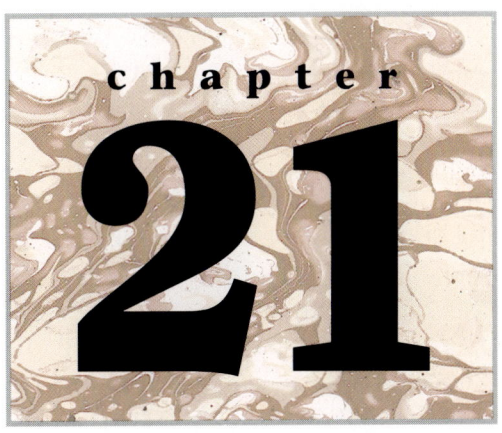

LENSECTOMY WITH IOL IMPLANTATION AND PHAKIC HYPERNEGATIVE IOLS FOR THE CORRECTION OF HIGH MYOPIA

W. ANDREW MAXWELL, M.D., Ph.D.

Most literature describes high myopia as a refractive error of more than 8.00 D due to an increase in axial length of more than 25.50 mm. Visual disturbance is great for the individual who suffers from this condition, although its incidence is relatively low. Visual disturbances include, but are not limited to, visual field restriction, decreased night vision, minification with spectacles, scotomata, and major loss of visual function without spectacle or contact lens correction. If myopic maculopathy exists, loss of central vision and distortion occur. Techniques to eliminate high axial myopia can significantly benefit high myopes. These patients are of special concern, however, because surgical risk and future pathology are related directly to an especially long axial length.

Surgical procedures currently available or under investigation include radial keratotomy, myopic keratomileusis, myopic epikeratoplasty, lensectomy with or without intraocular lens (IOL), and implantation of a hypernegative IOL in the phakic eye. Lensectomy and implantation of hypernegative IOLs primarily concern patients at the extreme of high myopia and will be the subject of this chapter. (The other techniques are described elsewhere in this book.)

Lensectomies with or without an IOL or implantation of a hypernegative IOL are used to correct significant ametropia because virtually all ocular surgeons who do anterior segment surgery are well trained in these procedures. Even so, special consideration needs to be given to these techniques in order to ensure a successful outcome. *Enthusiasm for these procedures must be tempered by the knowledge that vision-threatening complications may occur.* These complications will be detailed as each procedure is described.

Lensectomy and Intraocular Lens Implantation

Clear lens extraction is an appealing treatment for high myopia because most anterior segment surgeons are able to achieve excellent visual results with few complications after cataract/IOL surgery. However, compared to the other surgical techniques used to treat high myopia, lensectomy is the most invasive and may result in severe vision loss. Therefore, the surgeon and patient must ask: Are the risks worth the benefits?

The primary risk of the surgery is the increased propensity for retinal detachment in patients with high myopia. This has been reviewed by Neumann. Goldberg and Hyams et al have reported the incidence of retinal breaks to be twice as high in the phakic high myope compared to the phakic population. The incidence of retinal detachment on an annual basis in the aphakic population is 0.005% to 0.01% compared to about 1% in the high myope according to Goldberg, Hyams et al, Colvard et al, and Curtin. The lifetime risk of retinal detachment for a person with myopia greater than 5.00 D is 2.4% compared to 0.06% for the emmetropic patient, according to Ruben and Rajpurohit. Ashrafzadeh et al, Perkins, and Schepens and Marden have reported that the rate of retinal detachment in aphakic eyes correlates to the level of myopia. According to Perkins the annual rate of retinal detachment for eyes with a refraction from 0 to +4.75 D was 0.002%; from 0 to −4.75 D it was 0.02%; from −5.00 to −9.75 D it was 0.08%; and for greater than −10.00 D the rate was 0.68%.

Performing a clear lensectomy in the high myope deserves careful scrutiny because it not only results in an increased rate of retinal detachment, but it is generally felt that repairing retinal detachments in these individuals is more difficult and commonly results in loss of macular function.

Preoperative Evaluation

As with any cataract surgery patient, the high myope should undergo all necessary preoperative examinations. This includes a complete eye examination and an in-depth evaluation and discussion of the patient's needs and expectations as well as a detailed informed consent. Furthermore, a complete retinal evaluation with indirect ophthalmoscopy and scleral depression should be performed, probably by a retinal specialist. Any pathological area should be considered for preoperative treatment by photocoagulation or cryotherapy.

Surgical Procedure

The surgeon's usual method of anesthesia should be performed; however, great care should be exercised when performing retrobulbar or peribulbar anesthesia. The diameter of the globe is longer and larger in the myopic eye and the risk of perforation is significantly greater. Also, the sclera is frequently thinner and may predispose the eye to easier perforation. I use retrobulbar anesthesia and prefer to place the retrobulbar needle in position while the eye is in a straight-ahead direction to minimize damage to the optic nerve.

Phacoemulsification is recommended for lens removal for several reasons. First, because phacoemulsification maintains a basically closed system, the least possible fluctuation of pressure and disturbance of the posterior vitreous and retina will occur. Second, because phacoemulsification provides the surgeon with the greatest control and because most lenses are soft, only minimal phacoemulsification (primarily irrigation and aspiration) will be needed to remove them. Third, incision size will be kept to a minimum, resulting in less astigmatism and allowing more rapid wound recovery (since the procedure is refractive, astigmatism control should be considered). Fourth, because the procedure is extracapsular, the posterior capsule remains intact, which many surgeons feel reduces the incidence of retinal detachment.

If and when a posterior capsulotomy is performed, a low power IOL will provide additional stability to the vitreous initially and later on. If a capsulotomy is necessary, the opening in the posterior capsule should be as small as possible in order to ensure the desired result. This should be done using low YAG laser power and under optimal visualization and magnification. Dardenne et al reported a retrospective study of 1000 cases of Nd:YAG laser posterior capsulotomy. A high incidence of retinal detachment (12.3% in eyes with axial length greater than 26.10 D) was found, although it was not correlated with any laser parameters. Nevertheless, careful technique appears prudent.

It is recommended that the IOL power formula used be one that takes into consideration extremes in axial length (e.g., SRK II or Holladay) (Fig. 21.1).

A globe with average values of 43.50 D for the cornea and 23.50 mm for the axial length will require a posterior chamber IOL of about +19.00 D to obtain emmetropia, depending on the configuration of the IOL. This relationship is demonstrated nicely by the SRK I (Sanders/Retzlaff/Kraff) formula, in which P equals the power of the IOL necessary to obtain emmetropia, A equals a numerical constant assigned to each style of IOL based on its location in the eye, K equals the average dioptric power of the cornea established by keratometry, and AL equals the axial length of the eye in millimeters:

$$P = A - [(0.90K + 2.50AL)]$$
$$P = 117 - [(0.90)(43.50) + (2.50)(23.50)]$$
$$P = 117 - [(39.15) + (58.75)]$$
$$P = 117 - 97.90$$
$$P = 19.10 \, D$$

Generally, for each millimeter added to the axial length of the globe, the power of the posterior chamber IOL needed to obtain emmetropia is decreased by about 3.00 D, and for each millimeter subtracted, about 3.00 D is added. However, globes at the axial length extreme do not follow this rule precisely because of the nonlinear progression of focal distance relative to diopter power and because the IOL may settle in an unusual position in a very large or small globe. Also, the axial length measurements in a high myope are often inaccurate because of a posterior staphyloma. The clear lens of the adult eye has about +18.00 D of power. The phacoemulsification technique for removal of a clear lens is described in detail in Chapter 13.

Every effort should be made to place the implant in the capsular bag. Steps to help insure in-the-bag placement of the IOL include maximum pupillary dilation, optimal visualization by proper microscope adjustment and magnification, and capsulorhexis for an anterior capsulotomy. Pupillary dilation can be maximized by preoperative installation of flurbiprofen, 2.5% Neosynephrine, and 1% Cyclopentolate, three times, five minutes apart, starting 90 minutes preoperatively. About 0.50 cc of nonpreserved 1:1000 epinephrine added to 500 cc of irrigating solution helps maintain pupillary dilation during the procedure as does efficient nontraumatic phacoemulsification. The proper placement of the entrance incision into the anterior chamber is a key factor in minimizing iris trauma during phacoemulsification.

Results

Only limited results are available on a large series of high myopes in which careful preoperative evaluation and treatment and an optimal surgical technique (as described above) were performed.

Verezella reported the incidence of retinal detachment in 1,783 patients who had phacoemulsification lens extraction for myopia equal to or greater than 10.00 D. Clear lens extraction was

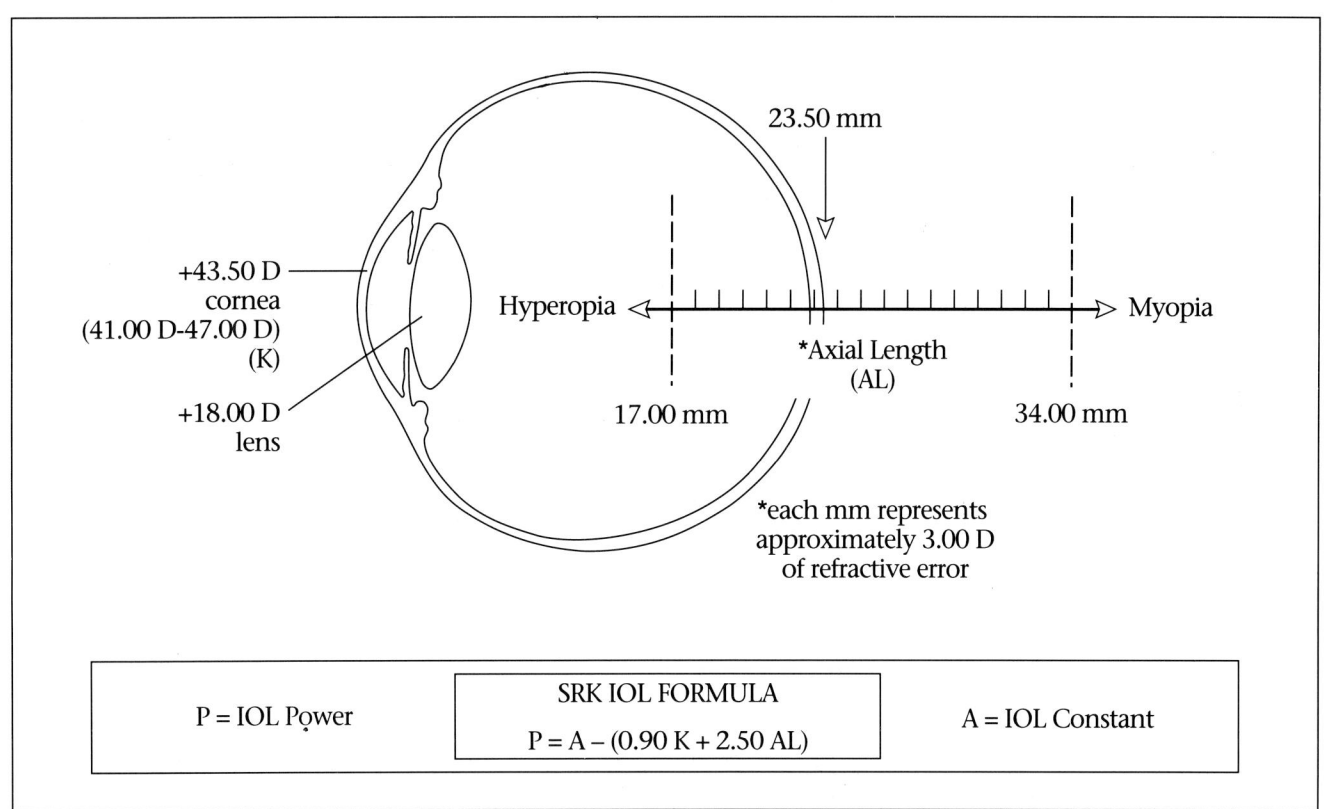

Figure 21.1 *This cross section of the globe illustrates average "refractive status" as well as axial myopia and hyperopia. The refractive status of an eye is determined by the relationship between the refractive power of the cornea and the length of the globe. A healthy cornea usually possesses a net refractive power in the range of 41.00 D to 47.00 D. The axial length of a healthy eye may range from about 17.00 mm to 34.00 mm.*

performed in 763 eyes and cataractous lens extraction was performed in 1,020 eyes. Of the cataractous group, 16 (1.56%) developed retinal detachments and in the clear lens group, five (0.65%) developed retinal detachments. Follow-up periods were not given in this report.

Livernois and Sinskey reported a 3% (one patient) incidence of retinal detachments in 32 patients with a preoperative mean refraction of −9.20 D. Neumann reported on seven eyes with high myopia after lens removal for cataracts. The mean preoperative refraction was −21.48 D with a short-term follow up (mean 11 months ± 8.60). The refractive results were good (5 of 7 within 2.00 D of emmetropia).

I have followed, for a minimum of four years, eight high myopes with preoperative refractions greater than −20.00 D, who underwent clear lens removal. All patients had thorough preoperative evaluation and no retinal pathology needing preoperative treatment. Two of the patients had planned extracapsular cataract extraction with posterior chamber IOL, and six had phacoemulsification cataract removal with posterior chamber IOL. One patient with a preoperative refraction of −22.75 D and a postoperative refraction of −0.75 D developed a temporal retinal tear nine months post cataract removal and four months after having the posterior capsule polished. The patient was referred to a retinal specialist who treated the retinal tear by cryopexy and argon laser photocoagulation. Within two days, the patient developed a retinal dialysis; within one week, the retina detached and was repaired successfully. After four additional procedures, the patient had hand motion vision. Prior to the retinal detachment, the patient had a corrected visual acuity of 20/25. While the patient may have developed retinal detachment without lens removal, this type of experience has led me to await a well-controlled prospective study before treating high myopia with clear lensectomy. *The risks of retinal detachment are simply too high to justify performing the procedure routinely on a young adult population.*

Hypernegative Intraocular Lens Implants

Although proposals have been made to use a negative powered implant in the phakic eye, only recently have studies begun on such a device. A multicenter trial from France (Baikoff et al) is the most comprehensive evaluation of this hypernegative IOL to date. The information contained herein was obtained from this group's reports and by personal communication with Baikoff, the originator of the lens design used in the study.

Lens Design

The lens is patterned after the anterior chamber implant design by Kelman. Its footplate design, vaulting, and optic design are unique. The footplates are designed to provide minimal angle contact while being large enough to prevent goniosynechae. The IOL is vaulted at 25 degrees, which provides a clearance of 1.00 mm from the central iris and lens while being positioned 2.00 mm posterior to the central cornea. A compression of 1.00 mm leaves a clearance of 0.30 mm from the optic zone to the peripheral cornea. The 4.50 mm optic diameter was selected to eliminate contact of the peripheral borders with the corneal endothelium. The optic is 0.70 mm thick for a −20.00 D lens. Figure 21.2 shows design characteristics of the lens used in the French multicenter study. Figure 21.3 shows a hypernegative IOL implanted in a patient.

Preoperative Evaluation

Preoperatively, patients were evaluated for anterior segment pathology, cataracts, corneal guttata, and ocular hypertension. Any patients with positive findings were excluded from the study. A complete retinal evaluation was performed, and retinal lesions having the potential to lead to detachment were photocoagulated prior to surgery.

The lens selection criteria were as follows. Diameter was determined by adding 1.00 mm to the horizontal white-to-white limbal measurement. Lens power selection was based on spectacle refraction powers. IOL powers equal to spectacle refractions from −10.00 D to −15.00 D were used. From −15.00 D to −20.00 D an IOL power of 1.00 D less than spectacle lens power was used. For spectacle corrections from −20.00 D to −25.00 D, an IOL power of −2.00 D less than spectacle lens power was used.

Surgical Procedure

To provide the best access to the anterior chamber, surgery was performed temporally. A corneal incision was made parallel to the iris plane. A viscoelastic was used to form the anterior chamber and coat the IOL. Following IOL implantation and suturing, the feet were properly positioned and pupil distortion was evaluated. Balanced salt solution was used to replace the viscoelastic, and subconjunctival antibiotics and corticosteroids were employed. No peripheral iridectomy was performed. Topical corticosteroids were used for six weeks postoperatively.

Results

Table 21.4 shows the refraction results for up to one year postoperatively and Table 21.5 shows the uncorrected and best corrected visual results of 41 consecutive cases reported by Baikoff. Myopia ranged from –9.00 D to –25.00 D with an average preoperative refraction of –14.58 D. As expected, the final refractive and visual results are good and relatively predictable. The results reported by Collin for a larger number of patients in the French multicenter study, in which surgery was performed by many surgeons, including Baikoff, were essentially equivalent to Baikoff's personal experience.

Complications

While the results are good, potential complications are of concern. Baikoff reports removing three lenses because of excessive residual refractive error. Two were replaced successfully. One patient chose not to replace the lens after removal. Baikoff reports no rotational or frontal plane displacement, although several patients experienced transient ocular hypertension associated with steroid use. Two cases of pupillary ovalization (presumed secondary to oversized lenses) and two cases of iris atrophy were reported. One late retinal detachment occurred in Baikoff's personal series but none in the 150 multicenter

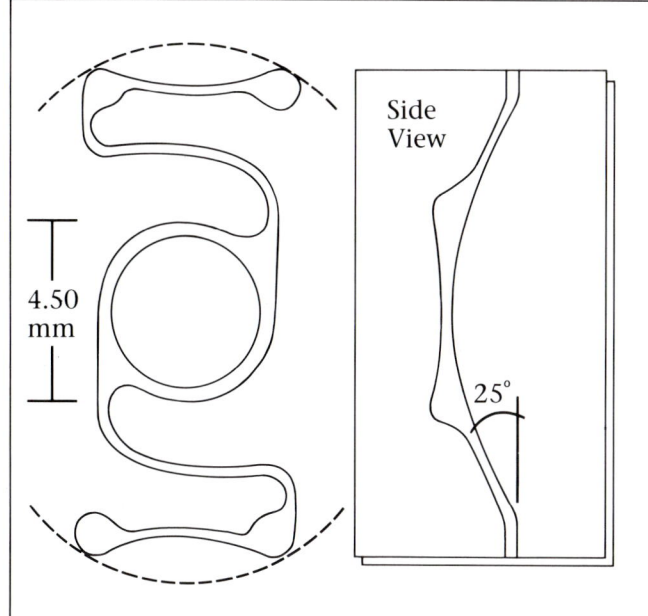

Figure 21.2 *The Baikoff hypernegative IOL. (Reprinted with permission of Domilens, Inc.)*

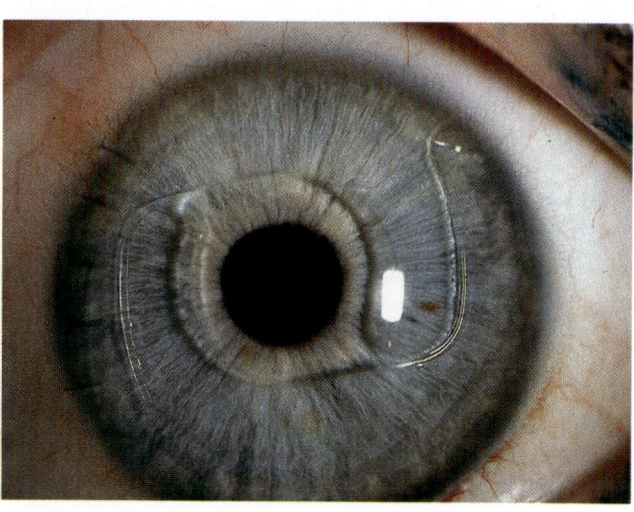

Figure 21.3 *The anterior segment with the Baikoff hypernegative IOL in place. (Photograph compliments of Dr. George Baikoff.)*

Table 21.4
Phakic Hypernegative IOLs: Refractive Results

	Preoperative	1 month	3 months	6 months	12 months
Number of Eyes	41	40	37	32	34
Mean Refraction	–14.95	+0.06	–0.05	–0.20	–0.13
Standard Deviation	±5.30	±1.05	±1.03	±1.06	±1.01
Range of Refractive Error	–9.00 to –35.00	–2.00/+2.00	–2.00/+2.00	–1.70/+2.00	–2.00/+2.00

study cases. The most consistent complaint was the luminous halo with pupillary dilation, which was probably related to the implant edges. No pupillary block, ocular hypertension, crystalline lens opacification, or corneal dystrophy was reported.

Baikoff retrospectively evaluated endothelial cell counts in a small number of patients and found an average cell loss of 5% at two to three months and 9% at one year.

Conclusion

While the early results of the French multicenter study and of Baikoff's study are encouraging, more in-depth evaluation of results and complications are necessary, as is a well-defined and controlled long-term study. There is little doubt that optimal refractive results can be obtained; the results described above confirm this. A controlled trial is needed to evaluate not only the visual results, including contrast sensitivity and glare problems, but more importantly, to objectively measure adverse reactions. This trial should include evaluation of possible long-term progressive endothelial cell loss, effects on anterior segment morphology and intraocular pressure, and an objective evaluation of chronic inflammation.

A 40-year-old patient who has had an anterior chamber IOL in place for 20 years has a good possibility of developing peripheral corneal edema. Will these patients need corneal transplants while still in their forties and fifties? Preoperative and postoperative cell counts need to be performed in order to evaluate endothelial cells and possibly warn of impending long-term problems. Inflammation can be assessed by quantitatively measuring the blood-aqueous barrier integrity with an anterior segment fluorophotometry or the laser flare/cell meter.

Summary

There is little doubt that the high myope can obtain an excellent visual result by either lensectomy with a low power posterior chamber IOL or phakic hypernegative lens implantation. The potential success and acceptance of these procedures depends on proof of their safety from well-controlled prospective studies. In other words, the benefit to risk ratio must be established.

Table 21.5
Phakic Hypernegative IOLs: Visual Acuity Results

	Preoperative	1 month	3 month	6 month	12 month
Number of Eyes	41	39	37	32	34
Mean Visual Acuity	(<20/200) <0.05	20/40– (0.46)	20/40 (0.50)	20/40 (0.51)	20/30– (0.60)
Standard Deviation		± 2 Snellen lines (± 0.20)	± 2 Snellen lines (± 0.25)	± 2 Snellen lines (± 0.21)	± 2 Snellen lines (± 0.26)
Range of Uncorrected Visual Acuity		20/200–20/20 (0.05-0.95)	20/200–20/20 (0.10-1.00)	20/200–20/20 (0.10-1.00)	20/80–20/20 (0.25-1.00)

Clinical Points to Consider

☛ Clear lens extraction may enable the high myope to obtain excellent vision as a result of accurate IOL power and multifocal IOLs, but the risks are serious.

☛ The long-term concerns relating to phakic hypernegative IOL implantation include progressive cataract formation and peripheral corneal edema.

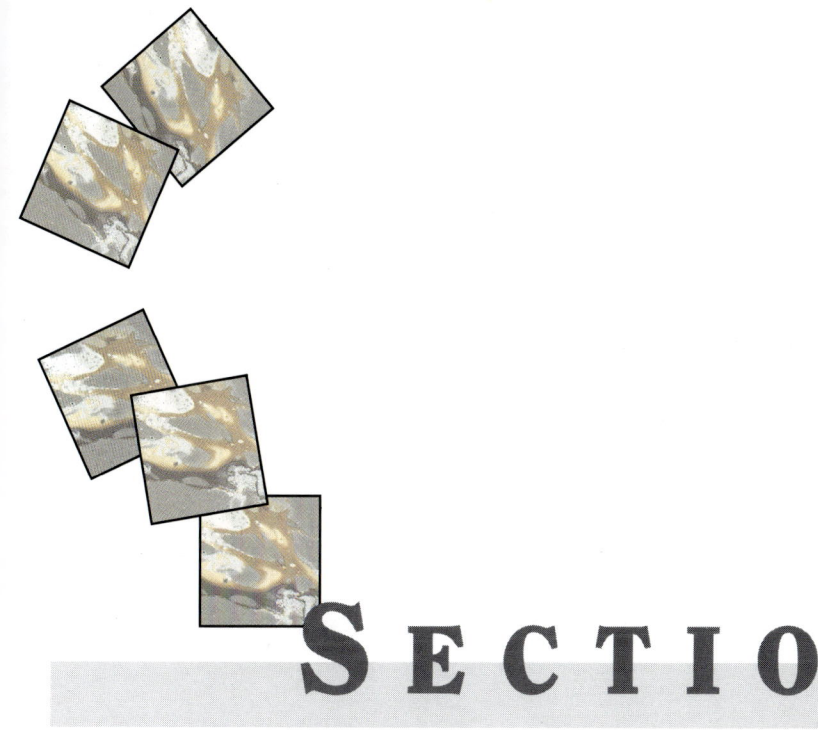

SECTION FIVE
SURGERY OF THE CORNEA

RADIAL KERATOTOMY
FREDRIC B. KREMER, M.D.

For more than a decade, I have routinely used refractive surgery when trying to correct refractive errors. Hyperopia as high as +15.00 D and myopia as high as –26.00 D have been amenable to surgical intervention. Virtually all forms of refractive surgery used for spherical corrections are combined with astigmatic keratotomy, as necessary.

The radial keratotomy (RK) procedure is based on a computer program derived from regression analysis, which is based on RK performed with intraoperative ultrasound corneal thickness measurements, a variety of exquisitely sharp diamond blades, and central optical zone sizes as well as the number of incisions and the degree to which they are deepened as they course toward the periphery.

RK appears quite easy, but it is extremely difficult. Surgeons who perform RK incorrectly and inappropriately conclude that the procedure does not work; however, those who do it correctly receive more appreciation from their patients than they have ever received in the past.

Mechanism of Action

The myopic eye possesses a mismatch between the refractive power of the cornea (too steep) and/or the axial length of the eye (too long) (Fig. 22.1). RK treats myopia by reducing the refractive power of the central cornea but it has no effect on the axial length of the eye, nor the associated pathologic retinal conditions.

This reduction in central corneal refractive power is achieved by weakening the dome-shaped corneal structure in the midperiphery, which bows out. The cornea is fixed at the limbus; the geometry of a dome dictates that the central portion of the cornea (including the visual axis) must flatten as a result of this bowing out, converting the central and para-central cornea from a spherical system to an aspheric system (Fig. 22.2). (The significance of an aspheric cornea is discussed at length in Chapter 2.)

Fyodorov, the founder of modern RK, originally performed RK incisions so that they extended beyond the cornea and crossed the limbus into the sclera. Because the limbus makes a less effective

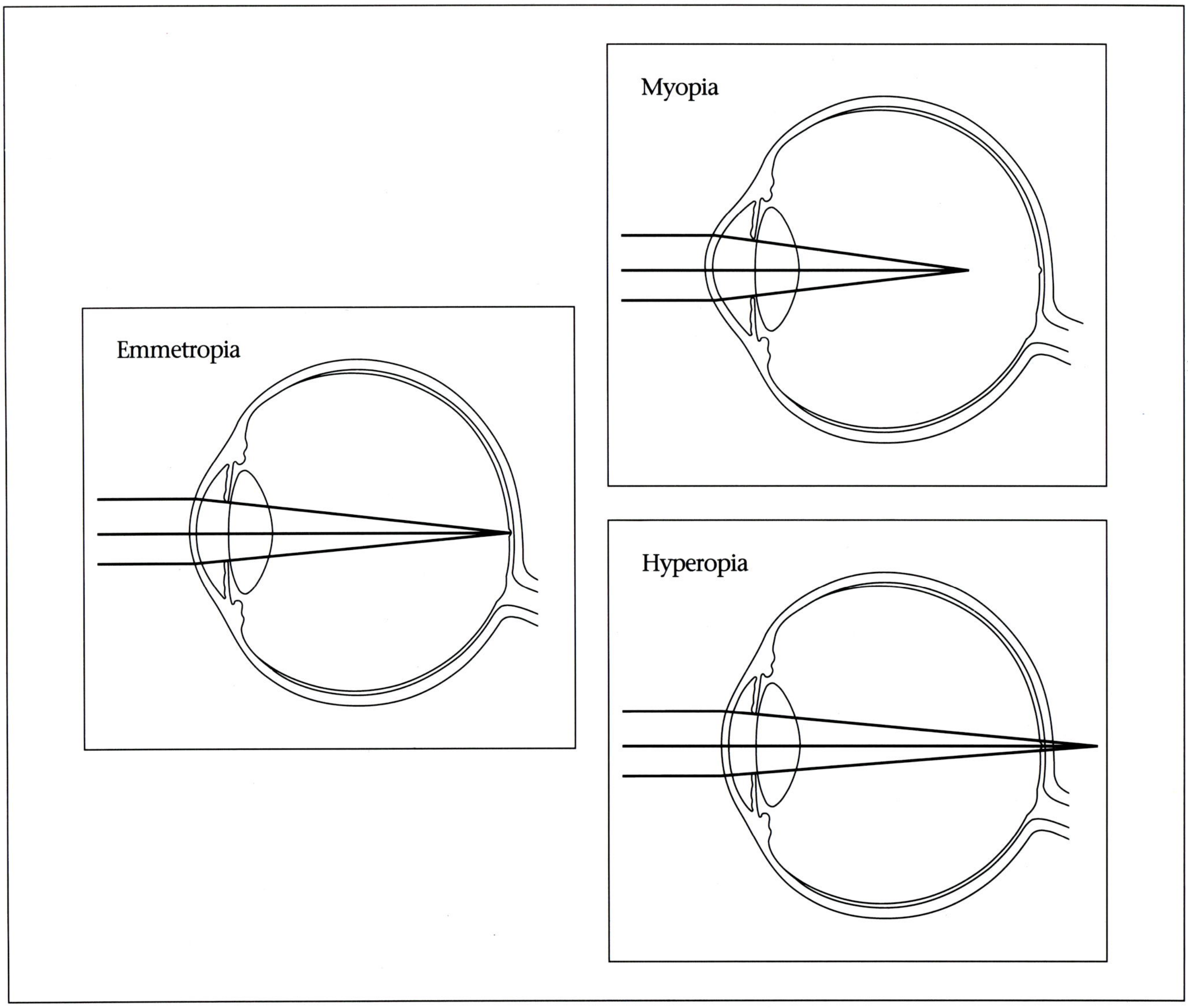

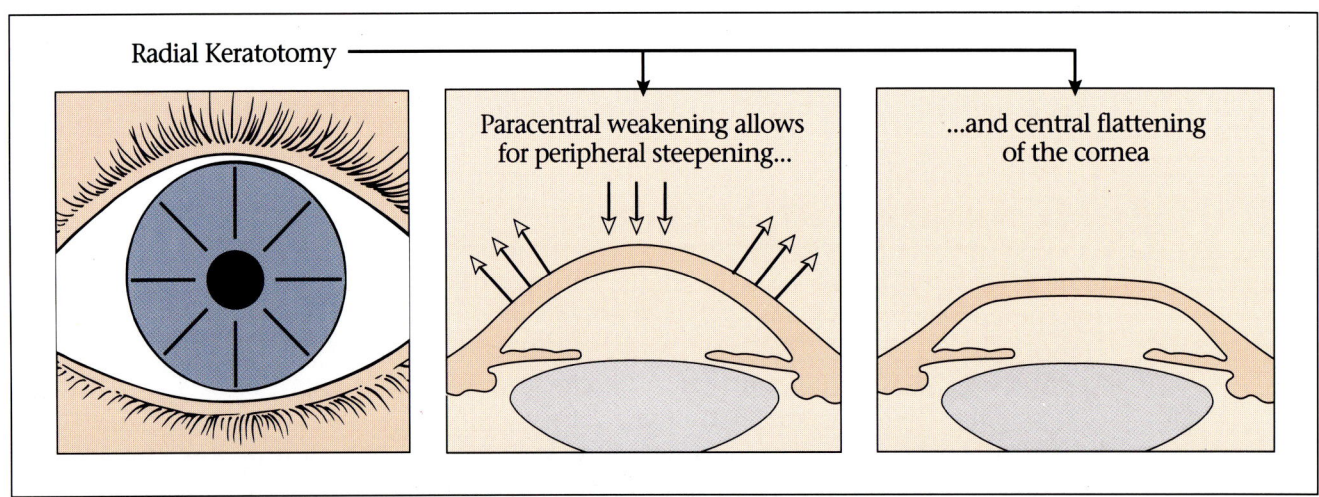

Figure 22.1 *Schematic depiction of emmetropia, myopia, and hyperopia.*

Figure 22.2 *The mechanism of action of RK.*

anchor for the cornea, this maneuver actually reduced the effectiveness of RK. The central 3.00 mm of an RK incision provides most of the effect; thus, the greater the weakening of the para-central cornea, the greater the flattening of the central cornea.

Although RK's mechanism of action is relatively simple, attention to preoperative and surgical details insures consistency of result. Three surgical factors are responsible for RK's effectiveness:

1. Optical zone (OZ) size
2. Number of incisions
3. Incision depth

It is important to consider these factors in detail.

Optical Zone Size

The OZ diameter generally ranges from 3.00 mm to 5.00 mm, although thinner diamond blades, which cause less central scarring, make a 2.75 mm OZ possible in certain cases. The OZ is usually smaller than the visual axis, which is limited by the pupil. Virtually all RK patients "look" through the central portions of their corneal incisions. The midcorneal knee occurs at about 7.00 mm and *does not* coincide with the diameter of the OZ (Fig. 22.3).

Incision Number

The greater the number of incisions, the greater the effect of the RK. Incisions should be symmet-

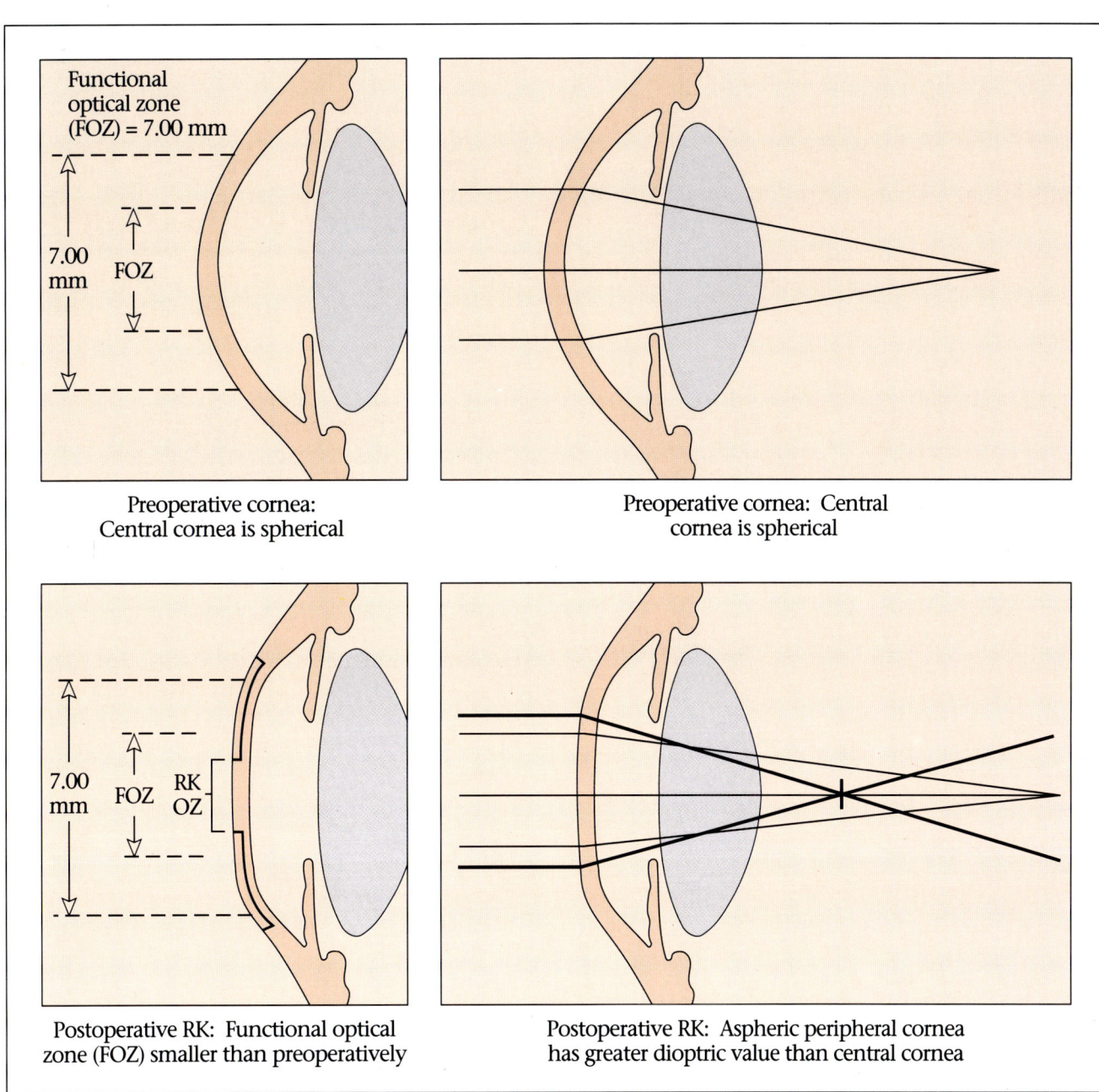

Figure 22.3 *Schematic depiction of the differences between the preoperative functional optical zone (FOZ), post RK FOZ, and the RK optical zone (OZ) which is used to determine RK incision length. Notice that the post RK FOZ includes the central portion of the RK incisions.*

rically placed about the OZ. Three, four, six, eight, 12, and 16 incisions are commonly used. Thirty-two incisions are not advocated because the surgical scarring and risk of creating irregular astigmatism outweigh the 10% increase in effect gained from doing a 16-incision RK under the same conditions. Table 22.4 depicts the approximate ratio of effect depending on the number of RK incisions assuming the same OZ and depth. The effect from eight incisions is considered 100%, because eight is the most commonly used number of RK incisions.

Depth

An achieved depth of 85% to 90% of corneal thickness is important for consistency. It is interesting to consider that a back-cutting blade, which is 10% longer than the cornea is thick, achieves 85% to 90% corneal incision depth. This 15% to 20% difference between blade length and achieved incision depth is due to the give of the cornea under pressure from the blade, i.e., the small but significant resistance offered to the penetration of the diamond blade, and the tendency of the back-cutting blade to "water ski" out of the cornea during the incision.

Bias

Bias is the percentage that must be added to the corneal pachymetry measurement in order to determine which blade length will achieve the desired result. This bias may be positive or negative and is determined by the diamond blade construction and direction of incision. For example, assume a corneal measurement of 0.60 mm. In order for a quality back-cutting diamond blade to obtain a 90% incision, the blade depth chosen might be 0.60 + 0.06 = 0.66 mm. The 0.06 refers to a +10% bias with a blade length of 110% of pachymetry readings.

For a front cutting (vertical) blade to obtain the same 90% incision depth, a –5% bias might be necessary. The blade length would be 0.60 mm – 0.05(0.60) = 0.57 mm. Front-cutting diamond blades usually create a corneal incision that is about 5% less deep than the length of the blade. Therefore, a front-cutting blade will produce a corneal incision about 15% deeper than a back-cutting blade of the same length, which equals 0.09 mm with an initial blade setting of 0.60 mm (Fig. 22.5).

A front-cutting blade offers the advantage of improved visibility for the surgeon and a perpendicular incision shape at the OZ limit; however, the drawbacks of a front-cutting blade are that it distorts the OZ line during a radial incision and, more importantly, can easily *cut through the patient's visual axis with inadvertent patient eye movement*. For this reason, front-cutting blades should be used for astigmatic keratotomy and redeepening of RK incisions but not for the primary RK incisions. The safety of the "American" (center to periphery) technique for RK incisions is undeniable and greater depth can always be achieved by increasing blade length.

Achieved corneal incision depths of greater than 95% can lead to greater effect but also *corneal instability* and fluctuating vision. Achieved corneal incision depths of less than 75% can lead to severe undercorrection or even *total regression* after a reasonable result for several weeks or months.

Preoperative Evaluation

Evaluation of the patient starts with a complete history and ophthalmic examination. Corneal surface regularity should be verified in order to identify and eliminate patients with subtle keratoconus. A stable cycloplegic refraction or manifest refraction is obtained. Contact lenses, if worn, will need to be discontinued until stable keratometric and refraction readings are obtained. Visual acuities with and without correction, pupillary function, extraocular muscle function, slit lamp examination, intraocular pressures by applanation, and dilated fundus examination are performed.

Ocular dominance is determined because patients usually prefer to use the dominant eye for distance vision should monovision be considered. It is important to review the patient's goals and expectations along with the risks and benefits of the procedure. An extensive informed consent is prepared, the patient's responses are reviewed by a member of the office staff, and the form is then signed by the patient. If a patient has unrealistic goals, surgery should be avoided.

Surgical Preparation

Surgery is performed in a sterile, completely equipped ophthalmic operating room. The patient is generally given 5.00 mg of Valium orally approximately one-half hour prior to the onset of the procedure. The patient wears a clean jumpsuit over street clothes, surgical cap, and shoe covers. After walking to the surgical suite with an escort, the patient is placed on the operating table. The patient's head is tilted somewhat more posteriorly, with the chin up, than is typical for cataract or other ophthalmic procedures. A neck support is used to obtain proper head position. The patient is then prepped and draped in a routine sterile fashion.

A printout from the computer program is taped to the operating microscope so that it can be seen clearly by the operating surgeon. This printout should include the patient's name, the opera-

Table 22.4 RK Incisions Approximate Ratio of Effect

No. of Incisions	Relative Effect (constant OZ and depth)
3	60%
4	65%
6	80%
8	100%
12	110%
16	120%

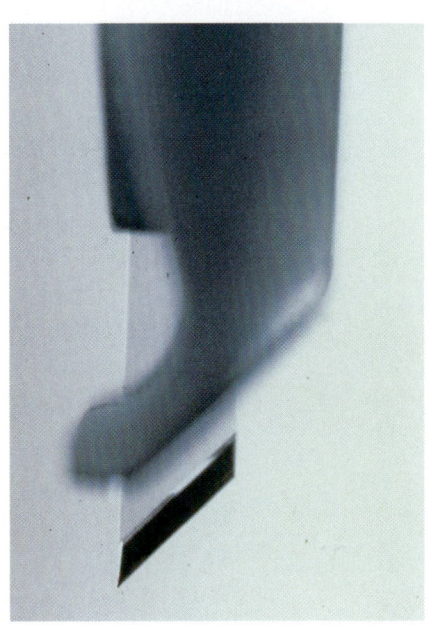
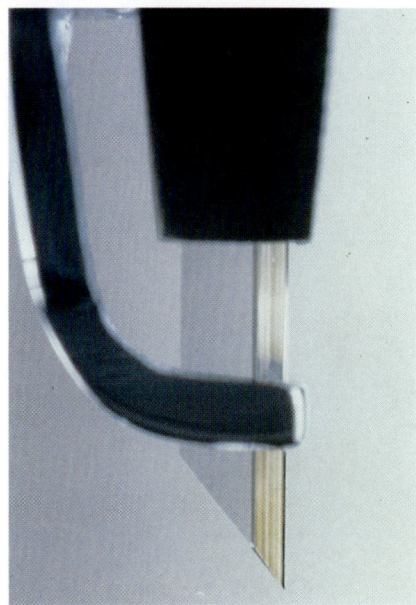
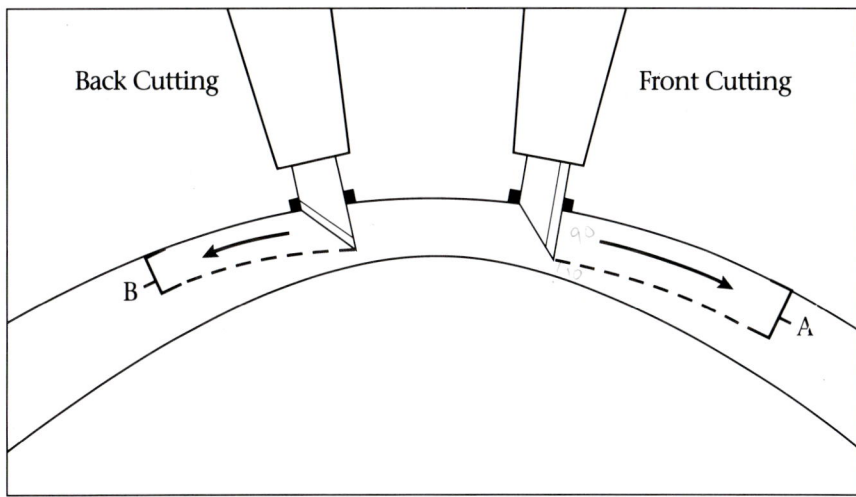

Figure 22.5 **(Left)** *A back-cutting diamond RK blade.* **(Right)** *A front-cutting diamond RK blade.* **(Bottom)** *A front-cutting blade makes a deeper incision than that made by a back-cutting blade of equal length.*

Table 22.6
Radial Keratotomy Nomogram: Nordan/Maxwell Methodology

Assumptions: 90% achieved depth; centrifugal incision; noncycloplegic refraction
Factors considered: refractive error; age; IOP; sex; corneal thickness; (the sum of these factors = working sphere)
Factors not considered: corneal diameter; keratometry

REFRACTIVE ERROR

Working Sphere	Number of Incisions	Optical Zone		
−0.50	3	5.00		
−0.75	3	4.50		
−1.00	6	4.50		
−1.25	6	4.25		
−1.50	6	4.00		
−2.00	8	4.00		
−2.50	8	3.75		
−3.00	8	3.50		
−3.50	8	3.25		
−4.00	8	3.00		
	8			
−4.50	8	3.00	5.00	
−5.00	8	3.00	5.00	7.00
−5.50	8	3.00	5.00	7.00
−6.00	16	3.00	5.00	
−6.50	16	3.00	5.00	7.00
−7.00	16	3.00	5.00	7.00
−7.50	16	3.00	5.00	7.00

AGE

Myopia	18–23	24–27	28–31	32–34	35–37	38–41	42–45	46–48	49–53	54–57	58 and above
0 to −2.00	−0.75	−0.50	0	+0.25	+0.50	+0.75	+1.00	+1.25	+1.50	+1.50	+1.75
−2.25 to −4.75	−1.00	−0.50	0	+0.25	+0.50	+0.75	+1.00	+1.25	+1.50	+1.50	+1.75
−5.00 + more	−1.50	−0.75	−0.25	0	+0.50	+0.50	+1.00	+1.25	+1.50	+1.50	+1.75

INTRAOCULAR PRESSURE

Add −0.25 D for every 2 mm Hg less than 15 mm Hg. If IOP is greater than 22 mm Hg, control IOP as appropriate and consider under correction.

SEX

Female, age 24–34, add −0.50 D to refractive error.

CORNEAL THICKNESS

If central corneal thickness is less than 0.49 mm, add −0.50 D to refractive error if original refractive error is −2.00 D or greater. If central thickness is greater than 0.75 mm, add +0.50 to refractive error.

tive eye, the patient's refraction, and the surgical plan. The multiple regression analyses performed on my patients have demonstrated that the results of RK depend on the following variables:

1. Refraction
2. Age
3. Intraocular pressure
4. Number of incisions
5. Central corneal thickness
6. Optical zone diameter
7. Incision redeepening
8. Sex

(Note that preoperative keratometry is not included as a determinant of RK effect.)

When performing RK, it is recommended that both the computer-derived regression analysis and the resultant surgical plan be followed as closely as possible (Table 22.6).

Anesthesia

RK is performed with a topical anesthetic. In general, the use of retrobulbar or peribulbar injection is contraindicated. While the surgeon is scrubbing, the patient is given drops of proparacaine, a topical anesthetic, and instructed to keep the eyes closed to avoid evaporation and thinning of the cornea. These anesthetic drops are used three or four minutes before the start of the procedure so that anesthesia will be total for the cornea and the conjunctiva. The anesthetic drops make the application of a lid speculum tolerable. Consideration should be given to the use of a Lancaster speculum, which cannot be forced closed by the patient's lid closure reflex. Proparacaine drops are instilled in the operative eye once again after the corneal pachymetry measurements and again prior to the placement of the incisions.

Surgical Procedure

After the speculum is placed, the patient is asked to fixate on the "coaxial" light of the operating microscope. The barrel of the microscope is vertical to the floor and perpendicular to the iris. A rheostat is used in order to provide a minimal level of light at this point in the procedure. The surgeon must be aware of the true angle of incidence of the "coaxial" light for the brand of microscope being used, since the corneal light reflex will vary according to the angle of incidence. A fixation device that is truly coaxial may be attached to the microscope. Generally, the visual axis is situated midway between the superior and inferior limbus; however, the position of the visual axis in the horizontal direction can vary considerably. Most of the time the visual axis is displaced somewhat nasally but it may be central or, on rare occasions, even displaced temporally (negative angle kappa).

In any event, *the most important reference relationship for marking the visual axis is the circular OZ mark, which should be concentric with the miotic pupil* (Fig. 22.7). For this reason, some RK surgeons use pilocarpine drops preoperatively since the visual axis is always located within the miotic pupil. In this case, the patient is instructed to look at the "coaxial" light, but less attention is paid to the corneal light reflex than to ensuring that the iris plane is perpendicular to the observor and that the epithelial OZ mark is

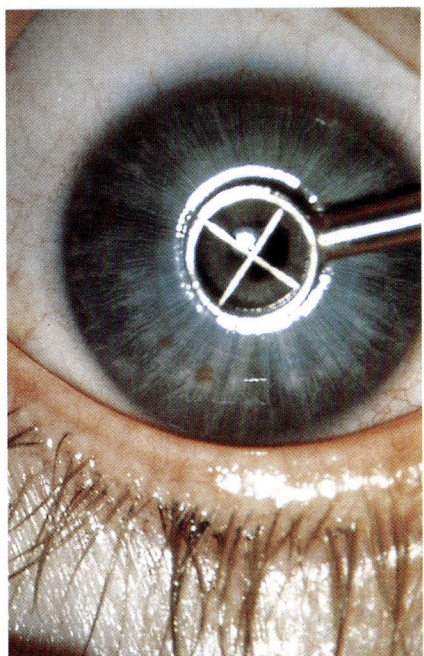 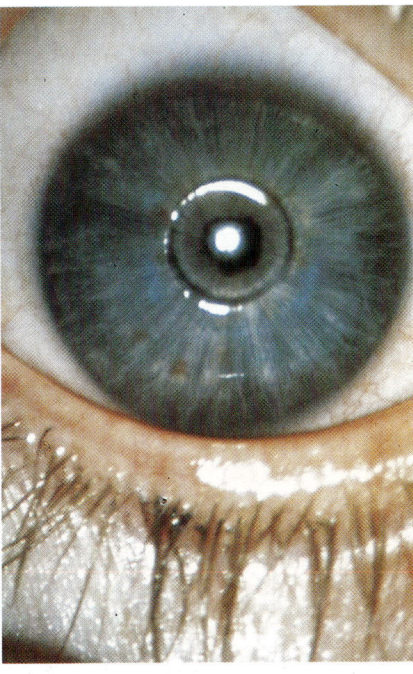

Figure 22.7 (Left) *A single OZ epithelial mark being made.* **(Right)** *An epithelial OZ mark.*

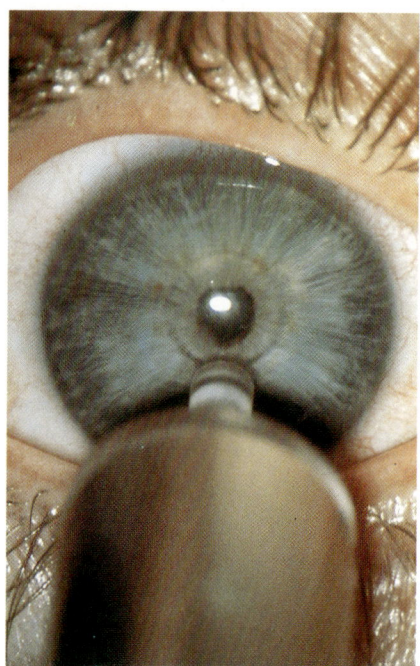

Figure 22.8 *Corneal pachymetry measurement being made.*

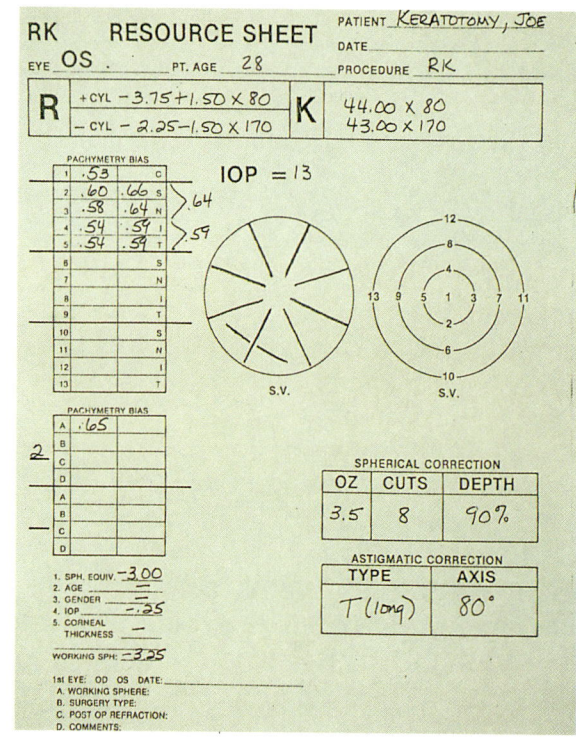

Figure 22.9 *Form used to record corneal pachymetry data, calculate blade length, and formulate the RK surgical plan.*

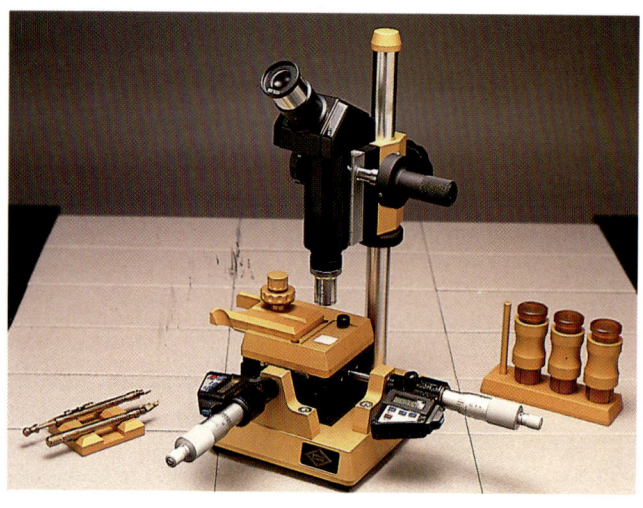

Figure 22.10 (Left) *Microscope used to determine RK blade length.* **(Right)** *The magnified view under the microscope allows the surgeon to evaluate not only blade length but also footplate and blade quality. The footplates pictured are in poor repair.*

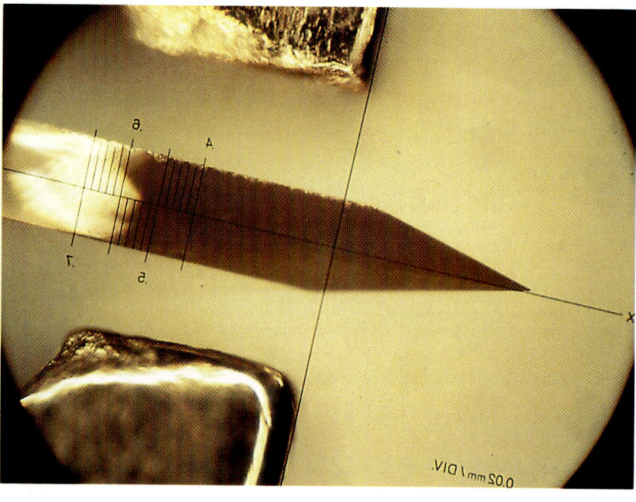

Figure 22.11 *Measuring the length of an RK blade using a gauge block viewed through the operating microscope at high power.*

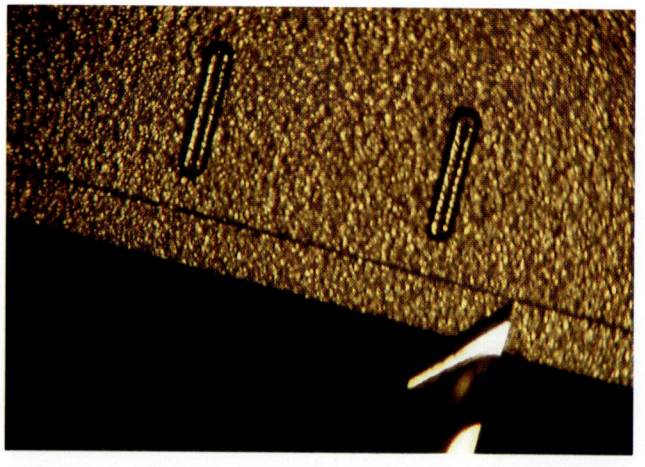

concentric with the pupil. An epithelial mark should not be placed in the center of the visual axis because it is time-consuming and a small scar may result. If the surgical plan calls for multiple depth zones, a marking trephine with multiple rings is used. An RK surgeon should develop a constant, accurate method for marking the visual axis because this is one of the most crucial steps of the entire procedure.

After the circles are in place, the tip of the ultrasonic pachymeter is used to take the corneal thickness measurements (Fig. 22.8). It is easiest to use the solid tip probe but a water-filled probe is equally accurate. In a one-zone case, on the epithelial OZ mark four measurements are taken in the cardinal positions. Multiple zones require additional thickness measurements. The bias measurement, which dictates the blade length for obtaining 90% incisional depth, is recorded directly on a linear table, rather than on a circular graph, which may be confusing (Fig. 22.9). Hand recording takes less time than the printer of the pachymeter. The circulating nurse repeats each measurement aloud as it is recorded so the surgeon can determine if there is a gross mistake. A 2- or 3- zone case always implies that the correction provided by a 3.00 mm OZ has been surpassed and that a 3.00 and 5.00 OZ (3,5) or a 3.00, 5.00, and 7.00 OZ (3,5,7) will be used.

Blade Preparation

Blade preparation for one-zone cases and for the first zone of multizone cases is the same. A back-cutting diamond blade is used. The length of the blade corresponds to the shortest of the bias measurements taken previously. A second preset blade will be used or the length of the first blade increased if the pachymetry for any zone varies by 10% or greater. The blade is advanced to its approximate length by using the micrometer handle of the blade holder. It is critically important that every length be verified with a gauge. This can be achieved with a separate microscope that has a built-in gauge (Fig. 22.10) or by using a graduated length gauge block and placing the operating microscope on its highest magnification (Fig. 22.11).

For one-and-one-half and two-zones cases, a second back-cutting diamond blade may be prepared. The length of this blade is arbitrarily chosen to be 0.05 mm longer than the length of the blade used for the first zone. The previously taken measurements are used as a map to determine where the deepening can be initiated relative to the 5.00 mm OZ. In a situation where the three-zone approach is planned, a third diamond blade may be prepared and this blade may be of the front-cutting (vertical) configuration. The front-cutting blade will have a length that is arbitrarily chosen to be 0.02 mm longer than the blade used for the second stage. Experience has shown that a vertical blade cuts about 0.03 mm deeper than a front-cutting blade of the same length and therefore, adding 0.02 mm to the length of the vertical blade creates an incision 0.05 mm greater than the second redeepening zone incision made by a front-cutting blade (Fig. 22.12). The blades should be completely prepared before surgery is begun so time is not spent changing the blade during the procedure.

Incision Placement

Anesthetic drops are again placed in the eye just prior to fixation of the globe. The bifixation forceps are used to fixate the globe either at the 6 o'clock and 12 o'clock vertical positions or in a position slightly temporal to the 6 o'clock to 12

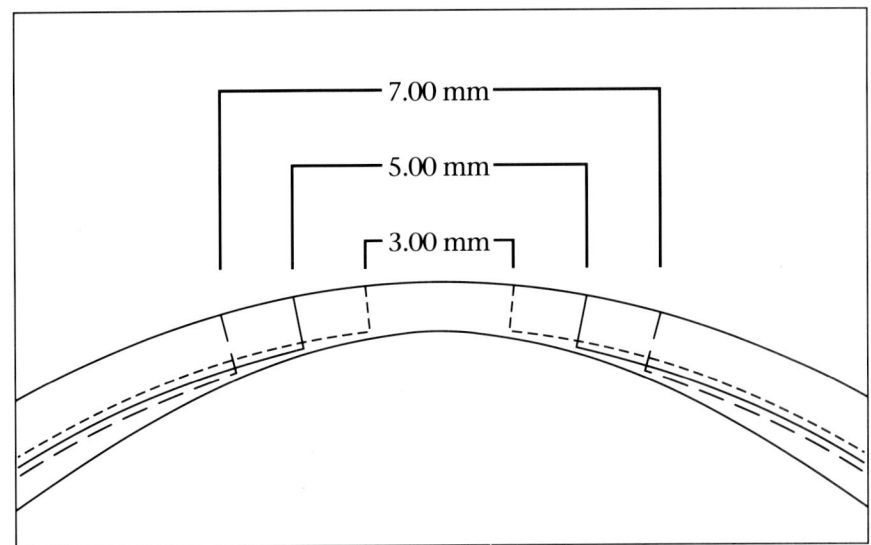

Figure 22.12 *Since the cornea increases in thickness from the center to the periphery, the increased blade lengths used for the second and third zones of an RK incision leave a constant amount of corneal tissue uncut.*

o'clock vertical meridian (Fig. 22.13). The forceps are then folded to the side of the nondominant hand of the surgeon and the appropriate blade holder is grasped in the dominant hand. All of the incisions on the same side as the surgeon's dominant hand are then made. The order of the placement varies with the number of incisions used, as shown in Figure 22.14. Then the forceps are flipped to the opposite side and the remaining incisions are placed with the nondominant hand.

In a two-zone case, the second blade holder is used to deepen the incisions from the 5.00-mm OZ to the peripheral edge of the incision. The corneal thickness measurements taken at the beginning of the case should be used to indicate at which incisions each stage of deepening should begin. For a one-and-one-half zone approach, only half of the incisions are deepened in an alternating fashion. If a two-and-a-half or three-zone approach is used, the third (vertical) blade will then be used to deepen the incisions from the limbus toward the 7.00-mm OZ circle. The previously taken corneal thickness bias measurements should also be used to indicate where each incision should stop.

The incisions are then irrigated with balanced salt solution *unless a microperforation has occurred*, using a special cannula with a blunt tip and a bottom port. A gentle washing motion should be used rather than a high pressure stream that might perforate the posterior stroma into the anterior chamber.

Broad spectrum antibiotic drops are instilled and the lid speculum is removed. A patch is not applied. I have not found any benefit from collagen shields after RK; in general, they cause blurry vision and are uncomfortable.

Postoperative Management

The patient is instructed to use broad spectrum antibiotic drops four times per day for one week. Immediately following surgery, the patient should return home and remain in a darkened room for eight to sixteen hours with both eyes closed. Listening to music or the television helps pass time. A light, cold compress applied to the operative eye may make the patient more comfortable. Demerol, Percodan, Darvocet, or similar medications may be taken postoperatively for pain.

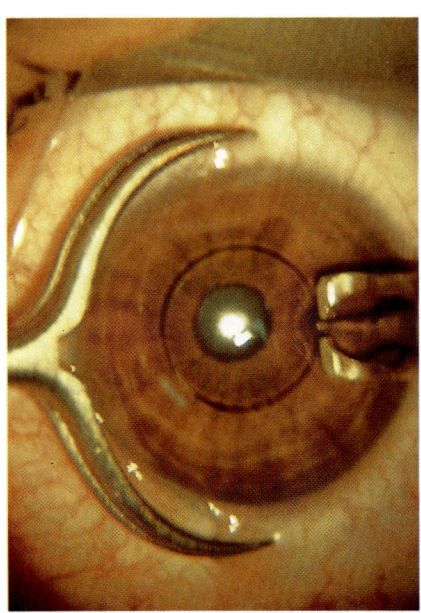

Figure 22.13 *Kremer bifixation forceps stabilize the globe while the first incision of an RK is performed.*

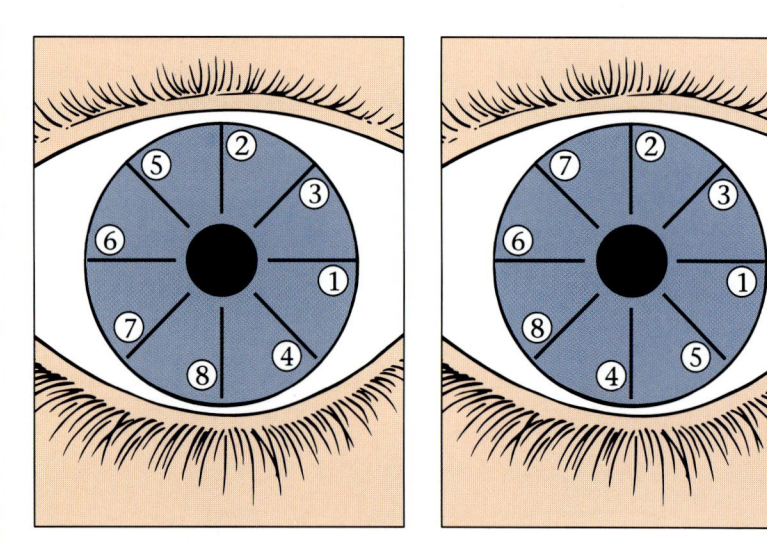

Figure 22.14 (Left) *The order of incisions for an RK performed on a right eye: if the superior incision (8) requires a longer blade length; incisions 1 through 4 are performed with the right hand, 5 through 7 with the left, and 8 again with the right.* **(Right)** *Incisions of equal depth : if all incisions are performed with the same blade length; incisions 1 through 5 are performed with the right hand and 6 through 8 with the left.*

On the first postoperative day examination, the patient typically exhibits a completely epithelialized cornea and has a refraction that is near plano. The patient is seen again one week postoperatively, at which time hyperopia is the norm. This hyperopia is frequently equal in magnitude to half the preoperative myopia.

One month postoperatively, the refraction continues to be somewhat hyperopic, such that a patient who required −5.00 D of correction before RK might now require about +1.00 D. The refraction generally stabilizes by three to four months at or near plano. However, some patients may take much longer to stabilize. When RK is performed well, incisions are virtually invisible at unmagnified levels of observation six months postoperatively (Figs. 22.15 and 22.16).

In 0.5% of the population, there will be essentially no improvement following RK. These patients may benefit from myopic keratomileusis at least six months post RK. Depending on the preoperative refractive range, there may be a 0% to 10% incidence of undercorrection that exceeds 1.00 D. This undercorrection is managed with additional RK surgery about four to six months after the initial RK, not by steroid drops or pressure patching. Significant, clinically relevant overcorrection occurs in approximately 0.3% of patients; they may then be treated by contact lenses, spectacles, homoplastic hyperopic lamellar keratectomy, or plano epikeratoplasty.

Conclusion

Radial keratotomy has become the most widely performed method of refractive surgery and has spawned the increased use of astigmatic keratotomy. Initial concerns about endothelial cell loss and corneal health following RK have not been borne out by follow-up of over a decade. The benefit/risk ratio of RK for an informed, appropriate patient and a skilled surgeon remains extremely high.

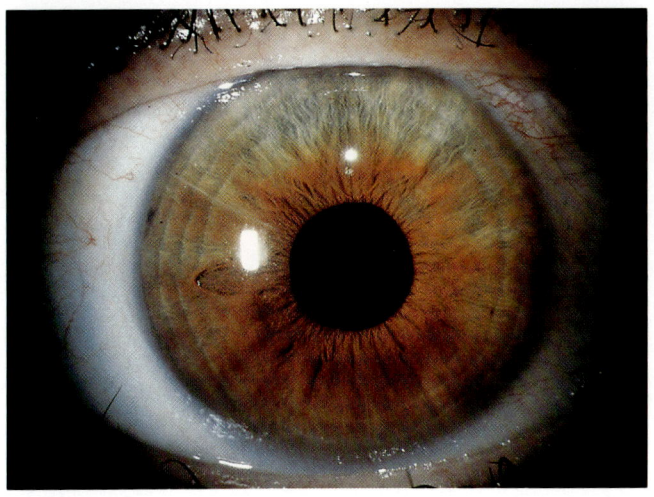

Figure 22.15 *The three RK incisions with a 5.00-mm OZ are virtually invisible six months postoperatively.*

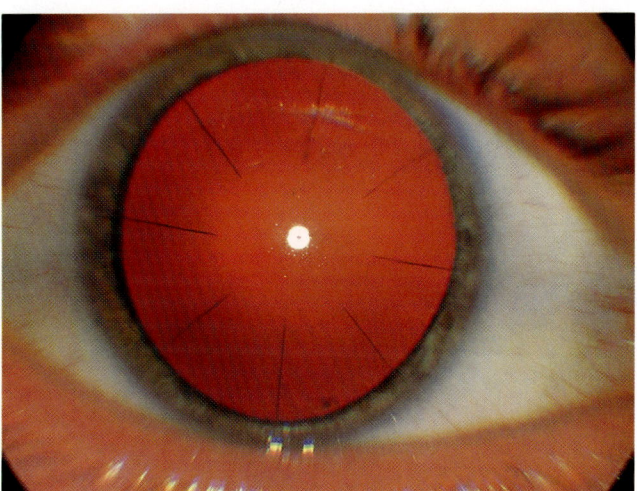

Figure 22.16 *The red reflex of this eye with dilated pupil highlights the eight RK incisions.*

Clinical Points to Consider

- ☛ Radial keratotomy creates a paracentral corneal knee with compensatory central corneal flattening.

- ☛ A back-cutting blade and a front-cutting blade of equal length create corneal incisions of different depths.

- ☛ The effect of RK is influenced by the patient's age, sex, intraocular pressure, and corneal thickness.

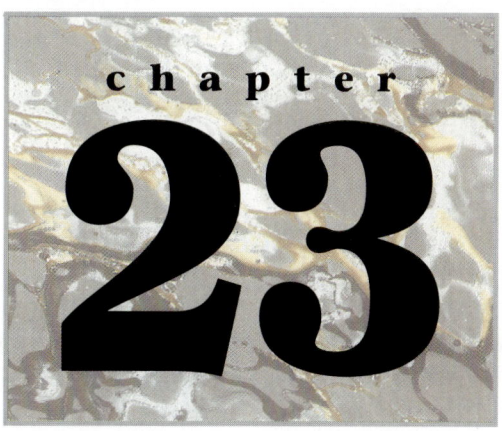

Astigmatism: Concepts and Surgical Approach

LEE T. NORDAN, M.D.   JOHN D. HOFBAUER, M.D.

Astigmatism is often the factor that prevents excellent uncorrected visual acuity. Along with refinements in phacoemulsification, small incision intraocular lenses (IOL), the YAG laser, and radial keratotomy (RK), the correction of congenital and acquired astigmatism and the prevention of surgically induced astigmatism must rank as two of the major accomplishments in anterior segment surgery in the 1980s. No longer should astigmatism be considered an inevitable postoperative occurrence or an unfixable congenital malady. Ocular surgeons can now approach astigmatism correction and prevention systematically.

The surgeon's attitude toward astigmatism correction is as important as the surgical techniques used to correct astigmatism. A cataract or corneal transplant surgeon must have the confidence as well as the knowledge needed to correct astigmatism. Of course, the results of astigmatism correction are never perfect, but if the surgeon invests time and energy in reducing astigmatism, the patient will often be rewarded by being able to function well without spectacle or contact lens correction. This chapter will present the basic concepts of astigmatism and a strategy for the correction of congenital astigmatism. These principles can be applied to the prevention and correction of astigmatism associated with cataract/IOL, corneal transplant, and RK surgery.

Concepts and Principles

Regular Astigmatism

Regular corneal astigmatism exists when the meridians of greatest and least refractive power of the corneal surface are perpendicular to each other (Fig. 23.1). The dioptric power (D) of the refractive interface along any meridian of the cornea is described by the formula

$$D = \frac{n_1 - n}{r}, \text{ in which}$$

n = the *index of refraction* of air, the medium from which the light is exiting (The index of refraction correlates to the velocity of light through a given medium. Air, with an index of refraction of 1.00, is the standard against which all other media are judged; n = 1.372 for cornea, and n = 1.330 for aqueous.)
n_1 = the index of refraction of the cornea, the medium being entered by the light
r = the radius of curvature of the interface measured in meters

The net dioptric power of the cornea along a meridian is created by the major convergent refraction of the light at the air/cornea interface and the minor divergent refraction of light at the cornea/aqueous interface (Fig. 23.2). Since this latter interface produces a relatively constant refraction of about –6.00 D throughout the entire central corneal surface, the change in corneal dioptric power is accurately reflected by documenting the change of curvature of the anterior surface of the cornea. It also follows that since regular corneal astigmatism exists when the meridians of greatest and least curvature are perpendicular, then each meridian must have a different refractive power since the radius of each meridian varies. The amount of regular astigmatism equals the difference in refractive power between the meridians with the shortest and longest radius of curvature. A lens (or cornea) that exhibits a regular astigmatic surface focuses a point of light into two perpendicular lines, which are separated by an interval determined by the dioptric difference between the meridians of greatest and least dioptric power. This is different from a spherical lens, which focuses a point of light to a single point. The derivation of the word astigmatism is Greek and means away from (*a*) a point or spot (*stigma*).

Astigmatism is often referred to as *cylinder* because a cylindrical lens can be used to correct astigmatism. A cylindrical lens is actually a portion of a geometric form known as a *torus* (a doughnut shape). A cylinder is a portion of a toric surface that has one finite radius and another radius equal to infinity, which describes a circle so big that it creates a straight line (Fig. 23.3).

The notation that denotes the power of a correcting cylinder is known as positive (plus) or negative (minus). This plus or minus terminology relates to whether the refractive power of the cylinder is convergent or divergent relative to the eye. A sphero/cylindrical lens combination, such as might be found in a spectacle lens, can be described equally well in either plus or minus notation. The relationship is as follows:

1. Algebraically, add the sphere to the astigmatism and use the result as the new sphere

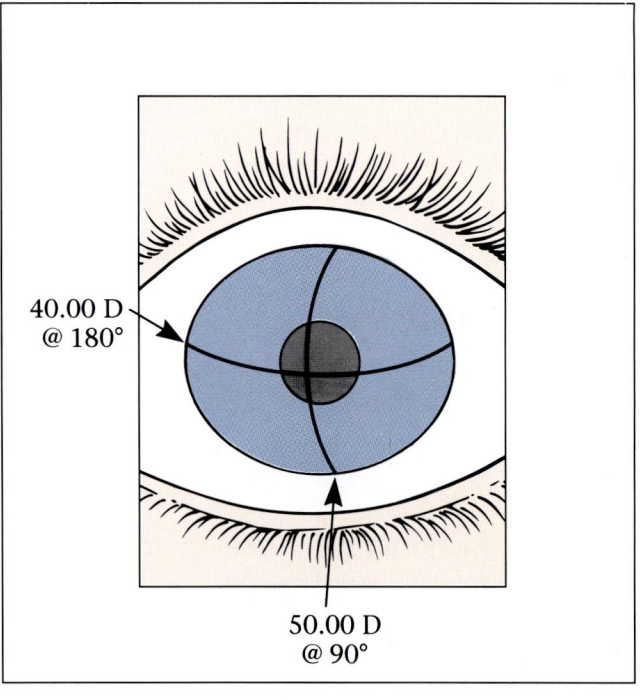

Figure 23.1 *Regular astigmatism exists when the meridians of greatest and least refractive power of a refractive surface are perpendicular to each other.*

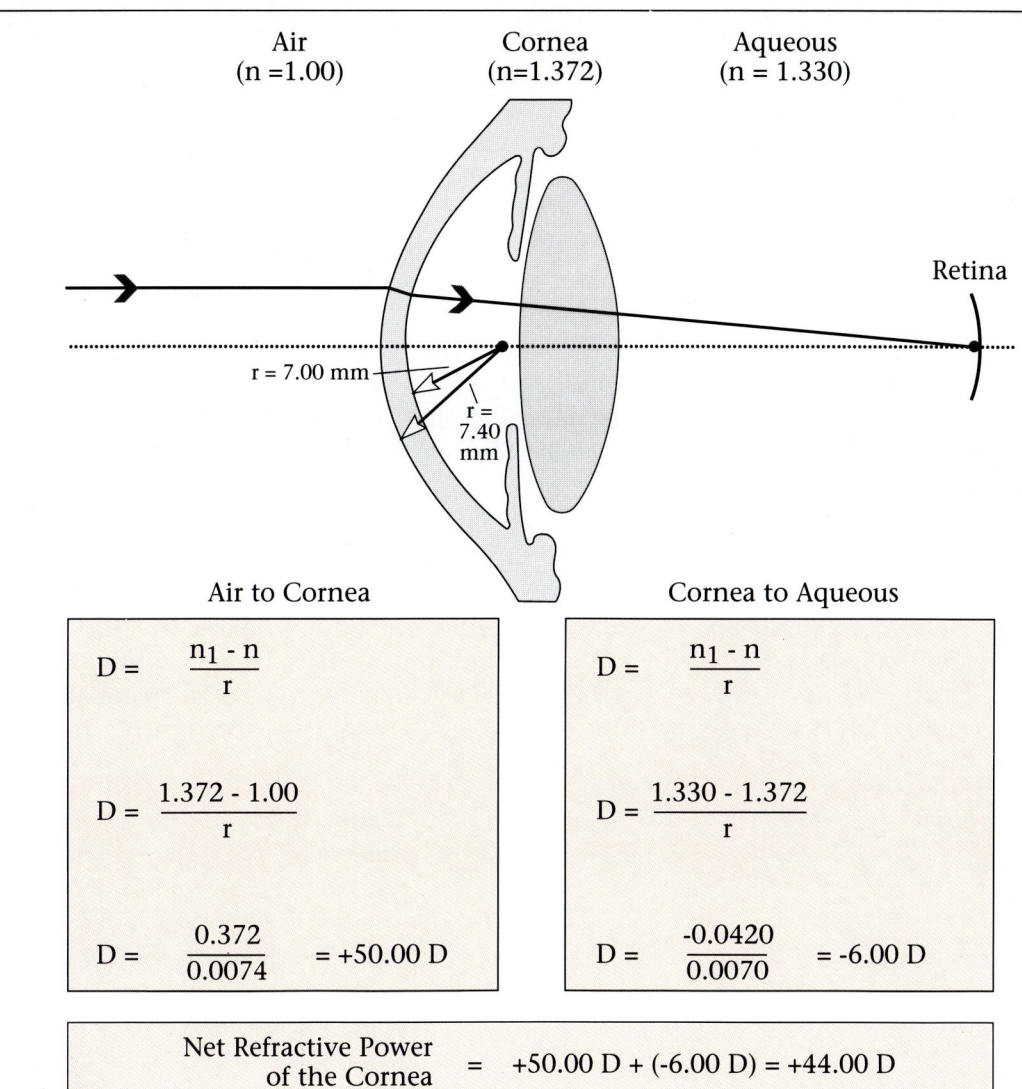

Figure 23.2 The net refractive power of the cornea is determined by the strongly convergent lens (+50.00 D) created by the air–cornea interface combined with the weakly divergent lens (−6.00 D) of the cornea–aqueous interface.

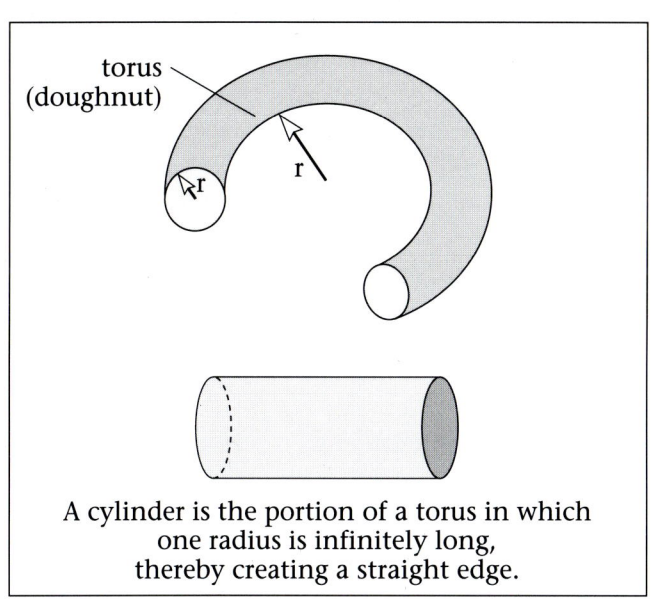

Figure 23.3 A torus is a geometric form that has two different radii of curvature, a doughnut shape. When one of the radii of a torus becomes infinitely long, it creates a straight edge and a cylinder is formed.

2. Change the power of the astigmatism and use this value as the new astigmatism

3. Change the axis of the original cylindrical lens by 90 degrees

For example:

+1.00 −3.00 × 80° = −2.00 +3.00 × 170°

Two cylindrical lenses of equal power placed with their axes perpendicular to each other produce a spherical refractive system, with all meridians having equal refractive power (Fig. 23.4). A spherical system is also created by two cylindrical lenses of equal but opposite power that are parallel to each other. Therefore, regular astigmatism can be corrected by employing a cylindrical lens to create a point focus and then, using a spherical lens that affects all meridians equally, moving this point of focus to or from the lens system so it falls on the macula (Fig. 23.5).

A patient's spectacles contain the lens necessary to correct the ametropia, and the patient's cornea is essentially the optical inverse of this corrective lens. The steeper meridian of the patient's cornea corresponds to the axis of the plus cylinder correction or 90 degrees away from the minus cylinder correction. When planning refractive surgery, it is useful to express the patient's refraction in minus cylinder form, since the sphere of the correcting lens correlates to the flattest meridian of the cornea. The primary effect of an astigmatic keratotomy (AK) is a flattening of the steepest meridian, so that, in essence, the minus cylinder portion of the correction is being removed.

Regular astigmatism may also be corrected by a spherical hard contact lens, which negates corneal astigmatism by the accumulation of tears between the contact lens and the cornea, as long as the astigmatism is not too large to affect the fit of the contact lens. Spherical soft contact lenses do not correct astigmatism well because they mimic the curvature of the corneal surface.

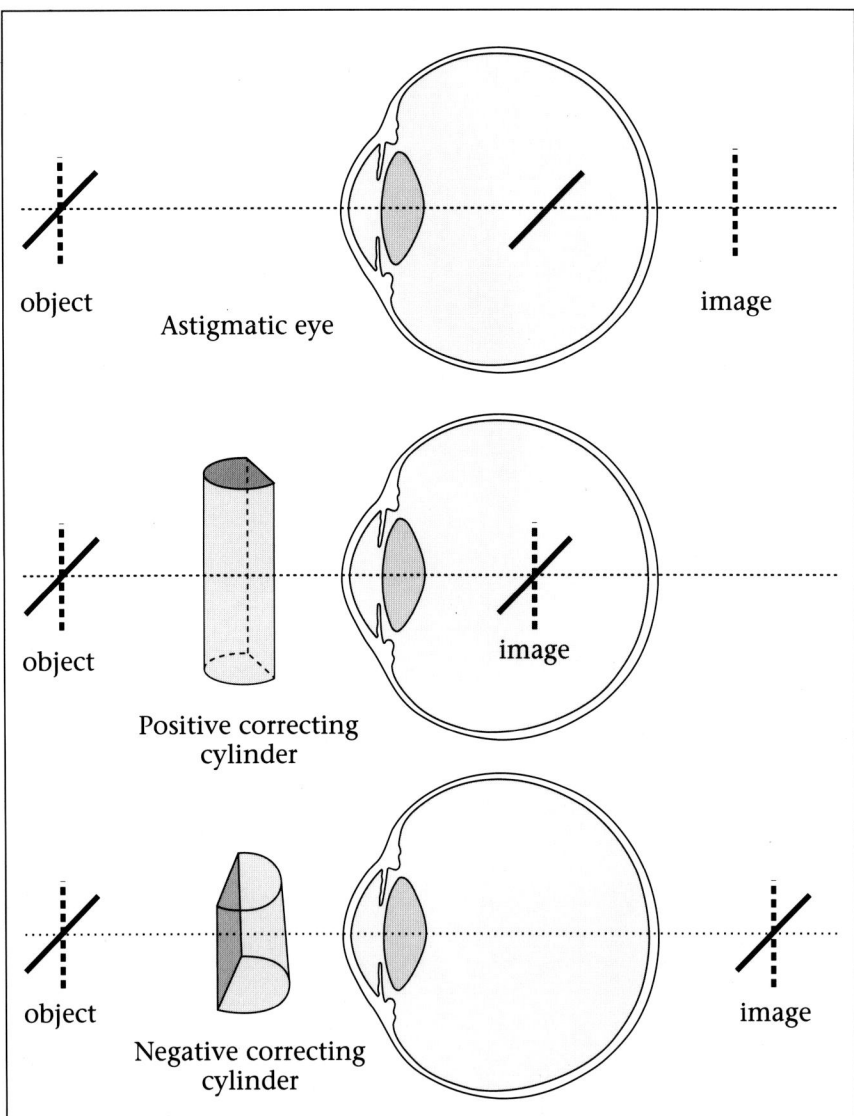

Figure 23.4 (Top) *The image of a point object that has passed through an astigmatic lens (cornea) is imaged as two focal lines, perpendicular to each other. In mixed astigmatism, one image line is focused in front of the retina and the other is theoretically focused beyond the retina.*
(Middle) *Two cylindrical lenses of equal power placed perpendicular to each other create a spherical lens system. Therefore, a correcting positive cylindrical lens positioned with its shortest radius of curvature perpendicular to the cornea's shortest radius of curvature will create a point image. Since a cylindrical lens only has refractive power perpendicular to its long axis, only one focal line will be affected. In this case, the distant focal line has been moved to join the other focal line in front of the retina.*
(Bottom) *A negative cylindrical lens with its shortest radius of curvature parallel to the shortest radius of curvature of the cornea will also convert the astigmatic cornea into a spherical lens system. In this case, however, the image line in front of the retina has been placed at a focus (theoretically) beyond the retina.*

The best approximation of an astigmatic patient's refractive status is expressed by the *spherical equivalent*, the algebraic sum of the sphere plus one-half of the astigmatism:

$$\text{Spherical Equivalent} = \text{Sphere} + \frac{\text{Astigmatism}}{2}$$

This resultant sphere represents the smallest blur circle in Sturm's conoid that allows for the best vision possible with spherical correction only. This concept is important when the surgeon must balance spherical and astigmatic values and their respective effects on uncorrected visual acuity (as will be discussed later) (Fig. 23.6).

With-the-rule astigmatism is astigmatism with the steeper meridian (+ axis of correcting cylindrical lens) vertical ± 30 degrees. *Against-the-rule astigmatism* is astigmatism with the steeper

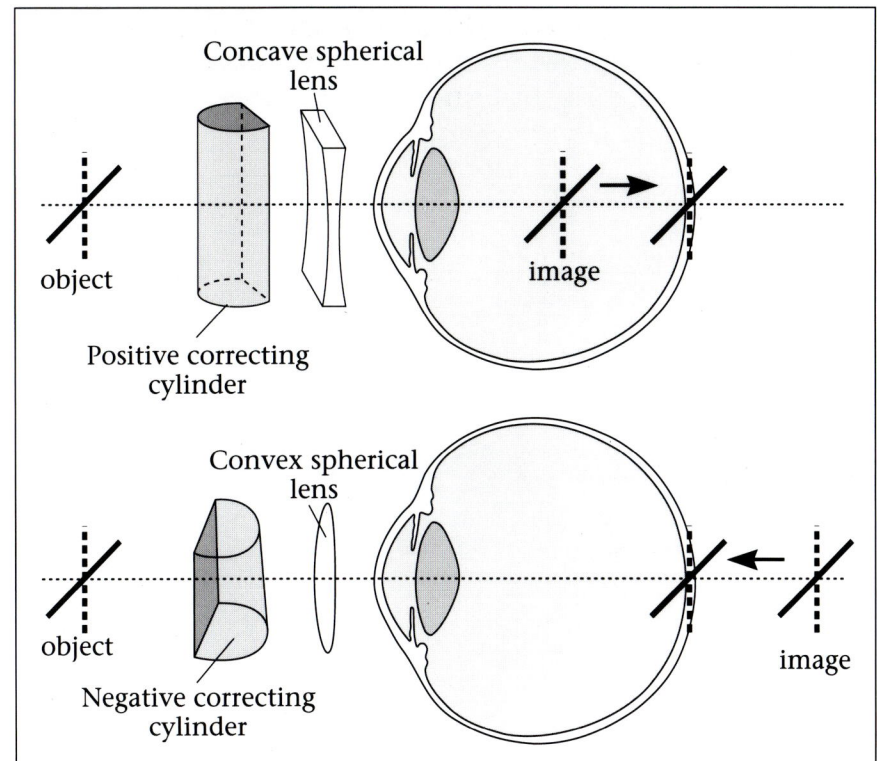

Figure 23.5 (Top) *A concave spherical lens can now be used to focus the point image created by the positive correcting cylindrical lens in Figure. 23.4 on the retina for clear vision.* (Bottom) *A convex spherical lens can now be used to focus the point image created by the negative correcting cylindrical lens in Figure 23.4 on the retina for clear vision.*

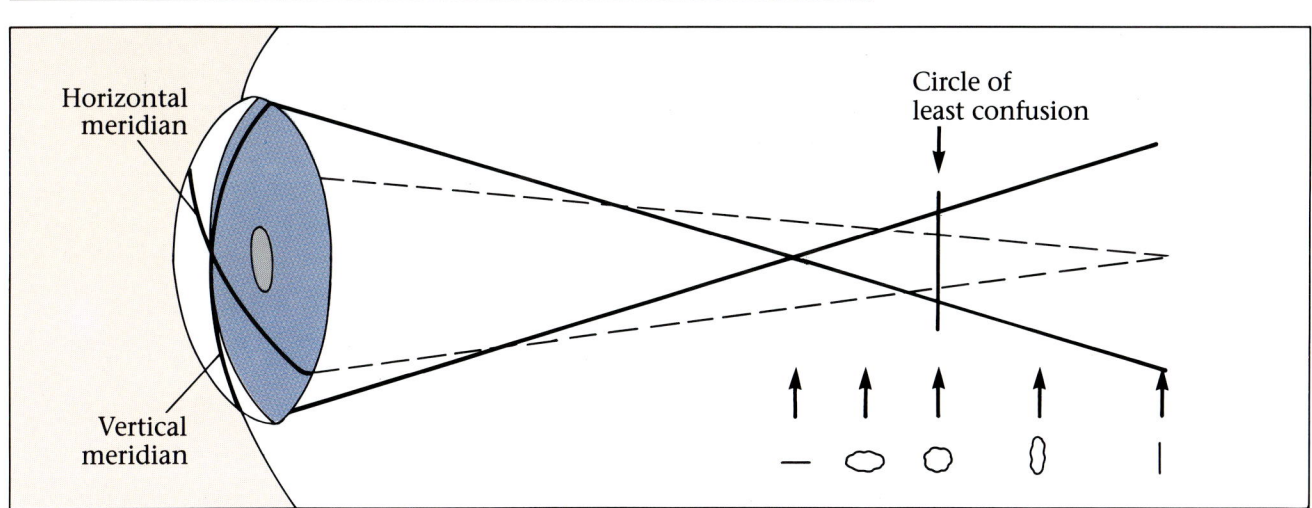

Figure 23.6 *Sturm's conoid is defined by the interval between the focal lines of an astigmatic image, which includes the circle of least confusion. The circle of least confusion is located dioptrically halfway between the two focal lines. The circle of least confusion represents the spherical equivalent of the eye and the point at which both focal lines are equally out of focus, thereby creating a blurry but circular image.*

meridian (+ axis of correcting cylindrical lens) horizontal ± 30 degrees. *Oblique astigmatism* is astigmatism that is neither with-the-rule nor against-the-rule (Fig. 23.7).

The term *meridian*, when used properly, refers to the orientation of the line created by the intersection of the corneal surface with an imaginary plane that passes through the center of the cornea, perpendicular to its surface. For example, the orientation of an AK could be described as a T-cut performed on the 80th meridian, commonly referred to as the 80-degree meridian, although the word *degree* is not truly applicable (Fig. 23.8).

The term *axis*, when used properly, applies only to the orientation of the cylinder of the correcting lens and is stated in degrees. In North America, the axis of the correcting cylindrical lens is measured in both the right and left eye from the observer's right, starting horizontally at 180 degrees and proceeding in a superior circular manner toward the observer's left to 180 degrees. However, the International method starts horizontally from the observer's right for the patient's right eye (as in North America) but from the observer's left toward the right in the patient's left eye. The right eye is measured identically in each system (Fig. 23.9). The astigmatism axis for the left eye, however, may

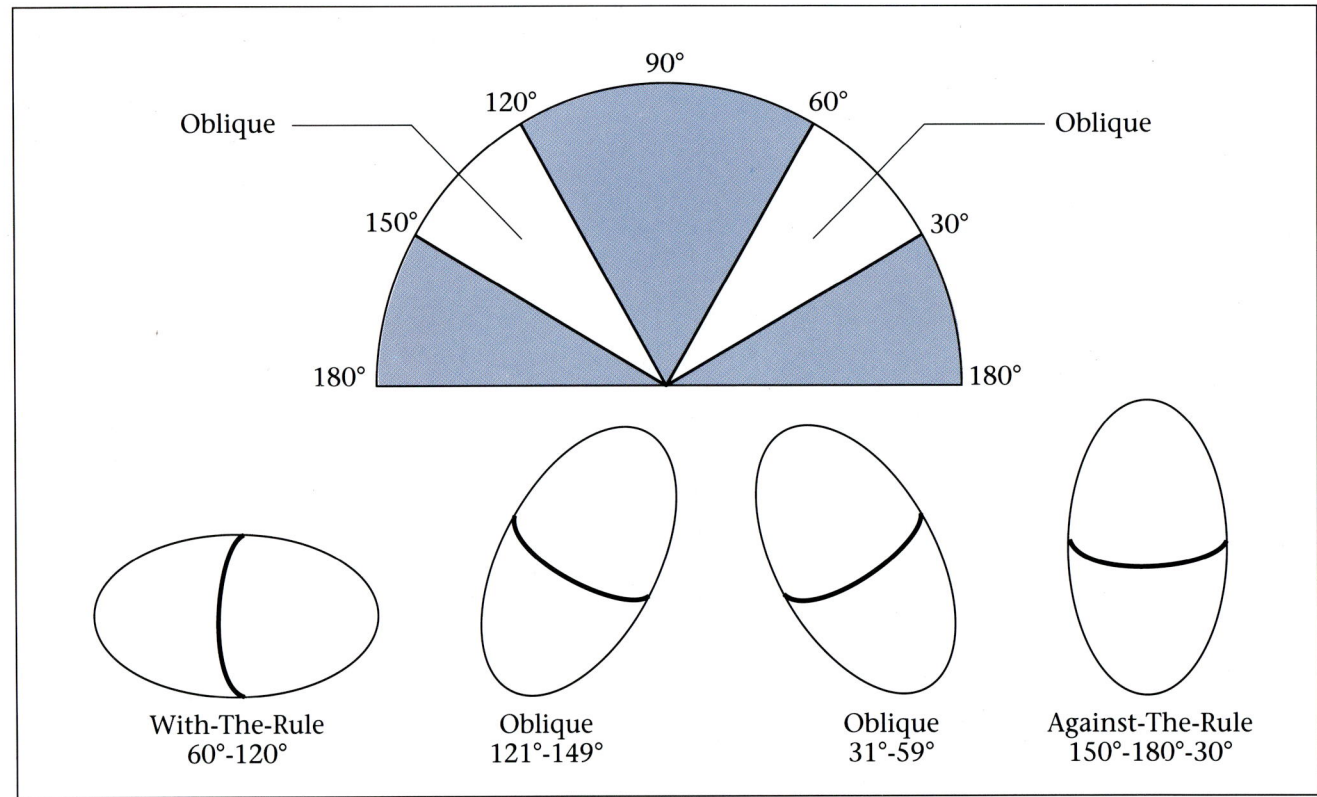

Figure 23.7 *With-the-rule, oblique, and against-the-rule astigmatism.*

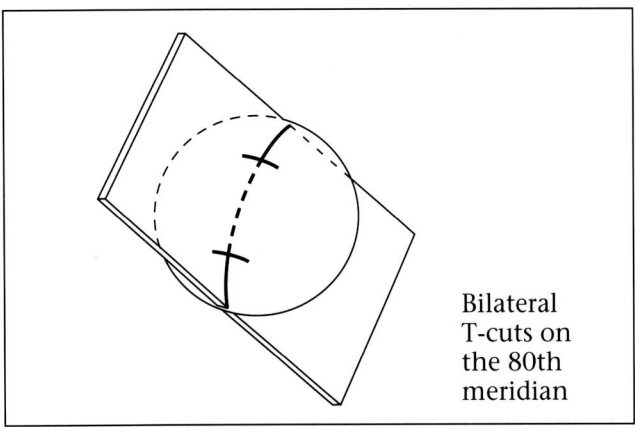

Figure 23.8 *The term* meridian *relates to position relative to the cornea. This diagram shows a cornea that has had an astigmatic keratotomy performed on the 80th meridian. The term* axis *relates to the orientation of the correcting cylindrical lens and is measured in degrees.*

be converted between the two formats by subtracting the given axis from 180 degrees.

Irregular Astigmatism

Often overlooked is *irregular astigmatism*, which is present when the refractive surface of the cornea exhibits variations in refractive power because the meridians of greatest and least power are not perpendicular to each other. This irregular optical surface is a microscopic phenomenon and may exist despite an apparently clear cornea. Irregular astigmatism may be caused by an epithelial phenomenon such as punctate keratitis or by a stromal problem such as keratoconus or scarring (Fig. 23.10). The stromal scarring may be adjacent to the visual axis and still cause significant irregular astigmatism of the central cornea (Fig. 23.11). In both cases, the air–epithelium interface is the site of irregular astigmatism, even though the pathology may be stromal since

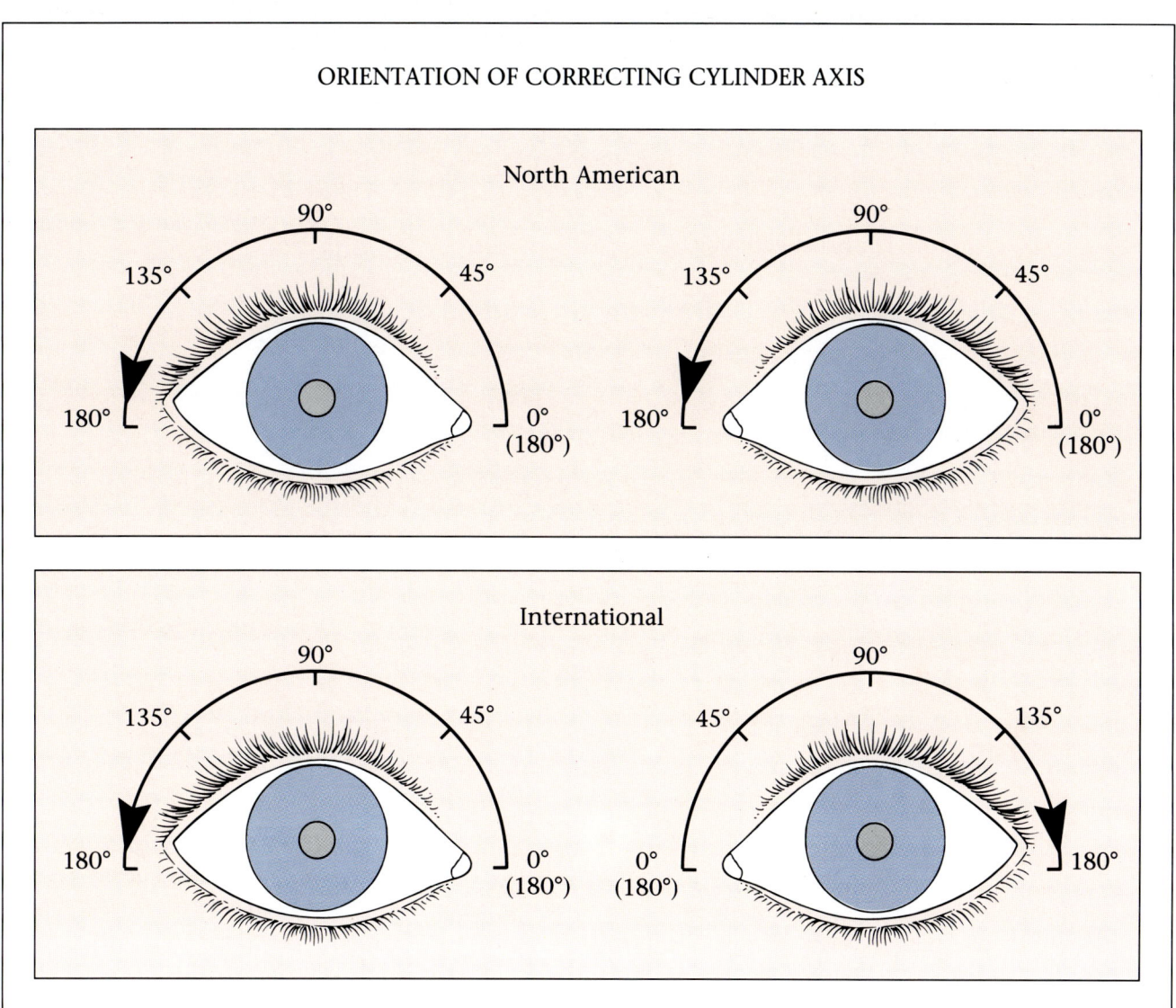

Figure 23.9 *The relationship between the North American and the International method of defining the axis of a correcting cylindrical lens. Note that the right eye is measured identically in each method but the left eye is measured differently.*

the normal epithelium undulates as dictated by the underlying stroma.

During an anterior segment examination, irregular astigmatism is one of the most overlooked conditions. Consider the following clinical examples:

• A cataract/IOL patient who is two weeks postoperative has best corrected visual acuity of 20/40 despite a normal preoperative exam and totally uncomplicated surgery. The surgeon suspects a mild maculopathy. Very often this patient has a subtle irregular astigmatism induced by a corneal wound that was not oriented with either the major or minor meridian of the preoperative cornea. Therefore, a "scissors action" takes place with resultant transient irregular astigmatism (Fig. 23.12).

• A patient sustains a penetrating wound to the cornea by means of a foreign body. A corneal scar adjacent to the visual axis results in a profound drop in visual acuity despite best attempts at correction. The patient is subjected to flourescein angiography, field examination, and repeated extensive indirect ophthalmoscopic examinations in an attempt to explain the decrease in vision. An astute anterior segment surgeon performs keratometry and diagnoses irregular astigmatism. Vision returns to 20/20 with a hard contact lens.

• Three refractive surgery patients, who have undergone myopic keratomileusis, laser corneal

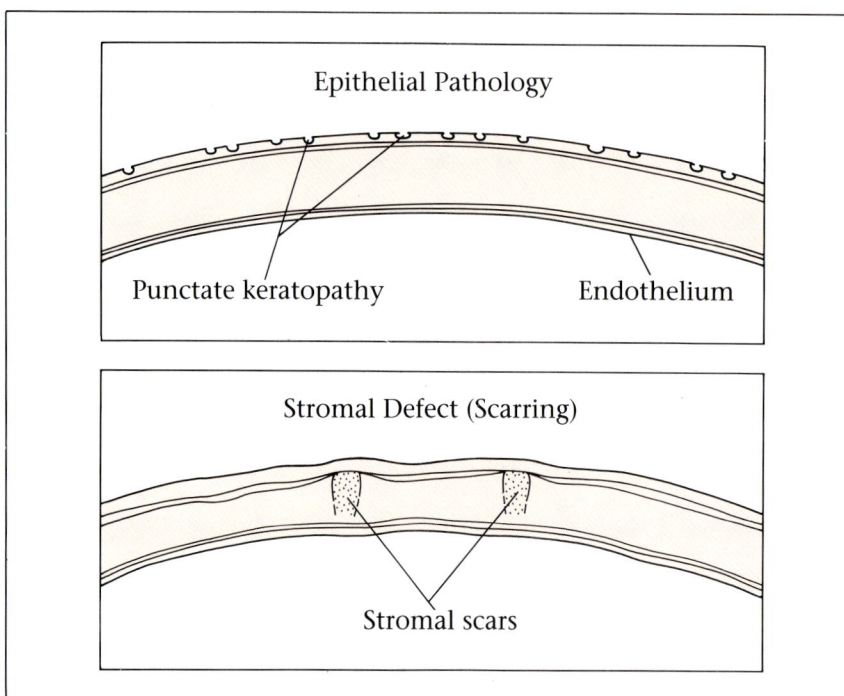

Figure 23.10 *Irregular astigmatism may have an epithelial or a stromal basis.*

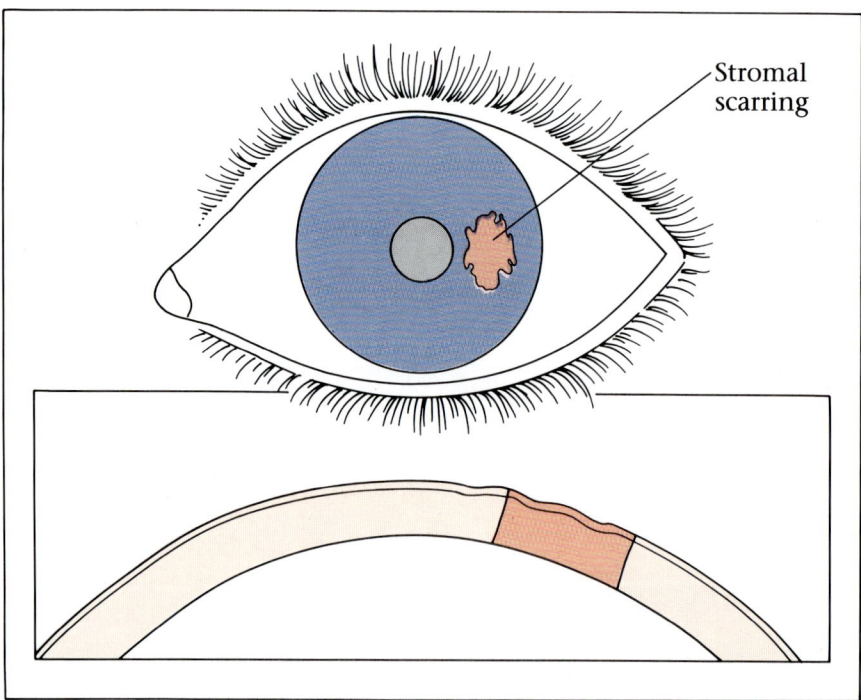

Figure 23.11 *The visual axis may be affected by irregular astigmatism caused by an adjacent stromal defect.*

ablation for myopia, and myopic alloplastic intracorneal implantation, respectively, are relatively satisfied with their results, but state that their uncorrected and best spectacle corrected acuity is not up to par with their preoperative spectacle correction. All operated corneas are crystal clear; however, keratometry demonstrates subtle irregular astigmatism in all cases. Improved quality of vision is achieved with a hard contact lens.

• An 18-year-old female has not worn hard contact lenses since they were lost three months ago. In each eye, uncorrected visual acuity is 20/70, which is correctable with glasses to 20/20− in the right eye and 20/30 in the left. Slit lamp exam reveals no corneal abnormality bilaterally but keratometry demonstrates barely irregular keratometric mires in both eyes. A diagnosis of mild keratoconus is made.

Diagnosis

Regular and irregular corneal astigmatism are best diagnosed using a keratometer. In the United States the B&L (Bausch and Lomb, recently renamed Reichert) keratometer is the most widely used and will be described here (Fig. 23.13), although other keratometers function in essentially the same manner. The B&L keratometer func-

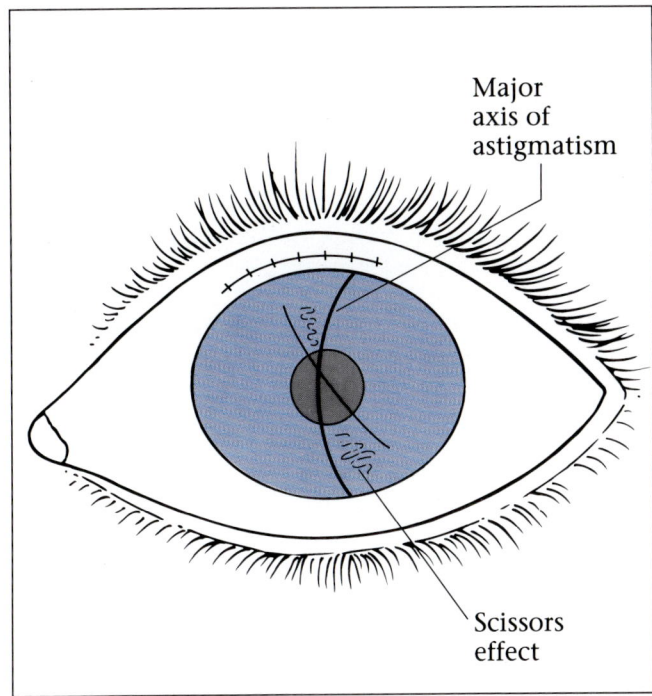

Figure 23.12 *A limbal wound that is not oriented on the steeper or flatter meridian of the cornea may cause transient corneal irregular astigmatism with a temporary reduction in visual acuity.*

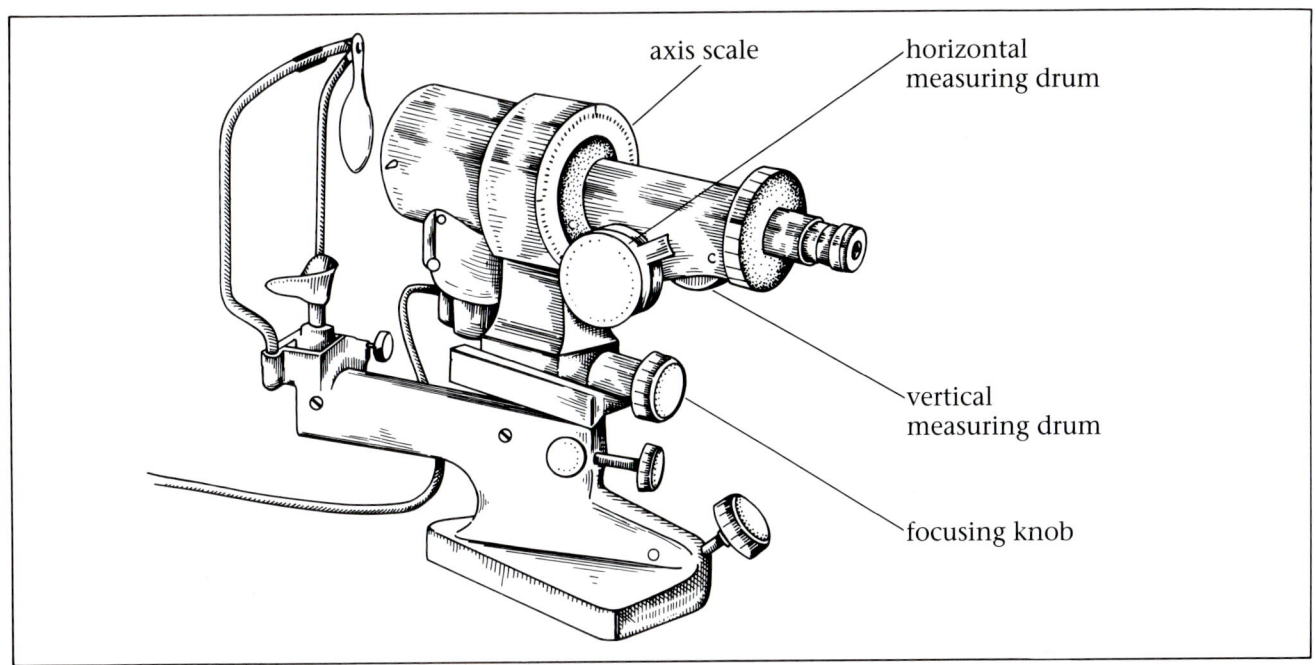

Figure 23.13 *The B&L (Reichert) keratometer and its components.*

tions by projecting a circular object onto the cornea and allowing the mirror-like qualities of the cornea to project the image mire back to the observer (Fig. 23.14). Doubling prisms offset the image vertically and horizontally. When the virtual image created by the reflective property of the cornea is brought into exact overlap and focus with the object circle, the keratometer is at the proper focal distance from the cornea.

The refractive power of the greatest and least powerful meridians are measured in diopters by aligning the perpendicular dioptric power indicators using the control knobs and rotating the barrel of the keratometer to insure that the meridians of greatest and least power are being measured (Fig. 23.15). The keratometer measures only the refractive power of the front surface of the cornea, then automatically subtracts an *assumed* negative dioptric value for the refractive power of the cornea-aqueous interface to yield a net diopter value for the cornea. Every keratometer manufacturer assumes a different value for the index of refraction of the cornea, so the assumed value is slightly different for each brand, with absolute values varying among them. The portion of the mire observed through the keratometer ocular correlates to the corneal topography 180 degrees opposite; i.e., a scar at the inferior border of the visual axis will cause an irregularity at the superior border of the circular mire.

Astigmatism quantification depends on the diopters of difference between the two meridians, rather than on the absolute readings. Remember, a keratometer measures only *corneal* astigmatism. If best correction is obtained with a spectacle that has a cylindrical component different from the keratometric astigmatism, this usually implies lenticular astigmatism or, possibly, astigmatism induced by a posterior staphyloma. In other words, the vector addition of lenticular astigmatism plus corneal astigmatism equals the best correcting cylinder (Fig. 23.16). The average lenticular astigmatism is –0.50 D against-the-rule.

The corneal surgeon should only perform an AK or wound recession on the steeper meridian of the cornea, since that is the only orientation

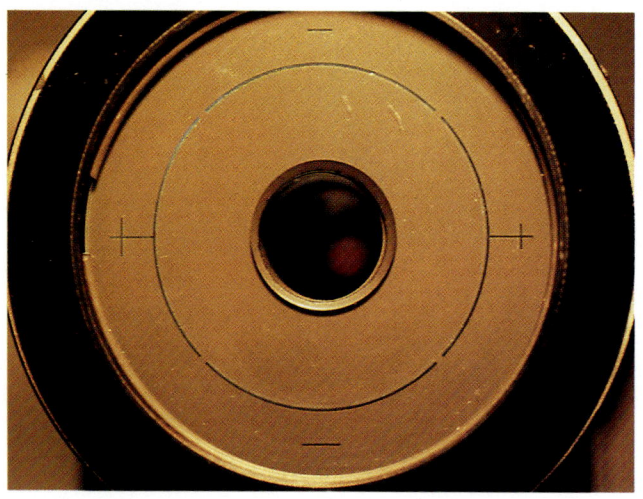

Figure 23.14 *When illuminated, this end of the keratometer projects a circular image onto the cornea.*

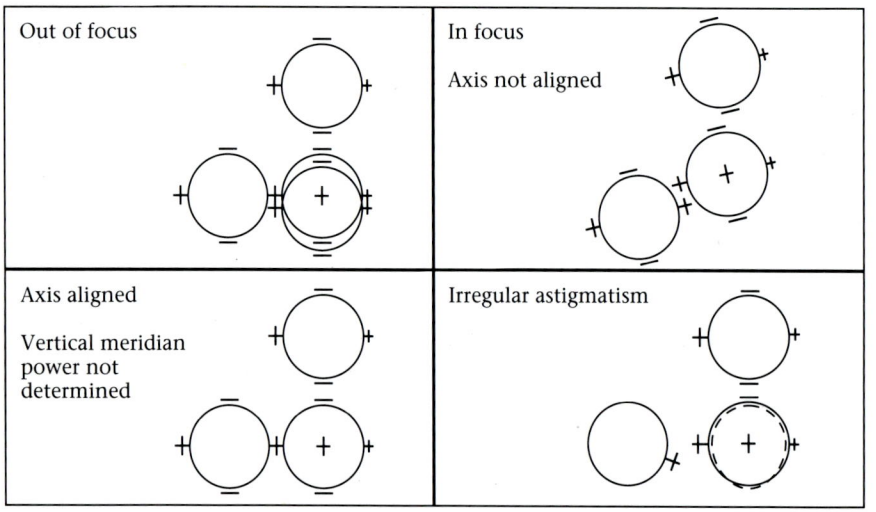

Figure 23.15 *Keratometry mires. (Top left) keratometer slightly out of focus (central circles not overlapping); (top right) keratometer in focus but not at the position of the axis of astigmatism; (bottom left) dioptric power of the cornea measured horizontally (overlap of central circle and + signs) but not vertically (– signs not overlapped); (bottom right) irregular astigmatism, in which the central circles and the + and – signs never coincide exactly.*

that produces quantifiable results. Therefore, when the keratometric astigmatism varies from the refractive astigmatism, the goal of astigmatic surgery should be to reduce the corneal astigmatism to a value that produces the least refractive cylinder. Creating no corneal cylinder would actually "bare" the lenticular astigmatism. To meet this goal clinically, plan surgery on the steeper *keratometric axis* for the amount of the *refractive cylinder*. The vector addition of the lenticular astigmatism plus the corneal astigmatism will then yield the best result, i.e., the smallest possible refractive astigmatism (Fig. 23.17).

As stated above, a mire is the light projected by the keratometer onto the cornea and reflected by the mirror-like quality of the cornea. A thin, con-

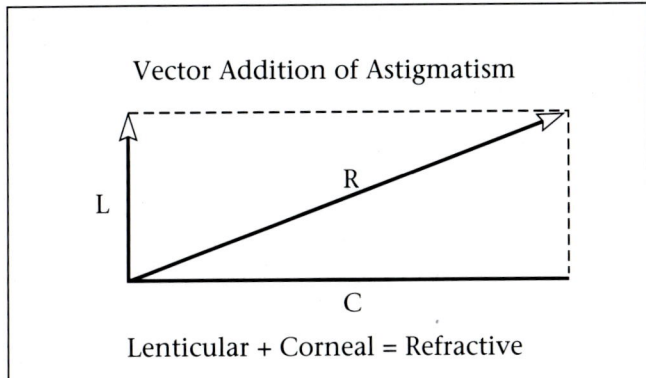

Figure 23.16 *By the laws of vector addition, corneal astigmatism plus lenticular astigmatism equals refractive astigmatism.*

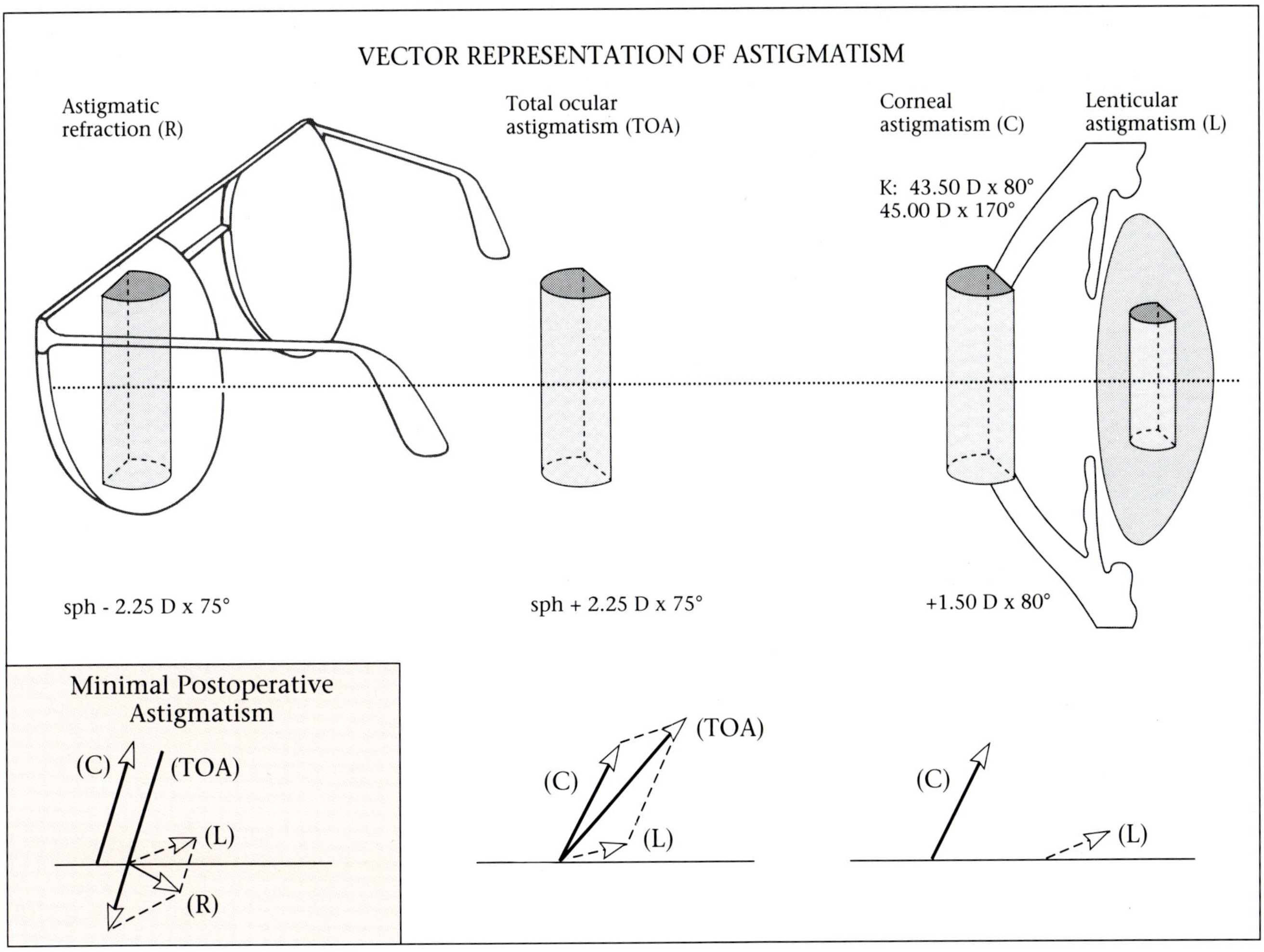

Figure 23.17 *The vector addition of lenticular astigmatism (L) plus corneal astigmatism (C) equals total ocular astigmatism (TOA). The refractive cylinder (R) is the optical inverse of the TOA. Astigmatic surgery performed on the steeper meridian of the cornea that corrects for the amount of refractive cylinder produces the least postoperative astigmatism.*

sistent mire that allows for exact overlap of the central circular or oval mires indicates regular astigmatism. A poor quality mire indicates an irregular epithelial surface. High quality mires that are not circular or oval and cannot be overlapped indicate irregular astigmatism of the cornea, which is caused by a stromal defect. All anterior segment surgeons should become experienced in judging the quality of keratometric mires. The mire's poor overlap can be graded from 0 to 4+, and an experienced observer can roughly correlate the loss in visual acuity with the loss of mire quality (Fig. 23.18). Only a slight irregularity of the mire can easily indicate a reduction of visual acuity to the 20/40 to 20/50 range.

A quantifiable measure of irregular astigmatism can be made by comparing best corrected spectacle and hard contact lens acuities. The hard contact lens acts as a perfect corneal surface with the tear film filling in the spaces between the back of

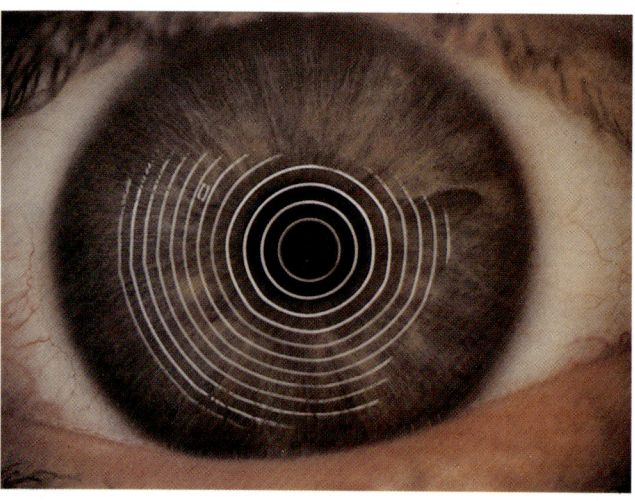
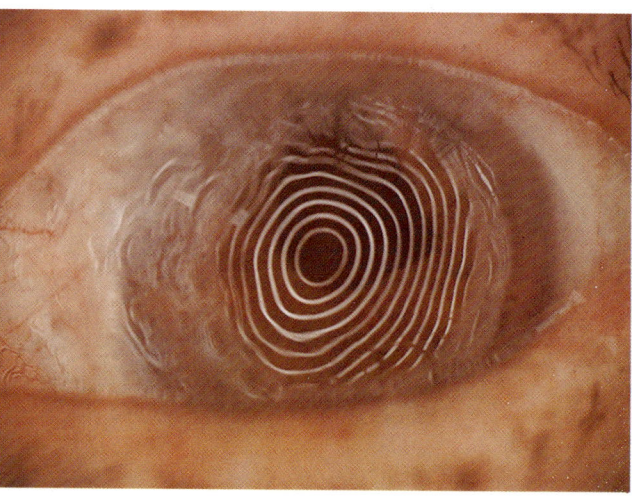

Figure 23.18 **(Left)** *Corneoscope photograph following an eight-incision radial keratotomy. The slight noncircularity of the corneal mires from the third ring outward indicates the presence of irregular astigmatism at these locations. The irregular astigmatism is not clinically significant in this situation.* **(Right)** *A Corneoscope study showing irregular astigmatism; inter-mire distance, mire shape, and mire thickness vary erratically. Irregular astigmatism caused by an epithelial abnormality, e.g. punctate keratopathy, produces a poorly defined keratometric mire and irregular astigmatism caused by a stromal abnormality, e.g., keratoconus, produces irregular central circles that cannot be overlapped.*

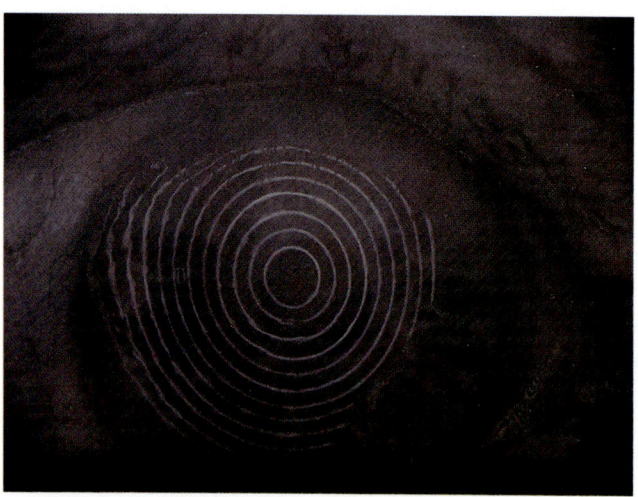

Figure 23.19 *Three year postoperative corneoscope photograph of a patient who had a preoperative cataract/IOL refraction with 2.50 D of against-the-rule astigmatism. Keratometry was 45.00 D @ 5° and 42.75 D @ 95°. Tight prolene sutures were used to close the wound in an attempt to correct the astigmatism. Keratometry readings three years postoperatively are 45.25 D @ 5° and 41.50 D @ 95°, as indicated by the horizontal ovality of the corneoscopic mires.*

the contact lens and the cornea. The difference in lines of visual acuity offers a quantification of the severity of the irregular astigmatism.

Irregular astigmatism = Snellen acuity (hard contact lens) vs. snellen acuity (spectacles).
For example:
Vision with hard contact lens = 20/30
Vision with spectacles = 20/100

Loss of six Snellen lines due to irregular astigmatism is demonstrated.

In addition to reduction in Snellen acuity, irregular astigmatism causes a reduction in the quality of vision by means of less contrast and more blur. It is akin to the image degradation caused by the mist on a mirror.

Corneal topography instruments are not nearly as sensitive as the keratometer in detecting irregular astigmatism because these instruments must attempt to quantify the corneal surface, despite minimal corneal surface irregularity. Also, the larger magnification of the discrete keratometer mire makes irregular astigmatism more noticeable. Corneal topography displays may appear normal while the keratometer demonstrates subtle irregular astigmatism that may account for the loss of several lines of vision. Corneal refractive surgery procedures should be evaluated with a keratometer, not only a topography instrument, which represents the general shape of the cornea by attractive color pictures but does not indicate the quality of the cornea's refractive surface with great sensitivity. Although the diameter of the keratometer mire varies slightly with the curvature of the central cornea, *the keratometer is still the best clinical method of assessing the functional status of the cornea in the visual axis.*

Irregular astigmatism is the factor that limits the success of virtually all corneal refractive procedures. If the postoperative patient is not able to be corrected by spectacles to within at least one-half of a Snellen acuity line compared to the preoperative level of spectacle vision, then the legitimacy of a given procedure must be questioned.

AK can correct regular astigmatism only, *not* irregular astigmatism. Both regular and irregular astigmatism may coexist. Therefore, AK on a keratoconic patient is not usually warranted because, despite the correction of regular astigmatism (if it remains stable), the patient will not see well due to the irregular astigmatism.

Correction

Now that astigmatism, in general, has been presented consider the realities of correcting regular astigmatism. Specific decisions concerning the risk/benefit and the surgical strategy must be made.

Theoretically, there are two ways to correct regular astigmatism: *steepen the flatter meridian of the cornea* or *flatten the steeper meridian of the cornea*. Clinically, however, the only quantifiable, long-term method of astigmatism correction is to flatten the steeper meridian, i.e., increase the radius of curvature of the stronger refractive meridian. Flattening the steeper meridian can be accomplished by *wound recession (slippage)* or *AK*.

Three methods of astigmatism correction that do not generally provide long-term quantifiable correction for structurally normal corneal and limbal anatomy were the best available for many years. These ineffective methods of astigmatism correction include steepening the flatter meridian by:

Wedge resection
Tight sutures
Collagen shrinkage by heat or diathermy

These methods require purposeful overcorrection and/or tissue compression by tight sutures. With time, the sutures must be removed, resulting in decompressed tissue; however, the intraocular pressure may stretch the wound, causing the astigmatism to gradually reappear. Consider the refractive status of 3.00 D against-the-rule patients who have undergone cataract extraction and have had no special treatment for their preexisting astigmatism, other than tight sutures. Virtually all of these patients will have regained their original against-the-rule astigmatism after several years, even though the nonbiodegradable suture may be in place (Fig. 23.19).

Astigmatic Keratotomy
MECHANICS

Consider the cornea to be a portion of a circle that represents the cross section of a globe. An AK or wound recession adds length to the circumference of the circle, causing an increase in the radius of curvature of the cornea and a decrease in refractive power. This model is a convenient way to remember the action of an AK as

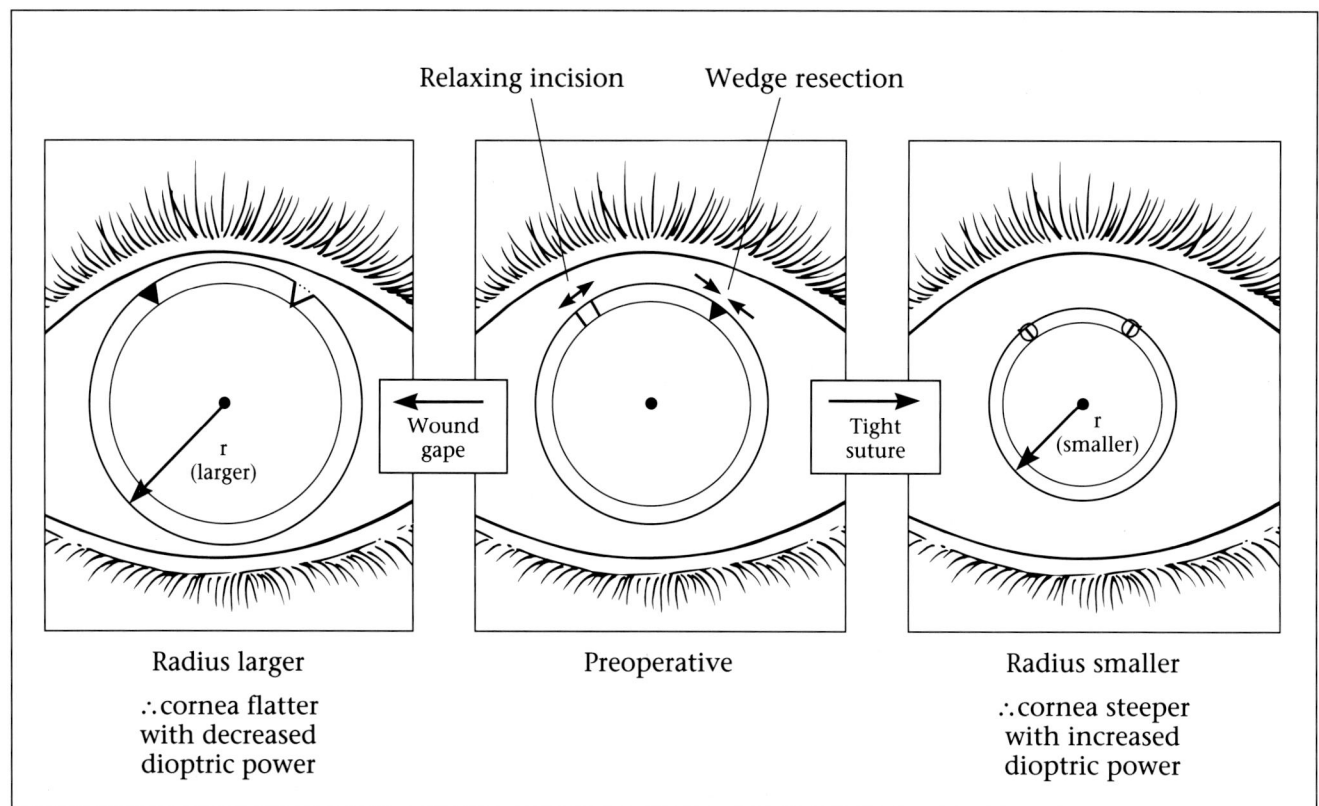

Figure 23.20 *Consider the cross-section of the globe as a circle when determining the effects of various procedures on the central cornea. Astigmatic keratotomy and wound recession create a circle with a larger diameter, thereby reducing the dioptric power of the central cornea. Tight sutures and wound resection create a circle with a smaller diameter, thereby increasing (transiently, at least) the dioptric power of the central cornea.*

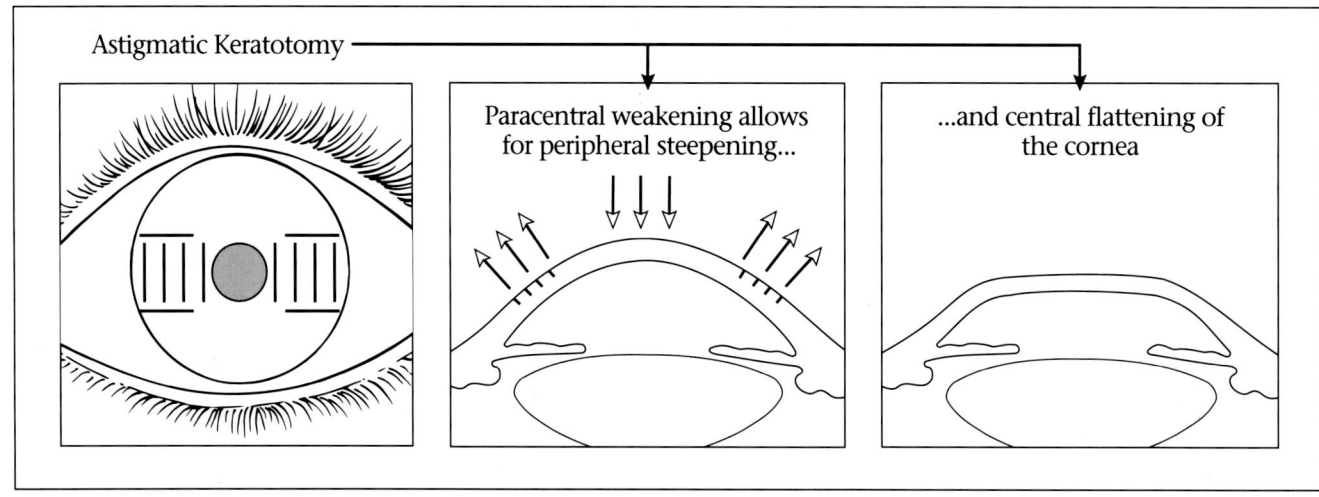

Figure 23.21 *An astigmatic keratotomy causes a steepening of the paracentral cornea with a compensatory flattening of the central cornea.*

well as the effects of a tight suture or resection, which causes the reverse phenomenon (Fig. 23.20).

In actuality, it is important to remember that only the central cornea is the area of concern. AK causes a steepening of the paracentral area of the cornea and a secondary central flattening because the dome-shaped cornea is anchored at the limbus (Fig. 23.21). The midperiphery is weakened by both radial and transverse incisions, thus creating the same qualitative effect on the central cornea. Transverse incisions are more effective than radial ones in flattening the central cornea because they allow for more gape of the wound with increased steepening of the midperiphery of the cornea. Similarly, a tight suture actually flattens the cornea at its point of application and causes a secondary central steepening (Fig. 23.22).

Wound recession or AK corrects astigmatism mostly by flattening the central portion of the corneal meridian in which it is performed. Concomitantly, however, a slight-to-moderate steepening of the meridian perpendicular to the involved meridian occurs. This phenomenon is analogous to squeezing a tennis ball and letting it regain sphericity by releasing pressure on the steeper meridian (Fig. 23.23); both meridians change simultaneously but in opposite directions. This concomitant but opposite change in perpendicular meridians during astigmatism is called *coupling*.

Therefore, a 6.00 D astigmatism with a keratometry reading of 40.00 D @ 180° and 46.00 D @ 90°, for example, is corrected by reducing the 46.00 D to 42.00 D and increasing the 40.00 D to 42.00 D, even though the AK was performed only at the 90th meridian (Fig. 23.24). AK does *not* correct this 6.00 D of astigmatism by reducing the 46.00 D to 40.00 D with no change in the flatter meridian. There is great significance in the amount of steepening of the flatter meridian because the shift of the flatter meridian represents the amount of myopia induced in the spherical component of the postoperative refraction (Fig. 23.25).

The *coupling ratio* is determined by the *length of the transverse incision* of the AK; that is, the

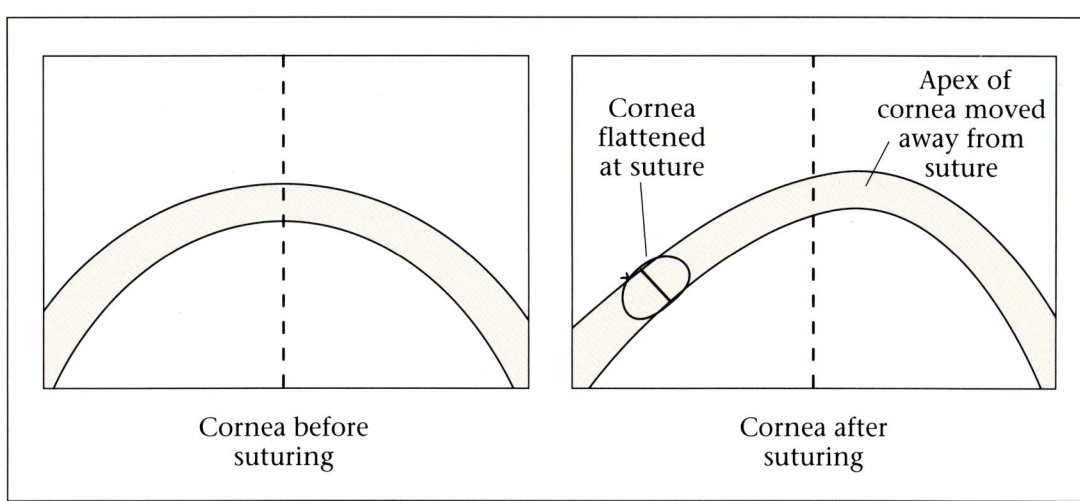

Figure 23.22 *A tight suture causes a flattening of the peripheral cornea with a compensatory steepening of the central cornea; however, the apex of the dome of the cornea has been shifted slightly away from the suture.*

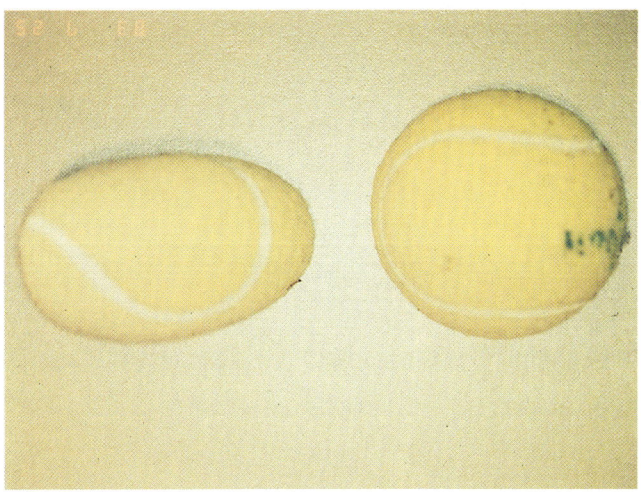

Figure 23.23 *A tennis ball model is useful in depicting the action of astigmatic keratotomy. As the tennis ball (cornea) becomes round (goes from astigmatic to spherical) both meridians change but in opposite directions.*

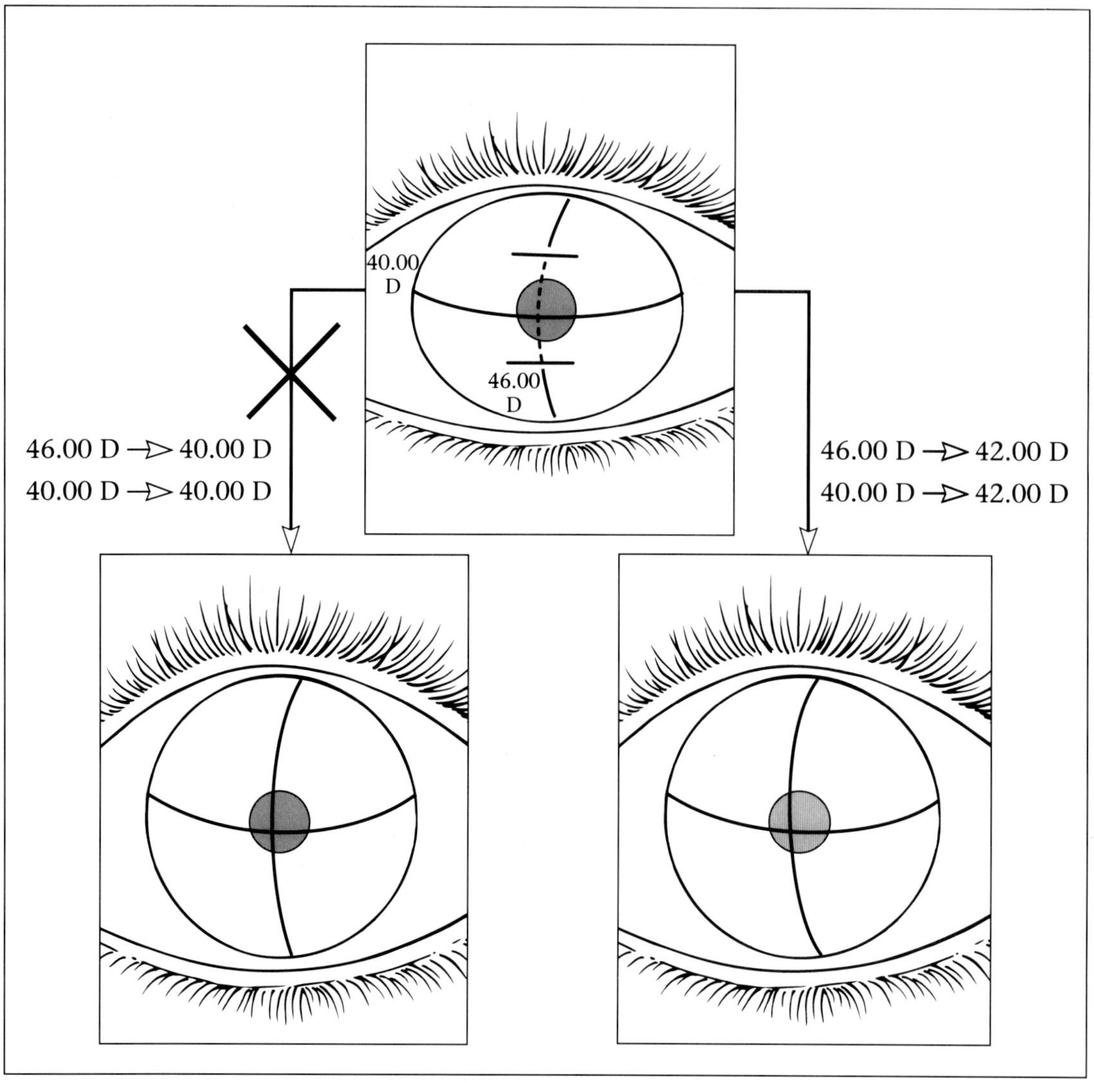

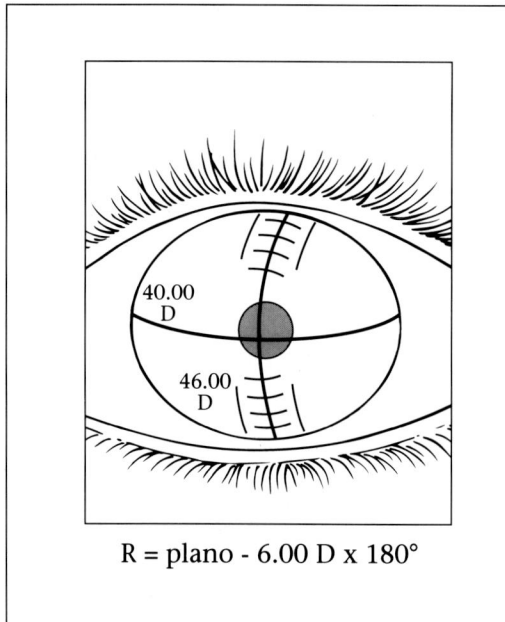

Figure 23.24
An astigmatic keratotomy on the 90th meridian causes central corneal flattening of its own meridian and some central corneal steepening of the 180th meridian.

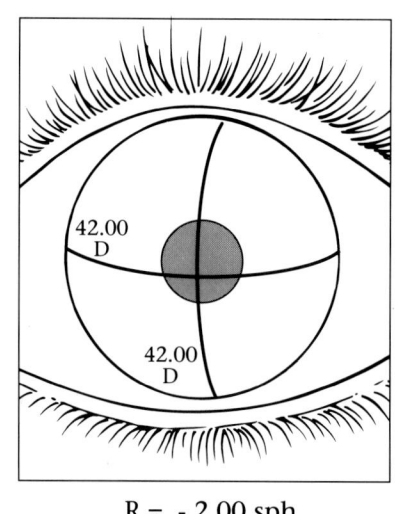

Figure 23.25
Following astigmatic keratotomy, the spherical equivalent becomes more hyperopic but the spherical component becomes more myopic.

longer the transverse incision, the more the flatter meridian will steepen. This principle can be used advantageously when correcting hyperopia that coexists with myopic astigmatism. Thus, the narrowest Ruiz procedure possible would be used to correct astigmatism in a compound myopic astigmatism case, when this configuration of AK is combined with RK in order to induce the least amount of extra myopia. Coupling is not quantifiable when performing an AK on a penetrating keratoplasty (PKP), since the circular corneal scar disrupts the normal dynamics of the AK relative to the limbus.

A successful AK causes the *spherical equivalent* of a patient's refraction to become more *hyperopic*, even though the *spherical component* is made more *myopic*. Consider the following example:

Preoperative:
  Plano $-3.00 \times 90°$ (spherical equivalent = $-1.50D$)
Postoperative:
  -1.00 sph (spherical equivalent = $-1.00D$)

  Spherical equivalent: $-1.50D \rightarrow -1.00D$

Also, AK performed with a flat blade on a domed cornea in a relatively straight line will not cause an equal amount of gape in the wound. Therefore, a certain degree of irregular astigmatism develops on both sides of a transverse AK incision. For this reason, a large optical zone (OZ) is very desirable for AK since the functional OZ is reduced by at least 0.50 mm (Fig. 23.26).

We favor a 7.00 mm OZ, when possible, as the best AK–OZ compromise between adequate effect and reduced symptomatology with pupillary dilation. A constant OZ and consistent incision depth allows the effect of the AK to be correlated to the only other variable—incision length.

ASPHERICITY

The AK incision creates a paracentral knee in the cornea with a resultant aspheric cornea, similar to that found with RK (Fig. 23.27). This concept of asphericity is discussed more fully in Chapter 2, but is nicely demonstrated by the following case.

A 37-year-old male eye surgeon had the following refractive error:

  OD: $+2.50 - 2.25 \times 165° = 20/15$; sc = 20/40
  OS: $+1.75 - 1.75 \times 15° = 20/15$; sc = 20/40–

The patient desired improved vision without correction; was uncomfortable with hard contact lenses because of dry eye; and, due to the presence of the $+2.00$ D cylinder, did not tolerate the poor quality of vision obtained from soft contact lenses.

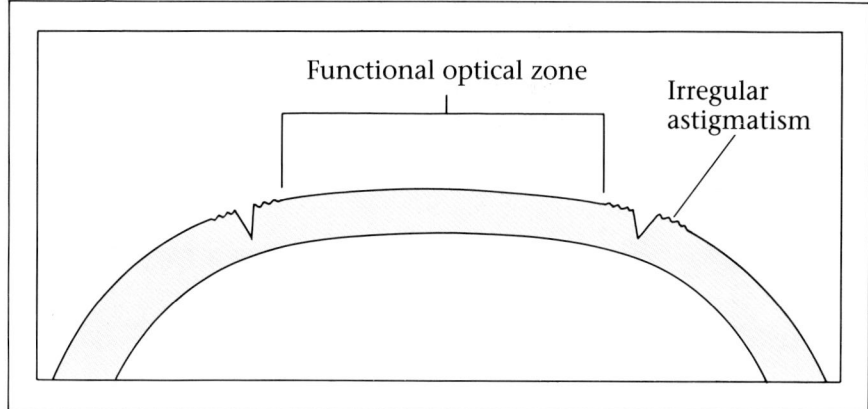

Figure 23.26 *Astigmatic keratotomy creates a functional optical zone that is smaller than the actual optical zone because irregular astigmatism surrounds the transverse corneal incisions.*

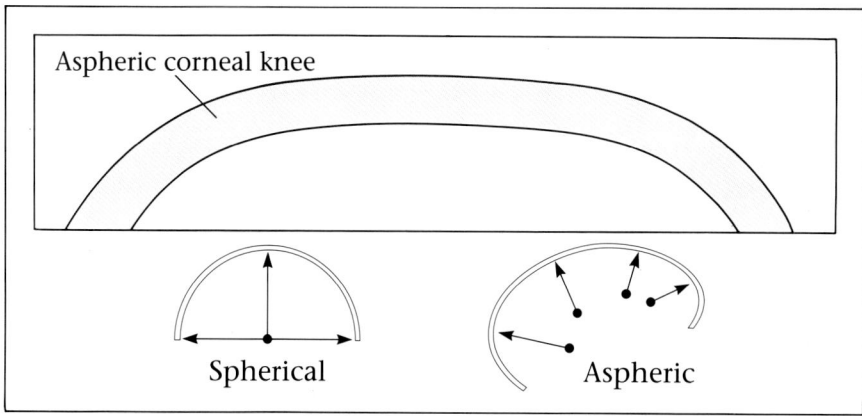

Figure 23.27 *Astigmatic keratotomy creates an aspheric paracentral corneal knee similar to the one created by radial keratotomy.*

Surgical Parameters:
3.50-mm T cuts; 7.00 mm OZ; achieved depth of 90%

OD: Double T cuts on 75th meridian
One year postoperatively:
   +1.75 − 1.00 × 145° = 20/15
   V sc = 20/20
   V (near) sc = 20/20

OS: Double T cuts on 105th meridian
Nine months postoperatively:
   +0.75 − 0.50 × 15° = 20/10
   V sc = 20/10
   V (near) = 20/15

One year postoperative photographs are shown in Figure 23.28. The one year postoperative keratoscopy for both eyes and the topographical analysis of the left cornea are presented in Figure 23.29. The patient has remained totally asymptomatic and is very pleased.

Notice the disparity between the patient's postoperative hyperopic refraction, yet excellent near and distance acuity. This uncorrected near and distance vision is better than would be expected from mild hyperopia in a 37-year-old pre-presbyope. A coupling ratio of about 2:1 has been achieved in both eyes since the steeper meridian has been flattened about twice the amount of flattening of the steeper meridian.

For the sake of simplicity, the above calculation of coupling was not done precisely; i.e., it did not consider pre- and postoperative keratometry, nor was true *induced* corneal astigmatic change by vector analysis computed, taking into account axis shift and lenticular astigmatism. Despite these limitations, the concept of coupling is well illustrated by the following calculations:

	Pre-operative		Post-operative	Change	
OD:	−2.25	→	−1.00	= 1.25	(steeper to flatter)
	+2.50	→	+1.75	= 0.75	(flatter to steeper)
OS:	−1.75	→	−0.50	= 1.75	(steeper to flatter)
	+1.75	→	0.75	= 1.00	(flatter to steeper)

Surgical Strategy for Astigmatism Correction

Presented below is a surgical strategy for the correction of astigmatism in congenital, cataract/IOL, and PKP situations. The requirements for AK are few, but demanding.

1. Corneal incision depth of 85% to 90%
2. Proper meridian alignment of AK
3. Proper OZ of AK
4. Transverse and radial incisions not intersecting

Congenital Astigmatism
1.00 D TO 4.00 D
T-cuts, combined with RK, as necessary (Fig. 23.30).

Diagram of T-cuts

A	B	C
1.00–1.50 D	1.75–2.50 D	2.75–4.00 D
(T = 3.50 mm)	(T = 3.50 mm)	(T = 4.50 mm)

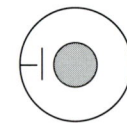 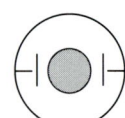 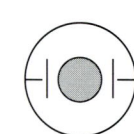

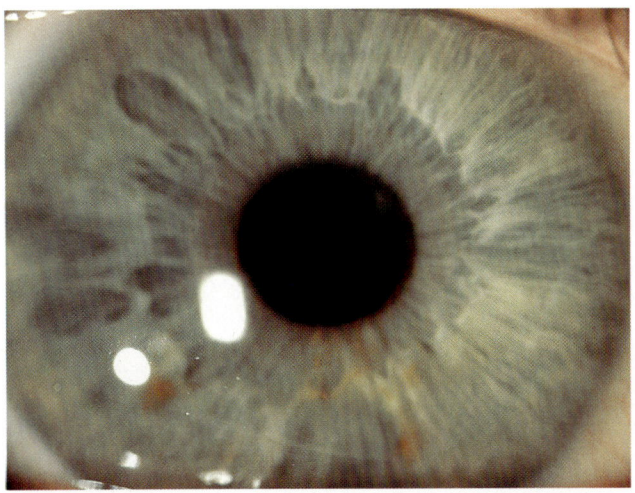
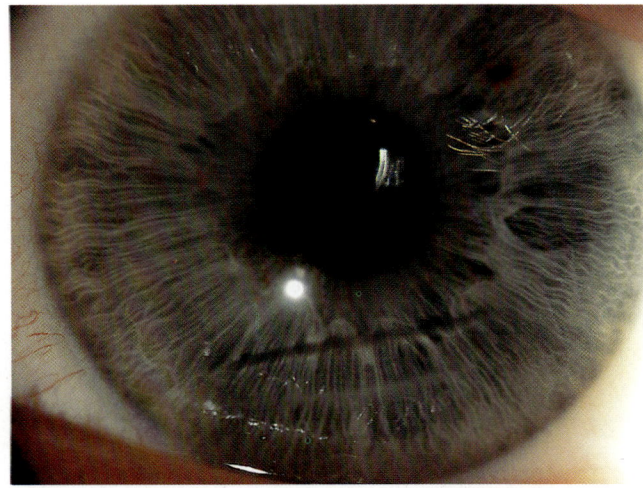

Figure 23.28 *One-year postoperative photographs following double T-cut astigmatic keratotomy;* **(left)** *the right eye with the astigmatic keratotomy on the 75th meridian, and* **(right)** *the left eye, with the astigmatic keratotomy on the 105th meridian. The dark black line on the lower iris is the shadow cast by the inferior transverse incision.*

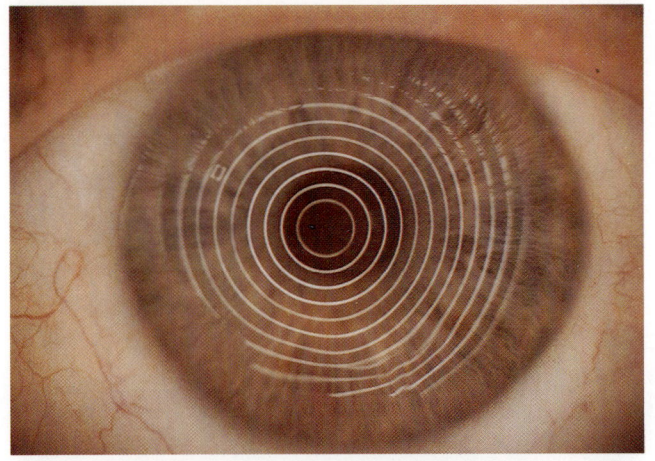
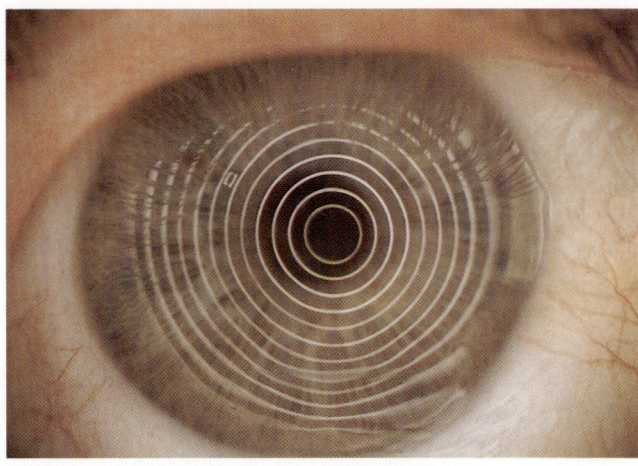

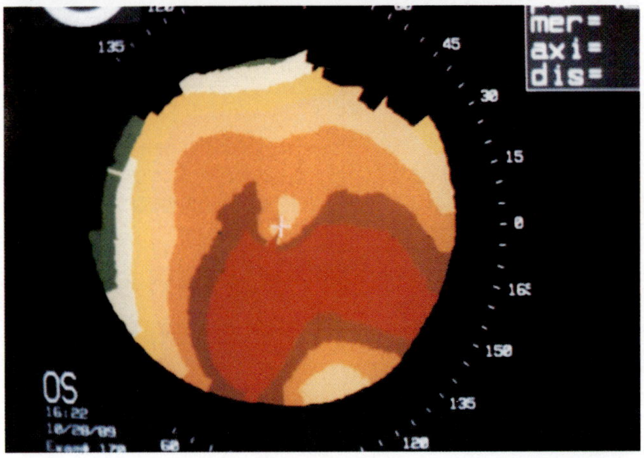

Figure 23.29 (Top left and right) *The one year postoperative corneoscope photographs of the patient also seen in Figure 23.28 show essentially spherical central corneal surfaces. The right eye is to the observor's left and the left eye is to the observor's right.* (Bottom left) *The one year postoperative Computed Anatomy topographical analysis of the central 6.00 mm of the left cornea shows numerous zones of varying dioptric powers. This cornea is aspheric as a result of the astigmatic keratotomy.*

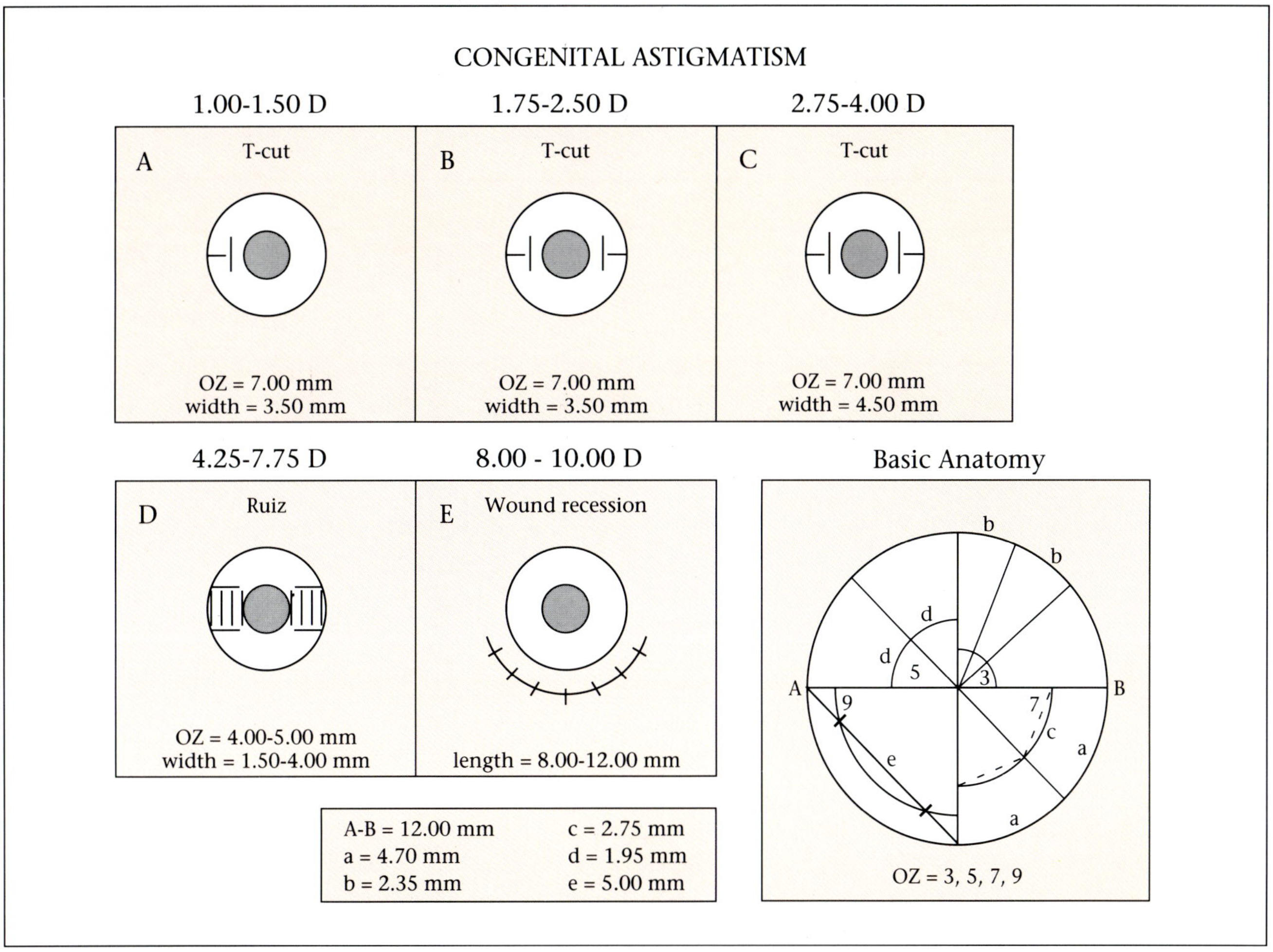

CONGENITAL ASTIGMATISM

A 1.00–1.50 D — T-cut — OZ = 7.00 mm, width = 3.50 mm

B 1.75–2.50 D — T-cut — OZ = 7.00 mm, width = 3.50 mm

C 2.75–4.00 D — T-cut — OZ = 7.00 mm, width = 4.50 mm

D 4.25–7.75 D — Ruiz — OZ = 4.00–5.00 mm, width = 1.50–4.00 mm

E 8.00–10.00 D — Wound recession — length = 8.00–12.00 mm

Basic Anatomy

A–B = 12.00 mm   c = 2.75 mm
a = 4.70 mm   d = 1.95 mm
b = 2.35 mm   e = 5.00 mm

OZ = 3, 5, 7, 9

Figure 23.30 *A method for correcting congenital astigmatism.*

The surgeon soon realizes that doing AK is like catching fish in a net—you only have to get the fish somewhere in the net, not in one exact spot. In other words, a 3.00 D astigmatism patient will have a satisfactory result if correction anywhere from 2.00 D to 4.00 D is achieved, since this range of correction leaves the patient with 1.00 D or less of astigmatism. This is a very broad range of permissible error. Also, the resultant aspheric cornea provides a wider range of available refractive power. Clinically, it is not realistic to expect AK surgery to produce an accuracy within ±0.50 D when preoperative starting values are higher than about 3.50 D. Fortunately, excellent clinical results are still likely despite our seemingly low level of sophistication.

T-cuts may be combined with RK when necessary (Fig. 23.31). In this situation it is extremely important that the surgeon plan the RK for the spherical equivalent, not the spherical component, if the goal is emmetropia. AK tends to make the flatter meridian of the cornea steeper due to the coupling effect, which negates the effect of RK on this meridian and keeps the eye more myopic. Adjusting RK for the spherical equivalent decreases the likelihood that this meridian will steepen. The disparity between planning RK for the spherical component compared to the spherical equivalent is not noticeable when there is a small amount of astigmatism but it becomes very significant if the astigmatism is above 2.50 D or so. For example:

Preoperatively: −1.00 −3.00 x 90°

To obtain emmetropia, the surgeon should perform RK for −2.50 D in order to obtain −1.00 D of spherical correction and AK for −3.00 D.

When combining RK and AK, either the T-cut may be made first so the radial incisions will jump over the transverse incision, or the radial incisions may be made first so the transverse incision jumps over the radials. A slightly greater effect will be gained when the transverse incisions are intact (Fig. 23.32). If a T-cut is to be performed on only one side of the visual axis, in order to correct a low preoperative astigmatism, it should be positioned under the upper lid to allow for faster healing and less glare.

4.25 D TO 7.75 D

Ruiz procedure, combined with RK as necessary (see Fig. 23.30).

Diagram of Ruiz Procedure

5.00 OZ	4.50 OZ	4.00 OZ
4.25–5.25 D	5.50–6.50 D	6.75–7.75 D

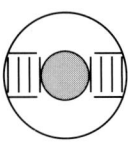

The Ruiz procedure, or a variant, is the most ef-

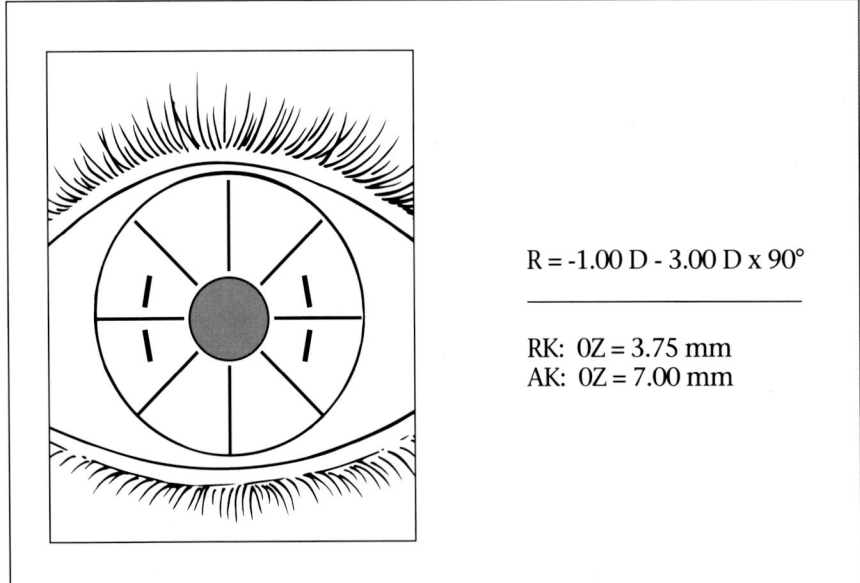

Figure 23.31 *Astigmatic keratotomy (T-cuts, in this case) may be combined with radial keratotomy when necessary. In this configuration, the radial incisions are performed first and the transverse incisions jump over the radials.*

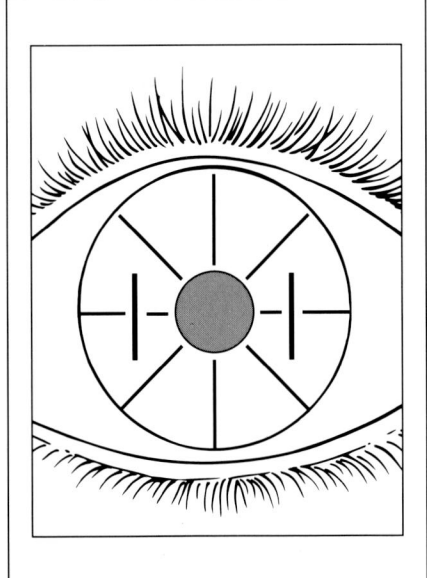

Figure 23.32 *The transverse T-cuts performed first with the radial incisions jumping over the transverse incisions. This technique provides increased correction and is valuable when correcting 3.00 D to 4.00 D of astigmatism.*

fective method for correcting high astigmatism; however, it is technically very demanding. The surgeon must remember:

1. No OZ smaller than 4.00 mm to avoid glare
2. OZ well centered and meridian located accurately
3. Ultrasound pachymetry at all incision sites to insure 85% to 90% incision depth
4. The most peripheral transverse incision (d) is placed very close to the limbus and the blade depth of the second most central transverse incision (b) is used as the blade depth for the pseudoradial incisions (r) (Fig. 23.33)

The width of the Ruiz procedure selected is based on the spherical portion of the patient's correction. The longer the transverse incisions of an AK, the greater the steepening of the opposite meridian with an associated increase in myopia. Therefore, a wide Ruiz procedure would be of value for a preoperative refraction exhibiting a mixed astigmatism, such as +2.00 −5.00 × 90° (Fig. 23.34). Notice that the spherical equivalent is *not* the determining factor when choosing the width of the Ruiz procedure for a mixed astigmatic case, but, rather, the ratio of the hyperopic spherical component of the refraction to the myopic astigmatic component of the refraction is most important.

Conversely a very narrow Ruiz procedure affects the opposite meridian minimally so it would be used to correct a compound myopia, such as −0.50 −5.00 × 90° (Fig. 23.35). If the goal is em-

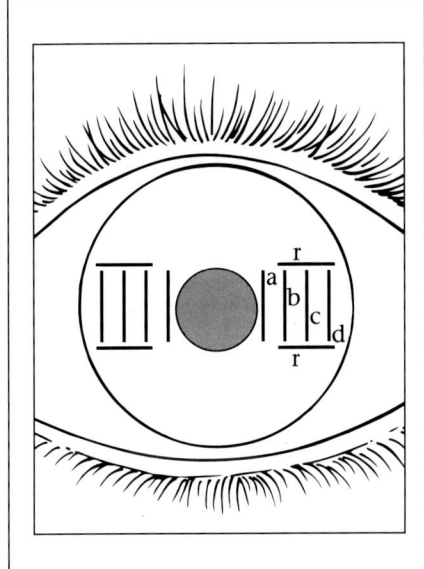

Figure 23.33 *In the Ruiz procedure, the blade depth of the second most central transverse incision is used for the pseudoradial incisions as well.*

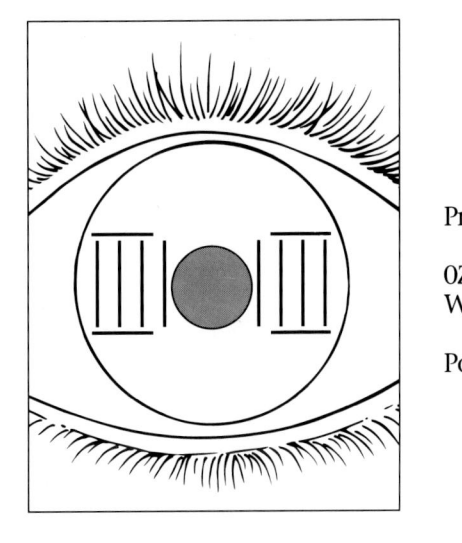

Pre-op: R = +2.00 D − 5.00 D x 90°

OZ = 4.00 mm
Width = 4.50 mm

Post-op: R = plano

Figure 23.34 *A wide Ruiz procedure causes increased steepening of the opposite (flatter) meridian and helps correct the hyperopic component of mixed astigmatism.*

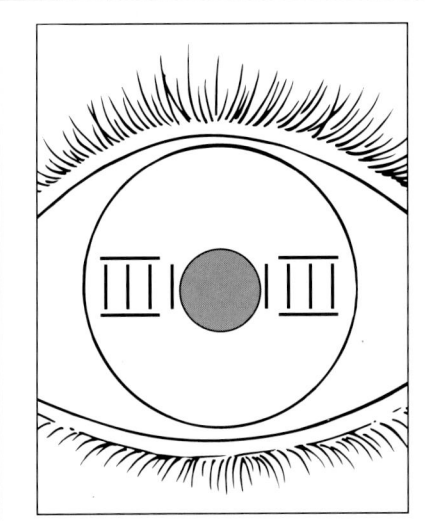

Pre-op: R = −0.50 D − 5.00 D x 90°

OZ = 3.75 mm
Width = 2.00 mm

Post-op: R = −1.50 sph

Figure 23.35 *A narrow Ruiz procedure is useful when the patient exhibits compound myopic astigmatism, since minimal myopic shift of the opposite (flatter) meridian is desired.*

metropia, the patient described in Figure 23.35 would need an RK, based on the spherical equivalent of –3.00 D, to actually correct the small amount of myopia (–0.50 D preoperative plus –1.00 D created) that would be present after the correction of the astigmatism (Fig. 23.36).

The width of a Ruiz procedure may range from 1.50 mm to 4.50 mm. The relationship between the width of the Ruiz procedure and the ratio of flattening to steepening of the principal meridians is summarized in Figure 23.37.

8.00 D TO 10.00 D

For large degrees of congenital astigmatism, which are quite rare, a limbal wound recession using a beveled wound or scleral flap of 10.00 mm to 12.00 mm and keratometric control is necessary (see Fig. 23.30). This procedure necessitates

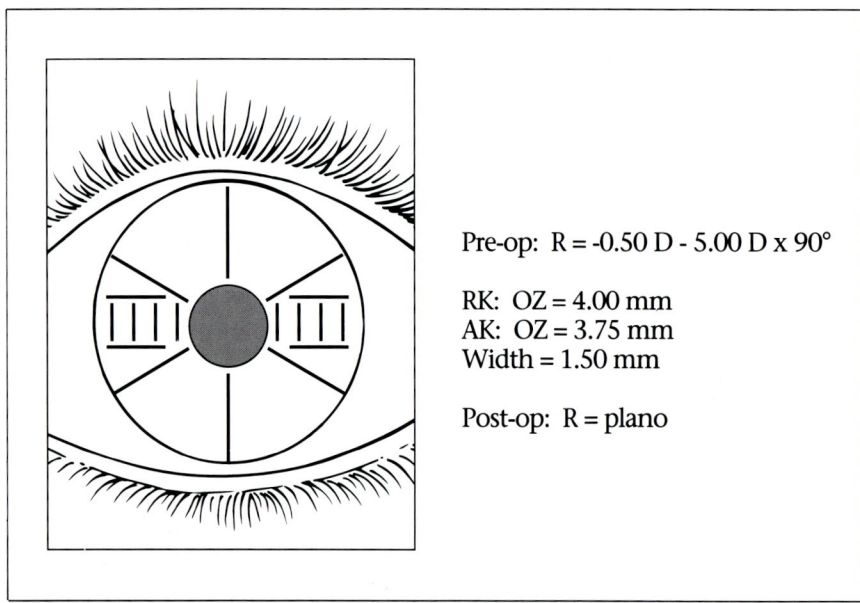

Pre-op: R = -0.50 D - 5.00 D x 90°

RK: OZ = 4.00 mm
AK: OZ = 3.75 mm
Width = 1.50 mm

Post-op: R = plano

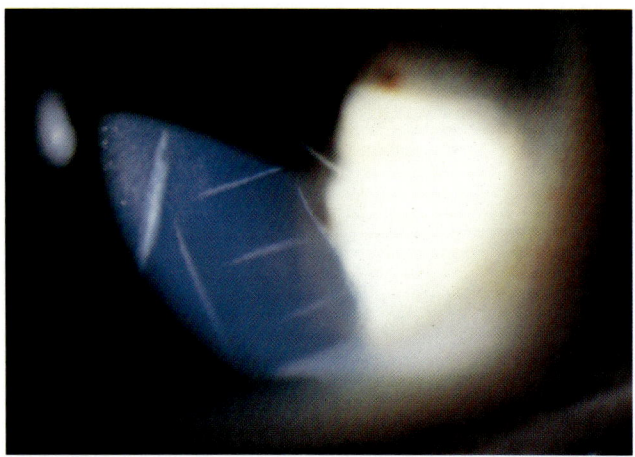

Figure 23.36 (Top) *A narrow Ruiz procedure combined with a six-incision radial keratotomy may correct compound myopic astigmatism to emmetropia. The radial keratotomy should be planned to correct the preoperative spherical equivalent.* **(Bottom)** *Combined radial keratotomy and Ruiz procedure.*

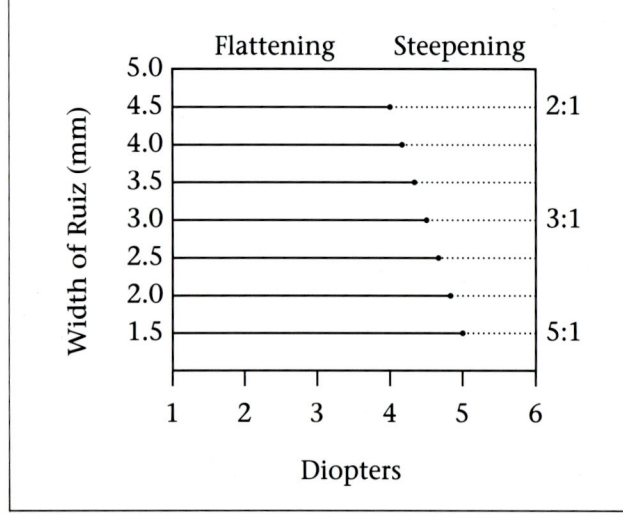

Figure 23.37 *The width of an astigmatic keratotomy affects the ratio of central corneal flattening in the meridian of the astigmatic keratotomy compared to the steepening of the opposite central corneal meridian. This graph demonstrates that a narrow Ruiz procedure (2.50 mm) causes about a 4:1 flattening/steepening ratio and a wide Ruiz procedure (4.50 mm) causes about a 2:1 flattening/steepening ratio.*

entry into the anterior chamber to achieve noticeable effect. If this large amount of astigmatism is not congenital, but rather the result of cataract surgery, PKP, or corneal trauma, different rules apply (see below).

Astigmatism Correction and Prevention During Cataract/IOL Surgery

If the surgeon accepts that permanent astigmatic correction is obtained either by wound recession or AK, the strategy for handling astigmatism during cataract/IOL surgery becomes rather straightforward.

First, let us review the scope of the problem. About 80% of cataract/IOL patients have a preoperative astigmatism of 1.50 D or less; approximately 13% have a preoperative astigmatism with-the-rule or oblique greater than 1.50 D and another 7% have an against-the-rule astigmatism greater than 1.50 D. *Residual permanent astigmatism of 1.50 D or less after cataract extraction is a reasonable and acceptable goal.* A patient with this amount of astigmatism can obtain an uncorrected visual acuity of about 20/30 with a spherical equivalent near zero.

Wound length directly relates to induced against-the-rule astigmatism. Therefore, one of the tenets of cataract surgery for those patients starting with low preoperative astigmatism is: The shorter the wound, the less possible effect on the resultant corneal astigmatism. Of course, a short wound must still allow for a safe surgical technique. It becomes obvious that small incision cataract/IOL surgery, if it does not affect the astigmatism due to its short length, solves the problems of possible postoperative astigmatism in approximately 80% of patients. Following is a summary of strategies for achieving low postoperative astigmatism following cataract/IOL surgery (Fig. 23.38).

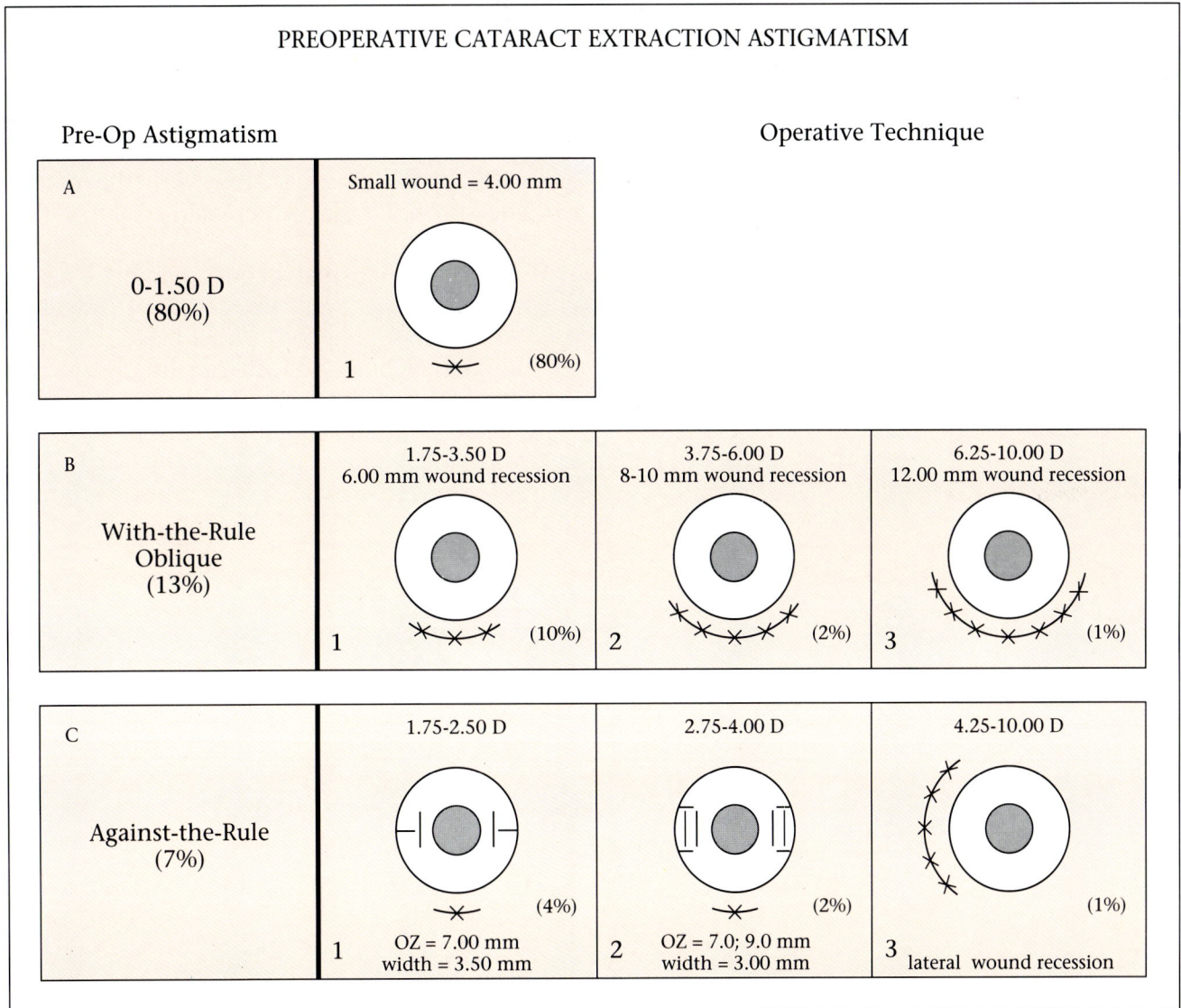

Figure 23.38 *A method for correcting preoperative corneal astigmatism during cataract/IOL surgery.*

Low Preoperative Astigmatism. Maintain low astigmatism (1.50 D or less) by using the shortest wound possible.

With-the-Rule Astigmatism and Oblique Astigmatism. In the presence of greater than 1.50 D of with-the-rule or oblique astigmatism, orient the wound on the steeper meridian. Create a wound long enough that *recession of the wound* will correct the preoperative astigmatism.

Therefore, if astigmatism is between 1.50 D and 3.50 D, use a 6.00 mm wound. If the astigmatism is 3.75 D to 6.00 D, use an 8.00 mm wound. If the astigmatism is 6.25 D to 10.00 D, use a 12.00 mm wound.

When a wound greater than 6.00 mm is used, a combined interrupted-running suture pattern is useful to allow for early postoperative cutting of the interrupted sutures.

A phaco surgeon should perform routine surgery and then enlarge the incision after the IOL has been implanted. Thus, the safest attributes of the smaller wound are present throughout most of the case. When it is surgically inconvenient to orient the wound on the steeper meridian, place the fixation sutures on the steeper meridian and torque the eye so that the surgery can be performed at 12 o'clock in the usual manner. This manipulation of the globe by the fixation sutures allows the surgeon to easily torque the globe 30 degrees in either direction (Fig. 23.39). When the fixation sutures are removed, the wound will be oriented properly.

A surgical keratometer (quantifiable or qualitative) must be used to insure that 0 to 3.00 D with-the-rule astigmatism remains at the conclusion of the procedure, depending on the surgeon's technique (Fig. 23.40). *Accurate keratometry can only be achieved with normal intraocular pressure.*

Against-the-Rule Astigmatism

1. If the astigmatism is between 1.75 D and 2.50 D, place the wound on the flatter meridian, and do an AK in the form of a bilateral T-cut at the steeper meridian using an OZ equal to 7.00 mm (see Fig. 23.38).

2. If the astigmatism is between 2.75 D and 4.00 D, place the wound on the flatter meridian, and do an AK in the form of a modified Ruiz procedure, which uses transverse incisions at the 7.00 mm and 9.00 mm optical zone (see Fig. 23.38).

Correction of against-the-rule astigmatism forces the surgeon to perform AK or create wound recession on the steeper meridian by operating from a lateral approach. This dilemma is created by the inability of tight sutures to permanently steepen the flatter meridian of the cornea, which is the accessible location when operating from above.

Since the acceptable goal is 1.50 D of residual astigmatism, an AK that only corrects 2.75 D of astigmatism can be used to correct a preoperative astigmatism of up to about 4.00 D. The wound must be closed in a neutral fashion. Relative to the correction of against-the-rule astigmatism, wound sizes varying from 3.00 mm to 12.00 mm when created on the flatter meridian contribute the same benefit—none. However, the smaller wounds run less risk of increasing against-the-rule astigmatism.

AK is performed just before placing fixation sutures for the cataract extraction. Ultrasound pachymetry should be performed before the prep so the correct blade length can be chosen. Be very careful to mark the proper corneal meridian. A notation at the preoperative slit lamp exam, regarding a landmark (e.g., a conjunctival nevus or iris feature) that indicates the proper astigmat-

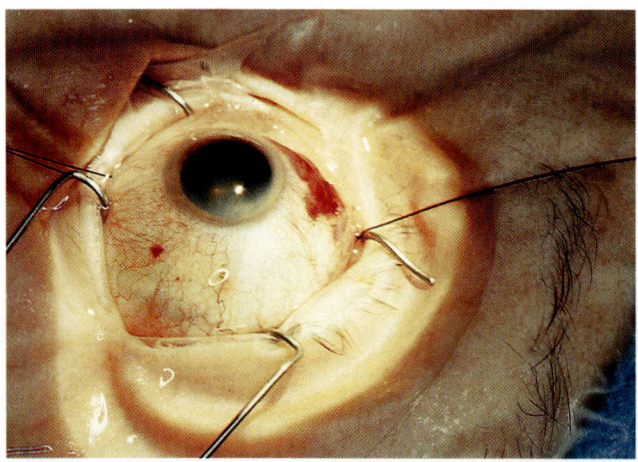

Figure 23.39 *Superior and inferior episcleral fixation sutures allow the globe to be rotated during cataract/IOL surgery so the surgeon may operate at 12 o'clock yet cen-*

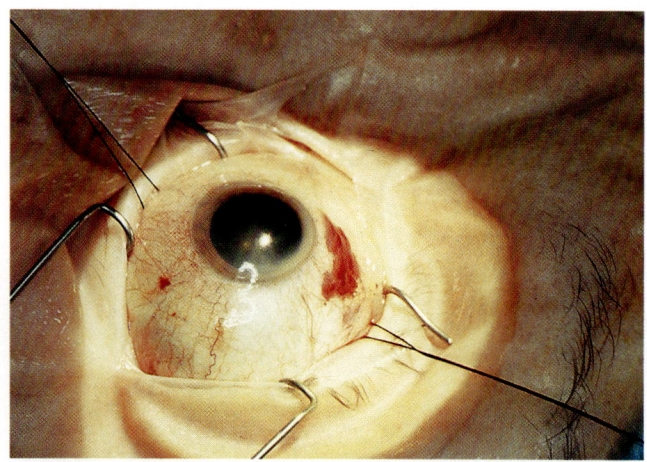

ter a wound at the proper meridian of the cornea. Notice how the globe in the photograph on the right has been rotated about 30 degrees compared to the globe on the left.

ic meridian, is very useful. A front cutting diamond blade with a bias of –5% (i.e., the blade length is 5% less than the pachymetry reading) in order to achieve a 90% depth incision is used for AK. The surgical procedure and technique for AK are similar to those for RK.

3. If the astigmatism is greater than 4.00 D, place the wound on the steeper meridian and operate from the side. Refer to the techniques described above for with-the-rule astigmatism in order to choose the proper wound length for any given preoperative astigmatism (see Fig. 23.38).

The coupling effect can be neglected when correcting low astigmatism; however, when the preoperative astigmatism is 4.00 D or greater, 25% of the total astigmatism should be added to the IOL calculation. This will take into account the change between the pre- and postoperative keratometry reading average, which is used in the IOL calculation. For example:

Preoperative keratometry:
  K: 40.00 D × 46.00 D (average = 43.00 D)
Postoperative: Coupling of 3/1 will produce a spherical cornea of 41.5 D
  46.00 D → 41.50 D (change = +4.50 D)
  40.00 D → 41.50 D (change = +1.50 D)

Therefore, the more accurate IOL calculation will take into account the *expected corneal shape* following the surgery, and use 41.50 D as the average keratometry reading rather than 43.00 D. This IOL power may be approximated accurately by using the normal preoperative routine and the actual keratometry readings, and then adding 25% of the preoperative astigmatism to the IOL power as calculated (Fig. 23.41).

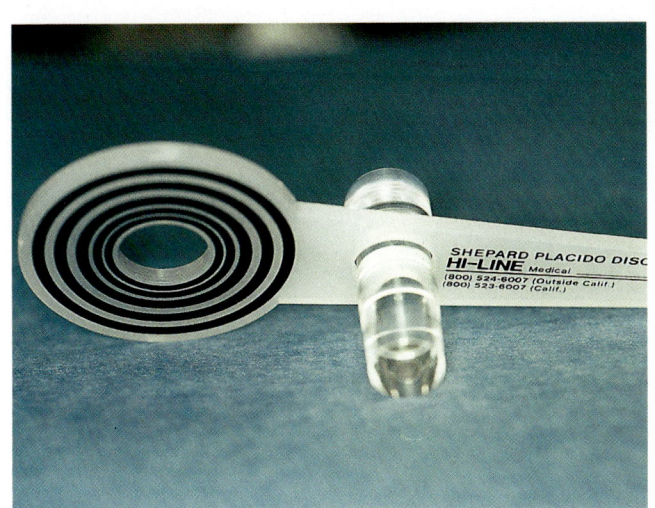

Figure 23.40 (Top) *A surgical keratometer with an applanation tonometer that insures proper intraocular pressure before using the keratometer.* **(Bottom)** *With wound lengths greater than 4.00 mm, a slight amount of with-the-rule astigmatism is desirable at the conclusion of a cataract/IOL procedure, since some recession (slippage) of the wound is expected. A horizontally oval mire indicates that the vertical meridian is steeper; therefore, with-the-rule astigmatism is present.*

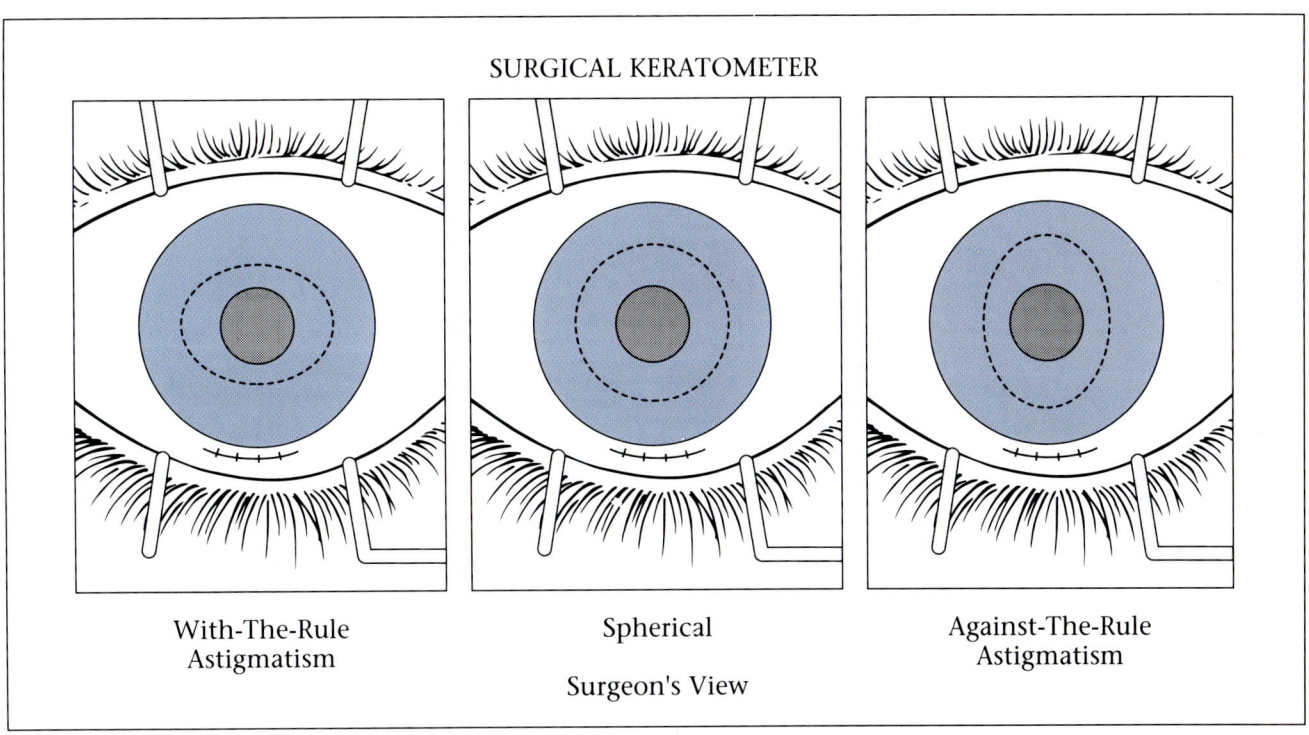

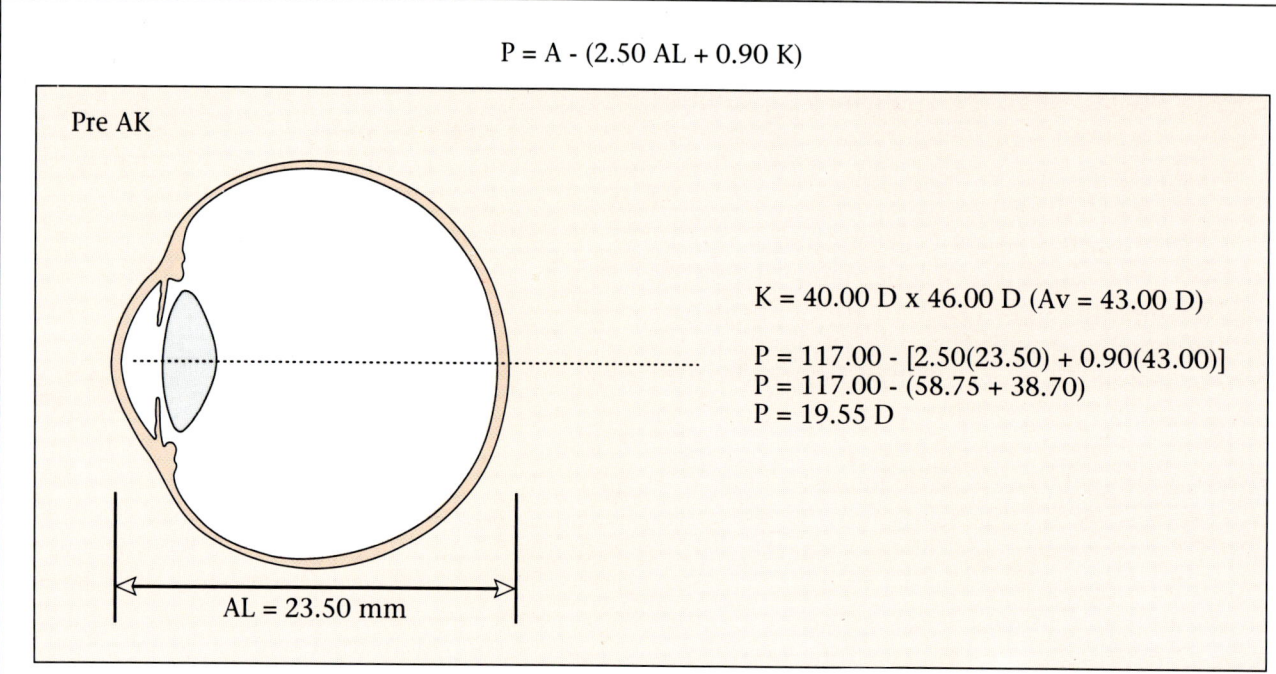

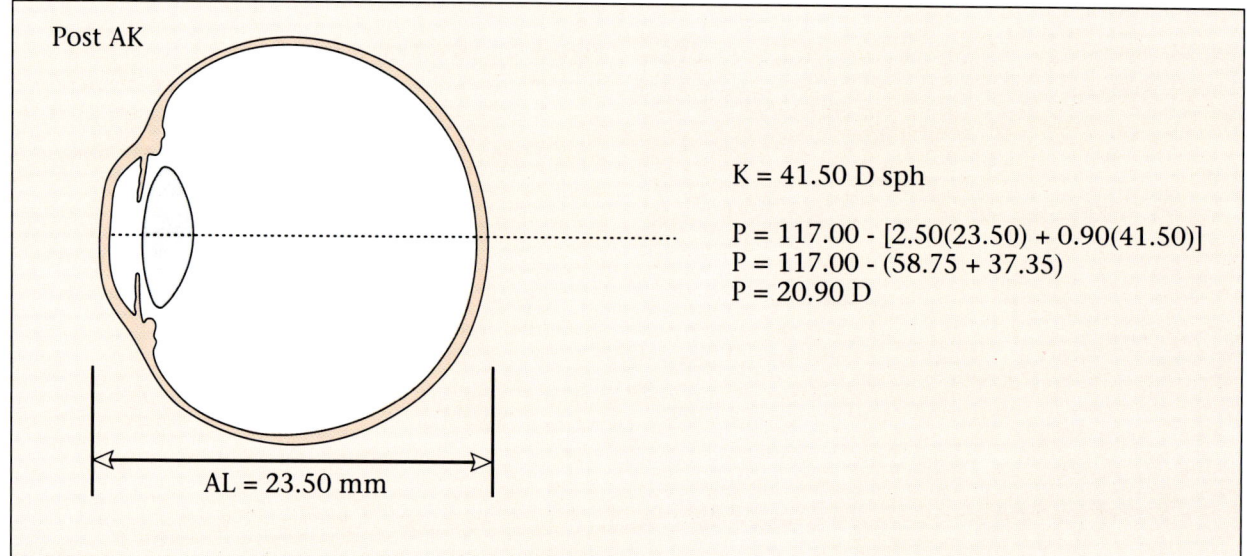

Figure 23.41 *If the surgeon plans to correct a large degree of astigmatism during cataract/IOL surgery, then the IOL power calculation will be affected. The preoperative IOL power calculation uses the average keratometric value (top). Following astigmatic keratotomy and cataract surgery, the postoperative central cornea will have an average keratometric value flatter than the preoperative average keratometric reading (bottom). An accurate approximation of the proper IOL power needed for a combined cataract/IOL and astigmatic keratotomy procedure may be ascertained by using the average preoperative keratometric value to calculate the power of the IOL and then adding 25% of the corneal astigmatism to determine the final IOL power.*

Correction of Postcataract Extraction Astigmatism

Almost invariably, astigmatism following cataract extraction that requires correction is due to wound gape from the incision above and is against-the-rule or oblique. The surgeon may use either AK or re-oppose the wound back to its original configuration. A wide blue-gray band concentric with the limbus at the incision site is reasonable evidence the wound has slipped and the original astigmatism was significantly less. Wound resection, which generally does not produce a long-term quantifiable result, is more effective when it corrects astigmatism created by previous surgery that has compromised the limbal anatomy.

Aphakia

If the eye is aphakic and a secondary IOL implant is necessary, re-opposing the wound is favored over an AK since the eye must be entered. Orient the wound on the steeper meridian and close it with interrupted 10-0 nylon under keratometric control, unless pathology at the site of the previous wound must be repaired (Fig. 23.42).

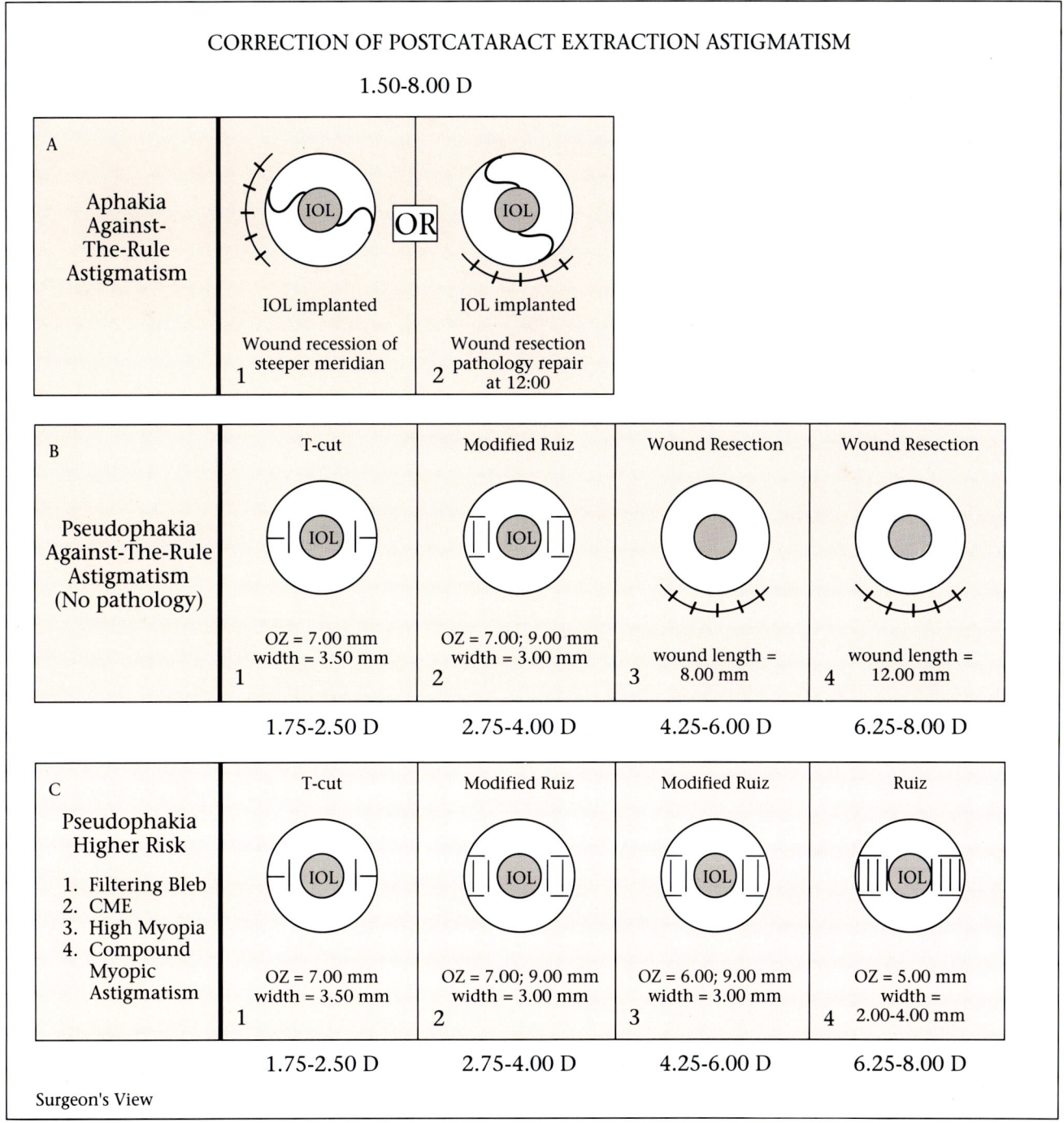

Figure 23.42 *A method for correcting aphakic corneal astigmatism.*

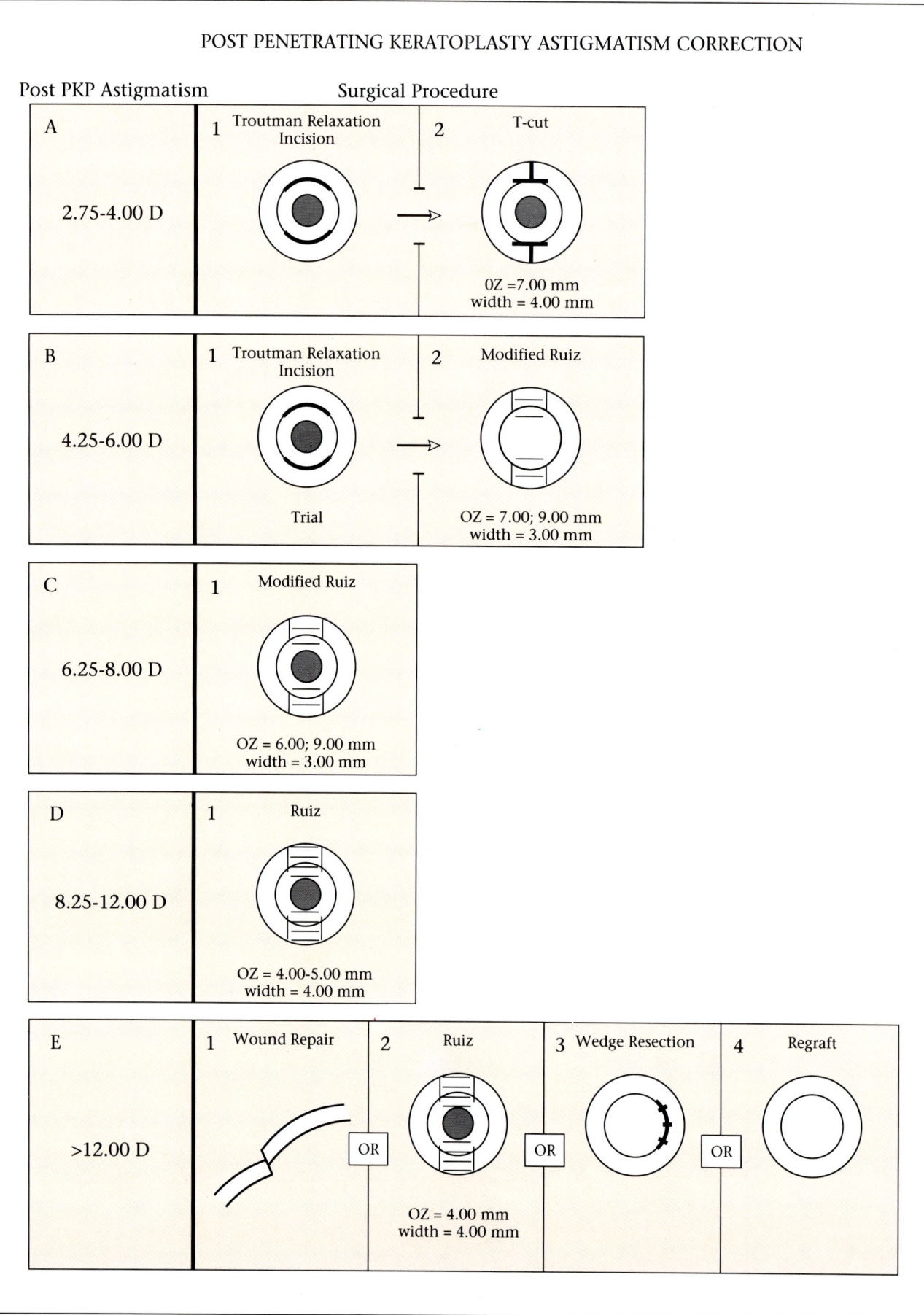

Figure 23.43 *A method for treating astigmatism associated with penetrating keratoplasty.*

Pseudophakia

If the eye is pseudophakic, the slipped wound may be reconstructed, especially if intraocular pathology requiring correction is present (i.e., vitreous to the wound, wound leak). Beware of the thinned sclera above, a result of the previous surgery. Create a scleral groove at the posterior limbus and enter into the anterior chamber in a beveled fashion, using a sharp 30-degree blade or keratome. Some degree of wound resection will occur during suturing and any irregular wound edges should be removed. However, large, round wound defects found beneath a conjunctival bleb cannot be closed by tight sutures without causing significant corneal distortion and may require a corneal patch graft for repair.

Wedge resection in this case will generally be effective because the patient most probably started with minimal astigmatism (80% chance), and the surgery is merely placing the corneal wound back to its original position (see Fig. 23.42).

Consider an AK if no intraocular pathology is present and the astigmatism is low or moderate. Only topical, not retrobulbar, anesthesia is necessary, and the risks associated with entrance into the anterior chamber are eliminated. Also, if the patient has a filtering bleb, high myopia, or has had cystoid macular edema or any other intraocular problem, then AK may well be the procedure of choice since no intraocular risk will be created (see Fig. 23.42). Also, if the pseudophakic refraction, such as plano $-3.00 \times 90°$, has a spherical equivalent that is significantly myopic, AK combined with RK is in order. In this case, if the astigmatism is corrected by wound reconstruction, the disabling myopia will still remain unless the IOL is exchanged as well.

If AK is performed following a cataract extraction, multiply the astigmatism by 70%. The value obtained will be the amount of astigmatism used when choosing the configuration of an AK. In other words, *postcataract procedure patients tend to get more correction from any given form of AK than congenital astigmatism patients.* This increased effect may be due to the altered structure of the limbal ring, a result of the previous surgery, and would not be expected with a wound of 4.00 mm or less. For example:

Pseudophakic postoperative refraction:
  $+1.00 - 4.50 \times 90°$.

Choose an AK that would produce only 3.00 D of correction in a congenital astigmatism case (4.50 D × 70% = 3.10 D). A bilateral T-cut with 4.50 mm transverse incisions and an OZ equal to 7.00 mm would be appropriate.

Astigmatism Correction Following Penetrating or Lamellar Keratoplasty

Currently, AK is the *only* lasting tool available to correct most astigmatism following keratoplasty. Since the *average* postoperative astigmatism following PKP is 4.00 D to 5.00 D, AK is a *mandatory* tool for the corneal surgeon. Five diopters of astigmatism often creates anisometropia, asthenopia, or a poor fit with hard contact lenses. The patient is not well served by a clear cornea and poor vision. The risk/benefit ratio of AK performed on a PKP is certainly very low, especially since high residual astigmatism is so debilitating. Corneal surgeons should pursue the goal of low post-PKP astigmatism vigorously. Thus, in most cases, *2.50 D residual astigmatism following PKP and AK is a reasonable goal.*

Corneal surgeons have tried in vain for decades to reduce post-PKP astigmatism with improved trephination and suturing techniques, but these attempts have uniformly failed. The hope that the corneal wound will "set" while it is being compressed by the 10-0 nylon is simplistic and incorrect. After the suture is removed, the compressed tissue and the wound change shape, dramatically or very little, for better or for worse. Also, it is not possible to correlate the shape of the trephination, the innate shape of the donor cornea, the innate shape of the recipient cornea, and the wound-healing process, and thus predict the curvature of the central cornea to within a few hundredths of a millimeter radius of curvature. If low regular astigmatism without irregular astigmatism is present with the sutures in place following PKP, leave them in position as long as possible.

Following PKP, there is both radial and circumferential tension created by the circular wound. Radial incisions that cross this wound will gape parallel to the limbus, which is not seen during routine RK. As stated with postcataract extraction, AK also tends to cause more correction of astigmatism following PKP, thus *astigmatism should be multiplied by 60% to obtain the value on which to base the AK configuration.* Following lamellar keratoplasty, this reduction in astigmatism is not factored in, but, rather, the same AK as would be used for congenital astigmatism is chosen.

When AK is performed following a PKP, all incision sites must be measured by ultrasonic pachymeter. The PKP wound tends to be thinner than the surrounding corneal tissue so the blade depth may have to be adjusted accordingly. Once again, achieved depth of 85% to 90% of corneal thickness is optimal.

Penetrating Keratoplasty Astigmatism Strategy

2.75 D TO 6.00 D
A trial of the Troutman relaxing incision in the wound (a form of AK) at the steepest meridian, on either side of the optical zone, for at least two clock hours may be performed. This procedure is performed under a topical anesthetic at the slit lamp. After the epithelium and Bowman's membrane are incised with a sharp blade, the wound is often extended more deeply by using the side of the blade to bluntly separate the stromal aspects of the wound down to Descemet's membrane. A wound leak may be treated by patching, bandage contact lens, or suture, as required.

Tight interrupted 10-0 sutures in the flatter meridian do not enhance the AK, but do provide control for about a year, during which time they are selectively removed.

As with all AK procedures, the eye is patched after application of antibiotics and steroids until the cornea is fully epithelialized. A bandage contact lens often creates a tight-fit syndrome when used immediately after AK.

If the Troutman relaxing incision is unsuccessful or regresses, the following strategy is employed (Fig. 23.43):

2.75 D TO 4.00 D.
Consider as about 2.00 D (3.25 D × 60% = 2.00 D). T-cuts on the steeper meridian with 7.00 mm OZ. Transverse incision length is 3.50 mm.

4.25 D TO 6.00 D.
Consider as about 3.00 D (5.00 D × 60% = 3.00 D). A modified Ruiz on the steeper meridian with 7.00 mm OZ. Transverse incision length is 3.00 mm.

6.25 D TO 8.00 D
Consider as about 4.50 D (7.25 D × 60% = 4.50 D). Trial of Troutman relaxing incision unlikely to work effectively. Modified Ruiz procedure with 6.00 mm and 9.00 mm OZ.

8.00 D TO 12.00 D
Consider as about 6.00 D (10.00 D × 60% = 6.00 D). Ruiz procedure with 4.50 mm to 4.00 mm OZ.

>12.00 D
When the corneal astigmatism following PKP becomes very high, the surgeon must look for wound apposition problems. A corneal donor may be pushed anteriorly by a bout of high intraocular pressure or a suture that has eroded from the recipient cornea and is no longer stabilizing the wound. This anterior movement creates a flatter meridian and the wound should be reopened and repaired (see Fig. 23.43).

A Ruiz procedure may be tried with an OZ smaller than 4.00 mm but significant glare may result (see Fig. 23.43). A wedge resection in the donor-recipient wound at the steeper meridian may be the only remaining alternative other than regraft. Of course, these cases are very difficult and moderate astigmatism may remain despite the best efforts of the surgeon.

However, some efforts should be taken to reduce this amount of astigmatism so that the patient can regain a functional eye. A monocular patient, obviously, will not warrant as aggressive an approach.

Reoperation After Astigmatic Keratotomy

Sometimes, an AK intended to correct astigmatism does not achieve its goal. The surgeon must consider using more transverse incisions to create a smaller OZ or redeepening the existing incisions if slit lamp examination reveals less than optimal depth. The surgeon's ingenuity and perseverance will undoubtedly be tested by treating these difficult cases as well as by performing repeat AK surgery (Fig. 23.44). Also, the surgeon must remember that *perfect is the enemy of good*. There will be situations in which it is better not to proceed, since the quest for perfection may bring the likelihood of failure to an unacceptable level (Fig. 23.45). Judicious boldness, honed by experience, should be the guiding philosophy.

Conclusion

Astigmatism is the factor that limits success in many anterior segment surgery cases. The ability to control and correct astigmatism is not perfect by any means, but significant strides have been made during the past decade to understand and cure it.

This chapter has provided the reader with a basic strategy for approaching congenital, postcataract/IOL, aphakic, and postkeratoplasty astigmatism. Most importantly, the surgeon must believe that the preservation of low astigmatism and the correction of high astigmatism is important enough to invest the time, care, and energy necessary to obtain good results.

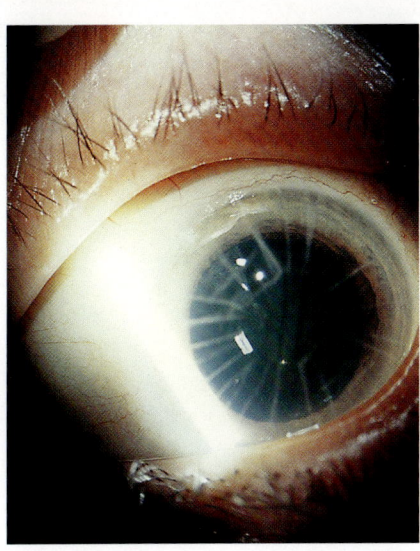

Figure 23.44 The cornea of a 65-year-old patient who underwent multiple Ruiz and radial keratotomy procedures in an attempt to correct his initial refractive error of –3.00 –4.50 × 40.00. Irregular astigmatism resulted.

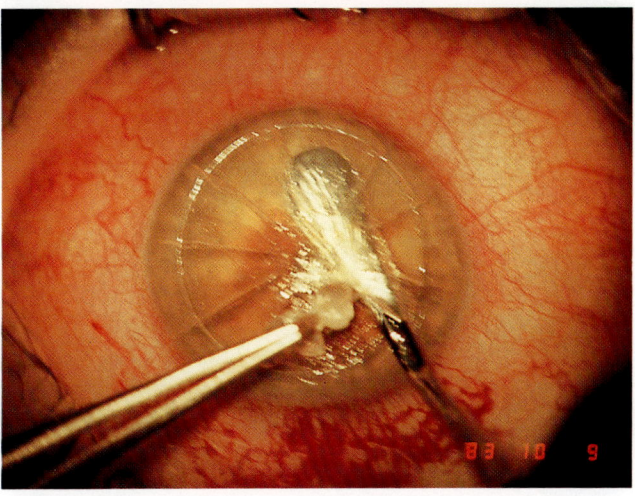

Figure 23.45 The patient described in Fig. 23.44 underwent a lamellar keratoplasty to correct the irregular astigmatism caused by the excessive amount of astigmatic and radial keratotomy incisions. A T-cut was performed after the lamellar keratoplasty to treat the residual regular astigmatism. The patient had 20/40 uncorrected vision, and two years later required cataract removal and IOL implantation. The patient's uncorrected visual acuity was 20/30 three months after the cataract/IOL procedure and correctable to 20/20–.

Clinical Points to Consider

☞ A surgeon's attitude toward the visual difficulties caused by astigmatism helps dictate the willingness to attempt a surgical cure for astigmatism.

☞ Astigmatic keratotomy and wound recession can provide quantifiable, if somewhat imperfect, long term correction of astigmatism.

☞ Residual astigmatism following cataract extraction/IOL surgery is, perhaps, the most important factor limiting best uncorrected vision.

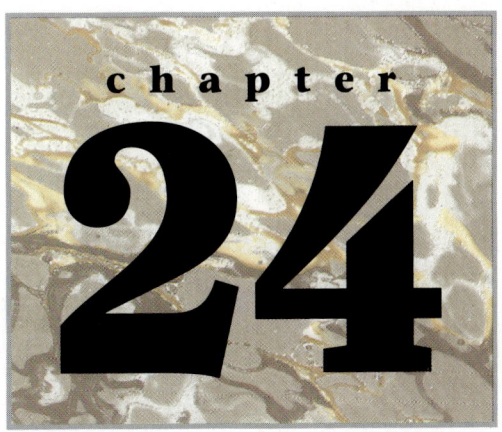

PENETRATING KERATOPLASTY

ROGER F. STEINERT, M.D.

Successful corneal transplantation requires meticulous technique to obtain a clear, optically functional, and long-lasting graft. Many postoperative difficulties can be avoided by appropriate surgical technique, preoperative recognition of potential healing difficulties, and early postoperative recognition of sometimes subtle incipient abnormalities. The complexity of corneal healing and surgery require that all but the most straightforward transplants are best handled by a cornea specialist.

Diagnosis and Evaluation

A successful transplant begins with a complete history of both the ocular disease and the patient's overall physical status, complete ophthalmic and physical exams, and a laboratory evaluation. Knowing the etiology of the corneal disease and its course determines not only the probability of successful transplantation but the surgical technique and the preoperative and postoperative maneuvers that can improve the prognosis. For example: A patient who presents with a scarred and thinned cornea that interferes with vision may have a bacterial ulcer, and the predisposing factor must be identified. Chronic blepharitis must be aggressively treated preoperatively as prophylaxis against perioperative infection and postoperatively because of the marked tendency of blepharitis to flare after operative stress, with secondary disruption of the ocular surface's new, delicate donor tissue. Examination of the patient's face may reveal acne rosacea, which requires systemic as well as topical therapy. A history of arthritis and an examination of the joints (hands) can alert the surgeon to rheumatoid arthritis, which predisposes the cornea to both infective and sterile ulceration, causing the dual corneal enemies, keratitis sicca and accelerated collagenase activity, once the surface is violated.

Table 24.1 categorizes the major elements that must be investigated when performing a preoperative evaluation and devising a

Table 24.1
Penetrating Keratoplasty: Evaluation and Treatment

Preoperative Risk Factor	Finding/Determination	Action
Eyelid		
Structural abnormality	Entropion	Preoperative surgical repair
	Ectropion	Preoperative surgical repair
	Scarring	Preoperative plastic reconstruction
Functional abnormality	Lagophthalmos/neuroparalytic dysfunction	Medial/lateral tarsorrhaphies
	Nocturnal lagophthalmos	Lid taping/postoperative moisture chamber
	Exposure keratitis	Dry eye therapy (keratitis sicca, see below)
Meibomitis/blepharitis	Staph colonization	Pre- and post-op lid shampoo, warm compresses, topical antibiotics; add topical steroids as necessary
	Seborrhea	
Tear film		
Conjunctival abnormality	Acne rosacea	Systemic tetracycline or doxycycline
Aqueous deficiency (keratitis sicca)	Decreased tear meniscus	Nontoxic lubricant drops and ointment
	Fluorescein and Rose Bengal staining	Punctal occlusion
	Low Schirmer test	Medial/lateral Tarsorrhaphies
Mucin deficiency (glycoprotein abnormality)	History of acid/alkali/thermal burn with conjunctival keratinization	Conjunctival limbal transplant from fellow eye, six months pre-PKP; avoid PKP, if possible
	Radiation	Intense keratitis sicca therapy (see above)
	Ocular cicatricial pemphigoid	Very poor prognosis, with or without mucus membrane grafts
	Stevens-Johnson syndrome	
Cornea		
Severe thinning	Active necrosis	Identify and treat etiologic factors. Defer PKP as long as possible
		If perforation, excise lesion; intensive topical and systemic antibiotic, anti-inflammatory medication
		If sterile lesion, immunology/rheumatology consult
		If peripheral corneal melt, conjunctival resection at limbus
		Corneo-scleral tectonic graft
		If infected lesion, topical antibiotics; consider corneoscleral graft with peripheral cryotherapy
	Severe keratoconus	Preparatory tectonic lamellar graft
	Keratoglobus	
	Pellucid degeneration	
	Prior inflammatory disease	Monitor for reactivation of old inflammatory process
Vascularization	Stromal vessels	Preoperative limbal argon laser treatment
		Prolonged postoperative steroids
		Monitor for rejection
		More interrupted sutures
Neurotrophic (e.g., herpes zoster, simplex, s/p acoustic)	Decreased or absent corneal sensation	Lubricants; tarsorrhaphies

treatment plan for penetrating keratoplasty (PKP). Such a list cannot be inclusive because of the nearly infinite possible combinations of medical factors and therapeutic alternatives, but it serves as a guideline when organizing the preoperative analysis. If risk factors are not stable and well controlled preoperatively, the prognosis for a successful transplant is greatly reduced.

Diagnostic Procedures

If the fundus cannot be visualized adequately, B-scan ultrasonography helps rule out retinal detachment or other anomalies such as tumor. More commonly, a hazy view of the posterior pole is obtained. If cystoid macular edema (CME) is suspected, a common occurrence in pseudophakic corneal edema, adequate corneal clarity for

Table 24.1 Continued
Penetrating Keratoplasty: Evaluation and Treatment

Preoperative Risk Factor	Finding/Determination	Action
Anterior Chamber/IOL		
Iris abnormalities	Synechia pupil deformation	Synechiolysis during PKP
Pseudophakia	Iris-supported IOL	Exchange IOL, unless good history of tolerance with good vision.
	AC IOL	If corneal clarity permits, obtain fluorescein angiography
		Remove all closed loop IOLs with careful dissection of peripheral synechia to avoid iridodialysis
		Leave only well-positioned solid and flexible Kelman Multiflex style AC IOLs
	PC IOL	Leave unless poorly positioned
Cataract	Optically significant	Combined open-sky ECCE/PC IOL
Glaucoma	History of steroid response uncontrolled preoperatively	Preoperatively, challenge with strong topical steroids
		Cyclocryotheraphy, cyclophoto-coagulation, filtering procedure are all best performed prior to PKP
		Argon laser trabeculectomy usually not possible
Orbit	Grave's disease	(See eyelid)
	Exposure keratopathy	Preoperative immunology consultation
Systemic Disease	Collagen-vascular disease	Preoperative systemic medication
	Peripheral ulcerative keratitis	Prolonged postop combined topical and systemic medication
	Uveitis	
Dermatologic Disease	Eyelid involvement	Maximal preop optimization
Acne rosacea		Continued postop support
Eczema		Dry eye treatment (see above)
Ichthyosis		
Allergy	History of atopy	Allergy consultation
	Vernal keratitis	Preoperative identification and treatment of allergen
	Chronic tarsal papillae	
Central Nervous System	Neuroparalytic/neurotrophic disease	Lubrication
	s/p acoustic neuroma	Tarsorrhaphy
	s/p closed-head trauma	Lid taping

fluorescein angiography or angioscopy may be present. If there is reason to hope for improvement in the CME after keratoplasty, the surgeon may elect to proceed, but the preoperative determination of the CME is nevertheless informative. Laser interferometry and, in cases of mild corneal edema, potential acuity meter determination helps verify a macular function level that justifies PKP. Other visual function tests, such as blue field entoptic imagery, entoptic phenomenon, two-point discrimination, and gross visual fields are also occasionally useful.

If a new intraocular lens (IOL) is to be implanted at the time of corneal surgery, the IOL power should be determined either from the previous IOL, if possible, or by A-scan biometry, calibrated for phakia, pseudophakia, or aphakia, as appropriate. The keratometry readings of the healthy eye may have to be used.

Many variations of PKP technique yield excellent results. This chapter describes one fundamental technique and several consistently safe, stable, and predictable options.

Preoperative Preparation

Antibiotic prophylaxis is administered as polymyxin/bacitracin (Polysporin) ointment at bedtime the night before surgery and gentamicin or tobramycin drops every 15 minutes for four doses beginning two hours preoperatively. At the time of the local anesthetic block, povidone iodine 5% (Betadine solution 10% diluted with an equal amount of physiologic saline) is dropped into the conjunctival sac.

If the corneal transplant is to be combined with cataract surgery, or if a posterior chamber (PC) IOL is to be implanted, the pupil is dilated. Maximal pupillary dilation can be achieved by instilling Cyclogyl 1%, Neo-Synephrine 2.5%, and flurbiprofen (Ocufen) every 10 minutes for four doses in the operative eye. Alternatively, if the crystalline lens or a (PC) IOL is to be retained, or if the replacement IOL is an anterior chamber (AC) IOL, the pupil should be constricted with pilocarpine 2% every ten minutes for two doses beginning about one hour preoperatively. If the eye is aphakic with vitreous prolapse into the anterior chamber, it may be advantageous to obtain mid-dilation of the pupil by the effects of the retrobulbar block. An open-sky vitrectomy can then be performed and the pupil easily constricted or further dilated with either acetylcholine (Miochol), carbachol (Miostat), or epinephrine (without preservative) 1:20,000.

Most corneal surgery can be performed under local block anesthesia. Peribulbar block is achieved with lidocaine 4% (Xylocaine) mixed equally with bupivicaine 0.75% (Marcaine) plus one mL of hyaluronidase (Wydase) per 10 mL of anesthetic. After administering the block, a pressure lowering device is applied at 30 mm Hg for at least 15 minutes. Cases such as keratoconus or combined extracapsular cataract extraction (ECCE) benefit from maximal preoperative ocular softening. An intravenous push of 50 mL of 25% mannitol is an appropriate dose for most adults without a medical contraindication (e.g.,- congestive heart failure or renal insufficiency). The mannitol should be administered at least 20 minutes before the eye is trephined in order to achieve maximal reduction of ocular pressure.

Surgical Procedure

In the operating room, the periocular skin and lashes are prepped with 10% povidone iodine (Betadine). The drape should include a solid plastic adhesive sheet applied over the eye. An assistant can hold the lids apart using the plastic handle of a disposable cellulose microsurgical sponge. The assistant must be sterile and the sponges should be discarded immediately to avoid any contaminants from the skin.

The plastic drape that stretches between the open lids is incised with scissors from the lateral to medial canthus, taking care to elevate the drape off the globe to avoid corneal injury. The edge of the plastic is then folded around the lid margins to the tarsal surface as the lid speculum is placed. This draping technique is highly effective in isolating the lashes and meibomian glands and their bacterial colonization from the surgical field and helps provide a smooth surface, reducing the likelihood of snagging and possibly breaking the long delicate nylon sutures.

The lid speculum should allow maximal adjustability in order to elevate both the lids and the blades of the speculum off the globe. During the highly vulnerable open-sky phase of PKP, pressure on the globe can be even more disastrous than it would be during cataract surgery. I prefer either the Smirmaul or Schott speculum, which are hybrids of the Jaffe and Maumenee-Park speculums.

In conventional keratoplasty technique, the surgeon next sutures a Flieringa ring to the globe (Fig. 24.2). If this is done, a strong suture on a spatula needle insures secure fixation of the ring to the episclera and superficial sclera. The ring is intended to stabilize the open eye, so a ring sutured only to the conjunctiva will fail to provide support. Five or six interrupted 6-0 silk or 7-0 Vicryl sutures spaced evenly around the ring will usually suffice. The ring should have a diameter approximately 4.00 mm greater than the total corneal diameter in order to provide a space of 2.00 mm for the ring peripheral to the limbus. Once the ring is secure, the globe can be positioned and supported by passing bridle sutures of 6-0 silk around the ring at 6 o'clock and 12 o'clock, then snapping the sutures to the drape. Most surgeons find that the ring can be omitted in eyes that will remain phakic because the crystalline lens provides good internal support for the globe and resists collapse. Conversely, globes with a predisposition to collapse especially benefit from a well-placed ring. Such cases include young patients, high myopes, and those affected with keratoconus.

I have found, however, that the ring can be omitted in virtually all cases, with the exception of children, who have highly collapsible sclera. Particularly when the marking technique described below is employed, the modest amount of scleral collapse that sometimes occurs with or without a ring is of no consequence. Operating without a ring shortens the time it takes to perform the procedure, causes less trauma to the globe, and removes another element that tends to snag the nylon suture or dull the needle during placement of the running suture.

As with the Flieringa ring, if good akinesia has been obtained from the anesthetic block, a superior and/or inferior rectus bridle suture can be omitted. I place bridle suture(s) only if the natural position of the globe will interfere with exposure for the keratoplasty. Before omitting the ring or positioning sutures, however, the surgeon must have enough experience to be able to perform keratoplasty smoothly and efficiently. Beginning or occasional corneal surgeons should place a ring and positioning sutures on all cases.

Next, a Castroviejo caliper is used to determine the maximum size donor that will allow an adequate host rim (Fig. 24.3). A typical rim is about 2.00 mm in width, but it may be wider or narrower to encompass or avoid vessels or other pathology. The narrower the rim, the more likely that postoperative vessel ingrowth to the sutures, premature suture loosening, peripheral anterior synechiae, glaucoma, and graft rejection may occur. Conversely, the larger the donor graft, the better the postoperative corneal optical performance,

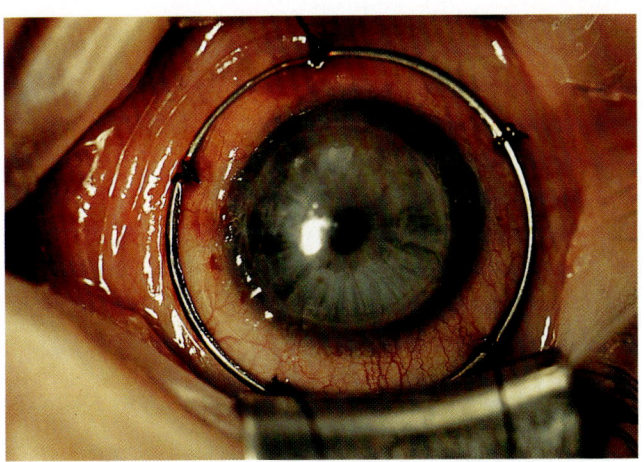

Figure 24.2 *A Flieringa secured to the globe with a combination of interrupted and bridle 6-0 silk sutures swaged to a spatula needle. The anterior segment of the globe is stabilized as well as lifted slightly, which allows*

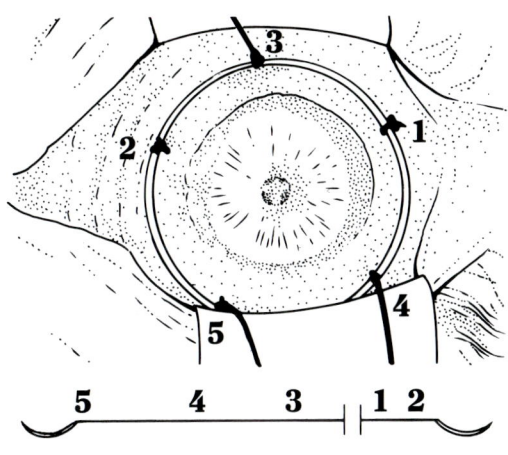

gravity to pull the vitreous downward away from the corneal wound. Five point fixation of the ring to the sclera, including three point bridle fixation, can be achieved with a 12-inch, double-armed suture.

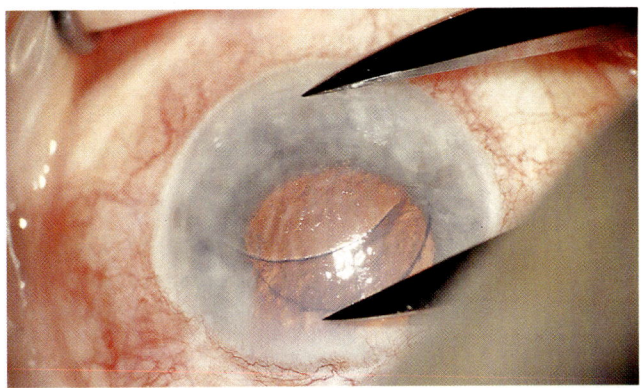

Figure 24.3 *Castroviejo calipers determine the size of the donor cornea for penetrating keratoplasty. Most recipient corneas can accept a 7.50 mm or 8.00 mm diameter trephination with at least 1.50 mm of clear recipient corneal rim in which to suture.*

the faster the recovery and the less chance that irregular astigmatism will develop. From the peripheral wound to the center, the corneal contour rapidly becomes more regular, and even a 0.50 mm increase in graft size will improve the average postoperative graft optical performance. Small corneal grafts, necessary for the techniques of past decades, are well known for high degrees of irregular astigmatism.

Most eyes cannot accept a trephination diameter greater than 8.00 mm, and many eyes allow only a 7.50 mm trephination. Occasionally, a large cornea will be able to accept an 8.50 mm trephination. The need to reduce the diameter to 7.00 mm or less is unusual in the absence of other peripheral corneal pathology.

Having determined the size of the host trephination, the donor button can be prepared on a separate sterile table. Most donors are now supplied as corneoscleral specimens. (If a whole globe is provided, first prepare the donor button by excising the corneoscleral tissue over the ciliary body/pars plana region, obtaining a 2.00 mm scleral rim while maintaining the anterior chamber until the specimen is stripped from the globe.) The donor is trephined from the endothelial side. A system that assures trephination, such as the Troutman punch, consists of a Teflon block, base support, sleeve guide, and universal handle. These punches are analogous to using a drill press instead of a hand-held drill, and result in a much more reliable and repeatable symmetrical donor buttons than a skilled surgeon can obtain with a hand-held trephine.

The corneoscleral donor is placed on the Teflon block and carefully centered by sighting down the trephine sleeve guide (Fig. 24.4). The trephine is advanced smoothly until it is in contact with the endothelial surface and firmly pushed straight downward without any rotary motion (Fig. 24.5). The cornea is typically cut abruptly and feels and sounds "crunchy". The scleral rim is grasped with a heavy toothed forcep and rotated around and slightly up the outside of the trephine blade while the blade is kept in firm contact with the block. This assures a full 360-degree section.

The trephine is carefully withdrawn from the block. The scleral rim usually remains on the trephine blade, but it must be observed for slippage, which might cause it to fall off and injure the donor endothelium. The donor button ideally remains on the Teflon block. The likelihood of adhesion is improved if the Teflon block is dry and the donor epithelium is dried with a cellulose sponge before the button is placed on the block. If the donor button fails to adhere to the Teflon block and remains fully inside the trephine blade without a presenting edge that can be grasped with a fine forceps, two maneuvers can be employed to safely deliver the button from the trephine blade: The trephine blade can be carefully removed from the handle. Using a dropper, the storage media fluid can be gently introduced down the inside wall of the blade. The fluid's weight may cause an edge of the button to protrude so it can be grasped by forceps. Alternatively, the dropper itself can be used as a suction device that, when applied to the epithelial surface, allows the button to be withdrawn from the barrel of the trephine.

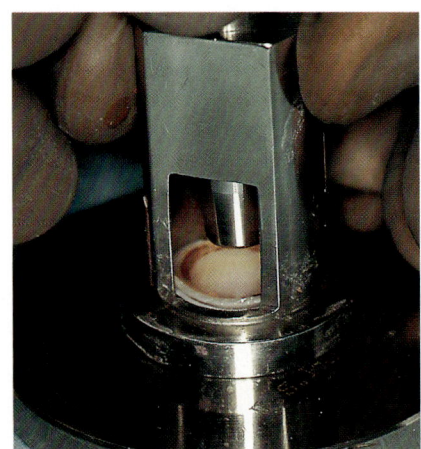

Figure 24.4 *The donor corneoscleral button is placed and centered in the Troutman punch. A Troutman punch creates donor buttons with perpendicular edges more reliably than hand held trephines, which often allow the donor to slide sideways during the cut.*

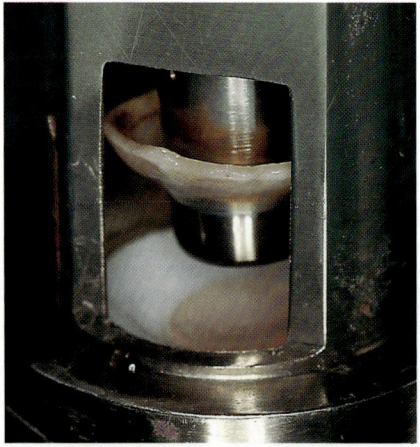

Figure 24.5 *Downward pressure on the punch handle cuts a donor cornea from the endothelial side. The donor corneoscleral rim has been moved up the trephine. After the trephine is withdrawn, the donor button will be left on the Teflon block.*

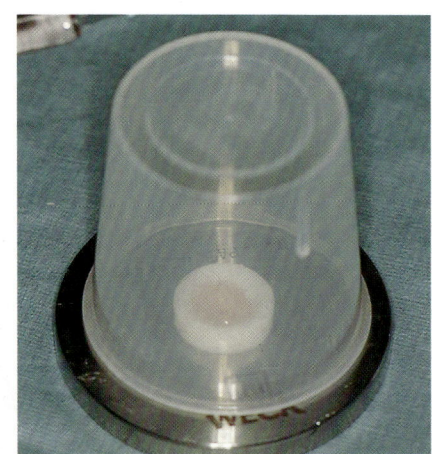

Figure 24.6 *Several drops of corneal storage medium or BSS are placed on the donor cornea, which is protected with a cover until needed.*

The donor button stays on the Teflon block on a separate sterile table until needed. The concave endothelial side faces up, and several drops of the corneal storage medium are gently placed on the endothelium to prevent dehydration and damage. A protective cover is placed over the block. This can be a small, sterile plastic or glass beaker (Fig. 24.6). If one is not available, half of the small plastic box that held the disposable trephine blade is suitable. Be careful that no bright, drying overhead operating lights are shining on the button.

With the technique described here, the best results are obtained with a donor that is 0.20 mm or 0.25 mm larger than the host trephination. For example, a 7.70 mm donor button is prepared for a 7.50 mm host recipient bed. The only exception is keratoconus, with its tendency for postoperative steepening and its frequent association with axial myopia. Some surgeons will employ undersized donors for keratoconus, particularly for higher degrees of myopia. Undersized grafts may be excessively flat, however, with poor optical performance. For keratoconus, I therefore recommend a donor and host of equal size.

Trephining the Patient's Cornea

The patient's cornea is prepared for trephination. If the iris is not diseased and the pupil is normal, the trephination should be centered over the pupil. Preoperative pilocarpine causes a miotic pupil, which makes centration of the trephine more accurate. Optical performance is maximal if the visual axis is as far from the wound as possible. The pupil is often decentered slightly nasally in the normal eye and accentuated by the ellipsoidal shape of the temporal limbus. If there is iris pathology, surgical manipulation of the iris is planned, or corneal opacity makes it impossible to visualize the pupil, the trephination should be anatomically centered relative to the limbus.

The center point, be it the pupil or the anatomical center of the cornea, is marked with a sterile surgical marking pen (Fig. 24.7). A radial keratotomy (RK) marker, its spokes coated by the surgical marking pen, is then applied to the cornea (Fig. 24.8). I prefer the Arrowsmith RK marker because it is relatively thin, easy to accurately center, and includes concentric rings at 3.00 mm and 6.00 mm, which help center the trephine. The radial marks later guide the accurate placement of the interrupted cardinal sutures.

Trephination is performed. The Hessburg-Baron suction trephine is easy to use (Fig. 24.9), only slightly more expensive than basic disposable trephine blades, and reliably achieves well-centered perpendicular cuts. In trephination, the most common errors are poor centration and oblique cuts, resulting in poor postoperative optical performance of the graft. The suction trephine helps to reduce the chance of such errors.

The most frequent difficulty with the Hessburg-Baron trephine is establishing suction. In most cases, difficulty in establishing adequate suction is due to redundant conjunctiva that slides under the trephine or because the pressure needed to keep the trephine perpendicular to the cornea is not uniform. By carefully stroking any redundant conjunctiva off the cornea and applying uniform pressure with an index finger over the barrel lumen of the trephine, usually satisfactory suction is readily achieved. Only highly irregular corneal surfaces prevent adequate suction. In those cases, stabilization of the trephine assembly by the thumb and forefinger of the surgeon's nondominant hand enables trephination. Each trephine is packaged with instructions for its use.

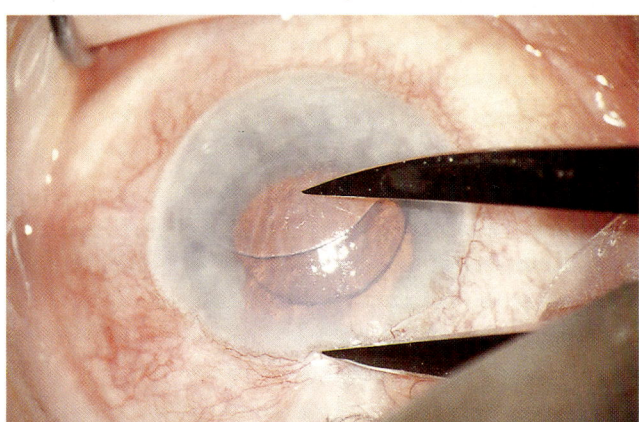

Figure 24.7 *Determining the geometric center of the cornea by calipers aids in positioning the graft. When possible, a miotic pupil effectively insures graft centration on the visual axis, rather than relying on the geometric center of the cornea.*

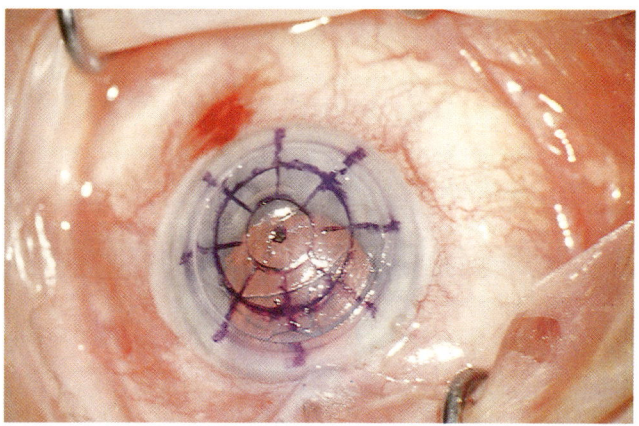

Figure 24.8 *An eight-blade radial keratotomy marker coated with gentian violet dye marks the position of the graft as well as the sites for cardinal sutures.*

A posterior lip of the recipient wound helps assure a watertight wound without overtightening the suture. In contrast, a through-and-through trephination and excision of the host button that results in perpendicular walls creates an end-to-end appositional wound. This type of "butt" joint is structurally weak and prone to leaks. It is for this reason that cataract limbal wounds are variously performed with bevels, steps, and flaps. If a posterior lip is left on the corneal host rim, much the same mechanical advantage can be obtained in PKP. As long as the lip is uniform over 360 degrees, and particularly if the lip is thin, it will not induce any net astigmatism. Moreover, the suction trephine has a tendency to "undercut" the host so that the endothelial diameter is larger than the epithelial diameter. The posterior lip counteracts this, as does the tendency of most donor punches to create a larger endothelial diameter than epithelial diameter.

The posterior lip is fashioned by trephining as deeply as possible but stopping short of perforation. The Hessburg-Baron trephine blade advances about 0.09 mm per quarter turn. Under direct observation through the operating microscope, the blade should initially be set parallel to the inner wall of the suction chamber. The blade is then retracted three, one-quarter turns. After the trephine is placed satisfactorily on the host cornea and good suction is obtained, the blade is steadily advanced three, one-quarter turns forward (clockwise) to the original setting. Next, deep cuts without perforation can be obtained using the following guidelines:

Typical keratoconus with moderate inferior thinning: four, one-quarter turns
Normal thickness periphery: five, one-quarter turns
Mild edema: six, one-quarter turns
Severe edema: seven, one-quarter turns.

The trephine assembly is stabilized in a neutral position by the thumb and index finger of the nondominant hand, taking care not to press down, lift up, or apply any rotating or lateral forces.

The anterior chamber is entered with a sharp blade in the depth of the trephination groove with the blade handle angled at about 45 degrees so the tip of the blade points toward the pupil. Care is taken to avoid the iris, lens, and other structures. After an opening of about 2.00 mm to 3.00 mm is made in Descemet's membrane, the blade is withdrawn. Viscoelastic is then injected. Corneal scissors are introduced and, with the blades at an angle, the button is excised (Fig. 24.10). I prefer the Castroviejo corneal scissors, which resemble the delicate Wescott scissors. A right-handed surgeon makes the stab opening to the right side at 9 o'clock and uses the right hand to cut with the scissors inferiorly around to 3 o'clock. The scissors are then returned to the 9 o'clock position and the host button excision is completed superiorly around to the 3 o'clock position. A left-handed surgeon performs the mirror image of this technique.

One blade of the scissors should remain in the anterior chamber from cut to cut, exiting only when the surgeon's hand needs to be repositioned. This enables a smoother, quicker cut, and the surgeon has a better chance of maintaining an even bevel. As the excision proceeds, the surgeon often will need to stabilize the host button by grasping it with a 0.12-mm Colibri forceps.

After completing the excision, inspect the overall result, particularly the bevel. Trim off any irregular tags or uneven portions of the posterior bevel lip. Inspect the area carefully to insure that no residual host Descemet's membrane remains in the bed. This membrane may be translucent, thus difficult to see. Also, because it strips off easily from the edematous host button, if it is not identified and removed, the new graft will fail.

At this stage in the procedure, the surgeon performs any other anterior segment procedures

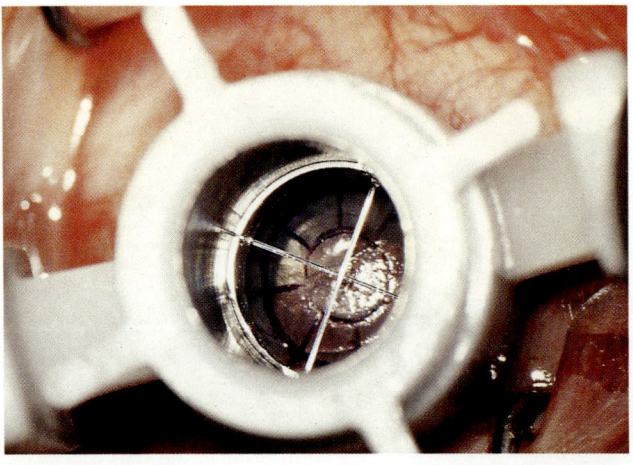

Figure 24.9 *The Hessburg-Baron suction trephine is centered by using the marker rings on the recipient cornea and the crosshairs inside the trephine shaft. A 90% depth trephination of the recipient cornea is attempted.*

dictated by the pathology of the particular case. (These auxiliary procedures are reviewed in other chapters.) The goal is to restore the anterior segment anatomy to as normal as possible, minimizing the time in which the globe is open and vulnerable to expulsive hemorrhage, and correcting abnormalities that will diminish the likelihood of a successful outcome.

Extracapsular Cataract Extraction and Intraocular Lens Implantation

The most important element to successful ECCE in the course of PKP is a soft eye. Mannitol is administered and at least 20 minutes of decompression with an ocular pressure-reducing device is required preoperatively. The lid speculum must be carefully adjusted to avoid pressure on the globe. The anterior capsulotomy is easily performed with Vannas scissors. A circular tear capsulorhexis can be attempted, and it may facilitate an elegant result. However, the surgeon must be aware that positive vitreous pressure may cause an anterior capsular tear to extend outward toward the lens equator.

If this extension begins, immediate conversion to a scissors capsulotomy is indicated. The nucleus is delivered by rocking, tilting, spearing, and looping maneuvers; I generally use an 18-gauge needle in one hand and a Simcoe lens loop in the other. Meticulous and complete cortical stripping and removal is then performed. Automated I/A units can be used with the irrigation bottle only several centimeters above the operative eye but may function erratically due to aspiration of air in the open-sky situation. Without a closed chamber, the tip tends to engage the anterior capsule and cause tears. The delicate control of a manual irrigation/aspiration (I/A) system in this setting (e.g., the gently curved "reverse" Simcoe I/A cannula) may be desirable. After completing cortical clean-up, the posterior capsule is polished centrally, if needed. With a viscoelastic opening the capsular bag, a relatively stiff all-PMMA PC IOL is inserted horizontally. The stiffness of the haptics helps resist any positive vitreous pressure. A 7.00 mm optic is preferred to smaller diameter optics to guard against optical problems if the pupil is eccentric postoperatively. The pupil is constricted with a miotic agent. A peripheral iridotomy at the 12 o'clock position is always made prophylactical-

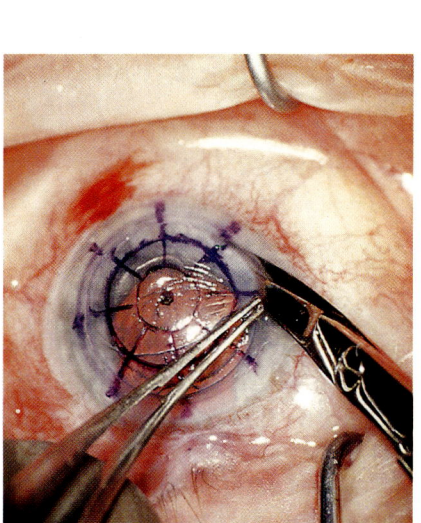

Figure 24.10 *The anterior chamber is entered with a microblade at 9 o'clock. Straight corneal scissors are placed at a 45-degree angle to the recipient cornea at the base of the trephine groove, and the central host cornea is excised.* **(Left and right)** *I prefer to create a posterior lip at the base of the recipient cornea that acts as a gasket and helps seal the keratoplasty wound. Other corneal surgeons use right and left cutting corneal scissors with angled handles to excise the central host cornea, leaving a perpendicular corneal edge that will abut cleanly against the perpendicular edge of the donor cornea.*

ly because of the complexity of these cases and the increased difficulty of achieving a laser iridotomy postoperatively.

Intraocular Lens Removal

Atraumatic removal of an IOL varies with the lens style and the adhesions that have formed. In general, iris-supported lenses will have adhesions at the pupillary sphincter. These are dissected by a combination of gentle traction with smooth forceps and excision with scissors and blades. AC IOLs, particularly the closed-loop variety, generally have peripheral anterior synechiae holding the haptic in the angle. If traction is applied to withdraw the haptic, a hemorrhagic iridodialysis will occur. In order to completely remove the haptic, it must be transsected and passed through the synechial tunnel. A special haptic cutting instrument helps the surgeon gain access to the haptic in the angle. If in doubt, it is usually better to cut off the haptic and leave the peripheral haptic stub buried in the angle.

Unlike iris-supported and AC IOLs, PC IOLs usually do not cause transplant failure. A PC IOL is left in place unless it grossly malfunctions (e.g., tilts or shifts laterally). Some PC IOLs can be removed by rotation. If adhesions resist rotation, the haptic is cut and only the central portion of the IOL is removed.

SECONDARY INTRAOCULAR LENS IMPLANTATION

If even fragments of posterior capsule remain, iridocapsular adhesions can often be dissected by blunt and sharp dissection and a PC IOL fixated in the sulcus. In the absence of a posterior capsule and with enough normal angle structure, the surgeon can select either AC or PC secondary IOLs. I have had excellent results with flexible Kelman three- or four-foot AC IOLs.

A PC IOL can be secured either by suturing it to the peripheral iris or by passing sutures through the scleral wall at the ciliary sulcus. Sulcus fixation after trephination can be obtained by passing a double-armed 10-0 polypropylene (Prolene) suture behind the iris into the bed of a half-thickness scleral flap prepared before trephination. The sutures should exit about 1.50 mm behind the posterior aspect of the limbus in order to be at the level of the ciliary sulcus. Each haptic is secured to the loop of the double-armed suture by a girth-hitch loop. The suture is then tightened and the two arms tied together securely. At the end of the case, the scleral flap is sutured over the external polypropylene suture and then the conjunctival flap is sutured. This diminishes the possibility of exposure of the suture ends, which could be inadvertently cut by another ophthalmologist or provide a tract for microorganisms leading to endophthalmitis (see Chapter 9).

Anterior Vitrectomy

Any prolapsed vitreous should be thoroughly removed to avoid its incarceration in the wound or around an IOL. Bulk removal of prolapsed vitreous can be sufficiently performed with cellulose sponge spears and scissors, and the cellulose spear should stroke the surface of the iris to insure removal of all strands from the anterior chamber. For a more complete vitrectomy, particularly if there are vitreous adhesions to the posterior iris surface of if a secondary PC IOL is to be implanted, subtotal vitrectomy with a mechanical vitrector is recommended.

Anterior Segment Reconstruction

Procedures such as goniosynechiolysis and iris suturing are helpful in selected cases. The surgeon must judge the merits of a prolonged operative time with an open eye versus the risk of iris hemorrhage in the search for anatomical normalization. Goniosynechiolysis can reduce synechial angle closure, which may cause severe postoperative glaucoma. Blunt and sharp dissection is performed either under direct visualization, while indenting the angle, or with a small dental or ear, nose, and throat mirror. Iris suturing, sometimes combined with sphincterotomies, can create a central pupil. This may help restrict the entrance pupil to the central graft and IOL optic, reducing glare and optical aberrations. Excessive traction on the iris root with iris sutures can deform the globe, however, leading to iridodialysis, bleeding, and iris tears. If the iris is sutured, a noncutting needle (e.g., the Ethicon BV 100) and permanent suture (e.g., 10-0 Prolene) are recommended.

Suturing the Transplant

The anterior chamber and IOL are coated with viscoelastic material to reduce trauma to the donor endothelium. The viscoelastic material should be carefully injected into the angle to help maintain an open angle postoperatively. The donor button is transferred onto the operative field with the Paton spatula. Cardinal sutures of 10-0 nylon are often placed sequentially at the 12, 6, 3, and 9 o'clock positions. However, when placing six cardinal sutures at the 12, 2, 4, 6, 8, and 10 o'clock positions, no sutures at the awkward 3 o'clock and 9 o'clock positions are required. To avoid torquing the graft when the first cardinal suture is passed, pass the needle directly under the teeth of the Colibri forceps rather than adjacent to the area being grasped. Alternatively, the double-toothed Pollack forceps can be used or the assistant can stabilize the button by grasping it with a second forceps at the 6 o'clock position.

The second cardinal suture at 6 o'clock is traditionally said to be the most important, because it will determine whether tissue is distributed equally to the two halves of the host. Unequal tissue distribution leads to severe irregular postoperative astigmatism and wound leakage. The proper placement of the 6 o'clock suture in the donor is best determined by placing gentle traction on the donor button with the forceps at 6 o'clock. The wrinkle that develops will bisect the donor button. One can determine if the two halves are equal fairly accurately by passing the needle through the donor and into the host rim at the mark made by the RK marker. Before passing the needle fully through the donor and host, inspect the location of the donor button relative to the host on both sides. With the rigid needle stabilizing the donor and host, the surgeon should manipulate the graft margins to the right and left. Although the apposition of the donor and host will be variable, one can usually determine whether the 6 o'clock suture is accurately placed. If it is not, backing off the needle from the host rim is easily done and another location determined and tested similarly.

After the first two sutures are passed, the 3 o'clock and 9 o'clock sutures are placed. The surgeon facilitates this by dividing the donor button into quadrants using the marks from the RK markers and the appearance of the wound as guides (Fig. 24.11).

The surgeon who performs PKP only occasionally will find the most reliable suturing technique for a patient with an avascular, uninflamed cornea is to place four more interrupted sutures. After the eight interrupted sutures are satisfactorily placed (i.e., there is just enough tension to appose the wound), the sutures are rotated to bury the knots. Most knots bury more easily from the donor side. The knot is then rotated until it is as far as possible into the host rim. A double throw, cinched, followed by two square single throws generally provides enough tension to appose the wound and a knot small enough to bury easily. An alternative is four single-throw slip knots. A 3-1-1 knot often is too bulky to bury easily, and it resists removal postoperatively.

After the eight interrupted sutures, a 16-bite running suture is placed (Figs. 24.12 and 24.13). By beginning the running suture in the depth of the wound and finishing with a pass through the donor cornea to meet the starting point, the knot will self-bury in the wound. Thus, the surgeon avoids the last fearful moment of trying to bury the running suture knot and the risk of breaking the running suture. There are two running suture bites between each interrupted suture. The run-

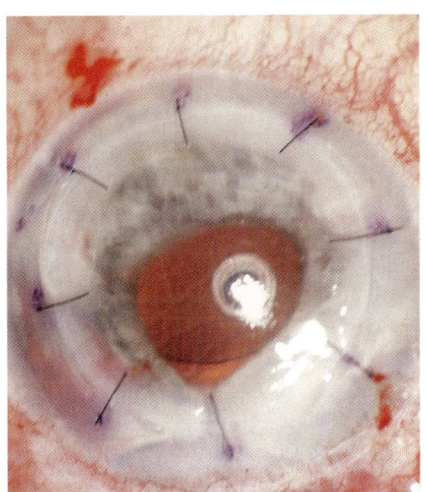

Figure 24.11 The donor cornea is initially secured in place with eight interrupted 10-0 nylon sutures with buried knots.

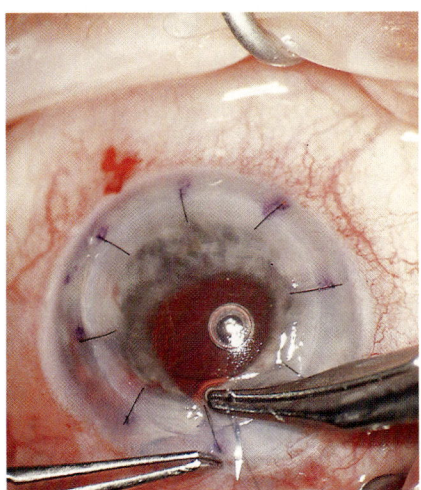

Figure 24.12 A running 10-0 nylon suture further closes the corneal wound, and begins inside the wound near 12 o'clock.

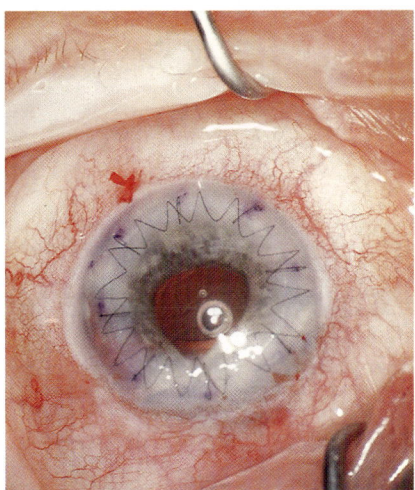

Figure 24.13 A completed PKP with eight 10-0 nylon interrupted cardinal sutures and a 16-bite 10-0 nylon running suture.

ning suture bites should be spaced equally, as if the interrupted sutures were not present, because the interrupted suture may be removed early postoperatively. In the space between the first two interrupted sutures, therefore, the first bite is 25% along the space and the second bite is 75% along the space. The third bite is then 25% into the space between the next two interrupted sutures, and so forth. When the interrupted sutures are later removed, the running suture bites will be evenly spaced. About four inches of running suture is required to comfortably complete the running suture for 360 degrees. Before tying the knot, the tension of the running suture is adjusted so the donor and host wound edges are apposed and the wound is watertight but tissue is not bunched. The tighter the wound, the more prolonged the visual recovery; this is due primarily to the irregular astigmatism caused by the tight suture.

If the cornea is vascularized or inflamed, it is likely that the sutures will loosen prematurely in the early postoperative period. In such cases, using 16 interrupted sutures instead of four or eight running sutures is prudent.

Buried knots may be more comfortable for the patient than externalized knots with suture ends that are not cut flush with the knot. Also, corneal wounds may heal faster as a result of deep, intrastromal neovascularization attracted by the buried knots. However, these buried knots may be difficult to remove at a later date without disrupting the corneal wound and the deep stromal neovascularization may increase the chance of graft rejection.

A third suturing method consists of placing a 24-bite running suture (four or six interrupted cardinal sutures) and removing the interrupted sutures at the end of the case. This technique allows adjustment of the running suture with the aid of an operative qualitative keratometer, to minimize astigmatism. To reduce astigmatism postoperatively, the running suture can be adjusted using the slit-lamp. This 24-bite technique may speed early visual recovery (Figs. 24.14 and 24.15). Wound integrity depends entirely on the running suture, however, and this suturing method is not recommended for surgeons who only occasionally perform PKP.

Before making the final adjustment of the running suture, the anterior chamber should be reformed to normal depth and pressure. This is done by injecting BSS through a 30-gauge cannula that passes through the wound. The surgeon should take care not to catch the cannula on Descemet's membrane and traumatize it. The suture ends are cut short with either a blade or a Vannas scissors. The knot is adjusted so the suture ends do not protrude. Stabilization sutures and rings, if used, are now removed. A steroid and antibiotic (e.g., Decadron and gentamicin) are injected subconjunctivally, a topical antibiotic ointment (e.g., polymyxin/Bacitracin), a light patch, and protective shield are placed. A cycloplegic is generally not required.

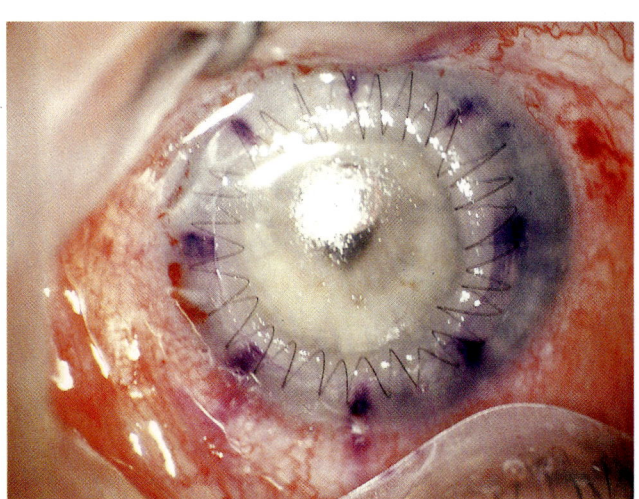

Figure 24.14 *A completed PKP with a 24-bite 10-0 nylon running suture.*

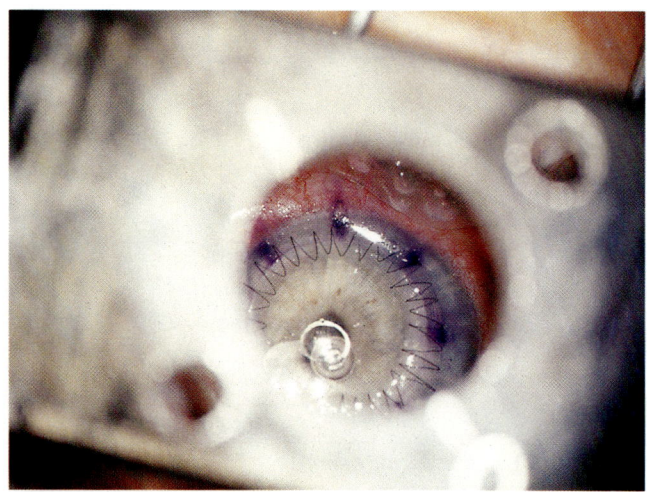

Figure 24.15 *A PKP closed by a 24-bite running suture without any interrupted sutures (and adequate intraocular pressure) can be examined for large amounts of corneal astigmatism with a qualitative keratometer. The suture tension can be adjusted until the mires are reasonably circular. Further adjustments of the suture can be made postoperatively.*

Postoperative Regimen

Patients are examined on the first postoperative day, at about week one, weeks three to four, and months three, six, 12, 18, 24, and yearly thereafter. This is only a minimum regimen. More frequent follow-up exams are common and should occur when indicated.

Routine postoperative medical regimens vary considerably among keratoplasty surgeons. Steroids, for example, enhance graft survival by decreasing postoperative inflammation and the risk of immune rejection. Intensive topical steroids may also delay wound healing, induce glaucoma in some patients, cause cataract in phakic patients, and may promote secondary bacterial, fungal, or viral infection.

Following is a regimen that appears successful in most cases. The ophthalmologist must monitor the patient vigilantly, however, and alter the regimens according to the patient's particular postoperative course, allergies, or contraindications.

OPERATIVE DAY
Subconjunctival cortisone
Subconjunctival antibiotic
Semipressure patch with overlying Fox shield
Oral carbonic anhydrase inhibitor (Diamox Sequel 500 mg, Neptazane 50 mg)

Topical
Dexamethasone 0.1% q2h 7 AM to 11 PM
Polymyxin/Bacitracin ointment qid
Beta-blocker (Timoptic, Betagan, Betoptic) 0.5% bid

Systemic
Analgesic tablets (e.g., Percocet q 6 hrs)

FIRST POSTOPERATIVE WEEK
Combination steroid-antibiotic (e.g., dexamethasone-tobramycin or prednisolone acetate-gentamicin) qid
Moderate pressure patch if epithelial defect is present
Discontinue lid patching as soon as epithelium is intact.

THREE TO SIX MONTHS POSTOPERATIVELY
The patient should taper steroid-antibiotic to qd as condition permits.

AFTER SIX MONTHS
Antibiotics are discontinued.
Steroid prophylaxis is continued in the form of dexamethasone 0.1% or prednisolone 1% qd for aphakic and pseudophakic patients.

Phakic patients are changed to prednisolone phosphate 0.125% qd for another three to six months and then steroids are discontinued completely.

Visual Rehabilitation

Rehabilitation can begin as soon as the corneal surface is sufficiently smooth to permit keratometry, keratoscopy, photokeratoscopy, and/or refraction. This may occur as early as the first postoperative week but more commonly occurs no sooner than about one month postoperatively, and often several months later. As soon as accurate data are obtained, the surgeon begins selective removal of individual interrupted sutures in the steep meridian(s). Only an experienced surgeon should consider removing more than two sutures 180 degrees apart at an exam. Measurements should not be taken until at least two weeks after sutures are removed so that new corneal contours can be established. Immediately measuring change after suture adjustment or removal can be educational but does not necessarily indicate the change in the corneal contour that will ultimately result. If no interrupted sutures remain in the steep meridian, the running suture can be adjusted by tightening it in the flat meridian and moving the slack suture material along to the steep meridians 90 degrees away. This maneuver requires a cooperative patient, good forceps, and carries some risk of breaking the running suture. It is better to be conservative rather than compromise wound integrity.

Using a suturing technique of all interrupted sutures allows for suture removal at three to four months because the knots promote faster wound healing than a running nylon suture. For patient comfort, the knots of an interrupted suture technique must be buried; consequently, they are more likely to induce deep neovascularization, which can promote graft rejection. After PKP, there is no valid way of assessing if adequate wound healing has occurred, and a small percentage of wound dehiscences will occur, even if nine to 12 months pass before the running suture is removed. These are some PKP suturing technique issues that must concern the surgeon.

Spectacles can be dispensed as soon as a stable refraction with a tolerable level of spherical and astigmatic correction is obtained. Generally this is between three and nine months postoperatively, and it should be at least two weeks after the last suture adjustment. Most patients can tolerate up to 4.00 D of cylinder in their spectacles, and it is wise to stop suture manipulation at this point. If there is reason to doubt a patient's ability to tolerate a new refraction, the patient may wear the proposed prescription in a trial frame in the office for about 30 minutes.

With these techniques, one rarely needs to resort to hard contact lenses after keratoplasty. Also, it is best to avoid the stress that a contact lens puts on a graft, particularly while the graft is relatively anesthetic and sutures remain in place.

Failure to achieve expected visual recovery with a clear and smooth transplant is usually due to irregular astigmatism or maculopathy. Irregular astigmatism can usually be diagnosed by keratometry or keratoscopy. Computer-assisted topographic analysis may be helpful if this sophisticated equipment is available. If doubt remains, a diagnostic hard contact lens with over-refraction will yield dramatic improvement in acuity by optically removing the irregular astigmatism. Careful fundus exam with a 90.00 D lens or fundus contact lens will reveal many maculopathies. Cystoid macular edema may be difficult to see through a graft; thus a fluorescein angiogram enables the surgeon to make the diagnosis and initiate topical and systemic anti-inflammatory therapy.

In the absence of irregular astigmatism or if the active cystoid macular edema is not sufficient to explain the diminished acuity, the usual exams for evaluating unexplained visual loss should be performed. This includes testing color vision, performing formal visual fields, and neuro-ophthalmic clinical and radiologic examinations. The keratoplasty surgeon should be aware that cystoid macular edema can cause permanent loss of visual function through photoreceptor damage. The leakage may resolve but leave no visible trace on examination or fluorescein angiography after PKP. Particularly when a patient has pseudophakic corneal edema with a high probability of accompanying cystoid macular edema, this phenomenon is a frequent cause of unexplained visual loss after otherwise successful PKP. This is a diagnosis of exclusion, however, and a thorough examination of other causes of visual loss is appropriate before making a final diagnosis.

Complications

Surface Disease

As outlined in the preoperative evaluation and in Table 24.1, surface keratopathy is an expected complication after keratoplasty for a number of disorders. Therapeutic alternatives to surgery include topical lubricating drops and ointment; punctal occlusion for dry eyes; systemic tetracycline or doxycycline for lid inflammation; occlusive lid taping; bandage therapeutic soft contact lenses; therapeutic gas permeable scleral contact lenses; lateral, medial, or central temporary or permanent tarsorrhaphy; and, in extreme cases, a conjunctival flap. It must be remembered at all times that topical medications and preservatives in persistent epitheliopathies are frequently toxic. Discontinuing medication is often the most important therapeutic step.

Glaucoma

Open-angle glaucoma may develop or worsen after PKP. Proper diagnosis and follow-up should not omit gonioscopy, disc exams, and formal visual field testing, even if the corneal graft makes these tests suboptimal. Steroid-induced open-angle glaucoma usually responds to reduced or discontinued steroid use, although persistent elevation of the pressure may occur even when steroids are discontinued. If steroids are necessary for graft integrity, concomitant antiglaucoma medication should be added to normalize the intraocular pressure.

Synechial angle-closure is a dreaded and common complication after PKP. If surgical technique is meticulous, the patient will not have adhesions to the wound after leaving the operating room; however, inflammation or wound leaks can result in postoperative progressive formation of peripheral anterior synechia. Surgical reintervention to lyse these adhesions may be helpful. In the presence of permanent synechia and an unacceptable intraocular pressure with patient using maximum tolerated glaucoma medication, surgery must be considered before severe optic nerve injury and visual field loss occurs. Conventional filtration surgery has a poor prognosis in many of these cases, but some reports indicate that techniques such as the Molteno valve may improve the prognosis. Cyclodestructive procedures (cyclocryotherapy, trans-scleral cyclophotocoagulation, focused ultrasound) are usually successful in lowering intraocular pressure. Unfortunately, visual prognosis is often poor after cyclodestruction, and long-term graft survival is reduced due to chronic inflammation.

Recurrent Disease

Some corneal diseases recur in the graft. It is well documented that some corneal stromal dystrophies recur many years after the keratoplasty and may eventually require regrafting. True keratoconus probably does not recur but may be present in the donor, or it may be confused with postoperative graft astigmatism. Also, the total extent of the keratoconus may not have been included in the original trephination of the host cornea. The most troublesome recurrence is often herpes simplex keratitis. The eye should be free of inflammation and recurrent disease for at least six months before elective PKP. I recommend prophylactic administration of topical antiviral medication postoperatively while the patient is on strong topical steroids (e.g., dexamethasone 0.1% or prednisolone 1%). Vidarabine or trifluorothymidine are given with the same frequency as the strong steroid. Oral acyclovir's usefulness as prophylaxis or therapy for severe recurrence of herpes simplex keratitis is currently being investigated.

Rejection

Immune rejection has a peak incidence between the third and eighteenth postoperative month, but it can occur at any time. The patient and physician must guard against a false sense of security; rejections can occur more than a decade after surgery. Each postoperative examination must include meticulous documentation of any deposits on the endothelium. New precipitates should be assumed to be impending rejections.

Acute onset of localized or generalized edema is also assumed to be a rejection unless some other cause for endothelial decompensation is evident. The presence of edema and new keratic precipitates, either scattered or in the classic Khodadoust line, is, of course, unequivocal evidence of immunologic assault on the endothelium. Pure stromal rejection is never seen. Pure epithelial rejection, recognized as clustered or linear inflammatory cells in the epithelium, usually occurs in the first postoperative months and does not require treatment unless severe.

One standard treatment for rejection is strong steroid drops (dexamethasone 0.1% or prednisolone acetate 1%) every hour while awake and dexamethasone ointment at bedtime. For florid rejection in a patient with good overall health, some surgeons administer a short course of high-dose oral prednisone with a rapid taper (e.g., prednisone 80 mg po for two days, 60 mg po for two days, 40 mg po for two days, 20 mg po for two days). Intensive treatment with topical steroids should continue for at least two to three weeks without improvement before a rejection is declared irreversible. If improvement does occur, steroids should be slowly tapered off over several months, and the patient should be checked often for relapses. Increased suspicion of recurrent rejections is appropriate.

Postoperative instructions given to the patient should include information regarding early recognition of the symptoms of rejection. If decreased vision, redness, pain, or photophobia lasts more than two hours, the patient should call the ophthalmologist's office immediately. The staff should be aware that these symptoms may indicate an emergency and need an immediate response. If the patient cannot be seen immediately, the physician should prescribe hourly steroid drops. Because other problems may produce symptoms identical to those indicating rejection (e.g., infectious keratitis), it is critical that the patient be seen by the ophthalmologist as soon as possible.

Conclusion

Although PKP enjoys an overall success rate of more than 90%, the prognosis for a given patient varies greatly, depending on factors specific to that case. The most significant determinant of success is the degree of stromal vascularization of the *recipient* cornea. Deep stromal vessels cause corneal rejection by providing a convenient means for exposing the donor's endothelial antigen to the body's immune system, as well as a means for carrying sensitized "attack" lymphocytes back to the endothelium. The incidence of endothelial rejection is about 8%, with about half of those rejections resolved by a short course of intensive topical, subconjunctival, and oral steroids.

The success rate of PKP improved from about 50% in the early 1960s to over 90% by the mid 1970s as a result of three major factors: 1) nylon suture (replacing silk) 2) the operating microscope (replacing loupes), and 3) topical steroids. The chances for a successful corneal graft are improved by excellent surgical technique and meticulous attention to detail, at the preoperative, operative, and postoperative stages. The surgeon must remember that the goal of a PKP is the best possible visual acuity, not only a clear graft. This means that appropriate attention must be given to the correction of postoperative astigmatism.

Since the early years of the 1900s, PKP has provided and will continue to provide the only chance for improved visual function for appropirate patients. Although not all patients can be helped, the rewards of penetrating keratoplasty can be exhilarating for patient and surgeon alike.

Clinical Points to Consider

☛ The major determination of PKP success is the degree of stromal vascularization of the recipient cornea.

☛ Excellent surgical technique, with good wound alignment and minimal trauma to the donor cornea during suturing, is an important factor for obtaining and maintaining a clear PKP.

☛ Glaucoma commonly accompanies PKP, either as a pre-existing condition or as a result of intensive, long-term topical steroid treatment.

☛ Following PKP, the treatment of postoperative astigmatism, which averages about 4.50 D, may be necessary to provide the patient with both a clear cornea *and* good vision.

☛ Epithelial and stromal rejection are self-limiting; endothelial rejection can cause graft opacity and failure.

LAMELLAR KERATOPLASTY

ROGER F. STEINERT, M.D.   LEE T. NORDAN, M.D.

Lamellar keratoplasty (LK) is performed to restore the structural or optical integrity of the cornea. Penetrating keratoplasty (PKP) is most commonly used to correct endothelial dysfunction as a result of dystrophy, repeated iritis, or sequelae of surgery and keratoconus; however, LK may be considered for other corneal opacities and irregularities as well as for tectonic corneal reconstruction, which may enable successful PKP at a later date. Although PKP is usually the surgeon's first choice when confronted with an eye that has a corneal opacity or decreased function, the need to transplant new healthy corneal endothelium is the only absolute indication for PKP instead of LK.

Overview

LK does not invoke a clinically significant graft-host rejection since an LK donor remains outside the body cavity and is not subjected to identification as a foreign antigen by the body's immune system. Despite this advantage, however, the number of LKs performed decreased dramatically in the early 1960s because topical corticosteroids, the operating microscope, and nylon suture raised the success rate of PKP (which provides an excellent chance of visual recovery) to well over 90%. Many corneal specialists may have seen but never actually performed LK for optical rehabilitation during their specialty training.

A lamellar graft contributes only *shape* to the host cornea. Endothelial function, epithelial function, and keratocyte function are ultimately supplied by the recipient cornea. Therefore, it is no surprise that several techniques to correct refractive errors (keratomileusis, epikeratoplasty, and alloplastic intracorneal implantation), all of which attempt to change the central corneal curvature, are based on the principles of LK. Interestingly, an LK donor cornea may remain totally clear—without functional keratocytes—as proven by observing the clear corneas of patients who have undergone keratomileusis and epikeratophakia with lenticules frozen on the Steinway-Barraquer cryolathe.

Indications for Lamellar Keratoplasty

LK is feasible as long as the recipient corneal endothelium is healthy, although most surgeons desire that an opacity or thinning not extend beyond 80% of the corneal depth. A lamellar procedure is preferred over PKP in most cases in which the risk of immunologic rejection is moderate to high (e.g., disciform Herpes keratitis) or in which the greater structural integrity of the globe following a lamellar graft may be important (e.g., an uncooperative child). Examples of good candidates for LK, as opposed to PKP, are presented in Table 25.1.

Potential Problems

Careful preoperative evaluation and management of risk factors is necessary for optimizing the outcome of LK. Both LK and PKP have many of the same healing problems postoperatively, yet certain differences should be noted (Table 25.2).

The surgical technique for lamellar corneal grafts (optical grafts) to restore visual acuity is slightly more difficult than PKP. When LK is properly performed, the stromal interface causes only a one line drop of acuity on the Snellen chart. This effect lasts about a year, gradually decreasing during successive years as the stromal interface disappears.

The most common significant complication of PKP is loss of optical clarity, which occurs because of endothelial graft rejection with associated endothelial failure; LK, however, does not cause endothelial rejection. Epithelial and stromal (keratocyte) graft rejections may occur, but they are self-limited and do not affect the final visual outcome.

Stromal neovascularization is a major problem for both PKP and LK. Stromal neovascularization abets endothelial rejection by facilitating antigen recognition and transporting antibodies closer to the donor cornea. In LK, deep stromal recipient neovascularization of the recipient may follow the path of least resistance, the stromal interface between recipient and donor cornea, resulting in loss of corneal optical clarity.

Epithelial healing is important in both PKP and LK because it prevents infection and provides an excellent optical surface. A smooth, well-aligned wound allows epithelium to cross the wound from the peripheral recipient to the more central donor. Wound leak is not a problem with LK, although it may be with PKP.

Healing and final optical correction are typically faster following LK than PKP, primarily because, in this nonperforating procedure, greater surface area contact and wound integrity allow for rapid suture removal. On the average, however, lamellar graft recipients seem to experience about the same amount of regular astigmatism as PKP patients, although a greater percentage of cases develop significant irregular astigmatism after suture removal.

The increased frequency of irregular astigmatism following LK compared to PKP are probably related mainly to two factors: First, the surface micro-undulations of the dissections of the lamellar bed of the donor and the recipient cornea may not match exactly. Second, a lamellar graft has two aspects to its wound—the vertical peripheral corneal junction, as in PKP, and the adherence of the lamellar graft donor to the underlying host cornea. Manipulation of the peripheral wound by suture relaxation or astigmatic keratotomy will have an effect on the regular astigmatism of the central cornea, but virtually nothing is known about how to manipulate the microscopic stromal healing interaction between donor and recipient, which may cause irregular astigmatism.

Surgical Procedure

Preparation

The preoperative and operative preparation of the LK patient is very similar to PKP. A Flieringa ring is not needed unless, perhaps, conversion to PKP during LK for deep corneal trauma in a child is necessary. Efforts to soften the globe are unnecessary. Fixation sutures of 6-0 silk are used, as necessary, to position the globe properly.

Recipient Lamellar Dissection

The patient's eye is addressed first to facilitate conversion to PKP, if necessary, without previously committing the donor. The first goal is to dissect a host cornea lamellar button to a depth below the stromal pathology. The shallower this dissection, the more recipient stroma available to provide a stable corneal shape. Host cornea dissection just above Descemet's membrane may provide a clear cornea postoperatively but cause severe steepening of the central cornea, indicative of corneal ectasia.

In order to achieve a lamellar dissection of the proper depth and location, a trephine diameter is selected, which leaves at least a 1.50 mm rim of recipient cornea as in PKP. A miotic pupil is invaluable for centering the trephination on the visual axis, usually slightly nasal to the geometric center of the cornea (Fig. 25.3).

An accurate, partial-depth trephination of the host cornea is needed, making the Hessburg-

Table 25.1
Lamellar Keratoplasty Candidates

Problem	Postoperative management problems	Stromal opacity with healthy endothelium	Increased PKP failure rate	Thin peripheral cornea
Example	Infants Mentally incapacitated patients	Disciform herpes simplex keratitis	Alkalai burn	Rheumatoid arthritis Trauma

Table 25.2
Lamellar Keratoplasty: Postoperative Concerns

Location	Problem	Cause
Epithelium	Delayed healing	Donor/recipient junction uneven; loose sutures External disease lids; conjunctiva; dry eye
Interface	Opacity Debris Neovascularization	Epithelial ingrowth Epithelial cysts Particulate matter (usually asymptomatic) Reaction to inflammation
Refractive	Regular astigmatism Irregular astigmatism Central corneal steepening	As with PKP Higher incidence than with PKP Recipient cornea too thin

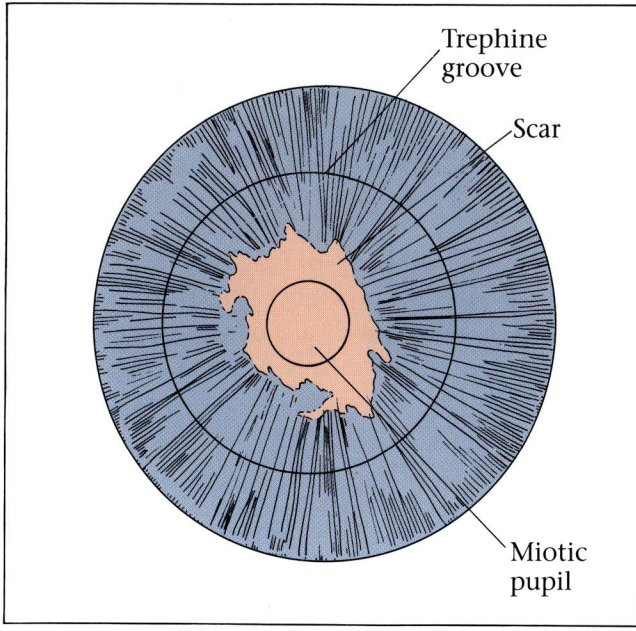

Figure 25.3 *The miotic pupil, usually located slightly nasal to the geometric center of the cornea, is an excellent landmark on which to center the partial thickness trephination of a lamellar keratoplasty.*

Baron trephine very useful (Figs. 25.4). Using this trephine, the technique is similar to that outlined for PKP (Chapter 24). The surgeon carefully adjusts the blade until it is aligned with the inner wall of the suction chamber. The blade is then retracted (rotated counterclockwise) by three, one-quarter (¼) turns (three-quarters [¾] of one turn, *not* 3¼ turns) of the handle. The trephine is applied to the patient's cornea, centered, and adequate suction is achieved by slowly releasing the syringe plunger. The blade is now advanced (rotated clockwise) three, one-quarter (¼) turns, (three-quarters [¾] of one turn, *not* 3¼ turns) back to the original position within the inner wall.

The blade is then advanced further to achieve the desired trephination depth. For a cornea of normal thickness, the blade is further advanced four-and-one-half (4½), one-quarter (¼) turns. As a rule of thumb, each one-quarter (¼) turn of the Hessburg-Baron trephine beyond the level of the inner wall will result in a trephination of 0.90 mm (90 μ) depth. Therefore, four and one-half (4½) one-quarter (¼) turns result in a trephination depth of about 0.40 mm (400 μ), approximately 80% of a 0.50 mm (500 μ) thick cornea. (The peripheral cornea is about 0.70 mm [700 μ] thick in the midperiphery. A lamellar dissection plane that starts in the periphery at a depth of 0.50 mm will achieve a depth centrally slightly shallower than this.)

The blade advance is reduced if the peripheral host cornea is thinner than normal (which requires that a detailed preoperative slit lamp exam be performed). Beware, however, because it may be very difficult to create a lamellar dissection if the residual corneal bed is very thin. Also, an old nonhealed perforating scar may allow leakage of aqueous from the anterior chamber through a latently patent corneal defect, even though the lamellar dissection has not broken the plane of Descemet's membrane. If a defect in Descemet's membrane is created, viscoelastic may be injected through the defect to keep the anterior chamber formed while the lamellar dissection is completed. For this reason, the most uncertain areas of the lamellar dissection should be performed last. The donor cornea will seal these defects but, if a central opacity develops as a result of endothelial damage, a PKP may have to performed later.

Even with the aid of pachymetry, judging the thickness of the cornea and the depth of corneal pathology can be very difficult. During trephination, the surgeon must carefully observe the junction of the blade's inner wall and the cornea. The blade should be advanced slowly and stopped at the first sign of fluid. The appearance of any moisture signals perforation. If a microperforation (less than 0.50 mm) occurs, it will usually be self-sealing and the procedure may continue as a lamellar keratectomy. If the perforation is larger,

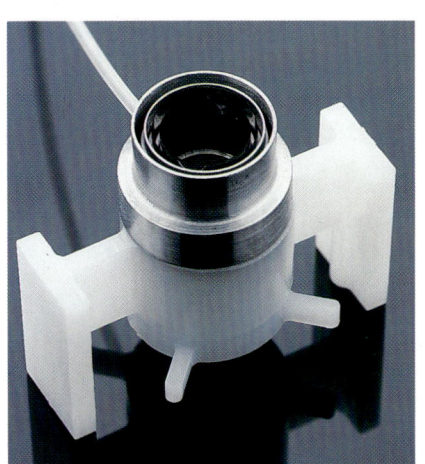
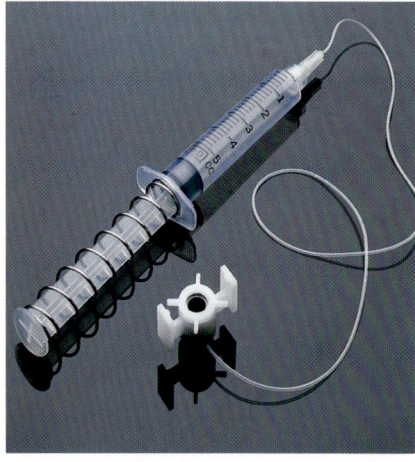

Figure 25.4 (Left) *Hessburg-Baron trephine. The double-walled outer cylinder firmly affixes to the peripheral cornea when a vacuum is created by releasing the springloaded syringe plunger, which is connected to the trephine cylinder by a thin silastic tube.* **(Right)** *Rotation of the handle advances and retracts the central trephine.*

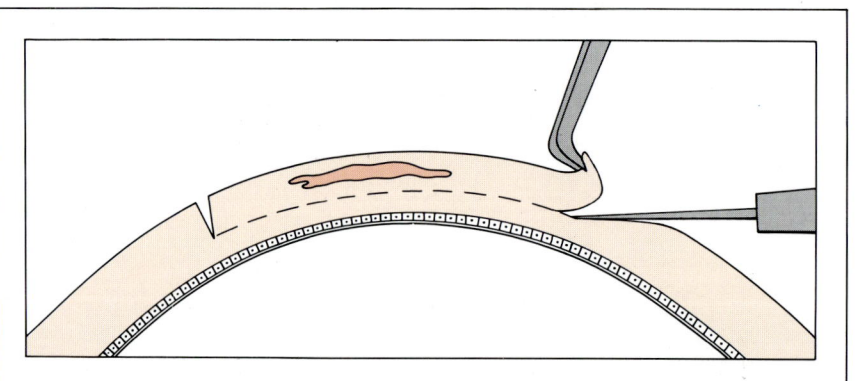

Figure 25.5 *The depth of the lamellar dissection is determined by the depth of the trephination, which is planned to be deeper than the corneal pathology. A sharp microblade is used to initiate the lamellar dissection plane and a semisharp spatula-knife used to separate, rather than cut, the stromal lamellae.*

it may be best to convert to a PKP, unless the corneal defect can be sutured to maintain the anterior chamber.

After completing the trephination of the patient's cornea, the groove should be inspected by separating the lips of the wound with 0.12 mm Colibri forceps (Fig. 25.5). If the trephination is satisfactory, the surgeon proceeds to the lamellar dissection of the corneal bed, using a Martinez spatula or Paufique or Tooke knife (Fig. 25.6). These spatulas are semisharp blades designed to divide the cornea by splitting and separating the corneal lamellae, rather than cutting collagen fibers. The depth of the lamellar dissection is chosen by grasping and everting the inner edge of the host cornea at 11 o'clock (for a right-handed surgeon; 1 o'clock for a left-handed surgeon) and starting the horizontal dissection plane with a sharp microblade (see Fig. 25.6).

The corneal lamellar dissection is begun by inserting the dissection spatula into the corneal pocket started by the microblade (Figs. 25.7 and 25.8). A circular or side-to-side motion of the spatula, rather than a fore-to-aft motion, is preferred since this technique encourages the spatula to create a single dissection plane. The bottom of the spatula should be kept parallel to Descemet's membrane, so the blade will not dissect more deeply. If the spatula begins to drag on the stromal bed, a drop of BSS will provide the needed lubrication. Excessive moisture, however, will cause stromal swelling and distort further dissection.

The dissection progresses until the entire bed defined by the trephination has been covered (Figs. 25.9 and 25.10). If the dissection has been precise, the host button will become free as the spatula intersects the last portion of the trephination groove. If the dissection is slightly deeper than the trephination groove in some areas, corneal scissors are used to complete the excision of the central cornea, leaving the recipient corneal edges as perpendicular as possible.

Once the host button has been removed, it is inspected for gross uniformity of thickness. The bed of the dissection is examined to determine that adequate amounts of scarring have been

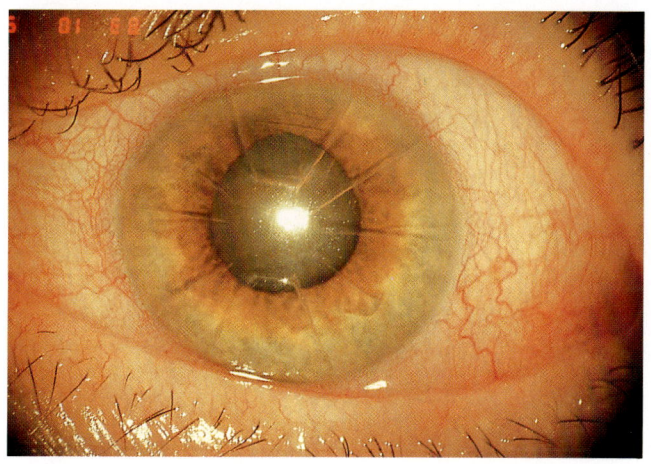
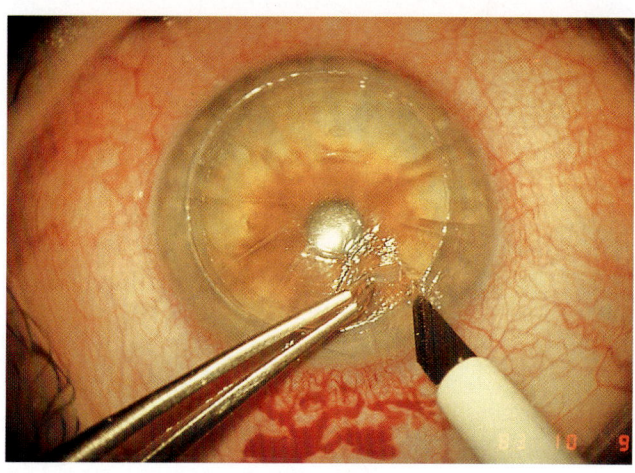

Figure 25.6 (Left) *The cornea of a patient who underwent several radial keratotomy and Ruiz (trapezoidal astigmatic keratotomy) procedures in an attempt to correct severe compound myopic astigmatism. Resultant glare and irregular astigmatism was successfully treated with a lamellar keratoplasty.* **(Right)** *A sharp microblade is used to determine the level of the corneal dissection by creating a stromal pocket into which the dissecting spatula is placed.*

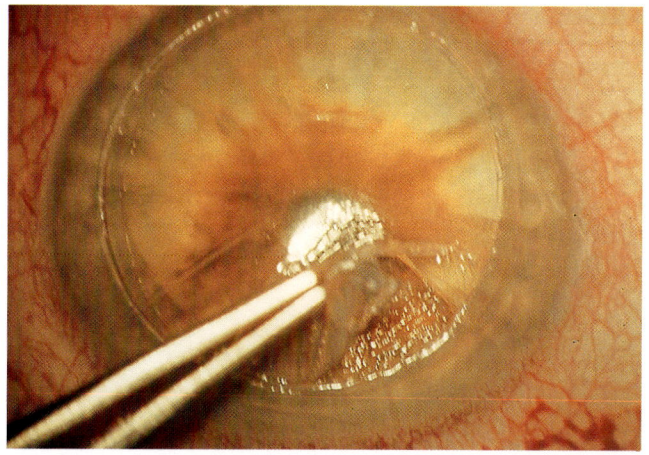

Figure 25.7 *Elevating a corneal sector created by the radial keratotomy incisions exposes the lamellar corneal bed, below; however, the tendency for the peripheral cornea to separate into sectors makes it difficult to achieve a lamellar keratectomy that remains in the same plane.*

removed as planned. If the dissection is too superficial, in whole or in part, a new lamellar plane may be defined initially by using a sharp, round tip disposable scarifier blade, such as the Grieshaber 681.01 or No. 69 Beaver. After a satisfactory deeper level is reached, the bed is redissected with the dissection spatula. Redissection is likely to cause perforation and should be attempted only if the original bed is obviously too superficial. A mild residual haze at the depth of the interface may have little or no optical effect postoperatively, and leaving this mild haze is preferable to perforating Descemet's membrane. This situation is a good time to remember the surgical adage, *Perfection is the enemy of good.*

Lamellar Donor Preparation

The exposed recipient lamellar bed is covered with a plastic corneal protector cap or a piece of lint-free instrument wipe so that no airborne debris will settle and stick on the stromal interface. The surgeon's attention is now directed to the donor cornea. Having a standard corneoscleral donor button in preservative or a donor globe

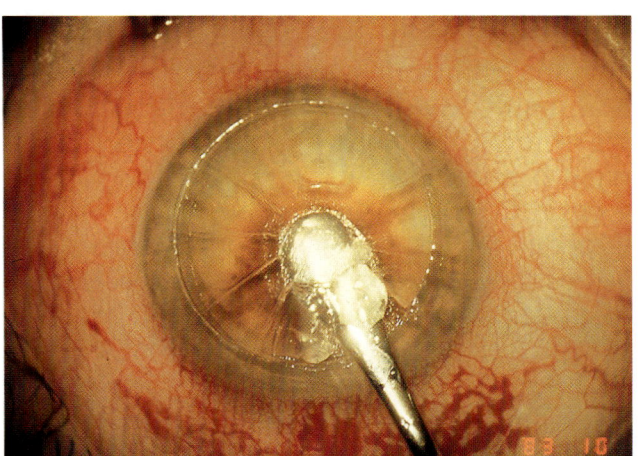

Figure 25.8 (**Top**) *The Paufique knife is advanced into the central cornea, which is free of incisions, and a circular motion insures that the corneal lamellae are separated, rather than cut, by the edges of this semisharp instrument.* (**Bottom**) *The lamellar dissection may be performed by a spatula that is either flat or mildly convex, and it should be moved in a circular motion to maintain the same intrastromal plane.*

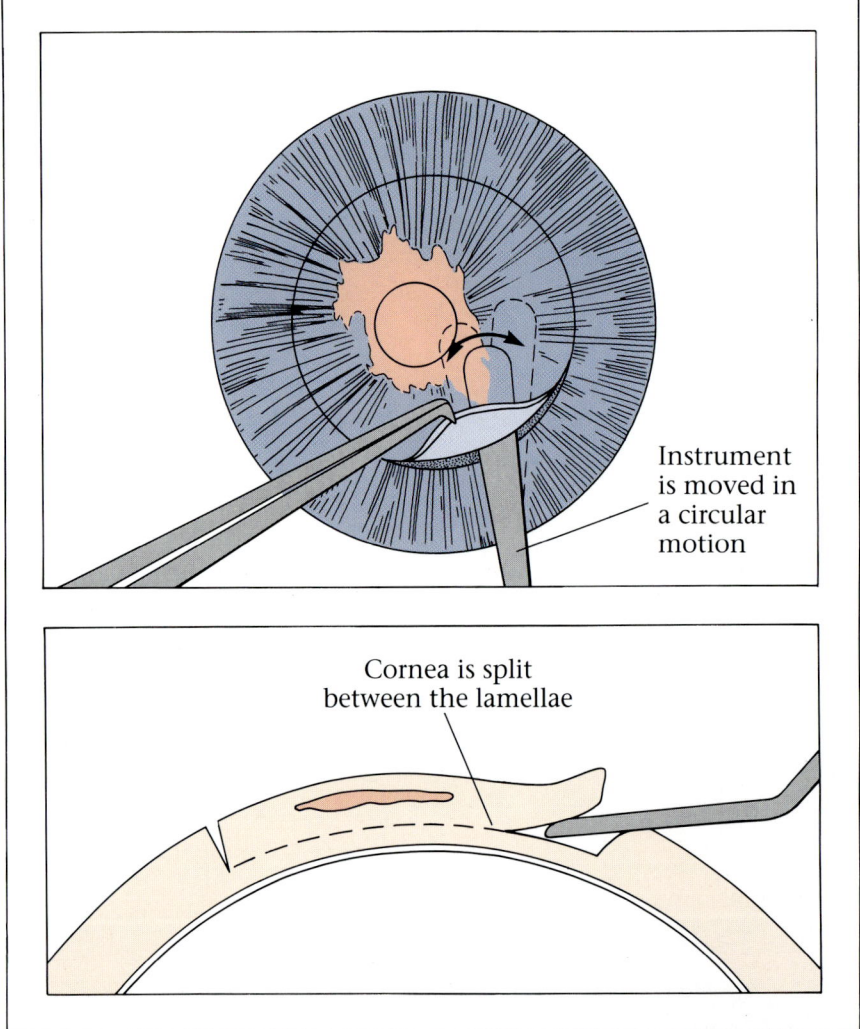

enables the surgeon to proceed with a PKP if the lamellar dissection has gone astray. A globe makes the lamellar dissection of the donor relatively easy. However, in order to perform a lamellar dissection on the corneoscleral button, it must first be fixated on a spherical surface, such as the silastic sphere of a prosthetic eye.

A full thickness donor cornea, after trephination and removal of the endothelium by rubbing with dry cellulose surgical sponge, may be used when the purpose of the lamellar graft is clearly tectonic. Remarkable clarity can be obtained, despite the presence of a double Descemet's membrane (Fig. 25.11). However, this thick donor may create a final central corneal thickness greater than 0.85 mm, which may compromise visual acuity. Also, care must be taken to insure that the donor does not project above the peripheral recipient at the corneal wound.

If a donor globe is available, it should be pressurized to normal IOP by injecting air through the optic nerve and clamping the optic nerve with a small hemostat. The globe may also be wrapped in gauze, which makes it much easier to handle. Ten to 20 drops of antibiotic (e.g., Tobrex, garamycin, chloromycetin, Polytrim) are applied to the cornea immediately before the globe is to be used. Healthy epithelium may be left on the donor, which can provide initial protection and rapid epithelialization. Under the operating microscope, a 4.00-mm to 5.00-mm vertical, peripheral corneal incision is made in clear cornea with a sharp microblade to a depth equal to the desired thickness of the donor (Fig. 25.12). The surgeon must be aware that the cornea of the donor globe is edematous and anticipate about 20% thinning of the donor after it has been subjected to the endothelial effects of the recipient.

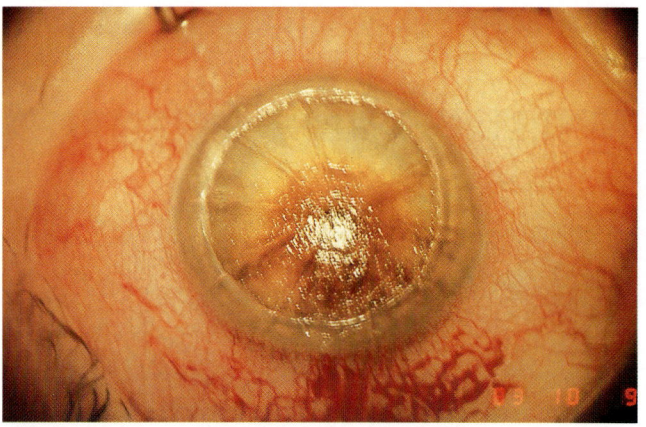

Figure 25.9 *The lamellar keratectomy has been completed, leaving a recipient lamellar bed, which awaits the donor cornea.*

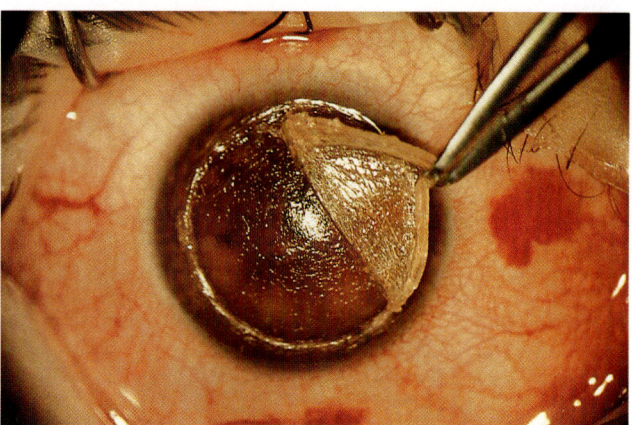

Figure 25.10 *The host cornea is removed after completion of the lamellar keratectomy.*

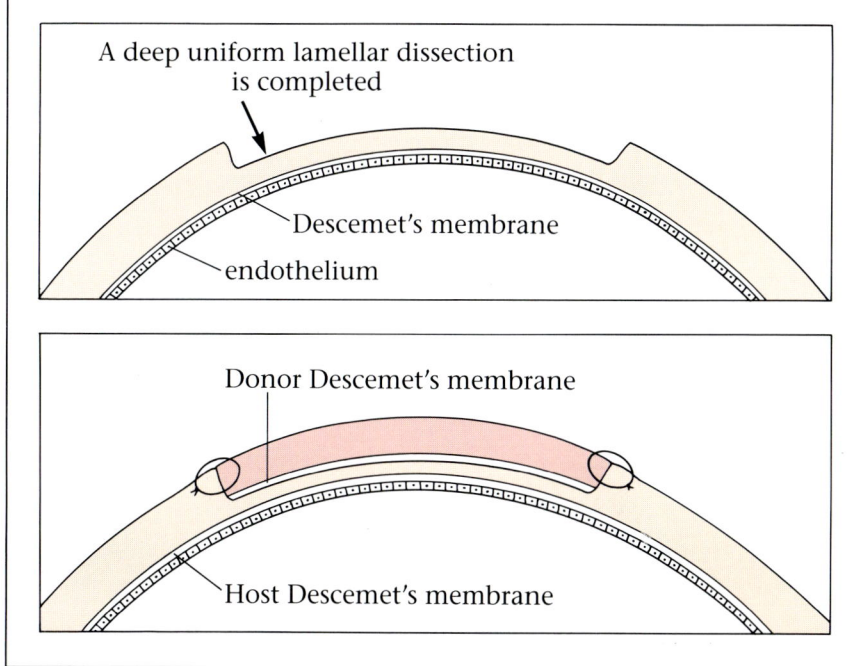

Figure 25.11 *A full thickness lamellar corneal donor with the endothelium removed results in a thick cornea that has two Descemet's membranes. This thickened cornea may provide an excellent foundation for a penetrating keratoplasty but may limit visual acuity.*

The same sharp microblade is now used to create the beginning of the lamellar dissection plane. The dissecting spatula creates the lamellar dissection in the donor cornea, as it had in the patient's cornea (Figs. 25.13 and 25.14). Dissection of the donor cornea progresses more easily than dissection of the recipient cornea since the donor cornea is edematous and the collagen lamellae are easily separated everywhere inside the limbus. A trephine of the desired diameter is used to create the donor corneal button by trephining from the epithelial side to a depth beyond that of the lamellar dissection. A donor diameter 0.25 mm larger than the recipient bed diameter is commonly chosen (Fig. 25.15). By first performing the donor lamellar dissection through a peripheral wound, the central trephination provides a donor with a smooth edge that has not been manipulated by forceps (Fig. 25.16).

The donor cornea is placed onto the recipient after meticulously inspecting the graft bed and removing all debris (Fig. 25.17). Retained epithelium has the potential to form progressive cysts in the lamellar bed, which may require removal but can usually be avoided by meticulous cleaning of the lamellar bed. The stromal surfaces donor and the recipient bed should be irrigated with copious amounts of BSS immediately before placing the donor onto the recipient cornea.

Suturing

Securing the donor into position can be achieved using a variety of interrupted and running 10-0 nylon suture patterns (Figs. 25.18 and 25.19). An excellent suture method involves four equally spaced 10-0 nylon cardinal sutures, which anchor the donor in position, followed by a running 16-bite 10-0 nylon suture with the knot cut extremely short, pulled to the scleral side of the wound, and buried just below the corneal surface (see Fig. 25.19).

Later, it is desirable to remove the suture knots through the scleral side of the trephination so as not to disrupt the freshly healing wound. The

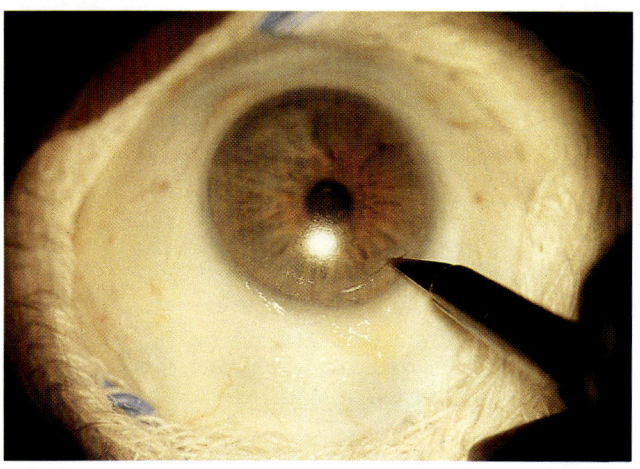

Figure 25.12 *A vertical, partial-depth peripheral corneal incision is made with a sharp microblade. The same blade is then used to start the lamellar dissection.*

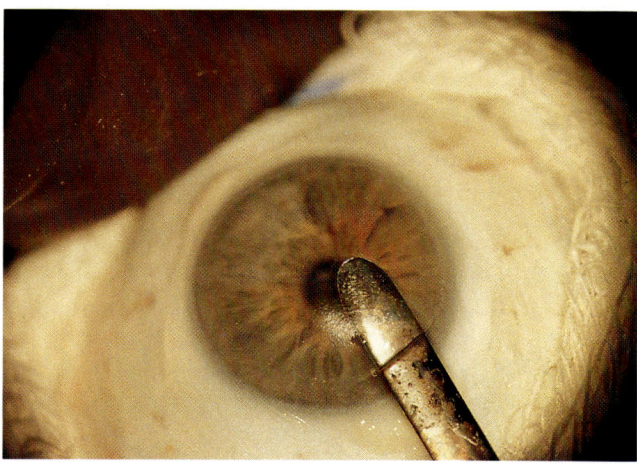

Figure 25.13 *The lamellar dissection of the donor cornea commences.*

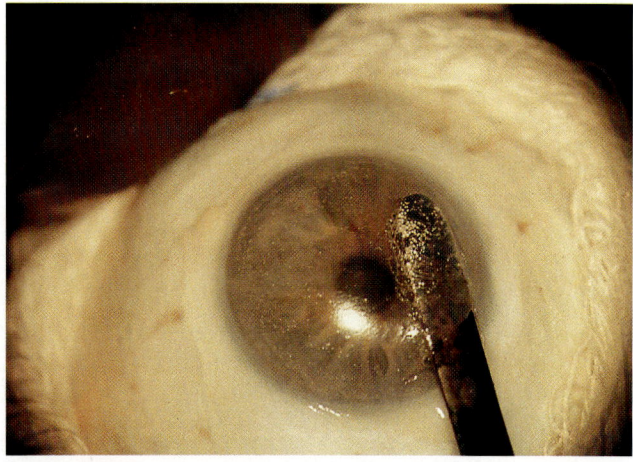

Figure 25.14 *Lamellar dissection of the donor cornea is extended to the limbus.*

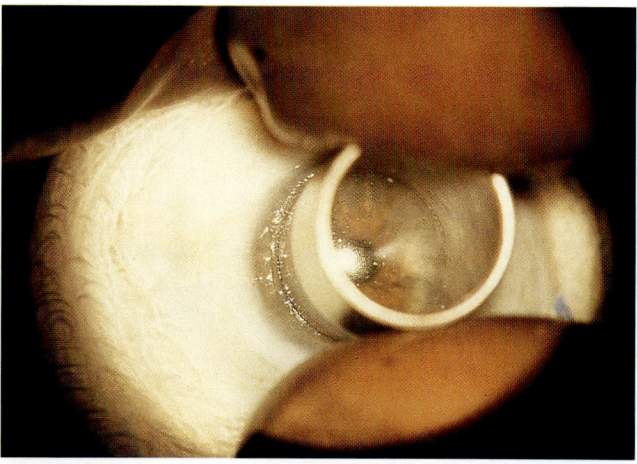

Figure 25.15 *Central trephination is used to create the donor for the lamellar keratoplasty.*

cardinal sutures can be removed at surgery. If the epithelium covers the wound overnight, the patient should be comfortable one day after surgery. For children and young adults, interrupted sutures may be advisable because of the unpredictable and frequently rapid loosening of sutures postoperatively.

In all cases, the goal of suturing is to approximate the edge of the donor and the host, avoiding gaps, bunching, and over-riding or under-riding of the wound, so the Bowman's layers on each side of the wound are aligned. Because the lamellar dissection has thinned and weakened the host cornea, the vertical edge of the recipient bed generally stretches outward. The donor button, consequently, appears "small," and the cardinal sutures must be placed quite tightly to achieve good wound apposition. Later in the suturing process, these early sutures may have to be replaced if they have loosened significantly.

After the completion of suturing, a subconjunctival injection of a steroid and antibiotic is given, sometimes followed by a drop of cycloplegic (Cyclogyl; scopolamine 0.125 %) and always by an antibiotic ointment and a pressure patch.

Postoperative care

Postoperative care of an LK patient is similar to that for a PKP patient. Several significant differences will be presented here. The reader is urged to review the PKP postoperative regimen (Chapter 24) for other details.

Steroid Management. Postoperative topical steroids are used in LK to quiet postoperative inflammation, discourage vascular ingrowth, and reduce sterile infiltrates and inflammation around sutures that tends to cause premature loosening of these sutures. Immunologic rejection is rarely an issue because the host endotheli-

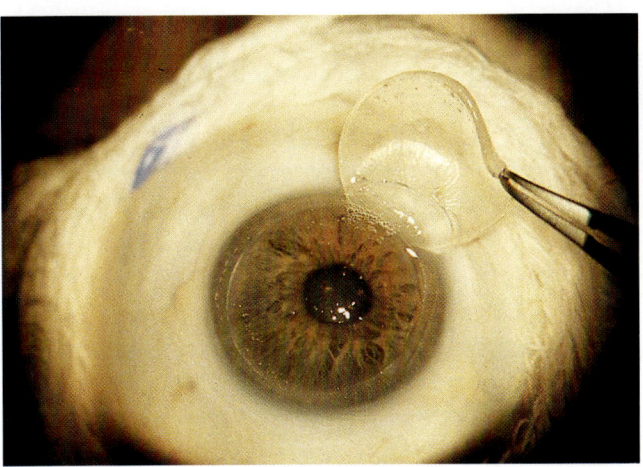

Figure 25.16 *The lamellar corneal donor is removed from the donor globe.*

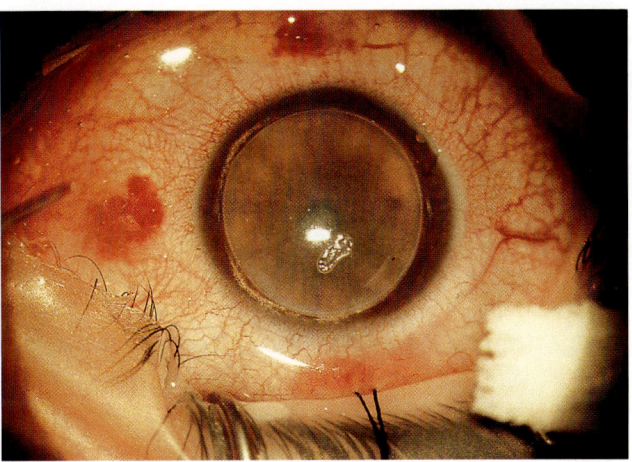

Figure 25.17 *A lamellar donor awaits suturing into the recipient corneal bed. The edematous donor is slightly opaque. The corneal clarity improves dramatically during the suturing process as the recipient's endothelium acts to dehydrate the donor cornea.*

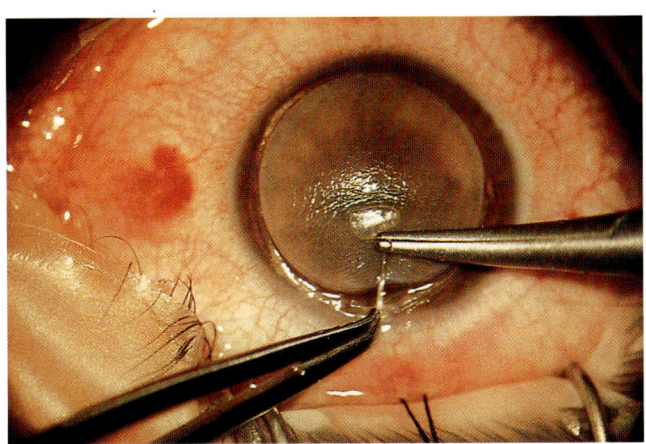

Figure 25.18 *The first cardinal suture is placed.*

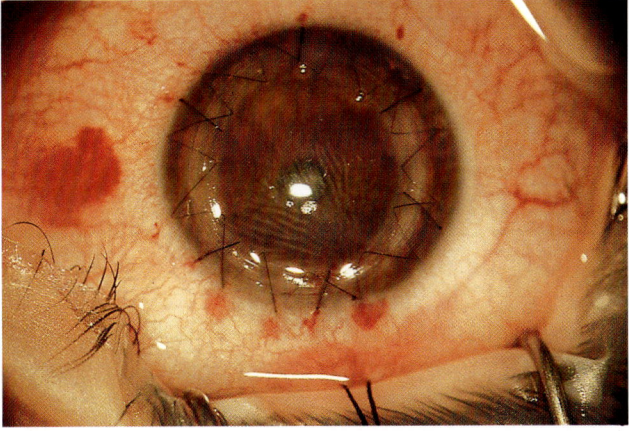

Figure 25.19 *This lamellar keratoplasty was secured in place with 10-0 nylon suture, using a combination of six cardinal sutures and a twelve-bite running suture.*

um is retained. Epithelial rejection rarely requires treatment and does not lead to graft failure as the recipient epithelium replaces the donor epithelium. Stromal rejection is exceedingly rare and usually presents as a central disciform area of corneal edema and optical haze, which resolves after six to eight weeks without topical steroid treatment and much more quickly with it. Because of the reduced incidence of corneal graft rejection, topical steroid use may be less intense and discontinued more rapidly following LK than following PKP. This reduction in steroid use has merit for phakic patients (who are often candidates for lamellar procedures) and for steroid responsive glaucoma patients. Typically, a strong topical steroid such as dexamethasone phosphate 0.1% or prednisone acetate 1% is prescribed four times per day for a week or two postoperatively and then a similar dosage of a weaker topical steroid is administered. All topical steroids are discontinued at the time of final suture removal.

Suture Management. As in PKP, loose sutures are removed promptly. If a running suture is present, elective interrupted suture removal, which improves astigmatism, can begin several weeks to a month after surgery. An interrupted suture is removed at the steepest meridian, determined by keratometry, refraction, photokeratoscopy, or computer-assisted topographical analysis. Adjacent sutures are never removed during the first two postoperative months because wound healing may be too weak to prevent frank wound gape. After the third postoperative month, wound integrity usually permits removal of all remaining sutures. Patients with known autoimmune collagen disease, such as rheumatoid arthritis, may be well served if the sutures are left in place longer to allow for even better wound healing. Several weeks after final suture removal, a stable refraction is expected. If the residual astigmatism is intolerably large and a hard contact lens cannot be fit, corneal relaxing incisions in the wound or astigmatic keratotomy usually reduce the cylinder to acceptable levels (Fig. 25.20).

Tectonic Lamellar Keratoplasty

Corneas requiring tectonic grafts are usually severely ectatic or are actively ulcerated. This degree of sight-threatening disease is best handled by referral to an experienced corneal surgeon, although the anterior segment surgeon may be faced with an imminent or frank perforation that must be addressed immediately. Fresh, frozen, or glycerin-preserved cornea or corneoscleral tissue may be used. A discussion of the many varieties of tectonic grafts is beyond the scope of this book.

Before surgery, the eye is protected with a patch and a Fox shield. The surgeon must decide whether local anesthesia with sedation or general anesthesia is indicated to prevent further prolapse of intraocular tissue by increased retrobulbar pressure. The ocular prep and draping should be done by the surgeon, since prolapsed ocular tissue may be encountered and undue pressure on the lids or globe may cause further intraocular damage. A dry cellulose sponge makes an excellent instrument for eliminating debris, mucous, and epithelium from within the perforating wound.

Any prolapsed vitreous must be excised using a sponge and scissors technique. Necrotic wound edges must be freshened back to viable stroma, usually with a fine forceps and Vannas scissors. The amount of tissue excised is minimal yet sufficient to yield a reasonably smooth contour and an edge that can retain suture. If the sclera is involved, a conjunctival flap is reflected to increase exposure, which enables complete repair.

Surgical Procedure

The Donor Graft

The size of the defect is measured with calipers, and a template that mimics the shape and size of the defect can be fashioned from a piece of drape, cellulose sponge envelope, cardboard, or any other material available. The surgeon uses a separate table to prepare the donor material under the operating microscope. At this point, the goal is to create a piece of donor tissue that approximates the defect, erring on the large size. The donor can be shaped in a variety of ways, but often a double trephination is a good starting point (Figs. 25.21 and 25.22). By using one or two of trephine sizes and double punching the donor, various size crescents can be obtained.

Securing the Graft

Returning to the patient, the donor is placed over the defect and inspected. If the edges can be accurately matched for at least one-third of the defect, the donor is held in place with several interrupted 10-0 nylon sutures. Once stabilized, the donor is trimmed with scissors to better match it to the defect. Ultimately, the donor is secured with interrupted 10-0 nylon sutures. The sutures should be spaced closely because some may loosen prematurely. In places where the structural integrity of the recipient cornea or sclera is questionable, a very long needle track insures an effective suture bite that will not loosen.

Other Forms of Lamellar Keratoplasty

Intrastromal Alloplastic Implantation

Changing Anterior Corneal Shape. As stated earlier in this chapter, autolamellar keratoplasty with reshaping of the donor is the basis for keratomileusis, an important refractive procedure. An autolamellar keratoplasty without reshaping the donor is also an important part of implanting alloplastic lenticules within the corneal stroma. A lenticule that changes refractive error by changing the shape of the anterior corneal surface, such as the hydrogel implant (Allergan Medical Optics Kerato-gel), must use a full lamellar keratectomy by an automated microkeratome with resuturing of the auto-donor over the lenticule. If the lenticule is inserted into a corneal pocket, the posterior surface of the cornea will protrude posteriorly into the anterior chamber, but the anterior surface of the cornea will not be changed enough to correct the refractive error.

These implants seem to work satisfactorily to correct hyperopia, since the convex dome of the cornea is made steeper, and irregular astigmatism is not a common problem (Figs. 25.23 to 25.25). However, these cases are generally amenable to treatment by secondary anterior chamber IOL implantation or hyperopic epikeratoplasty, neither of which necessitates a lamellar keratectomy by microkeratome. Treating high myopia by flattening the convex dome of the cornea by introducing a concave intrastromal lenticule have been rather unsuccessful because of irregular astigmatism, which results in poor quality in uncorrected and best corrected spectacle visual acuity (Fig. 25.26).

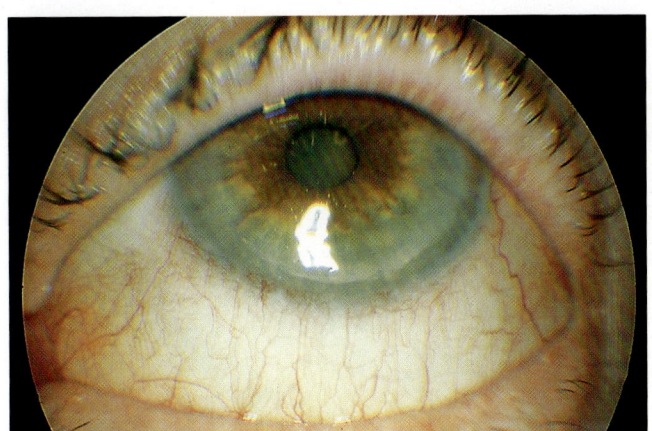

Figure 25.20 *Two months after suture removal a relaxing incision, 90% of the total corneal depth, was made in the keratoplasty wound to control postoperative regular astigmatism.*

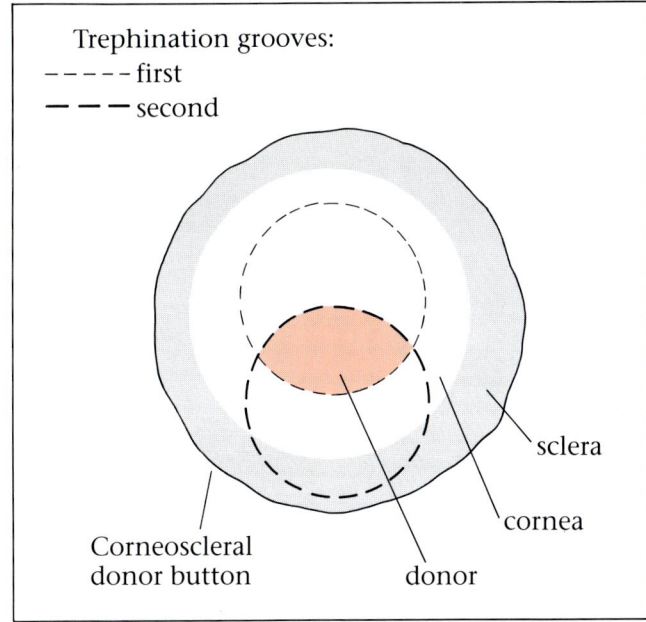

Figure 25.21 *A tectonic lamellar graft may be shaped by using intersecting trephinations of the same diameter.*

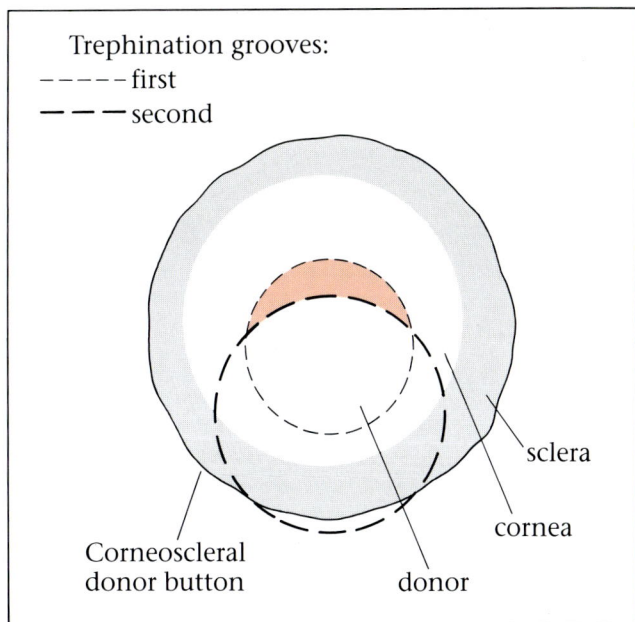

Figure 25.22 *Shaping a tectonic lamellar graft using trephinations of different diameters.*

Changing the Corneal Index of Refraction. Peter Choyce, M.D., developed an intrastromal refractive alloplastic implant of polysulphone that effectively changes the refractive capability of the cornea by increasing or decreasing its index of refraction, depending on the shape of the implant (Fig. 25.27). This concept is appealing because of the precision with which it seems a refractive error could be

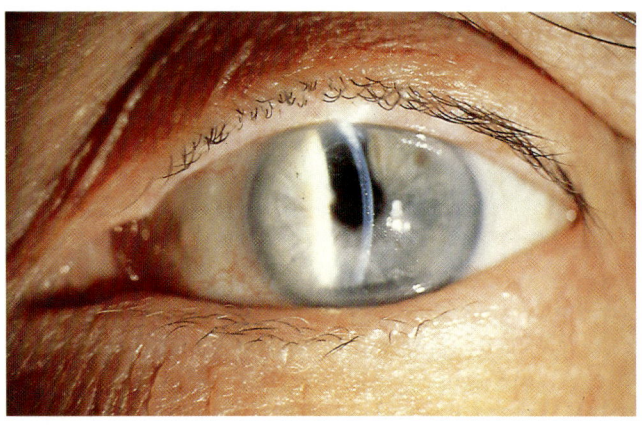

Figure 25.23 *An aphakic hydrogel alloplastic (AMO Kerato-gel) implant six months postoperatively. The patient has 20/25 uncorrected visual acuity in that eye.*

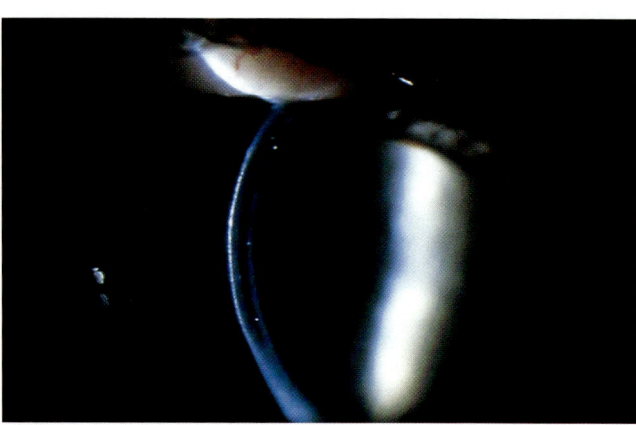

Figure 25.24 *A slit lamp view of the cornea in Figure 25.23. The clear intrastromal zone is the hydrogel implant.*

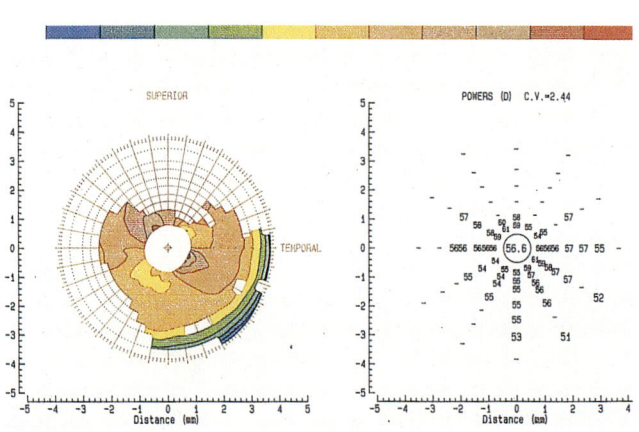

Figure 25.25 *A topographical analysis of the cornea of the patient presented in Figures 25.23 and 25.24. The central cornea's curvature has been increased to about 56.00 D.*

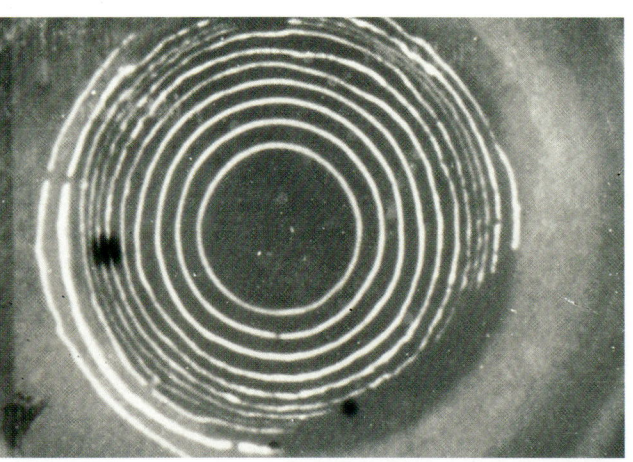

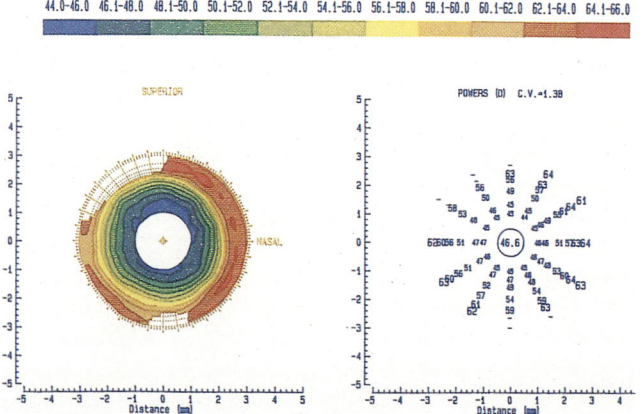

Figure 25.26 **(Left)** *A photokeratoscope of a primate's eye with a well centered minus power hydrogel alloplastic implant. The mires show a definite flattening of the central cornea (wide spacing between mires) with a steepening of the peripheral cornea (narrow spacing between mires). Close examination of the mires of the cornea, however, shows a definite irregularity of the mires, indicative of irregular astigmatism.* **(Right)** *The color-coded topographical representation of this cornea demonstrates the flat central cornea and the steep peripheral cornea. This symmetrical color-coded topographical map is based on specific digital values assigned to the photokeratoscopic mires. This digitalization process produces a study that fails to adequately alert the observer to the irregular astigmatism of the corneal surface and the consequent loss of visual function.*

changed. In addition, the thin, rigid polysulphone lenticule can be inserted into a corneal pocket, without the need for a total lamellar keratectomy. However, the polysulphone, which is rigid enough to possess a high index of refraction, is also rigid enough to erode through the stroma with globe movements and eyelid pressure. Hydration and nutrition of the stroma anterior to the implant, which is impermeable to water and nutrients, has also been a source of concern.

Lamellar Keratoplasty for Hyperopia

Luis Antonio Ruiz, M.D., has popularized the use of automated lamellar keratectomy as a surgical correction for hyperopia. The diameter of this deep keratectomy is varied; the smaller the keratectomy, the greater the effect. This keratectomy allows limited corneal ectasia with resultant central aspheric corneal steepening (Fig. 25.28). Although there is sufficient evidence that this

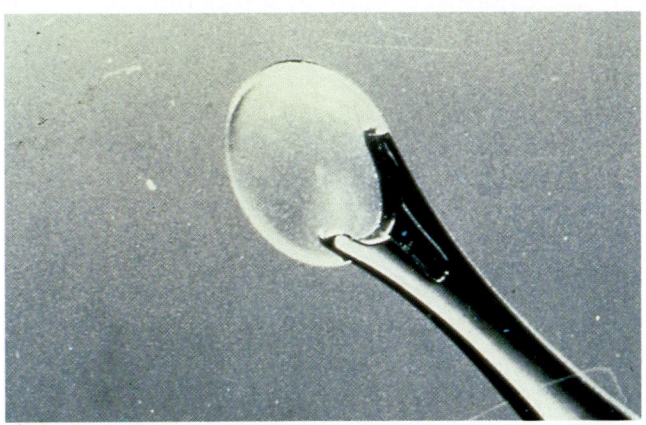 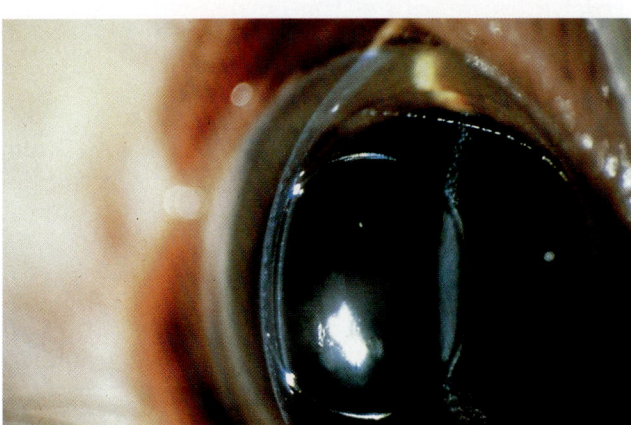

Figure 25.27 **(Left)** *A polysulphone alloplastic corneal implant.* **(Right)** *The polysulphone implant after intrastromal implantation.*

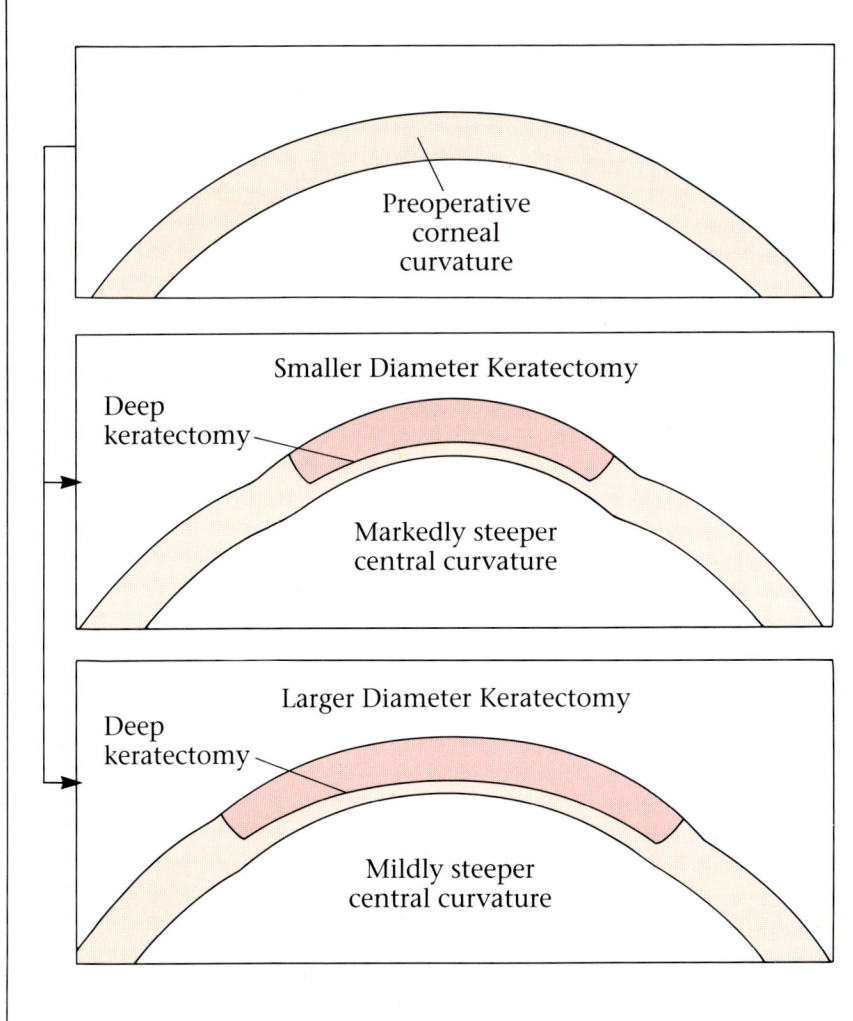

Figure 25.28 *A deep stromal keratectomy creates limited ectasia of the central cornea. The smaller the diameter of the keratectomy, the steeper the curvature of the central cornea.*

procedure can be effective, concerns remain about its predictability and long-term stability.

Oblique Peripheral Keratotomy

Epikeratoplasty is a form of LK. Most epikeratoplasty lenticules can be secured by implanting the peripheral edge of the lenticule into the shallow stromal pocket created in the recipient by an LK, without a keratectomy (Fig. 25.29) (see Chapter 28). The depth of this lamellar dissection is intended to remain less than 0.25 mm so the structural integrity of the cornea will not be affected by resultant ectasia if the epikeratoplasty lenticule must be removed.

This keratotomy can be performed with a No. 69 Beaver blade, Alcon Crescent blade, or a similar semisharp rounded blade. Initiation of the LK by a sharp microblade makes the LK easier (Fig. 25.30). A sharp diamond or pointed blade is not used since these knives can create a multiplane dissection by cutting corneal lamellae, rather than separating them. An occasional drop of BSS on the blade provides lubrication, as needed.

Conclusion

LK is an important surgical procedure for the corneal surgeon concerned with the structural and optical aspects of corneal function. A general familiarity with the principles of lamellar corneal surgery is valuable, since these principles allow the surgeon to treat many intrastromal corneal opacities, emergencies, and refractive cases in a relatively safe and effective manner.

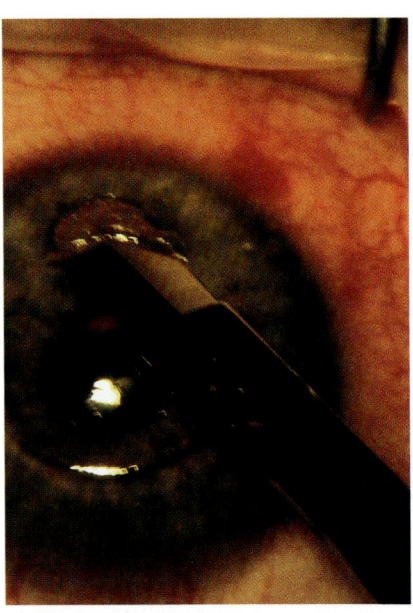

Figure 25.29 *An oblique peripheral keratotomy is performed using a No. 69 Beaver blade. The periphery of the epikeratoplasty lenticule will be inserted into this intrastromal pocket.*

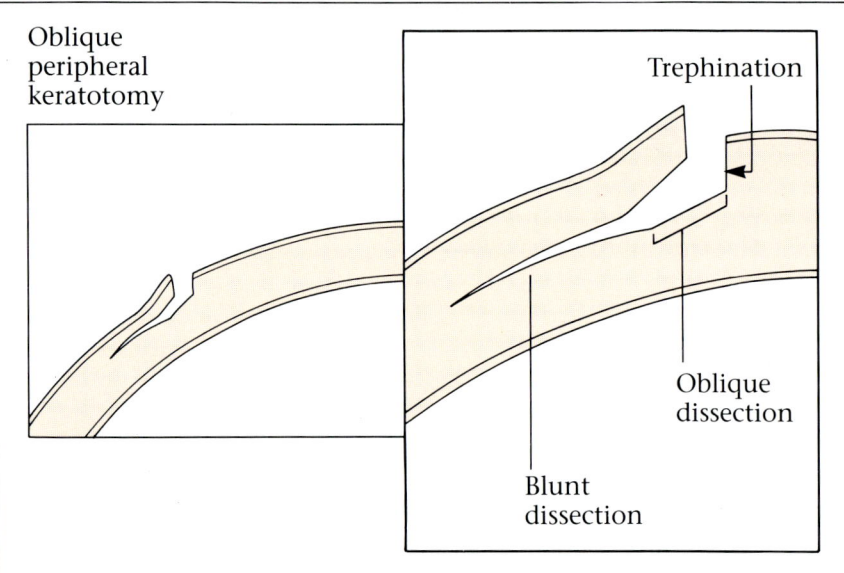

Figure 25.30 *Anatomy of an oblique peripheral keratotomy. The oblique keratectomy is easier to perform if it is started with a sharp microblade.*

Clinical Points to Consider

☛ The donor corneal tissue for lamellar keratoplasty contributes only shape to the host cornea, while the recipient cornea provides endothelial function, epithelium, and keratocytes.

☛ Lamellar keratoplasty does not elicit a clinically significant graft rejection.

☛ An eye may be optically rehabilitated by various forms of lamellar keratoplasty, such as a standard lamellar graft, a tectonic lamellar graft that allows for a PKP at a later time, and keratomileusis.

☛ The incidence of irregular astigmatism is higher with lamellar keratoplasty than with penetrating keratoplasty.

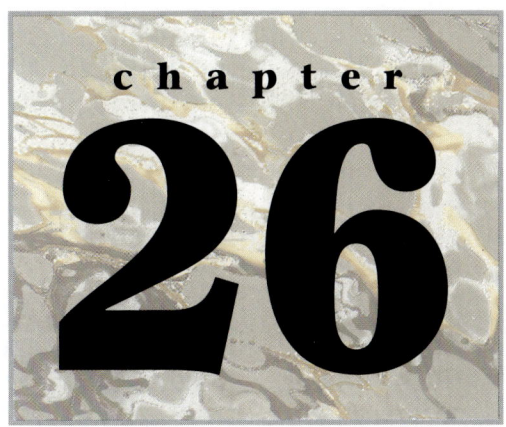

chapter 26

LASER CORNEAL SURGERY

ROGER F. STEINERT, M.D.

The laser and computer are probably the paramount symbols of current high technology. It is not surprising that lasers are important for treating many forms of ocular disease. The argon laser has been used for many years to treat diseases of the retina and choroid, angle closure glaucoma by peripheral iridotomy, and open angle glaucoma by trabeculoplasty. The Nd:YAG laser is used routinely for posterior capsulotomy and peripheral iridotomy, and attempts have been made to use it to fragment the lens nucleus before phacoemulsification. This chapter will discuss corneal surgery by laser.

Laser Basics

Laser stands for light amplification by stimulated emission of radiation. In brief, a laser functions as follows: Energy is added to the atoms of a crystal, solid, or gas by causing ionization of the molecules within the given medium. The impact between two excited atoms results in a release of monochromatic light energy, which then excites more atoms, causing the creation of even more light. This reaction is contained within a mirrored tube so the light produced can be reflected back into the medium to strike more atoms, causing a larger production of light. The light rays produced by each atom are of the same frequency and are vibrating together (in phase) to form a "coherent" light beam of very great intensity. When the laser light beam achieves a critical amount of energy, it is released from the tube through a semisilvered mirror, which continues to reflect a portion of the light while transmitting the remaining portion. Lasers are identified by the crystal, solid, or gas phasing medium used to create the monochromatic light (Fig. 26.1).

When the coherent laser light strikes an object, it is absorbed by the atoms of the object (tissue), thereby creating heat. The tremendous concentrated energy imparted by the laser light to the object disrupts its molecular bonds and causes the object to vaporize.

Since laser light is monochromatic, it passes through tissues of a color similar to itself and is absorbed only by tissue of a different color. Therefore, the potential exists for various types of lasers to be used to treat selectively the different colored ocular structures.

The area of effect created by a laser is known as a plasma field. Since *power = energy/time*, it can easily be ascertained that a laser pulse of a shorter duration and a smaller spot size will require lower energy (and cause less damage to surrounding tissue) to achieve the same degree of power as a longer duration, high-energy laser pulse. Lasers used in ophthalmology typically use the following energy levels (26.2):

Argon:
$$\text{watts} = \frac{\text{Joules}}{\text{seconds}}$$

Nd:YAG:
$$\text{megawatts} = \frac{\text{milliJoules}}{\text{nanosecond}} \quad \text{(pulsed)}$$

Picosecond Nd:YLF:
$$\text{megawatts} = \frac{\text{microJoules}}{\text{picosecond}} \quad \text{(pulsed)}$$

The cornea is clear; thus it must be given special consideration when undergoing laser treatment. Clear cornea absorbs very little laser energy, so high amounts of laser energy may be necessary to achieve the desired effect. Heat production must be minimized in order to minimize deforming the surrounding collagen fibrils. A laser that is used to cleanly incise the cornea must create a plasma field that is small enough to cause only localized damage and not create significant scarring.

Excimer Laser

Ultraviolet laser energy can be delivered to remove a given amount of corneal tissue over the entire corneal surface each time a laser pulse is applied to the cornea. The tissue must remain within the effective delivery zone of the excimer laser. Since the excimer laser's light is delivered as a broad beam, corneal templates must be used to limit tissue removal to the desired configuration. Adequate fixation of the globe during excimer laser treatment of the cornea is important during the repetitive application of laser pulses.

Nd:YAG and Nd:YLF Laser

In contrast to the energy delivered by an excimer laser, an Nd:YAG (neodymium, yttrium, aluminum, garnet) or related laser uses a crystal of four elements to create a very discrete laser energy plasma field. By stringing together the local-

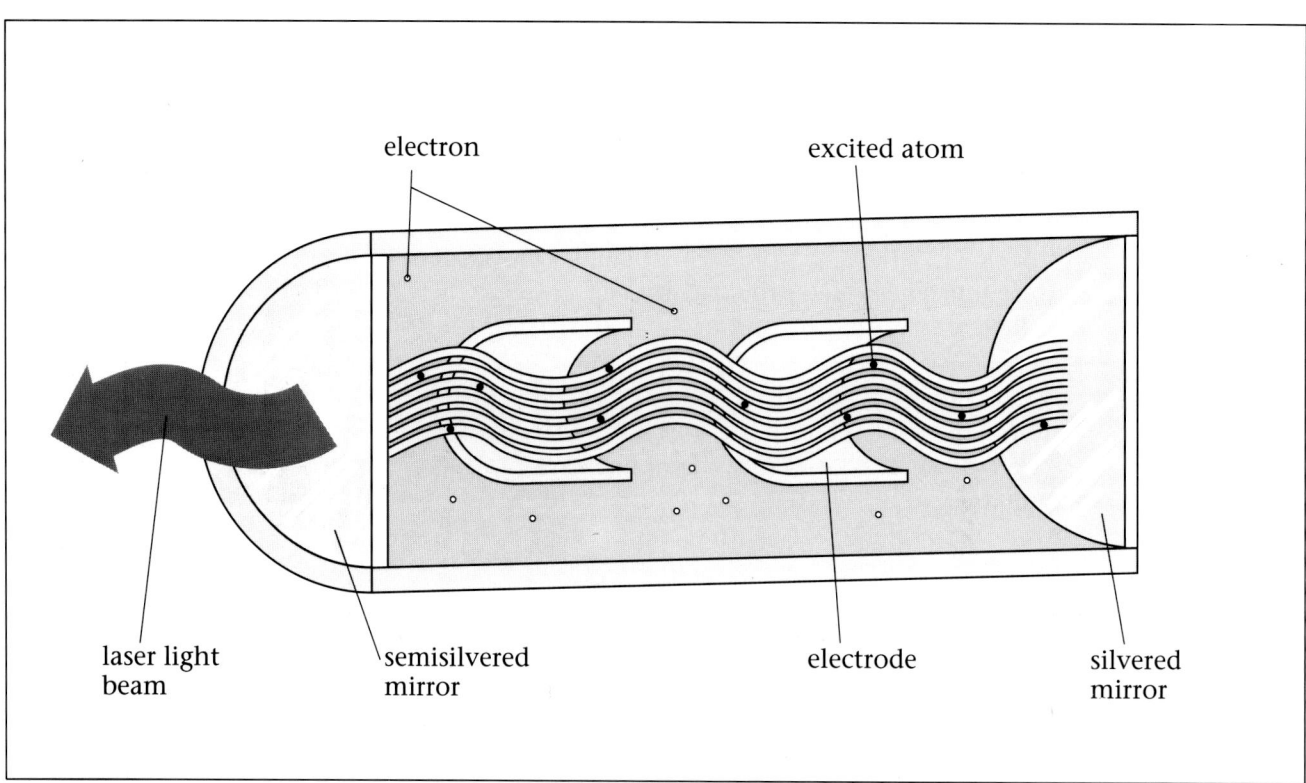

Figure 26.1 *Very basically, a laser works as follows: Energy is added to a medium creating ionization, which causes the production of monochromatic light. The monochromatic light is confined within a mirrored con-* *tainer, which causes additional atoms to be excited by the light and the light to become "in phase." When the laser light has enough energy, it escapes as a laser light beam through a semisilvered mirror at one end of the container.*

ized areas of tissue destruction caused by the small plasma fields, small holes and linear incisions may be created. However, achieving a precise depth may be difficult since the cornea must remain at an exact distance from the YAG laser. Also, tissue density and hydration, tissue destruction, and gas bubbles may affect the delivery and effect of the laser energy.

Excimer Laser Refractive Surgery

The excimer (excited dimer) laser, filled with argon and fluorine gases, is the best source currently available for high-powered short wavelength ultraviolet light energy. Emitting at 193 nm, the laser pulses remove layers of corneal tissue with submicron accuracy. Many researchers believe that the principal laser-tissue interaction represents a newly recognized mechanism, which has been termed *photochemical decomposition* or, more commonly, *photoablation*. The short wavelength ultraviolet light is hypothesized to be heavily absorbed by the carbon-nitrogen bonds in the peptide backbone of all proteins. Each photon at 193 nm has enough energy to lyse the chemical bond directly, thereby minimizing thermal injury to adjacent tissue. Some researchers believe that the principal tissue interaction is ultimately thermal; in any case, photoablation of the cornea at 193 nm produces a zone of structural damage to the adjacent protein substantially less than 1 μ in width. The precision of this process is superior to either mechanical keratectomy or longer wavelength ultraviolet, visible, or infrared laser tissue ablation. The argon-fluorine excimer laser has the potential to alter the corneal curvature, leaving a smooth surface and clear stroma.

Some early studies of excimer laser corneal surgery examined the ability of the laser to obtain linear keratectomy, analogous to radial keratotomy and astigmatic keratotomy. Because the laser *removes* tissue, rather than simply *incising* it as does a gemstone knife, the resultant epithelial plug is wider. This probably results in a more prolonged healing phase and wider scar. Despite an early encouraging report by Theo Seiler, M.D., and coworkers, astigmatic keratotomy is not under active investigation at more than a few centers, and investigations of excimer laser radial keratectomy have been suspended while attention is directed toward large area recontouring of the optical zone.

Photorefractive keratectomy (PRK) or, perhaps more precisely, anterior laser keratomileusis (ALK), are the terms most commonly applied to the process of excimer laser ablation used to flat-

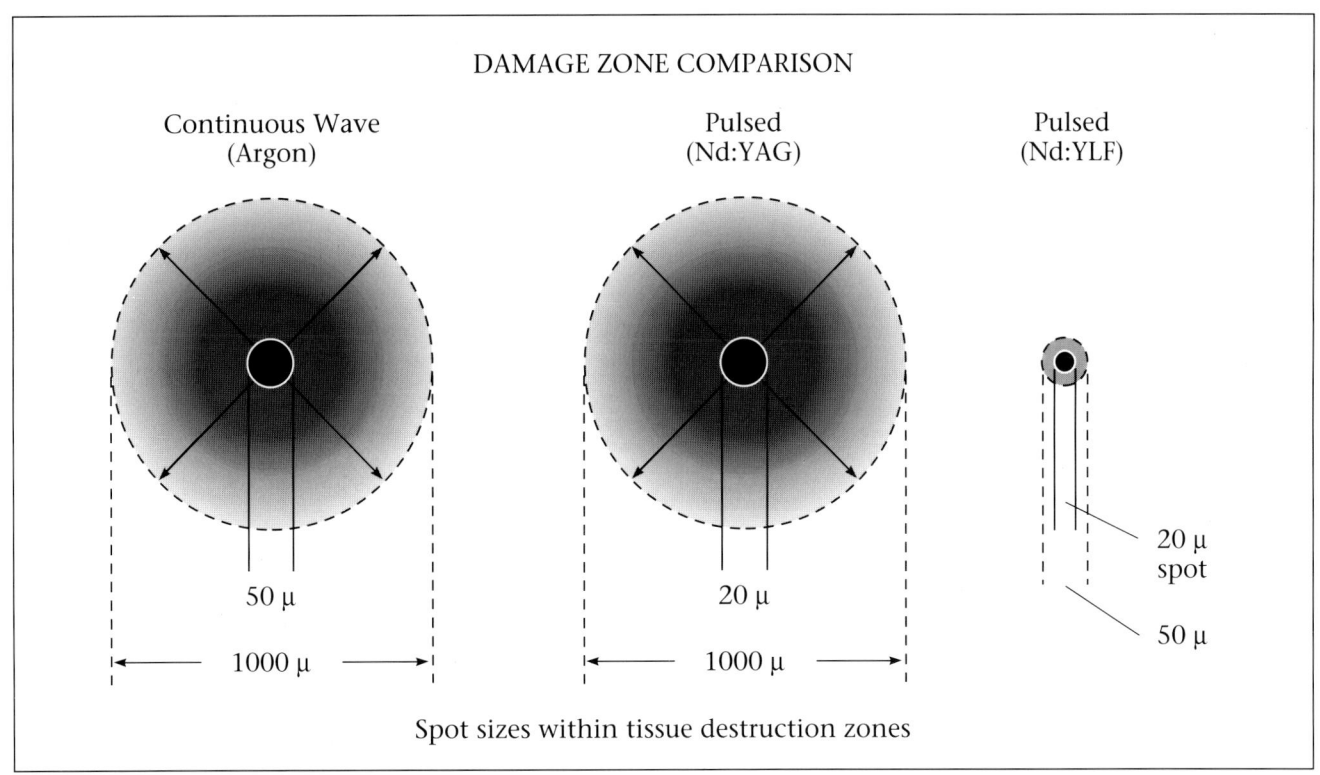

Figure 26.2 *A size comparison of the zones of effect created by argon, Nd:YAG, and Nd:YLF lasers. With the argon laser, the tissue destructive zone of effect caused by a shock wave is much larger than the spot size. With the* Nd:YAG and Nd:YLF lasers, the zone of effect is much larger than the spot size and plasma field, which, essentially, overlap.

ten the cornea's optical zone to compensate for myopia. The excimer laser has several unique features that facilitate this new approach to the correction of myopia. The laser is computer-controlled and, in principle, any size and shape of ablation can be performed reliably and repeatedly. The laser light impact on the cornea causes high-frequency, transient shock waves but no persistent deformation of the cornea, therefore, no tissue damaging stabilization technique such as freezing is required. The bed of the ablation zone remains optically clear. Extensive animal and human studies have demonstrated that rapid and stable re-epithelialization occurs, with reformation of normal basement membrane structures. The newly ablated surface may have a smoothness with less than 1 μ of variability. Studies thus far have largely supported a lack of mutagenesis or carcinogenesis by the 193 nm wavelength light.

Delivery Systems

Several companies in the United States and Europe have ongoing human investigations of first generation commercial devices. Several other companies, including ones in Japan, are expected to enter the market over the next few years. All systems have several common elements. Fluorine gas is both toxic and highly corrosive. Elaborate gas handling safety mechanisms, such as double containment systems and/or external venting, are required. The excimer beam is typically highly inhomogeneous. Both the laser itself and the subsequent optical system include devices to enhance the homogeneity of the beam and, hence, the smoothness of the subsequent ablation. A computer system is required to control the laser cavity and the resultant exposure. Fluctuation in pulse-to-pulse laser energy will also result in unpredictable ablation. The computer must monitor laser output in order to stabilize the energy density. Most units operate between 100 mJ and 250 mJ per square centimeter for large area ablation.

Units differ considerably in their optical systems, computer controls, size, electrical, and venting requirements, and interaction with the patient. For example, one system employs a diaphragm that gradually opens with each successive pulse, another system employs a diaphragm that closes in a stepwise fashion, and a third employs a linear beam that scans the cornea. All are ultimately designed to remove more tissue centrally and less tissue peripherally, thereby flattening the cornea. Maximum spot size and, therefore, optical zone varies, as does any requirement for a fixation pressure or suction ring on the globe. Some units include a flow of air or external gas (such as nitrogen) across the cornea to remove the ablation debris between pulses. At this time, it is not known which, if any, of these technical variations will affect the success of the procedure.

Procedure

Many aspects of the technique will depend upon the specific laser keratoplasty device used. ALK also has aspects common to any form of laser keratoplasty, and many of these aspects are common

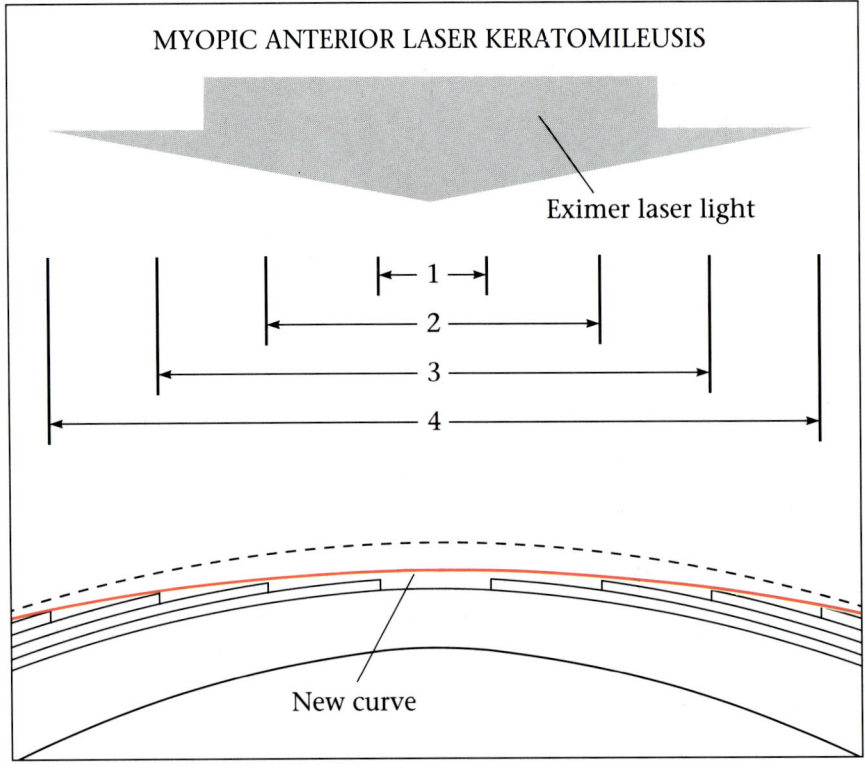

Figure 26.3 *A diagram depicting anterior laser keratomileusis by excimer laser. Each pulse of excimer laser energy removes about 0.25 μ of tissue wherever it strikes the cornea. By using a variable diaphragm that limits corneal exposure to the laser beam, more corneal tissue is removed centrally than peripherally. A new flatter central curve is created and then covered by the epithelium.*

to other types of keratorefractive surgery, such as the interaction between excision depth and optical zone diameter.

Preoperatively the precise optical axis is determined and marked. Pilocarpine drops are usually employed to facilitate this process. Only topical anesthetic drops, such as tetracaine, are needed for patient comfort. The cornea is mechanically de-epithelialized in a zone slightly larger than the intended ablation; the back edge of a knife blade or curette is employed. Epithelial toxic chemicals are avoided. Meticulous attention is placed on removing all debris (epithelial and other) from the ablation zone.

The amount of ablation is determined by the patient's baseline optical error and desired end point of correction (Fig. 26.3). For a diaphragm-controlled ALK unit, the program typically assumes an ablation depth rate of about 0.25 µ per pulse. There is a slight but relatively insignificant difference between the ablation rate of Bowman's layer and the underlying stroma. In contrast, epithelial ablation rates may differ substantially. It is for this reason that the epithelium is mechanically removed prior to the laser ablation. Depending on the unit, as well as the degree of myopia, ALK is typically completed within 10 to 60 seconds.

Immediately postoperatively, topical cycloplegic drops and an antibiotic ointment are applied along with a pressure patch. Strong oral narcotics for pain control are often needed during the one to three days it takes to complete re-epithelialization. Although some investigators do not use topical steroids, most currently favor the intense use of topical steroids for two to three months after ablation. Typically, between five and ten drops per day of a strong topical steroid are used initially, then rapidly tapered off over the first postoperative month and then more gradually over the ensuing one to two months. The potential for a steroid-induced rise in intraocular pressure must be carefully monitored and treated as indicated. Frequent postoperative visits are required to monitor both corneal healing and patient compliance.

Results

To date, formally analyzed and reported results are limited to the early experience of a few investigators. Advancements in the laser systems, the PRK technique, and postoperative anti-inflammatory medications as well as more experienced laser surgeons, may contribute to improvement of these results.

Most investigators currently feel that the best results are obtained in patients with no more than 5.00 D to 6.00 D of myopia. For between 60% and 90% of patients under this limit, the refractive status six months postoperatively is within 1.00 D of emmetropia. Typically, most investigators report an early overcorrection of 1.00 D to 2.00 D (hyperopia) that regresses during the first several postoperative months. Haze in the anterior stroma of the ablation zone can be seen upon slit lamp examination in more than half the patients (Fig. 26.4). This haze is typically maximal one to two months postoperatively and improves or totally resolves by six to twelve months. In most cases the haze is minimal and not apparent to the patient. Most patients are highly satisfied with the results, but their perceptions may be biased by their motivations for undergoing an investigational procedure. Series with large numbers of patients are being accumulated, but results have not yet been reported. A detailed analysis of issues such as glare, contrast sensitivity, computer assisted topographic

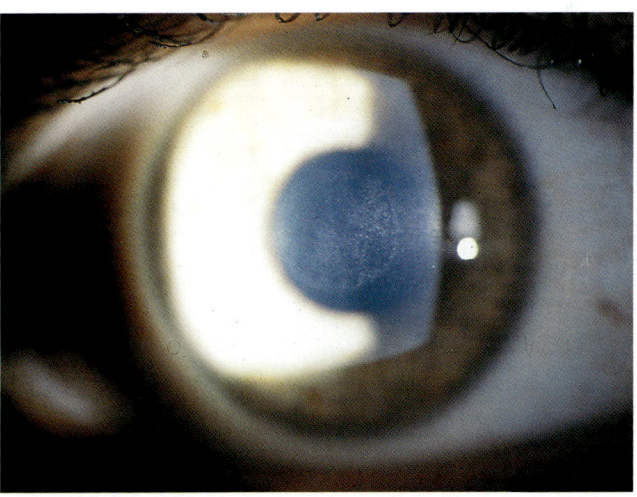 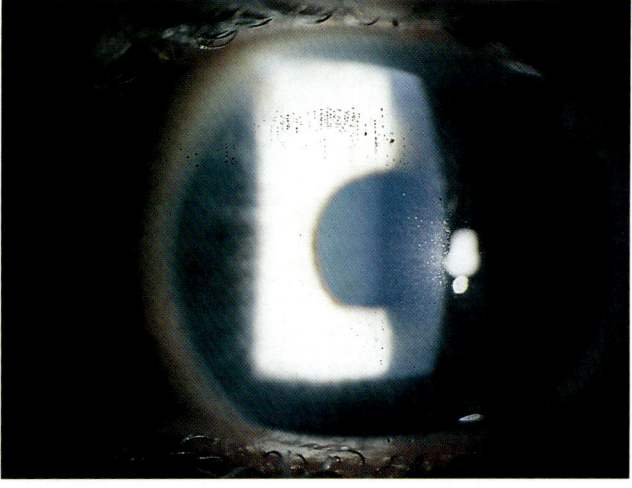

Figure 26.4 (Left) *Significant stromal haze following ALK is evident two months postoperatively.*
(Right) *A clear cornea following ALK is evident one year postoperatively.*

analysis (Fig. 26.5), and endothelial morphology are currently pending.

Complications

Numerous morphologic and immunohistochemical studies in both rabbits and monkeys have demonstrated a characteristic wound healing response after PRK. New collagen formation occurs in the bed of the ablation, consisting of disorganized layers of type III collagen with an absence of normal keratan sulfate in monkeys and type IV collagen in rabbits, as well as deposition of fibronectin and laminin even after re-epithelialization has occurred. The anterior stroma adjacent to the ablation zone shows an increased number of keratocytes with a high degree of metabolic activity. In addition to the new collagen deposition, there is hyperplasia of the overlying epithelium, sometimes exceeding a doubling of the normal epithelial thickness. Both the epithelial hyperplasia and new collagen deposition contribute to regression of the initially induced corneal flattening by the PRK procedure. The anterior stromal collagen alterations and new collagen deposition presumably account for at least part of the haze observed in the months after ablation. Perhaps the tendency for partial to complete clearing of the haze three to six months after ablation correlates with remodeling of the initial collagen reaction.

In human trials thus far, the amount of regression has been dramatically higher on the average and more variable from patient to patient when the intended initial ablation exceeds 5.00 D to 6.00 D. The mechanisms responsible for higher levels of regression and variability at this particular level of correction are not well characterized at the current time. Charles Munnerlyn derived a formula stating that the maximum thickness of ablation in the center of a myopic PRK is approximately the product of the square of the diameter of the optical zone, multiplied by the dioptric correction, and divided by three. Thus, a 5.00-mm optical zone and a 5.00 D to 6.00 D correction requires an approximate, central ablation depth of 42 μ. In theory and according to some clinical investigations, however, an increased wound healing response has been encountered after penetration of Bowman's layer, which is only 10 μ to 15 μ thick.

The mechanism of epithelial hyperplasia for an ablation zone as large as 5.00 mm is also not understood. In general, epithelial healing is rapid. Minor amounts of punctate keratitis clear within several weeks. Recurrent erosions or filamentary keratitis is rare. The surgeon must be alert, however, for patients predisposed to epitheliopathy. This especially includes patients with surface disorders such as keratitis sicca or blepharitis. One case of severe sterile ulceration in a noncompliant patient with a persistent epithelial defect has been reported.

Undesirable optical performance can occur. An optical zone smaller than the pupil, particularly a problem at night, can result in the perception of haloes around light sources. Decentration of the optical zone increases the likelihood of this problem. Decentration also can result in undercorrection and induced astigmatism. Early series have reported an occasional patient with a loss of one or two lines of best corrected visual acuity due to irregular astigmatism, haze, or both. The role of pharmacologic agents in the reduction or prevention of both the haze and the regression of the initial ablation remains controversial. Most investigators are using intense topical steroids in human trials. Premature discontinuation of topical steroids, either because of steroid-induced intraocular pressure elevation or poor patient compliance, has correlated with a tendency for increased anterior stromal scarring. At least one group of investigators, however, is avoiding routine use of steroids altogether. Further investigation is required to resolve this important question as well as to investigate other agents that may be useful, such as antimetabolites.

Directions for Future Development

Photorefractive keratectomy for myopia is the most straightforward application of excimer laser large area ablation to correct refractive error. If these investigations progress satisfactorily, attention will turn to more difficult applications. In principle, astigmatism can be addressed with the ablation of a compensatory toric surface on the anterior corneal optical zone. Hyperopia requires ablation of the midperiphery in order to steepen the central corneal curvature. Preliminary animal investigation shows a strong tendency for this type of partial "doughnut" ablation to fill in with epithelial hyperplasia.

Ultimately, broad irregular astigmatism may be addressed through computer-driven algorithms or by ablating a mask or mold shaped to fit the astigmatic curvature in a lock and key fashion.

Other therapeutic applications of the excimer laser for corneal pathology are currently under active investigation. Corneal pathology amenable to excimer laser therapy can be placed into two broad categories. First, local irregularities can be smoothed. Examples are irregularity after pterygium excision, trauma, band keratopathy that recurs despite conventional EDTA (ethylenediaminetetracetic acid) chelation, and the microscopic irregularity that characterizes recurrent corneal erosions. The second category is anterior stromal scarring. Ideally such scarring would not extend below approximately 50 μ. Otherwise the reactive scar formation of the treated cornea may be as bad or worse than the original pathology. Examples of candidates for this treatment are patients with opacity from superficial herpetic keratitis or superficial dystrophies such as Reis-Buckler's dystrophy.

The Picosecond Nd:YLF Laser

The standard Nd:YAG laser is not a practicable means of shaping the cornea because its milliJoule energy output and 1.00 mm diameter plasma-generated shock wave field create a large pit rather than a controllable surface or intrastromal change. Intelligent Surgical Lasers Model 4001 CLS, a picosecond Nd:YLF (neodymium, yttrium, lithium, fluoride) crystal laser that operates at wavelengths of 1053 nm and 527 nm, is capable of photodisruption of clear ocular tissues, such as cornea and vitreous, and photocoagulation of the choroid and vascular retina (Fig. 26.6). A plasma-generated shock wave field of 50 μ in diameter is created. The 4001 boasts eye alignment, eye tracking, and corneal topographic and pachymetric capabilities.

This picosecond Nd:YLF laser is capable of generating 1000 pulses per second in any three-dimensional array desired. Radial and astigmatic keratotomy incisions are possible. Current investigations indicate the possibility of achieving quantifiable intrastromal ablation with predictable change of the corneal surface. By leaving the epithelium intact, this intrastromal process would allow corneal refractive change quickly and without pain or the potential for infection. In order to achieve this goal, however, intrastromal ablation of corneal tissue must be accomplished despite the creation of intrastromal gas bubbles and the need to ablate a very large area consistently (Fig. 26.7).

Other areas under investigation include cataract fragmentation, anterior capsulotomy, donor and recipient corneal incisions for keratoplasty, internal sclerostomy for glaucoma control, microretinal photocoagulation, vitreous and epiretinal membrane discission, as well as the established uses of peripheral iridotomy and posterior capsulotomy.

Conclusion

Although the argon laser has been used to treat choroidal and retinal pathology for at least several decades, and the Nd:YAG has been invaluable for performing posterior capsulotomy and peripheral iridotomy, attempts to treat corneal pathology and change refractive error by means of laser are relatively recent. The excimer ultraviolet laser, limited by a template, reshapes the cornea by photoablation of the corneal surface. A picosecond Nd:YLF laser can make corneal incisions to a prescribed depth and may someday be capable of quantifiable intrastromal ablation. Certainly, the future will reveal both the benefits and limitations of laser technology as further attempts are made to modify successfully the corneal surface and treat a larger number of ocular diseases.

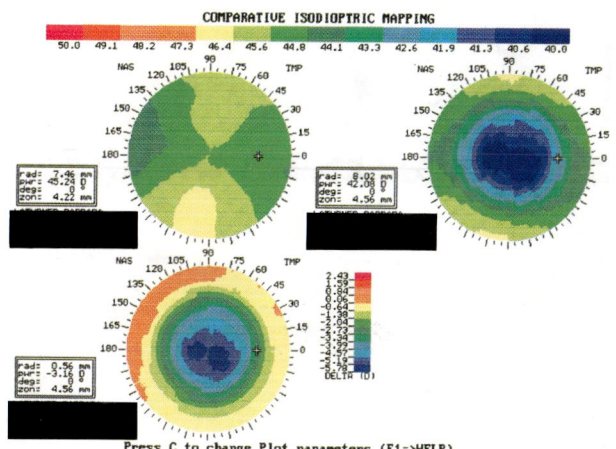

Figure 26.5 *A topographical study of the cornea of a −6.00 D myope who underwent myopic ALK. A comparison of the preoperative and postoperative topography is highlighted by a subtraction display that shows the change in curvature at each point. Notice that postoperatively the periphery of the optical zone is steeper than the center. The cornea is aspheric.*

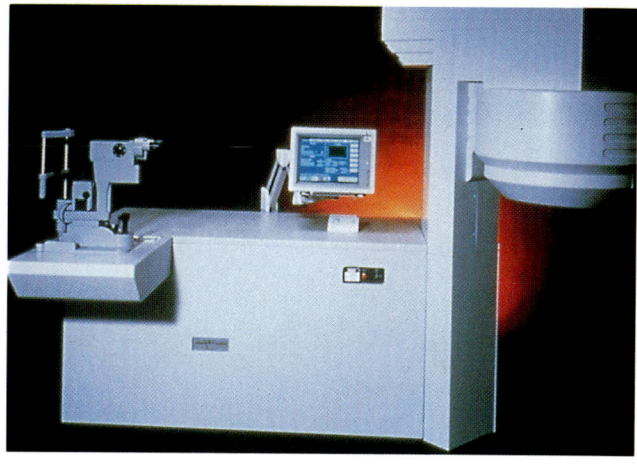

Figure 26.6 *The ILS Model 4001 CLS Nd:YLF laser.*

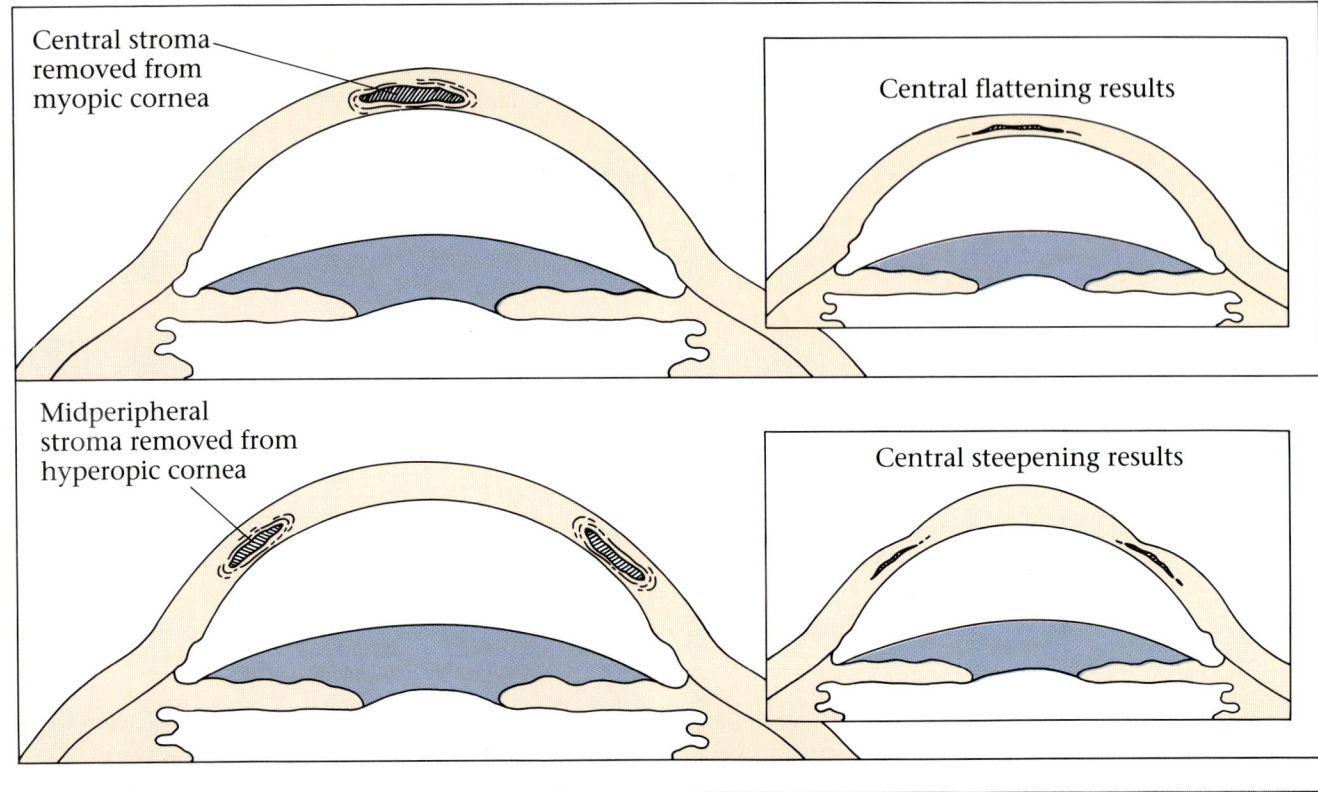

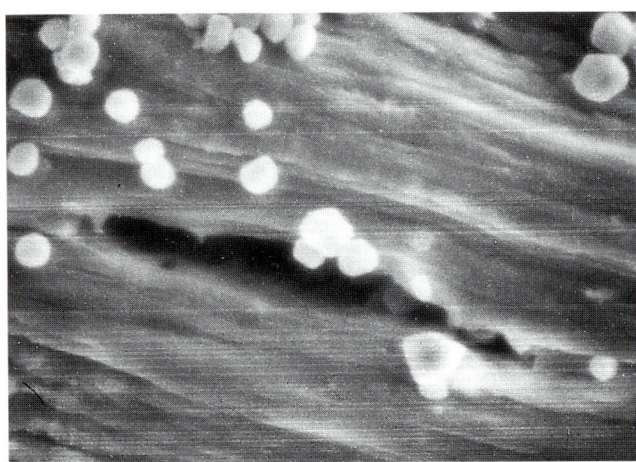
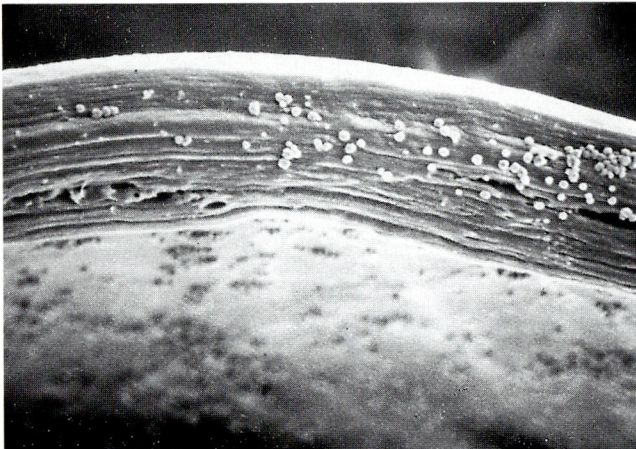

Figure 26.7 *(Top) The concept of intrastromal ablation to correct myopia and hyperopia.* **(Bottom left)** *Intrastromal ablation in a human cornea. The clear space that indicates tissue removal is 500 μ long and 10 μ wide, the thickness of one cornea lamella.* **(Bottom right)** *An overview of the cornea shows intrastromal ablation with collapse of the intracorneal cavity and flattening of the overlying cornea (right side of photo).*

Clinical Points to Consider

☞ Anterior laser keratomileusis by excimer laser is capable of consistently correcting myopia up to about –5.00 D with an adequate optical zone and limited corneal scarring.

☞ Anterior laser keratomileusis requires re-establishment of a smooth epithelial surface in the visual axis.

☞ Excimer laser photoablation below Bowman's membrane often causes significant corneal opacification.

☞ Refractive surgery by corneal intrastromal ablation may offer significant advantages.

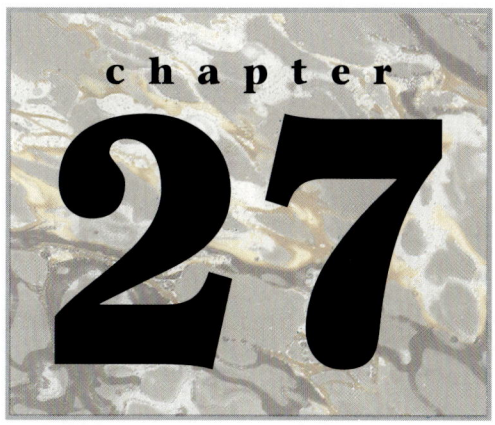

KERATOMILEUSIS

FRANCIS W. PRICE, M.D.

Keratomileusis is an exquisite surgical procedure capable of dramatically changing the lives of those with large refractive errors. The concentration necessary to perform a microkeratectomy combined with the sound of carbon dioxide gas blowing through the cryolathe during freezing makes keratomileusis the most dramatic of all anterior segment procedures. It is the only refractive surgery in use today with over 25 years of follow-up, yet it is a procedure practiced by few surgeons. Its limited availability is the result of three factors:

1. The preconceived complexity of the procedure and the equipment
2. The initial expense of the equipment and training necessary for its use
3. The possibility of postoperative irregular astigmatism

Despite these problems, keratomileusis should be more readily available to patients because its tremendous ability to improve vision and quality of life can not be matched by any other current procedure. The changes that occur for patients going from –15.00 D to plano are immeasurable. For the first time in their lives they can go swimming without glasses, use the bathroom in the middle of the night without glasses, and live without the constant fear of losing or misplacing their glasses.

Preoperative Considerations

As with all ophthalmic surgery, before doing keratomileusis the patient should be examined thoroughly. Those who have external diseases of the eye and lid, which can cause difficulties with corneal healing or clarity, are not appropriate candidates for this surgery. Individuals with developing cataracts should have extracapsular cataract extractions with placement of posterior chamber lenses, not keratorefractive surgery. Individuals with retinal deterioration should be advised that postoperative results may be limited. All patients need to be advised about the potential to develop postoperative irregular astigmatism. The possibility exists that hard contact lenses may be necessary to improve their postoperative best-corrected vision to a level of 20/40 or better, as occurs in 10% to 15% of individuals undergoing this surgery.

Autoplastic keratomileusis is generally effective for myopes from –6.00 D to –16.00 D and hyperopes from +4.00 D to +10.00 D (Fig. 27.1). Homoplastic myopic procedures may be effective for patients up to –20.00 D. The upper limits of correction have been set by Jose Barraquer, M.D., to avoid either flattening the cornea to less than 33.00 D or steepening it to more than 57.00 D. In myopic procedures, the central cornea thickness must stay greater than 0.30 mm or ectasia may result.

Instructional videotapes are quite helpful because they introduce the patient to surgical concepts prior to discussing them with the surgeon. A clear and comprehensive informed consent form is imperative.

After the patient has been counseled and surgery scheduled, a backup donor globe should be available. Although I have never needed to use backup tissue for a keratomileusis procedure, donor tissue provides a fail-safe feature in case there is a problem with the patient's own cornea in autoplastic keratomileusis procedures.

Performing keratomileusis using the Barraquer technique requires either of two easy to understand computer programs. One program, developed by Barraquer, uses an Apple computer format; the other, developed by Ophthalmic Prediction Software, works on IBM-compatible personal computers. Laptop computers work well with the IBM program.

The preoperative measurements that must be entered into the computer program include: spec-

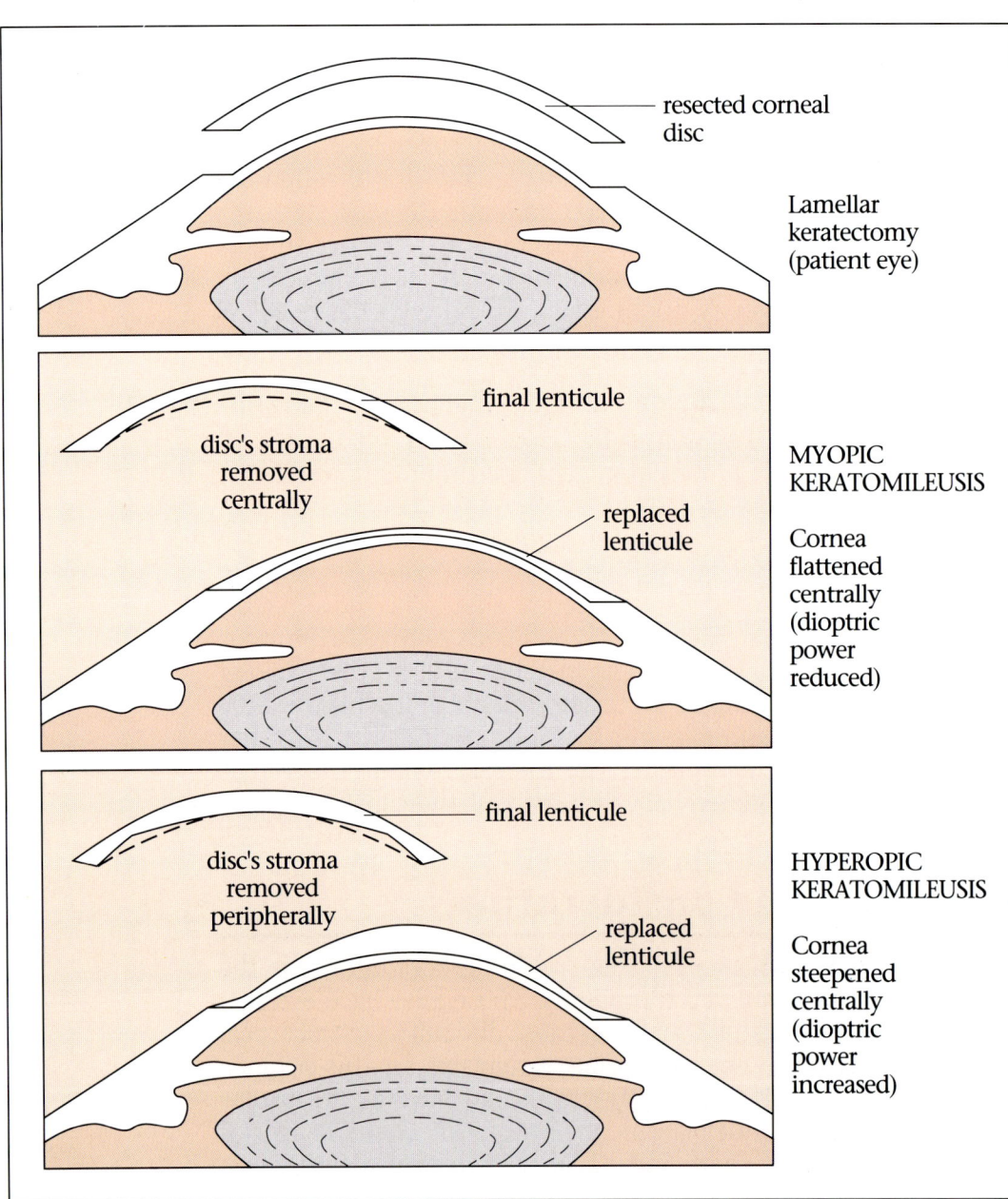

Figure 27.1 *Myopic keratomileusis removes corneal tissue, thus the central corneal surface is flatter and the refracting surface is less powerful. Hyperopic keratomileusis removes corneal tissue from the paracentral area of the cornea, thus the central cornea is steeper and the refracting surface more powerful.*

tacle correction at 12.00 mm, keratometry, age of the patient, and the desired refractive result. The surgeon should conduct a preoperative review of the program using the patient's data to make sure the planned resection will not leave the cornea too thin or lead to parameters incompatible with a good result. For instance, the program may suggest the cornea will be flattened too much or that the planned resected depth of the tissue will cause the remaining central thickness (EC) of the disc to be too thin.

The surgeon should be familiar with the program's proposed operation prior to surgery. During surgery, the surgeon should be able to anticipate each step so that there will be no prolonged waiting. For example, once the drape is cut and the speculum placed between the eyelids, leaving the cornea exposed for an inordinate amount of time can lead to drying and a decrease in the central corneal thickness. This causes an inappropriate resection depth by the microkeratome. The same drying effect can occur if after the disc of tissue has been placed on the lathe, the surgeon realizes that the computer program has projected inappropriate end results. The surgeon must then halt the procedure and change the optical zone or the diopters of correction to obtain appropriate parameters.

Surgical Procedure

Lathing surgeries are most commonly performed under local anesthesia. Retrobulbar anesthesia should be used, with the tip of the needle carefully directed in order to prevent perforation of highly myopic eyes. Approximately 5.00 cc of fluid is needed for retrobulbar anesthesia. This amount of fluid, compared to the 3.50 cc usually used for other procedures, provides for a moderate prolapse of the globe and increases pressure behind the globe, both of which facilitate the microkeratectomy. After the patient is prepped, the physician is gowned and gloved, although gloves are optional. A 1018 steridrape is placed on the surgeon's chest, the microkeratome is placed in one pouch and the appropriate suction ring in the other pouch.

The suction ring should be checked for adequate suction by placing the thumb and forefinger over the top and bottom of the ring and checking the change in suction from "closed" to "open". At this point, the microkeratome must be passed through the suction ring before it is placed on the patient's eye (Fig. 27.2). This insures that no debris is present, and there is no difficulty with the grooves on either the microkeratome or the suction ring, either of which could impede the progress of the microkeratome during surgery. The pass of the microkeratome across the eye is the most critical portion of the procedure. This pass must be effortless and unimpeded. If a different suction ring is used later on, the microkeratome should be passed through it prior to placing the new ring on the patient's eye.

Prior to bringing the patient into the operating room, 2% pilocarpine should be administered to constrict the pupil. The steridrape is incised in the palpebral fissure area, and the Kratz/Barraquer eye speculum E4106K (Storz) is placed so the edges of the plastic curl back under the lid margins. The conjunctiva should be inspected; if the retrobulbar injection has caused chemosis, an incision should be made over the bulbar conjunctiva laterally, approximately 5.00 mm to 6.00 mm posterior to the limbus. Wescott scissors can be used to press the conjunctiva against the globe in order to express fluid and eliminate chemosis. At this point, using the miotic pupil as a reference, the surgeon can see where the visual axis should be,

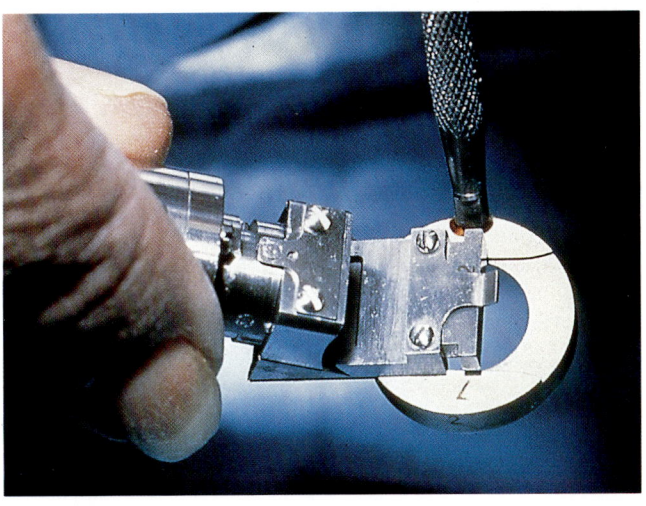

Figure 27.2 *The microkeratome, which creates the lamellar keratecomy and provides the corneal disc for reshaping, is checked by passing it through the suction ring prior to the actual procedure.*

and it can be marked with a 3.00 mm optical zone marker that has been dyed with gentian violet.

Traditionally, a needle is used to mark the epithelium nasally so the removed lenticule can later be repositioned appropriately; however, I have found the needle mark may cause difficulty with the epithelium. I prefer to use a straight marker dyed with gentian violet for the nasal meridian. The result should be a circle delineating the visual axis, which is intersected nasally by a straight line going to the limbus. The suction ring is then brought into the operative field and placed on the limbal area (Fig. 27.3).

When the suction ring is placed on the eye, the resected portion of the cornea should be centered on the visual axis. Usually, for proper orientation of the suction ring, small angled forceps are needed to grasp the inferior portion of the bulbar conjunctiva and manipulate the eye so the cornea is oriented properly within the suction ring. If the bulbar conjunctiva is edematous, it will obstruct the suction port within the ring and lead to inadequate suction. The cornea is applanated to check the intraocular pressure developed by the suction ring (Fig. 27.4). If an inappropriate suction results from conjunctival chemosis, a 360-degree peritomy should be performed and the suction ring placed on the bare sclera. If this happens, care must be taken to prevent the conjunctiva from coming up over the top of the suction ring. If the tonometer shows that the pressure is adequate but the sizing is shown to be inappropriate by the applanation lens, the suction ring must be changed in order to obtain the proper diameter of the corneal resection (Fig. 27.5). This is especially important when performing homoplastic procedures where the resected diameter on the donor eye is matched to the resected diameter on the patient's eye. Changing the suction ring to a larger number decreases the diameter of the area to be resected on the cornea.

After appropriate readings with the tonometer and applanation lens have been obtained, the microkeratome is brought into the operative field. It is placed in the grooves of the suction ring and brought forward so the razor blade is directly on the peripheral portion of the ring (Fig. 27.6). The on/off control of the microkeratome should be operated by an assistant. After the microkeratome has made a smooth continuous pass across the cornea, the assistant should immediately turn off and disconnect the microkeratome so it cannot be inadvertently turned back on, causing damage to either the underlying cornea or the resected disc of tissue. Once the microkeratome is turned off, the surgeon should turn off the suction. Then the suction ring and microkeratome should be lifted from the patient's eye and the two instruments disengaged.

After the resected disc of tissue is removed from the microkeratome and inspected, the resected bed is checked (Fig. 27.7). If the resection appears to have a normal contour, diameter, and depth, and the central bed is uniform, the cornea is irrigated with balanced salt solution and covered with a protector. If the resection is markedly abnormal (e.g., it is very shallow, the edges are very thin and ragged on one or more sides, the diameter is inappropriate, or the resected bed has marked irregularities from an inconsistent pass), the resected disc of tissue must be placed back on the eye and resutured. Surgery should be reattempted in three to six months. When performing the keratectomy, one of the most common problems is failing to pass the microkeratome in a smooth and continuous manner. Changes in

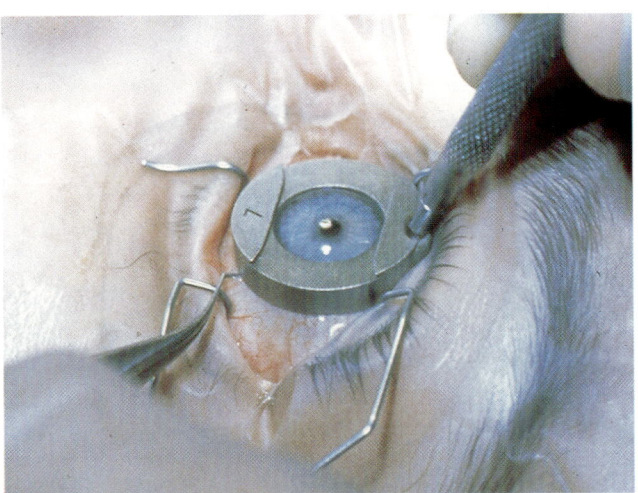

Figure 27.3 *The suction ring is placed on the globe and centered according to the visual axis.*

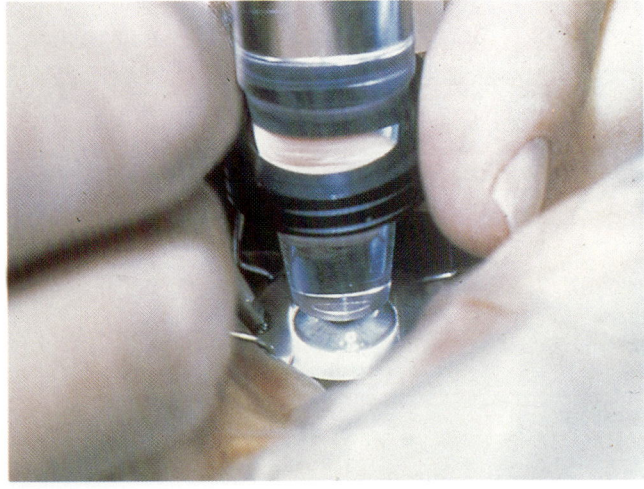

Figure 27.4 *The intraocular pressure is checked with an applanation tonometer. The intraocular pressure will reach about 65 to 80 mm Hg.*

the speed of the pass can cause irregularities in the resection depth, which are commonly manifested as vertical dips or divots in the resected bed. If these are significant, especially in the visual axis area, it is best to resuture the disc and do the surgery later. A resection that begins appropriately thick and ends up very thin and has ragged edges nasally is often an indication of poor initial suction between the suction ring and the globe or loss of suction during the microkeratoming phase.

If any of the above problems in the resected bed are noted but ignored (e.g., the cornea is lathed despite the poor bed), the result will be a significant amount of irregular astigmatism proportional to the degree of irregularity in the bed. Because the cryolathe (Fig. 27.8) resects tissue from the disc relative to the anterior surface of the disc, any portions from an area of deeper resection will end up having more tissue removed than those that were thinner, and all irregularities of the disc's posterior surface will be lathed out, leaving a uniform posterior surface. When the disc is placed back on the patient's eye, all the irregularities in the bed will become irregularities on the anterior surface of the cornea, whereas, if the disc of tissue had been sutured down without lathing, the irregularities in the disc and the bed would fit together like a "tongue and groove" and heal normally.

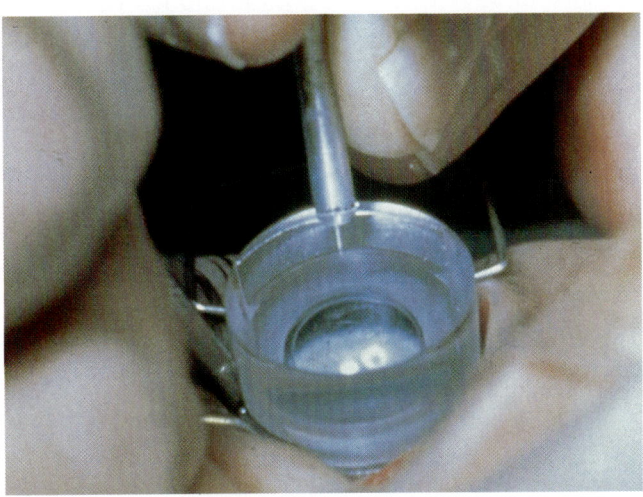

Figure 27.5 *An applanation lens can predict the diameter of the corneal disc that will be resected.*

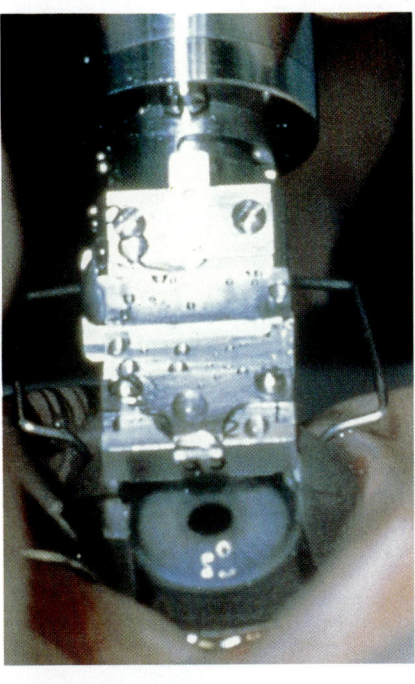

Figure 27.6 *The microkeratome is positioned.*

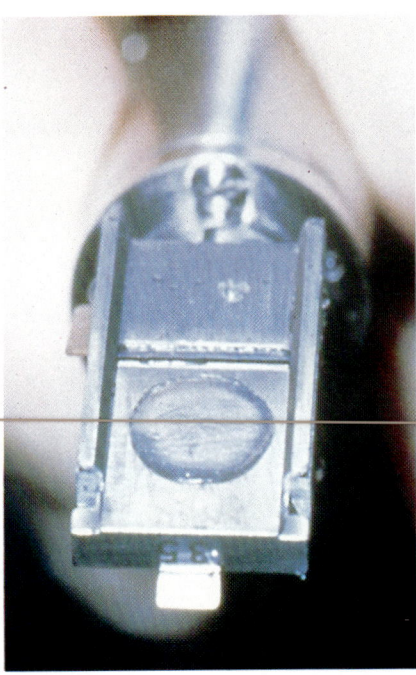

Figure 27.7 *The corneal disc is displayed on the microkeratome.*

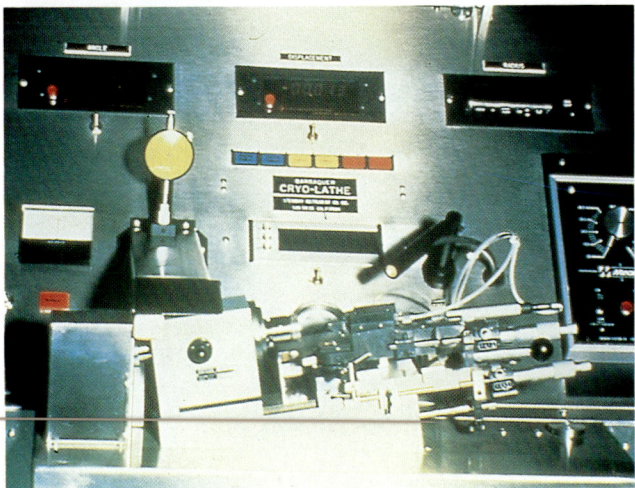

Figure 27.8 *The Steinway Barraquer cryolathe.*

Once the recipient cornea and disc have been inspected and found appropriate, the disc is placed on the cryolathe's thickness-measuring device. The measurement is recorded and entered in the computer program, which labels this quantity *ED*. The disc of tissue is placed in Kitton Green (a cryo protectant and dye) and its thickness remeasured and entered into the computer, which labels it *EDP*. The tissue is then put aside in a special container to protect it from drying and thinning from exposure or swelling from continuous immersion in Kitton Green.

At this stage the computer provides a variety of measurements. It gives the new radius of curvature for the tool and a new displacement, which is set on the lathe's micrometer. The "real displacement" should now be advanced on the lathe until it encounters the stop. As the displacement is advanced, the tool should not cut into the Delrin plastic base on which the corneal disc will sit. If the tool cuts into the Delrin, it indicates inaccurate settings for the radius of curvature and displacement. Ideally, when that stop is encountered, the displacement found on the digital readout should be very close to the displacement provided by the computer program. If all is well, the displacement is taken back to 10.00 mm, the cutting tool is angled out to the side, and the disc of tissue is placed on the Delrin. Care should be taken to place the corneal disc firmly against the Delrin. There should be no bubbles underneath the disc; bubbles under the central portion will increase the amount of resected tissue, which will adversely affect the refractive result for the patient. Some surgeons even use a balloon to place the corneal disc of tissue firmly against the Delrin. However, placement is routinely done with Weck-cel sponges only, making sure the fluid is drawn from behind the disc and is firmly in contact and centered on the Delrin. When the disc is positioned correctly, the CO_2 for the head of the cryolathe is turned on and the start button is pressed to activate the time readout. After 30 seconds of freezing, the cooling button for the tool is pushed and the angle of the tool set to the appropriate degree.

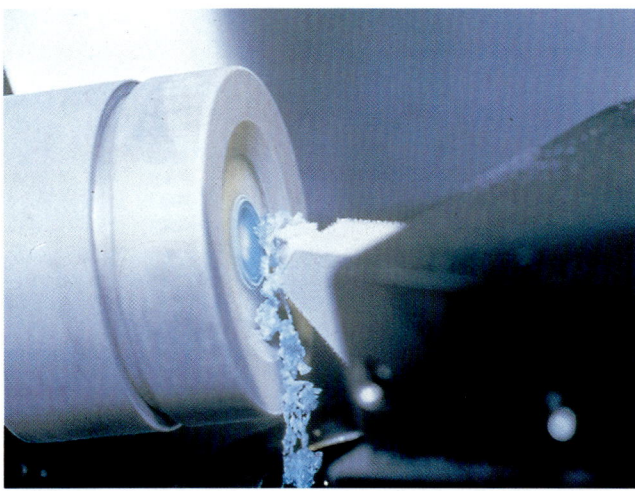

Figure 27.9 *The corneal disc is placed on the cryolathe. After freezing the disc and tool for about one minute and 15 seconds, a lenticule is created.*

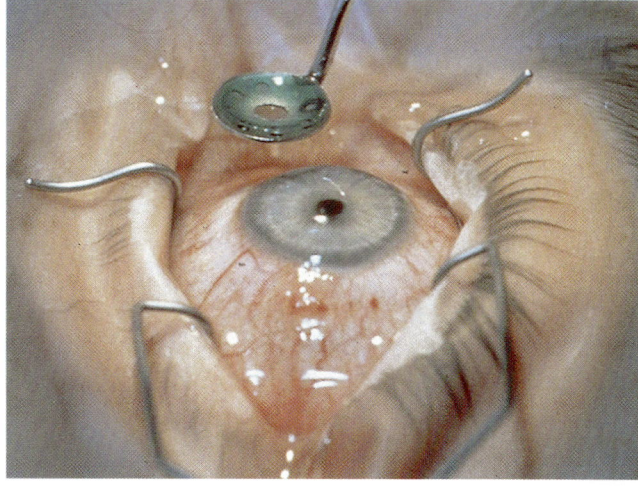

Figure 27.10 *The lenticule is transferred to the recipient with a spatula.*

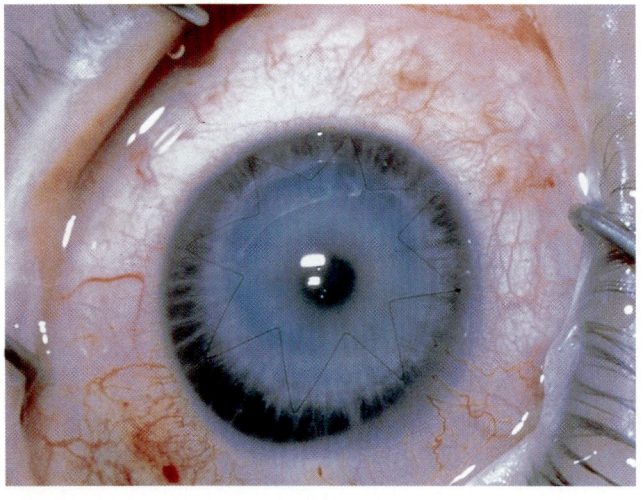

Figure 27.11 *Conclusion of a myopic keratomileusis. Note the eight-bite antitorque Barraquer suture.*

Occasionally, as the disc of tissue freezes, the edges may curl outward. If this happens, an instrument such as a curved Tubingen tying forceps can push it back. Remember, however, that a hand-held instrument is much warmer than frozen tissue, so the instrument will temporarily melt the tissue, causing it to change shape and go back against the Delrin. The tissue edge must be checked for a full 360 degrees. Once the tool is frozen, the angle is placed at zero, and the tool is advanced to the appropriate "real displacement" and used to make a slow continuous cut out to the appropriate angle (Fig. 27.9). The tool is then backed up, and both the tool and head are turned off. At that point, the resected disc of tissue is examined. If severe difficulty is noted, such as inadvertent cutting into the Delrin, a donor cornea for the new homoplastic disc will be needed to repeat the cryolathing. (It will take approximately 20 minutes for the cryolathe to warm so that the measurements will be accurate, i.e., offset the contraction of the metal during freezing).

During the lathing process, an operating microscope is used to monitor the freezing process and the orientation of the tissue. To insure a smooth procedure, it is advisable to perform the surgery with a video hookup so the surgeon can watch the controls on the cryolathe and the assistant can observe the lathing. For example, if the tissue were to come off the Delrin base during lathing, the assistant could alert the surgeon.

Once lathing is completed, the tool is backed up as far as it will go and angled outward so the tip points away from the reshaped lenticule. The fixation ring is loosened and the Delrin base is removed and placed on the sterile instrument table, defrosted with balanced salt solution, and covered with a protector. The microscope is then focused on the patient's eye.

When the microscope is in position, the corneal protector is removed from the patient's eye, and the resected bed is irrigated with balanced salt solution and cleaned with Weck-cel sponges. Be extremely careful during this process. The side of the Weck-cel sponge is never used more than once. Be careful not to drag any epithelium into the wound and carefully remove any debris or epithelium that may be there. Leaving debris or epithelium can cause postoperative problems but is usually not a problem for the experienced surgeon. After the bed is prepared, the lenticule is placed on the Barraquer spatula (the Barraquer spatula was also used to transfer the lenticule onto the cryolathe). The lenticule is then brought to the eye, irrigated with balanced salt solution, and inspected under the microscope. If all looks well, it is transferred onto the patient's eye and oriented according to the previously placed gentian violet straight mark (Fig. 27.10). Weck-cel sponges are used to orient the lenticule into the proper position, and a 10–0 nylon interrupted suture is placed at the 12 o'clock position. The suture bite is taken through the peripheral edge of the lenticule, into the peripheral bed, and out through normal cornea. Care is taken not to penetrate into the anterior chamber during this suturing process. I use the CU5 needle (Alcon) for suturing.

Next, sutures are placed at the 6 o'clock and 9 o'clock positions. When placing the first suture, the forceps grasp the peripheral-most edge of the resected bed and the suture is passed through the lenticule, into the peripheral bed, and out through the peripheral cornea. Never grasp the lenticule itself with the forceps. When placing the second and third sutures, the forceps must grasp only the limbal area or bulbar conjunctiva, but never the lenticule or the edge of the resected bed. Placing the forceps into the wound may introduce epithelial cells into it, which could lead to epithelial nests. This suturing method, in which the lenticule or bed is not grasped with forceps, is also applied during the next step, placing the running suture.

An eight-bite nontorque suture is placed. Afterward, the three interrupted sutures are removed and the running suture is tightened slightly, with the knot being buried in the superior recipient cornea (Fig. 27.11). If the suturing is done properly, the straight line of gentian violet should still be appropriately oriented on both the lenticule and the recipient cornea. Obviously, in a homoplastic procedure, a donor lenticule would not be marked and no attempt is made to align it with any special orientation relative to the recipient corneal bed. It should also be noted that prior to using a microkeratome on a donor eye, the epithelium is removed with Weck-cel sponges.

Once the lenticule is sutured in place, antibiotics and corticosteroids are injected subconjunctivally. The eyelids are shut with one interrupted 6–0 silk suture, and an eye patch is placed on the eye. The patient is allowed to remove the patch at home, where an ice pack that will not drip water can be placed over the eye to reduce swelling. The head should be kept elevated.

The sutures are removed from the lids approximately 48 hours after surgery, at which time the epithelium probably will have spread over the lenticule. During the cryolathing, all epithelium is destroyed and even though it is in place during the suturing process, it will slough off and have to repopulate. The corneal suture is removed ten days to two weeks postoperatively in autoplastic myopic cases and two to three weeks postoperatively in hyperopic or homoplastic cases. Patients will usually notice an improvement in their vision within a few days after the eye is unpatched, with significant visual improvement continuing anywhere from one to six months after the procedure. At six months the retractions are relatively stable, with some small changes occurring, possibly for up to a year (Fig. 27.12).

Surgery may be performed on the second eye as soon as the patient demonstrates that the first eye is totally functional (i.e., the patient should be able to read, drive, and perform all routine activities with the eye that received surgery). Occasionally, the patient may need a contact lens in order to carry out some of these activities.

It is very important to make sure the patient can function with the first eye before surgery is done on the second eye. If for any reason the first eye is nonfunctional, serious consideration must be given to whether surgery should be performed on the second eye. A second poor result could leave the patient with two nonfunctioning eyes.

Non-Freeze Keratomileusis

Non-freeze keratomileusis (NFKM) is an alluring concept that requires a special microkeratome and suction ring set (Fig. 27.13). NFKM was attempted originally by Barraquer and then abandoned and was redeveloped by Casimir Swinger, M.D., and Jorg Krumeich, M.D. Potential advantages include reshaping the cornea without causing freeze damage to the tissue (i.e., destroying all the epithelial cells and probably most of the keratocytes), which may delay healing. Also, the freezing that can occur irregularly throughout the tissue may cause irregular astigmatism. However, it may be hard to cut non-frozen corneal tissue as precisely as solid frozen tissue.

The resected disc of tissue must be 9.00 mm to 9.50 mm in diameter. It is removed from the patient's eye and placed epithelial side down on a special die on a corneal bench. The diameter of the resected disc must be large enough to drape over the edge of the die and be clamped down with a fixating ring. The microkeratome is then adjusted on the corneal bench for the second pass over the disc of tissue, in which a portion from the stromal side is resected. The amount of resected tissue and its shape is determined by the die underneath the tissue as well as by the height of the microkeratome from the die's surface. Once the resection is completed, the disc is removed from the bench, placed back on the patient's eye, and sutured in place.

Theoretically, NFKM should be easier to perform than the procedure that uses the Barraquer cryolathe. In my experience, however, it is more complicated and time consuming, routinely taking two or three times longer than the cryolathe procedures. In a clinical study done in the United States, surgeons had significant difficulty with the functioning of the microkeratome when it passed over the patient's eye, causing poor final refractive results. Smaller optical zones and a higher incidence of irregular astigmatism occur with the non-freeze method of keratomileusis than with the Barraquer cryolathe techniques. Nonetheless, the NFKM corneas heal extremely well and an excellent refractive result may be obtained within just a few weeks.

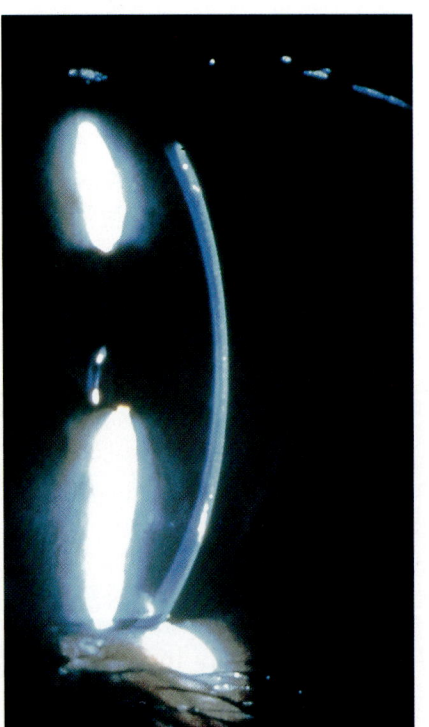

Figure 27.12 *A slit lamp photo of a cornea that has undergone myopic keratomileusis. The surgery has made the central cornea slightly thinner and flatter than normal.*

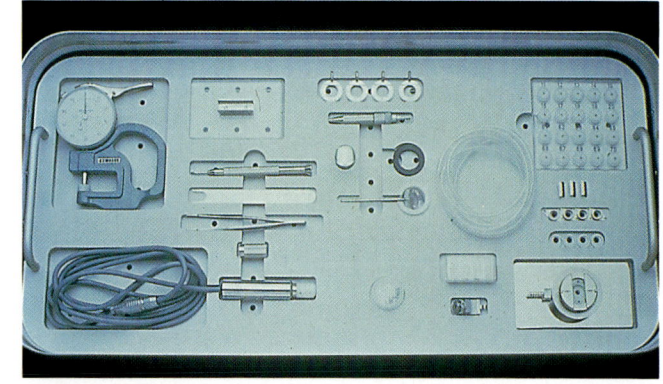

Figure 27.13 *The BKS (Barraquer, Krumeich, Swinger) non-freeze keratomileusis intrumentation.*

New Developments

Luis Ruiz, M.D., of Bogota, Columbia, has popularized *in situ* keratomileusis, in which an initial keratectomy creates a corneal disc and then the recipient corneal bed undergoes a second keratectomy (Fig. 27.14). The disc is then sewn into position in the standard method using an eight-bite, 10-0 nylon antitorque suture. A microkeratome that passes across the suction ring automatically has been developed; however, the most difficult aspect of using the microkeratome, creating adequate suction between the ring and the globe, must still be insured by the surgeon (Fig. 27.15).

Difficulties with *in situ* keratomileusis are caused by the tendency to obtain small diameter lenticules after resection by the second keratectomy and the high incidence of irregular astigmatism.

Draeger has developed a keratome that uses a rotary blade rather than the oscillating mechanism used with the Barraquer microkeratome. Clinical trials have yet to determine if the apparent advantages of the Draeger system, i.e., reduced vibration of the blade and direct visualization of the cornea, will produce an excellent keratectomy.

Complications

Probably the most common postoperative complication of keratomileusis that limits its use is the occurrence of irregular astigmatism. In the myopic procedures, this is usually offset by the magnification in image size that occurs when the

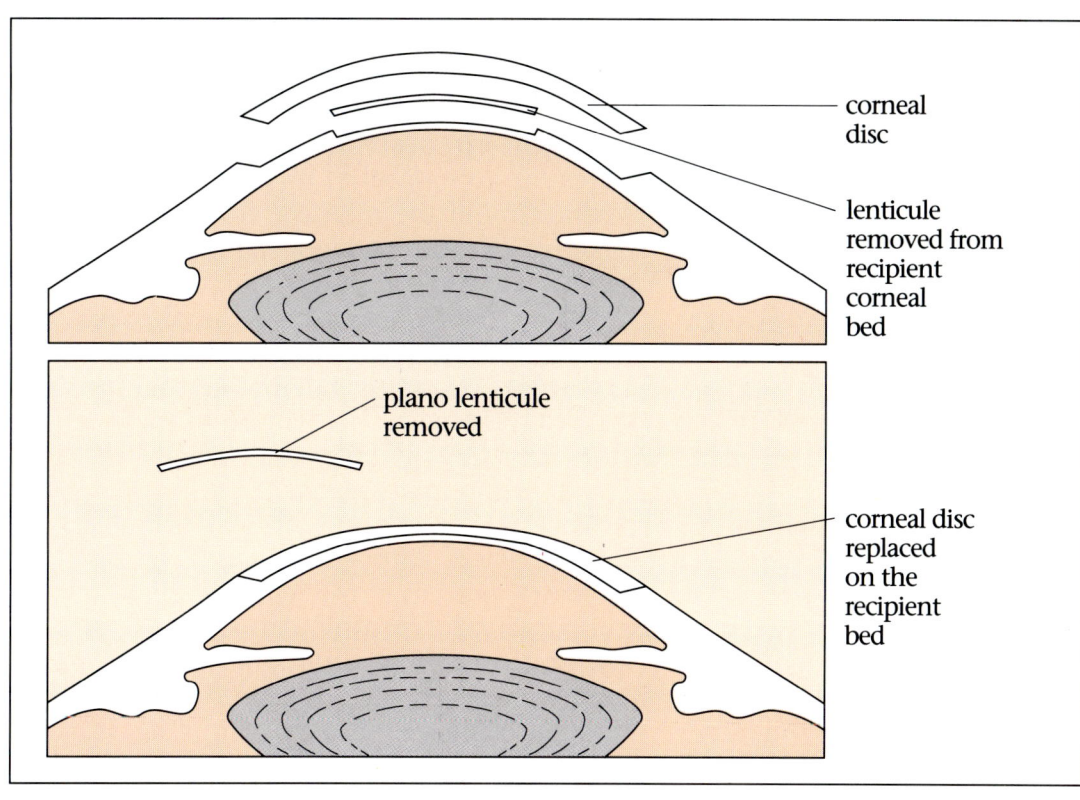

Figure 27.14 *A diagram of* in situ *myopic keratomileusis. Note that the keratectomy, which determines the postoperative refractive power, is performed on the recipient cornea, not the donor cornea.*

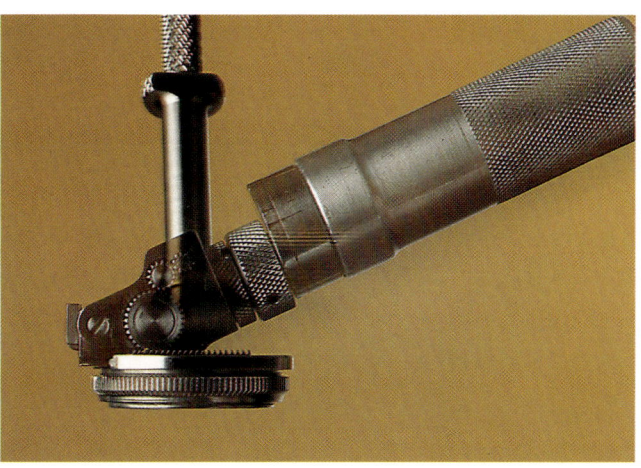

Figure 27.15 *An automated microkeratome.*

patient goes from being a high myope with spectacle correction to being an emmetrope with minimal or no correction. It appears that close to 10% of eyes undergoing keratomileusis may develop an unacceptably high rate of irregular astigmatism, but this is relative; it seems to be more of a problem in the United States where patients expect and demand a high degree of visual recovery.

The purpose of keratomileusis is to provide a functional improvement in uncorrected vision so the patient is able to perform without glasses activities that are taken for granted by others (e.g., going to the bathroom at night, being able see the lines on the bottom of a pool when swimming, driving, or just finding a doorway). Occasionally, the degree of irregular astigmatism is severe enough so that an individual must wear hard contact lenses to see clearly. (A soft contact lens would not correct the irregularity encountered.) Most patients need to wear a contact lens if their glasses cannot correct their vision to a level of 20/40. I have a patient whose uncorrected vision is 20/25 but wears contact lenses routinely in order to improve her vision to 20/20. Nonetheless, she is quite happy because the procedure has dramatically improved her functional vision and thus her quality of life.

As with any refractive procedure, a small overcorrection or undercorrection is expected, and anything within two diopters of emmetropia is usually considered a good refractive result for high myopes. If the patient is left myopic, radial keratotomy can be performed six to twelve months after surgery. Making the incision will be more difficult because of the varying thickness of the cornea, but it will fine-tune the visual result. Contact lenses can also be worn to improve vision. Fitting these contacts is more difficult than fitting standard contacts because the corneal surface is not shaped as it was previously. Often, the lenses move to the side. One difficulty with individuals who wear contact lenses following NFKM is that the cornea can mold beneath the contact, worsening their uncorrected vision. Within a few hours to a few days after removal of the contact, the cornea will return to the flattened state created by the myopic keratomileusis. Frequently, if a contact lens is necessary, patients can wear their presurgical contacts. Essentially, the contact is fitted on the midperipheral cornea, which is unchanged from the preoperative level. To correct the axial refractive error of the eye, the lens must have the same surface curvature centrally as it had preoperatively.

Infections can occur with this surgery as with any other surgical procedure, although I have not encountered this problem. I treat all my patients with Maxitrol drops or ointment four times a day for four days after the suture is removed from the eyelid and then twice a day until the sutures are removed from the cornea. Any combination of steroids or an antibiotic alone would probably suffice.

A bigger problem than infection is debris in the interface, but this should not be a problem if meticulous attention is paid to the surface of the lenticule and the resected bed. The stromal surfaces appear to attract foreign debris so care should be taken that none comes in contact with these surfaces. This is more of a problem with the non-freeze technique than with the cryolathing technique, although in no cases have I encountered enough debris to cause any visual loss. Also, epithelium can become lodged in the interface and cause an epithelial nest. This can lead to opacification of the interface or a change in the refractive effect because of induced changes on the anterior surface. These nests are very easily treated by finding the edge of the disc, partially elevating it from its bed by gentle traction with fine forceps, scraping out the epithelium, and resuturing the edge. Epithelium in the interface is actually a rare difficulty and may be more common for beginning surgeons.

I had one case of apparent cryo-damage to the lenticule where an opacified scar formed within the central portion of the lenticule a few months after surgery. Interestingly, it was evenly spaced between the anterior surface of Bowman's membrane and the posterior stromal surface of the lenticule. This scar caused a mild decrease in vision but was not severe enough to necessitate removal of the lenticule. The other eye was done using a non-freeze technique and no similar scarring occurred.

As with any other refractive procedure, a patient may have very good daytime vision but difficulties at night when the pupil dilates. This is not a significant problem in most patients, but if the resected disc is not centered, it can have the same effect as an incorrectly centered IOL. At night the patient looks through the central area, which has good correction, and the peripheral area, which has no correction. If the patient is significantly bothered, the only solution is wearing a hard contact lens.

If wearing a contact lens for high astigmatism or significant overcorrection or undercorrection is not viable, consideration should be given to repeating the surgery. Surgical records should be kept regarding the quality of the keratectomy and lathing. If the keratectomy was of exceptionally good quality, the lenticule can be peeled off and an applantation lens used to check the diameter of the lenticule. A donor globe can be used from which a disc of cornea of the appropriate thickness and diameter is resected. This disc is lathed and sutured onto the patient's eye. If there is significant irregular astigmatism, which may have been the result of the microkeratectomy, the surgery can be repeated by making a new pass across the cornea and then lathing a homoplastic donor disc. During a second myopic surgery, the central corneal thickness will be much thinner and a plate should be used to make a thin resection on the recipient eye. Usually a 0.20-mm plate is used.

Proper patient selection is the most important method of minimizing difficulties with irregular astigmatism. Patients who are extremely compulsive or need to have excessively fine vision for very detailed work should seriously consider whether they want to undergo a procedure that may cause them to need hard contact lenses. Most patients can tolerate a loss of one or two lines of best-corrected visual acuity and still function quite well. Those whose profession requires a large volume of detailed work could have some significant problems if irregular astigmatism occurs.

Probably the most catastrophic complication of keratomileusis is perforation of the cornea into the anterior chamber caused by not placing the depth plate in the microkeratome. This results in the microkeratome cutting extremely deeply—through the cornea and into the anterior chamber—and resecting the iris and lens as well. This problem can be avoided by only placing the head of the microkeratome on the handle only when the depth plate is in position.

Some surgeons believe that the interface created by keratomileusis may lead to decreased vision. I have found this to be totally inaccurate. I have had only one case of postoperative irregular astigmatism that could not be corrected with a hard contact lens; the decreased vision was caused by scarring within the stroma of the lenticule and was not associated with the interface. In fact, over a year after surgery, patients who have had a cryolathe myopic keratomileusis have minimal, if any, definition of the interface or peripheral scarring. Often, it is difficult to tell that surgery was done on the eye.

Theoretically, postoperative irregular astigmatism is more of a problem in hyperopic cases because the minified image size may lead to a mild loss of vision in addition to the loss arising from irregular astigmatism. Fortunately, in hyperopic cases there is minimal lathing to the central cornea, the majority of which occurs in the midperiphery of the lenticule.

Conclusion

Currently, Barraquer's keratomileusis is the best method for correcting severe hyperopia and myopia. Keratomileusis can offer an alternative to those patients severely handicapped by poorly fitting contact lenses or spectacles.

Clinical Points to Consider

☛ Keratomileusis can be used to correct refractive errors in the range of –5.00 D to –15.00 D and +4.00 to +10.00 D.

☛ Keratomileusis changes the anterior shape of the cornea by removing stromal tissue.

☛ The most difficult surgical step in keratomileusis is the keratectomy, not the lathing.

chapter 28

EPIKERATOPLASTY: PATIENT SELECTION AND SURGICAL TECHNIQUE

DANIEL S. DURRIE, M.D.   VANCE THOMPSON, M.D.

Epikeratoplasty was introduced by Herbert E. Kaufman, M.D., in 1979. The idea of an optical onlay lamellar keratoplasty was an exciting concept, and it was easily accepted in theory both by surgeons and patients. Taking donated corneal tissue, which was unacceptable for penetrating keratoplasty (PKP), and using it to surgically improve or correct various eye disorders was certainly an idea worth pursuing. The concept of a central distribution center for processing donated corneal tissue needed to be evaluated because of the potential impact on corneal tissue supply. Since 1979, epikeratoplasty has been studied by numerous individual surgeons, has been evaluated in a large national clinical trial, and has come under the scrutiny of the FDA and other third party agencies. The procedure has survived as a viable treatment for certain eye conditions and has not lived up to expectations for other conditions.

When epikeratoplasty was initially developed, it was considered a therapeutic procedure by the FDA and successfully used for uncorrected aphakia and keratoconus. Attempts to develop epikeratoplasty into a viable refractive procedure were then made. The ability of epikeratoplasty to change the anterior corneal curvature can be very dramatic, and the short-term correction of refractive errors as large as –39.00 D to +22.00 D has been achieved (Fig. 28.1). In cases where large refractive errors are considered pathologic (hyperopia resulting from monocular aphakia and significant myopia above –12.00 D), epikeratoplasty may be indicated as a therapeutic procedure. In spite of the technical feasibility of using epikeratoplasty as a refractive procedure, however, the common occurrence of irregular astigmatism, power inaccuracy, and poor quality of vision have limited its success in correcting myopia, hyperopia, and astigmatism. Thus, at the present time, epikeratoplasty should be used as a therapeutic, not a refractive, procedure.

The interest of one of the authors [DSD] in epikeratoplasty increased after attending one of the first surgical training courses in June 1984 at Louisiana State University in New Orleans. Because of the conservative nature of ophthalmology in Omaha, Nebraska, during the late 1970s and early 1980s, numerous aphakic individuals did not have simultaneous intraocular lens (IOL) implantation during cataract surgery. DSD performed 20 aphakic epikeratoplasty procedures with good initial success in the latter half of 1984, and DSD was asked by American Medical Optics (now Allergan Medical Optics) (AMO) to become a medical monitor for epikeratoplasty. Over the past six years we have performed over 300 epikeratoplasty procedures and have been closely involved with the monitoring and development of this procedure.

This chapter will present suggestions for patient selection for epikeratoplasty, describe the preferred surgical technique for each indication, and review some complications. The applications of epikeratoplasty will be discussed as well as present and future technologies that may complement or compete with epikeratoplasty.

Concepts

Epikeratoplasty, originally introduced as epikeratophakia, is a derivative of Jose Barraquer's keratomileusis. Herbert Kaufman, M.D., and Ted Werblin, M.D., devised epikeratoplasty to eliminate the most difficult and dangerous step of keratomileusis, the keratectomy of the patient's central cornea (Fig. 28.2).

The epikeratoplasty lenticule is created by placing a donor corneal button on the Steinway-Barraquer cryolathe, fashioning a plano lenticule while the donor cornea and cryolathe tool are frozen, introducing the appropriate dioptric power into the lenticule by changing the radius of the tool of the lathe, and establishing the diameter of the lenticule with the tool. The lenticule is then thawed and freeze-dried so it can be stored almost indefinitely. A plano epikeratoplasty lenticule can be used in keratoconus since it causes central cornea flattening.

It was hoped that attaching the donor cornea to the recipient cornea by means of a peripheral circular keratotomy (with keratectomy and peripheral undermining) would prove to be stable yet reversible. The interface between the smooth Bowman's membrane of the recipient and the stroma of the lenticule was not expected to be the limiting factor to excellent visual acuity. Oversizing the diameter of the epikeratoplasty donor relative to the recipient's circular keratotomy allowed the donor to be tucked into the stromal pocket of the recipient cornea and sutured into place with 16 interrupted 10-0 nylon sutures.

Before 1985, the Kaufman-MacDonald epikeratoplasty (KME) technique was the standard method. The main problems with the KME technique are delayed epithelialization, prolonged stromal haze, inaccuracy of predicted refractive power, and irregular astigmatism, especially following myopic epikeratoplasty. The first two problems relate to freeze-drying of the donor lenticule.

In 1985, Lee T. Nordan, M.D., introduced the Nordan epikeratoplasty technique (NET), which presented several new concepts: The edges of the epikeratoplasty donor are beveled to match the shape of the recipient's stromal pocket, in which no keratectomy has been performed (Fig. 28.3). The plano donor lenticule is obtained by using the microkeratome on a donor globe and then it is cryolathed, an attempt to mimic the corneal hydration factors and formulas used with Barraquer keratomileusis. The epikeratoplasty lenticule is greatly oversized, 8.50 mm, relative to the 6.50 mm trephination on the patient's cornea. The donor, without freeze-drying, is stored in the same

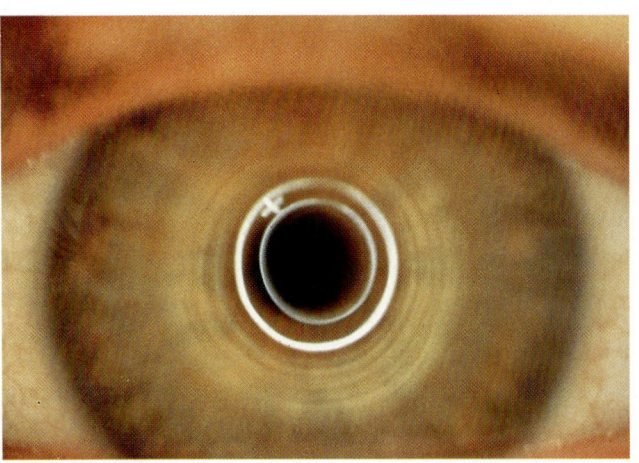

Figure 28.1 *Corneoscope study of myopic epikeratoplasty two years postoperatively shows dramatic central flattening of the central cornea. The patient was –22.00 D preoperatively.*

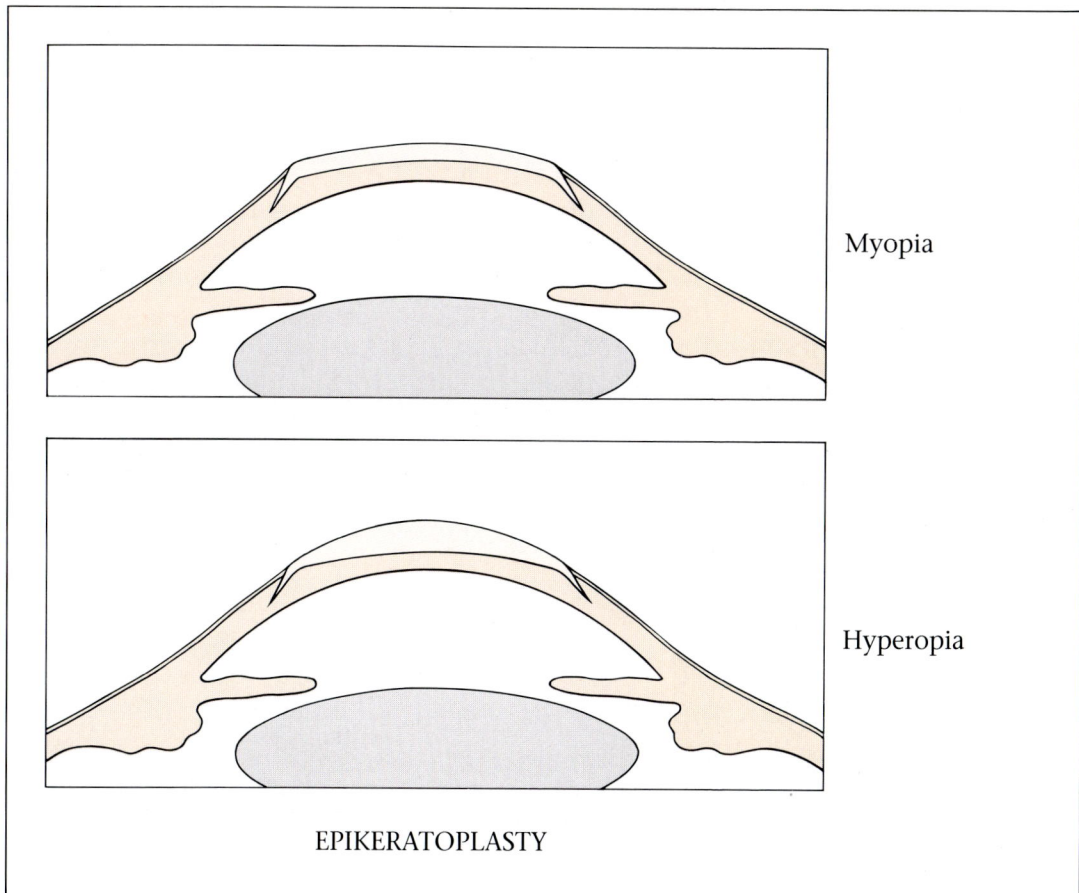

Figure 28.2 *Myopic epikeratoplasty creates a flatter central corneal curvature. Hyperopic epikeratoplasty creates a steeper central corneal curvature.*

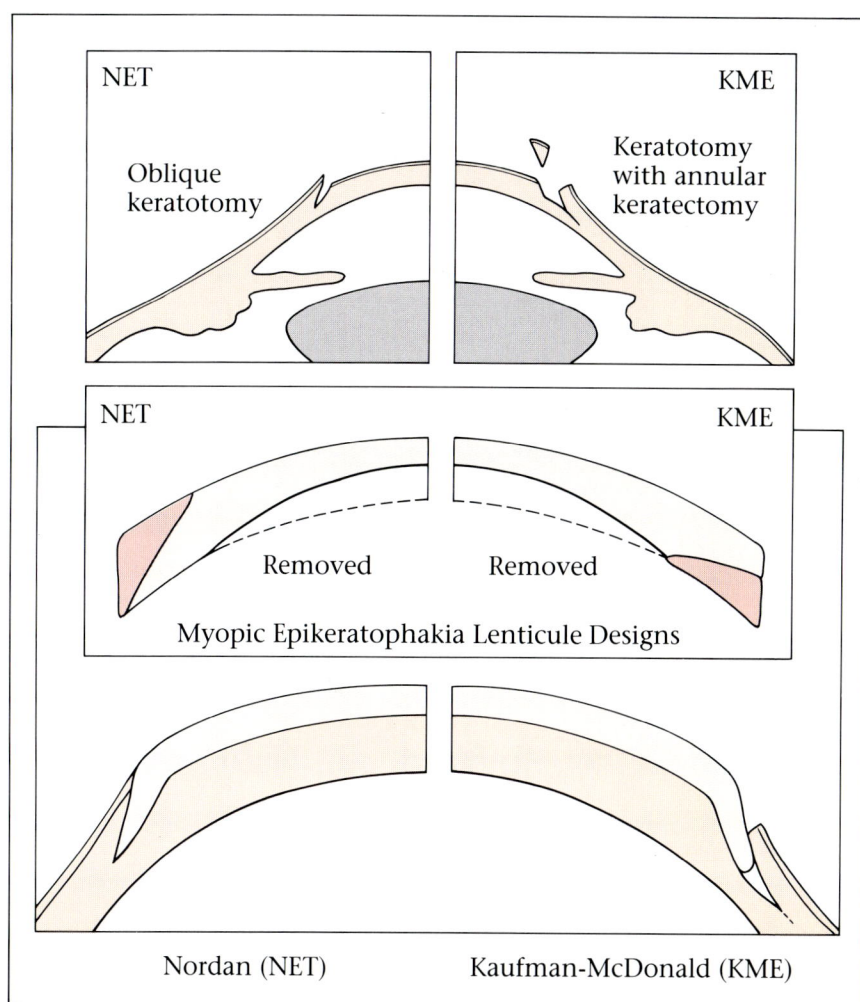

Figure 28.3 *The Nordan epikeratoplasty technique (NET) uses an angled keratotomy without a keratectomy. Also, NET donor lenticules have a beveled edge that fits into the recipient's corneal pocket, causing minimal distortion of the lenticule. The original Kaufman-McDonald epikeratoplasty (KME) technique uses a keratotomy and a keratectomy of the recipient cornea.*

corneal storage medium used to store donor corneas for PKP (Fig. 28.4). The donor cornea is sutured onto the recipient cornea using eight interrupted 10-0 nylon sutures, tucked into the stromal pocket, and further anchored with an eight-bite Barraquer anti-torque suture (Fig. 28.5).

NET allows for rapid epithelialization and establishment of donor clarity because the beveled edges of the donor make the contour of the wound very smooth, eliminating the need for the donor cornea to bend into the recipient keratectomy, and the tissue is healthy (i.e., nonfreeze-dried). However, irregular astigmatism, the result of the geometric difficulties inherent in placing a concave donor cornea onto a convex recipient cornea without a firm bond between the stroma of the donor cornea and Bowman's membrane of the recipient cornea, is a major problem following myopic epikeratoplasty with both techniques. Similarly, irregular astigmatism is a significant problem when a minus-power alloplastic implant, designed to correct high myopia, is implanted

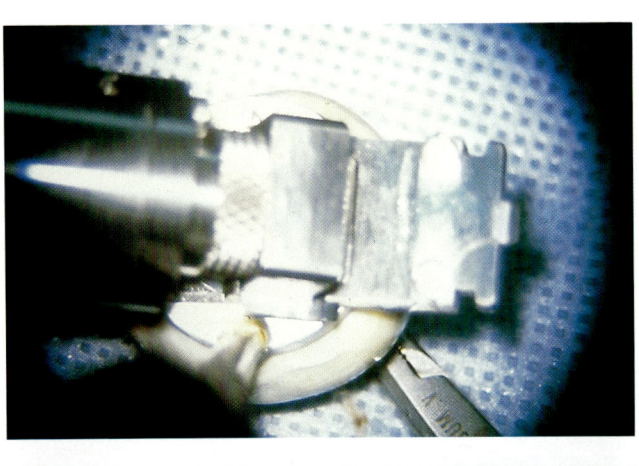
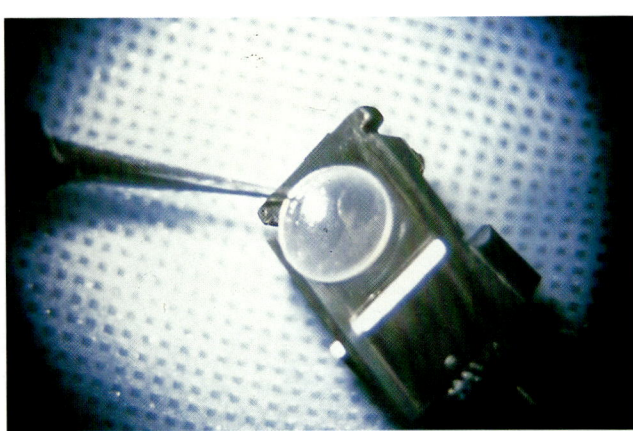
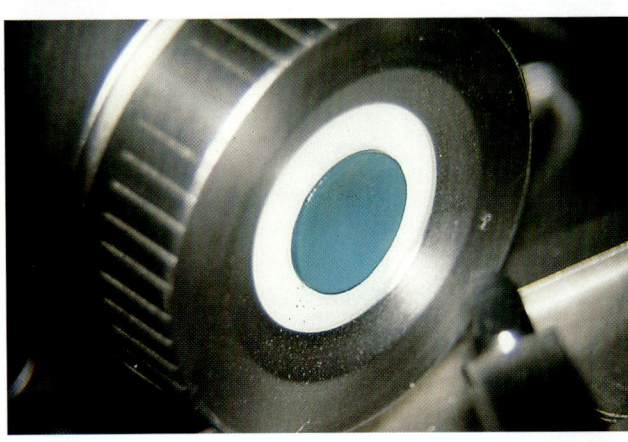
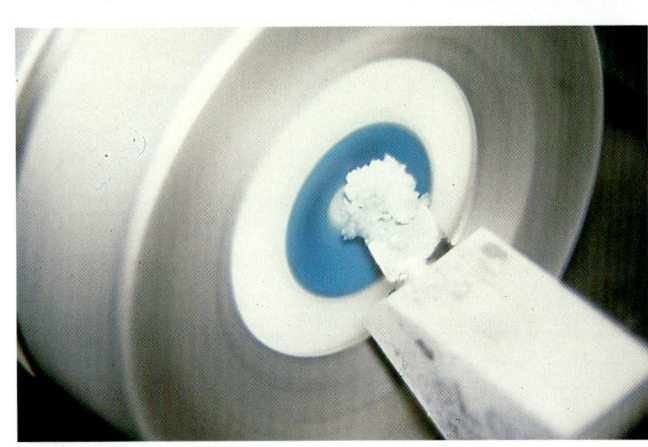
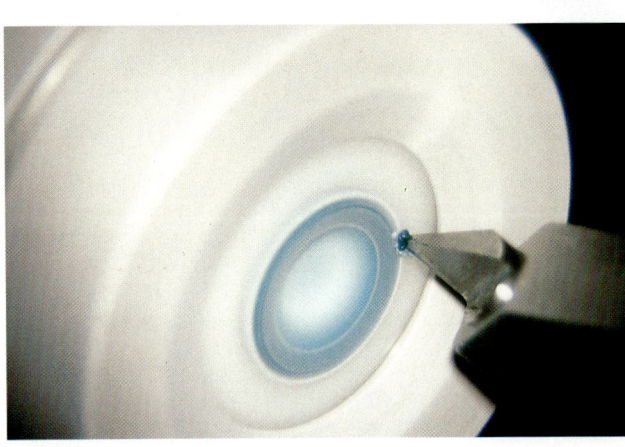

Figure 28.4 (Top left and right) *A corneal disc, removed from the donor globe by a microkeratome, will be shaped into a NET lenticule.* **(Middle left)** *The corneal disc is dyed and placed on the Delrin base of the Steinway-Barraquer cryolathe.* **(Middle right)** *The disc is frozen and an epikeratoplasty lenticule is fashioned by determining the lathe settings for lenticular diameter, curvature (dioptric power), and edge design.* **(Bottom left)** *The beveled edge of the NET lenticule is created.* **(Bottom right)** *The NET lenticule is remarkably clear immediately after defrosting.*

intrastromally following keratectomy of a recipient cornea.

Aphakic Epikeratoplasty

Patient Selection

Aphakic epikeratoplasty patients may be either unilaterally or bilaterally aphakic, but they must be contact lens and spectacle intolerant (Fig. 28.6). Certainly monocular aphakic patients, both pediatric and adult, are spectacle intolerant because of significant anisometropia and, if they cannot wear a contact lens, have a visually useless eye because of their uncorrected refractive error.

Patients selected for epikeratoplasty should have contraindications for IOL implantation. These contraindications may include anterior chamber disorganization due to either previous injury or surgery, chronic iritis, or uncontrolled glaucoma (Fig. 28.7). It is our opinion that secondary anterior chamber lenses should not be used in pediatric or young adult patients because of the tendency for late corneal decompensation and increased intraocular pressure. Therefore, epikeratoplasty is the treatment of choice in this patient group. In the older adult monocular aphakic patient, a secondary anterior chamber IOL probably affords more rapid and accurate visual recovery, but epikeratoplasty is an acceptable alternative. Endothelial function is a consideration in both a secondary anterior chamber IOL implantation and epikeratoplasty.

It is also important to note that the healing of an epikeratoplasty relies on epithelialization over Bowman's membrane of the donor; thus, candidates for epikeratoplasty should have minimal external disease and an adequate ocular surface to promote good healing.

Surgical Procedure

It is important that the epikeratoplasty lenticule be well centered over the visual axis. Many aphakic patients cannot hold fixation well enough for

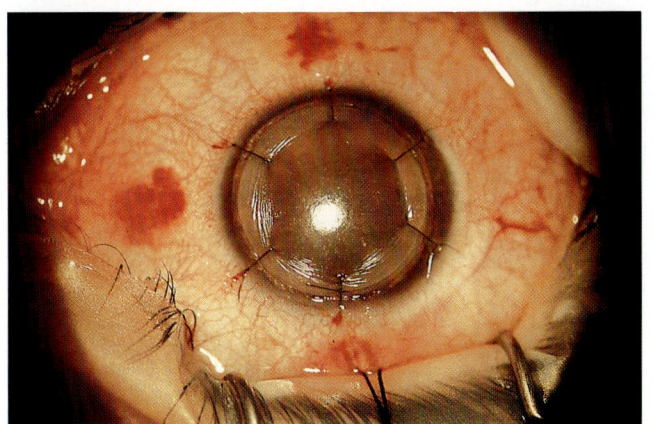 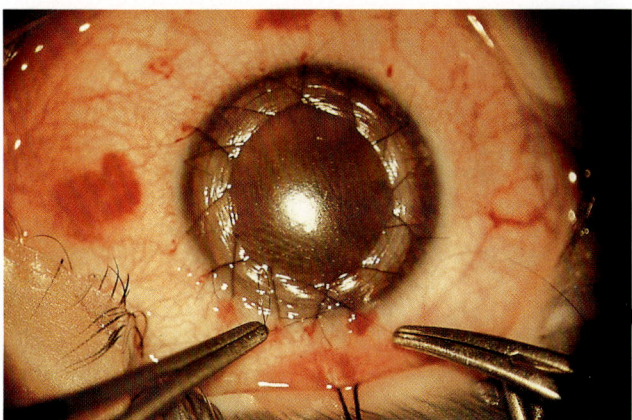

Figure 28.5 *The donor cornea is sutured onto the recipient cornea* **(left)** *and anchored in place with an eight-bite Barraquer anti-torque suture* **(right)**.

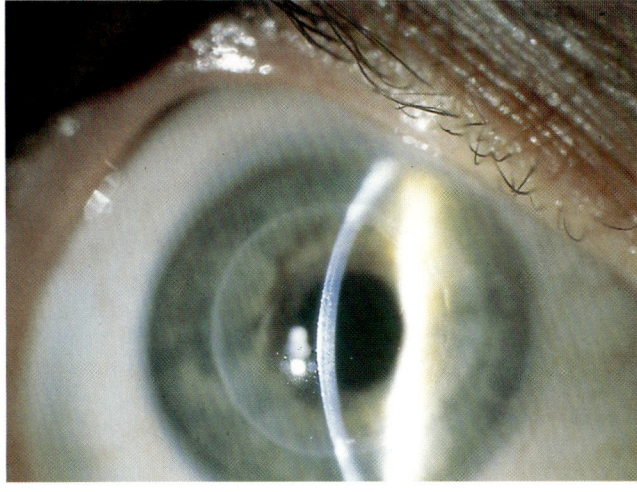 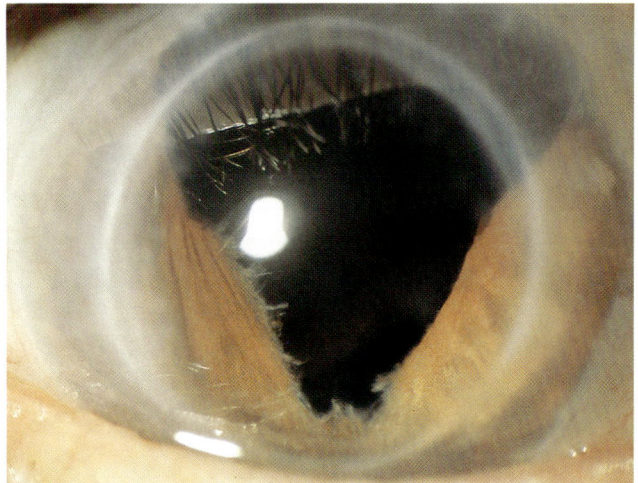

Figure 28.6 *Slit lamp photograph of a successful aphakic epikeratoplasty one year postoperatively.*

Figure 28.7 *A disorganized anterior chamber made this patient a poor candidate for anterior chamber IOL implantation.*

the standard optical centering techniques used in radial keratotomy. Also it is common for patients who are candidates for epikeratoplasty to have a disorganized anterior segment; therefore, the pupil cannot always be a guideline for centration during surgery. If the pupil is round and constricted, it should be used as a guideline for centration. If the pupil is not reliable, the epikeratoplasty lenticule is positioned in the geometric center of the cornea. Aphakic epikeratoplasty has a relatively large optical zone, thus centration is not as critical as it is for myopic lenticules.

At the beginning of the procedure, the epithelium of the recipient is removed by mechanical debridement alone. We use a light application of absolute alcohol with a Weck-cel sponge just before placing the epikeratophakia lenticule to kill residual epithelial cells. This step should be done very lightly and irrigated quickly to insure no adverse toxic effects. We have found that removal of epithelium by cocaine has no advantages over absolute alcohol or mechanical debridement and may impair re-epithelialization.

A circular keratotomy is performed to a depth of 0.25 mm using either a standard Hessburg-Baron trephine or a customized version with a stop at 0.25 mm (see Chapter 25).

The depth of the trephine cut should be checked after the trephine is removed and deepened manually with a blade if it is too shallow. Although an annular keratectomy was used in the initial aphakic epikeratoplasties, most surgeons have abandoned this part of the surgery, making for a less invasive procedure and easier removal or exchange of the donor if necessary. If the keratectomy is omitted, 1.50 D of hyperopic power must be added to the epikeratoplasty lenticule to compensate for the resulting decreased corneal curvature. The keratotomy is undermined peripherally for 1.00 mm to allow the wings of the epikeratoplasty lenticule to be placed easily into the corneal stromal pocket (Fig. 28.8).

Sixteen interrupted sutures are placed in the epikeratoplasty lenticule before the edges are tucked. This suture pattern allows for improved centration, improved postoperative topography, and less chance of inducing astigmatism.

If the epikeratoplasty lenticule is left on the surface during suturing, it is very easy to align the round lenticule with the underlying circular

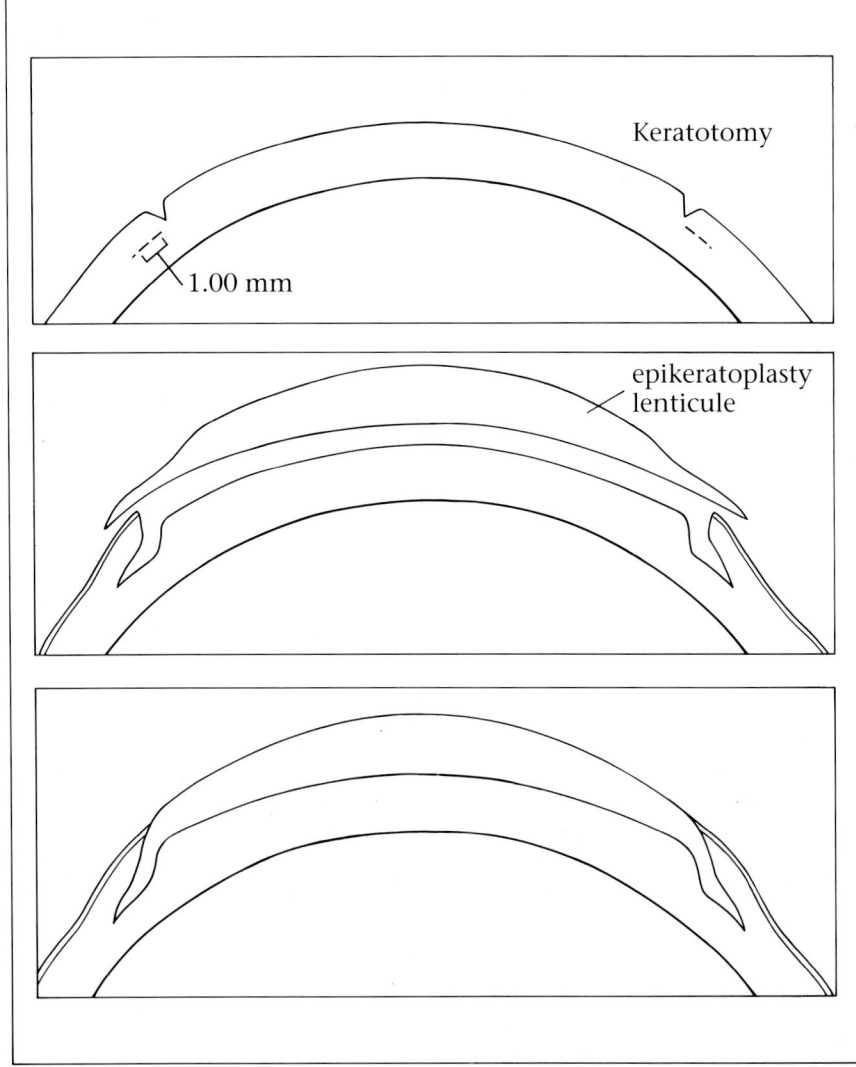

Figure 28.8 *Peripheral extension of the recipient cornea's keratectomy allows for insertion of the donor lenticule's wing.*

keratotomy mark on the cornea. After the 16 interrupted sutures have been placed, the edges of the epikeratoplasty lenticule are tucked into the previously undermined dissection with a cyclodialysis spatula. A combined antibiotic/steroid ointment and eye patch are applied.

The most important part of successful epikeratoplasty surgery is the postoperative regimen. Patching usually yields an epithelialized corneal surface within three to four days. Bandage contact lenses cause a tight lens syndrome and are not used. If the epithelium is not intact in one week, temporary lid adhesion should be used and if the lenticule is not totally epithelialized by two weeks, it should be removed. If an epikeratoplasty lenticule is left in a de-epithelialized state for longer than two weeks, the chance of infection and underlying scarring increases greatly.

In a well epithelialized epikeratoplasty lenticule every other suture is removed at one week and the remainder of the sutures at two weeks postoperatively. This early suture removal shortens the recovery period and does not cause wound dehiscence or lost lenticules. In infants, all sutures should be removed at one week if the epithelium is intact, which decreases the incidence of suture abscess and allows for earlier amblyopia therapy.

With proper patient selection and good surgical technique, epikeratoplasty can be extremely rewarding in the aphakic population. Patients who are candidates for this procedure have, by definition, no functional vision in the operated eye prior to surgery since they are contact lens and spectacle intolerant. The power of predictability of aphakia epikeratoplasty is only 34% within 1.00 D and 78% within 3.00D. This is quite acceptable in patients whose only choice is having a nonfunctioning eye or a partially useful one. Power predictability does not have to be highly accurate for epikeratoplasty to be valuable in aphakia, but this lack of power predictability precludes epikeratoplasty from being a viable refractive surgical procedure, as noted previously. Also, patients who undergo epikeratoplasty for aphakia may have a one to two line loss of best corrected visual acuity due to increased corneal thickness and topographical changes. Again, this is acceptable as therapeutic surgery for eyes that have no functional vision but is not acceptable as a refractive procedure.

Epikeratoplasty for Keratoconus

Patient Selection

Patients undergoing epikeratoplasty for keratoconus should be spectacle and contact lens intolerant and, according to FDA guidelines, PKP should be contraindicated (e.g., patients who have had multiple graft rejections in the other eye or are incapable of or unavailable for the long-term follow up necessary for PKP, such as institutionalized patients). Younger patients have better results and experience earlier clearing of their onlay lenticule after epikeratoplasty for keratoconus than do older patients. Patients considered for this procedure should have minimal corneal scarring, with any existing scars being at least 1.00 mm from the visual axis. A paracentral corneal scar may be moved centrally by the posterior pressure that an epikeratoplasty lenticule applies to the anterior surface of Bowman's membrane.

The purpose of epikeratoplasty for keratoconus is to improve the anterior corneal topography. Keratoconus patients with central corneal pathology are ideal candidates for this procedure because the lenticule is sutured in an area that has relatively normal topography (Fig. 28.9).

Widely spread keratoconic corneas in which peripheral portions of the cornea are involved in the

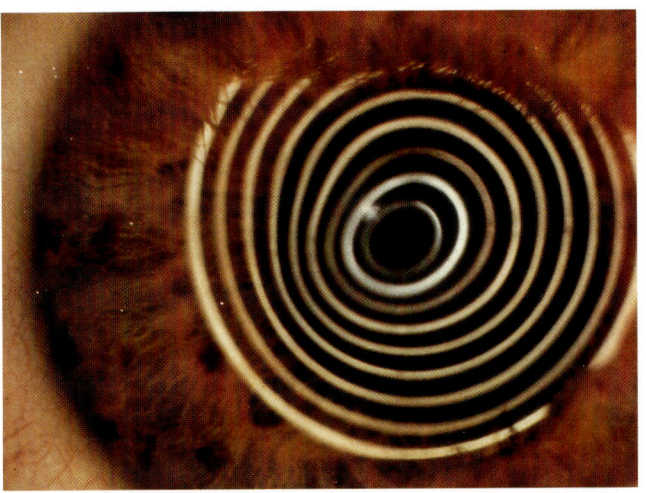

Figure 28.9 *Photokeratoscopic display showing a central "nipple" cone of keratoconus with normal peripheral cornea. This form of keratoconus is best suited for treatment by planar epikeratoplasty.*

cone, are more difficult to treat with epikeratoplasty lenticules because the circular keratotomy, keratectomy, and suturing is done in an area of peripheral distortion (Fig. 28.10). Although keratoglobus patients can be candidates for onlay lamellar keratoplasty techniques, the most successful patients are younger keratoconus patients who have central, nipple-shaped cones and minimal or no corneal scarring.

Surgical Procedure

The procedure flattens the anterior surface and pushes the ectatic cornea back into a more normal position. Intraoperative keratometry is helpful in directing suture placement.

The surgical technique of epikeratoplasty for keratoconus has essentially remained unchanged since the early development of the procedure in 1981 and 1982. Whether the epikeratoplasty lenticule should be centered over the apex of the cone or in the geometric center of the cornea is a point of debate. We feel that it is important to center the epikeratoplasty lenticule in the geometric center of the cornea if at all possible since an equal distance from the limbus to the sutures allows for more even healing. Epithelium is removed with blunt dissection. A small amount of absolute alcohol is applied to the de-epithelialized area to prevent epithelial inclusion cysts. The circular keratotomy is performed with an 8.50-mm trephine, either a single or twin bladed, custom-made. The twin blade trephine makes an inner and an outer cut and eases creation of a smooth and symmetrical annular keratectomy.

An annular keratectomy, which allows for an area of peripheral scarring, is performed. We prefer this keratectomy in epikeratoplasty for keratoconus (Fig. 28.11), although the keratectomy stage of the procedure has been abandoned in aphakic and myopic epikeratoplasty. The suturing technique uses 24 interrupted 10-0 nylon sutures with the sutures placed under significant tension.

Postoperative management differs little from a standard lamellar keratoplasty procedure. A topical antibiotic and steroids are started the first postoperative day. By the first postoperative week, the epikeratoplasty lenticule should be completely epithelialized. Sutures should be left in at least three months. If they become vascularized or loose, they should be removed. Postoperative topography analysis by corneoscopy is helpful in directing suture removal. Selective suture removal for excessive astigmatism can begin as early as one month. If the sutures are left in place too long or if they loosen, vascularization of the interface may occur and cause loss of graft clarity.

Visual Results

The ability to achieve acceptable uncorrected vision postoperatively with epikeratoplasty for keratoconus depends on the ability to control not only the regular and irregular astigmatism but also the underlying myopia. Because of the marked flattening induced by the epikeratoplasty lenticule, many patients have acceptable uncorrected vision after the procedure, equal to or better than PKP patients (Fig. 28.12). The best corrected visual acuity after keratoconus epikeratoplasty is slightly less than one would expect after PKP. Also it has been shown that contrast sensitivity is decreased with these optical onlay lamellar grafts. Older patients who have keratoconus or patients with extremely steep corneas may have persistent corneal folds that decrease visual acuity. Also, patients with significant topography changes outside the area of the annular keratectomy have significant astigmatism postoperatively. Although corneal relaxing incisions can be made, the results after keratoconus epikeratoplasty are as unpredictable as after PKP.

Excellent stability of best corrected visual acuity without recurrence of keratoconus has been the rule. Epikeratoplasty patients with a four to five year follow up do not show a tendency towards

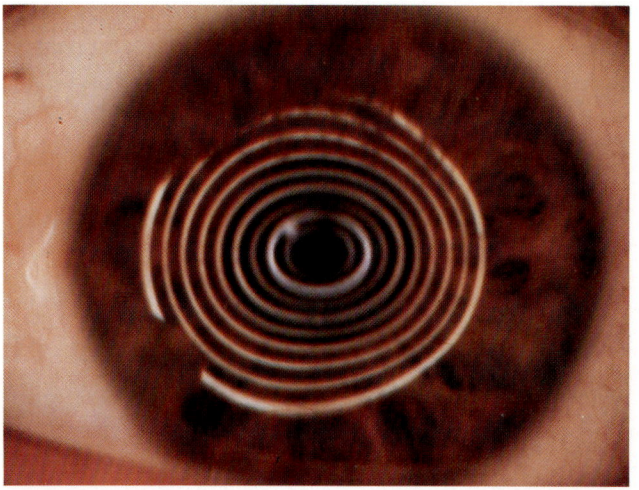

Figure 28.10 *Keratoscopic photograph of keratoconus showing a wide-based cone with paracentral corneal involvement. This form of keratoconus is poorly suited for correction by planar epikeratoplasty because the donor lenticule cannot cover the entire area or recipient corneal keratoconus. However, a planar epikeratoplasty can be used as a tectonic lamellar corneal graft to prepare an extremely thin peripheral cornea for a PKP, which will be performed at a later date.*

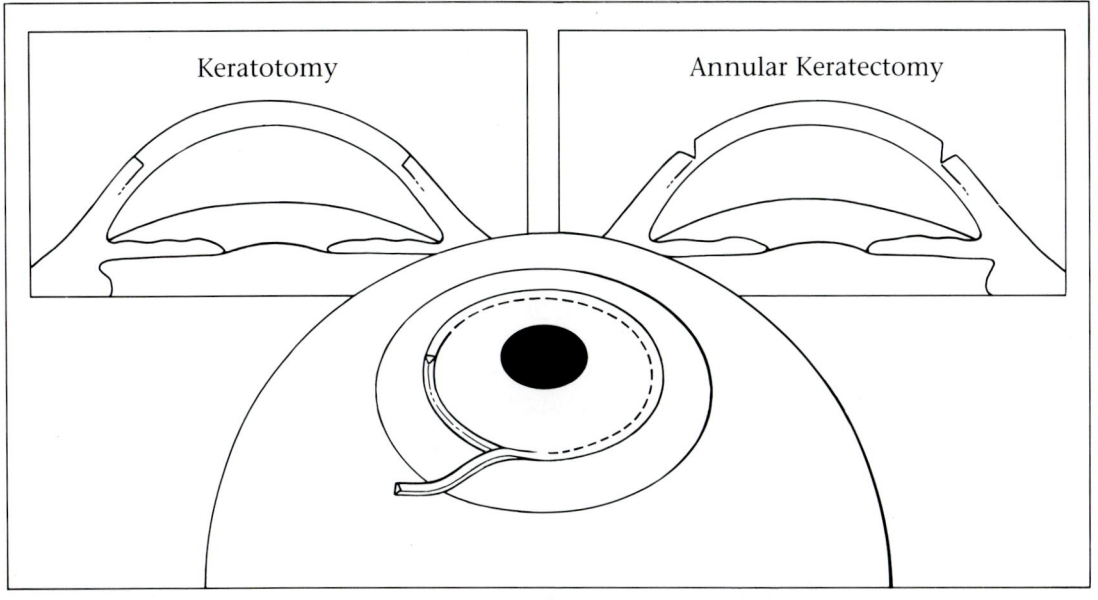
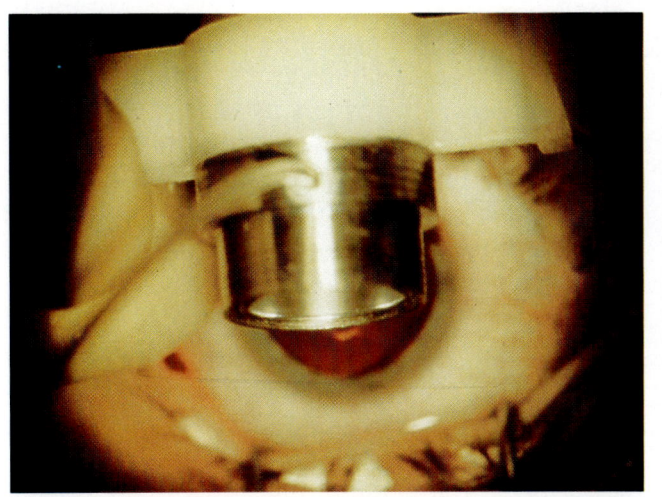
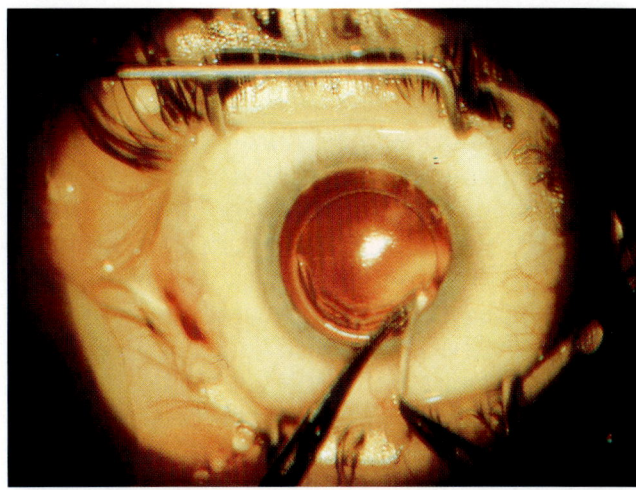
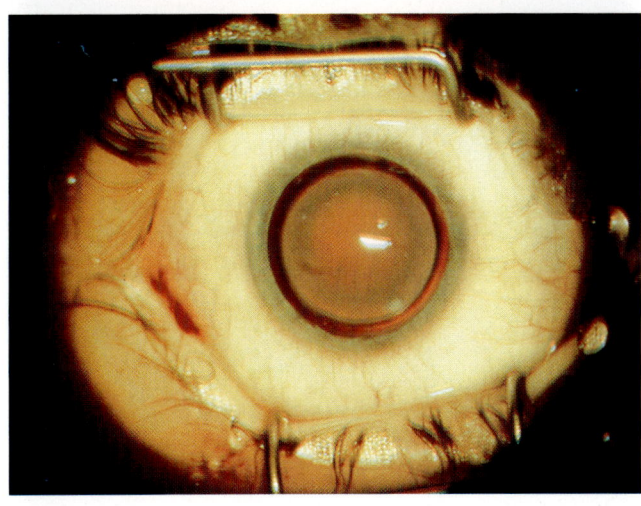
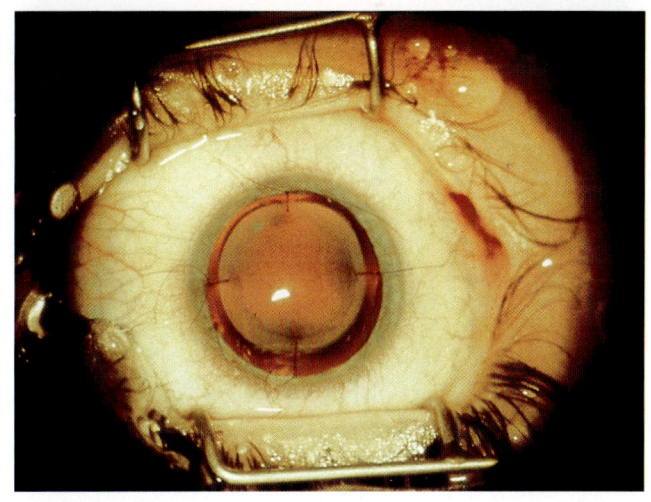

Figure 28.11 (Top) *Epikeratoplasty surgical overview. The KME surgical technique uses a peripheral keratotomy with or without a circular keratectomy to anchor the donor corneal in place.* **(Middle left)** *A double-bladed Hessburg-Baron suction trephine establishes the confines of the peripheral keratectomy.* **(Middle right)** *Vannas scissors create a 0.50 mm wide annular keratectomy.* **(Bottom left)** *The donor epikeratoplasty lenticule is in position, awaiting the interrupted sutures.* **(Bottom right)** *Four interrupted sutures anchor the lenticule in position.*

increased myopia or astigmatism. Complications have mainly related to poor epithelialization, vascularization, and irregular astigmatism.

Good patient selection and close adherence to appropriate surgical technique and the postoperative follow-up regimen may reduce the incidence of most complications.

As with mild keratoconus, plano epikeratoplasty may be a valuable treatment for severe keratoconus or keratoglobus in patients who have lost functional vision in the other eye because of corneal perforation or the sequelae of repeated penetrating graft rejections. Following epikeratoplasty, adequate visual acuity may still be gained with spectacles or contact lenses, despite the presence of scarring secondary to corneal hydrops in the visual axis (Fig. 28.13).

Potential Advances

As long as epikeratoplasty for keratoconus is used only for the conditions currently recommended, there will continue to be a low number of procedures performed. The potential for developing a safe extraocular alternative to PKP for young adults with keratoconus is certainly an attractive alternative. Because younger patients with small central based cones are the best candidates for epikeratoplasty, a controlled clinical trial of thinner epikeratoplasty lenticules in contact lens tolerant patients has been proposed. This procedure, unlike contact lenses, which only serve as an optical aid, might halt the progressive thinning seen in keratoconus.

Epikeratoplasty for High Myopia

Most of the initial excitement and interest regarding epikeratoplasty was based on its potential for alleviating myopia. The concept of having a "living contact lens" replace spectacles and contact lenses for moderate to severe myopia was an exciting concept for both patients and ophthalmologists. Over the past five years the results of epikeratoplasty as a refractive surgery for myopia have been disappointing, but it has found a valuable place as a therapeutic procedure for pathologic myopia and severe anisometropia.

Patient Selection

Patients selected for myopic epikeratoplasty should have no therapeutic alternative. We limit patient selection to children with unilateral high myopia, those with myopia greater than 12.00 D and contact lens and spectacle intolerance, and patients who have problems associated with high myopia, such as nystagmus, posterior staphyloma, and/or macular pathology. Even if myopic epikeratoplasty could be developed into a viable refractive surgery procedure, the expense of using human tissue for optical onlay will always be a major deterrent to wide-spread acceptance.

Surgical Procedure

Centering of the epikeratoplasty lenticule on the optical axis is more critical in myopic epikerato-

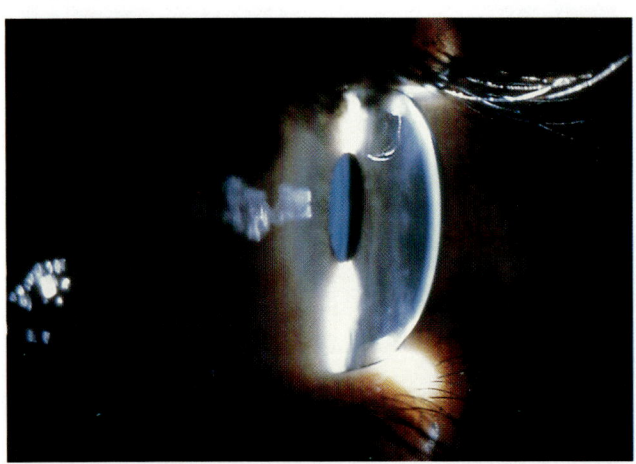

Figure 28.12 *Marked central corneal flattening is noted following epikeratoplasty for keratoconus.*

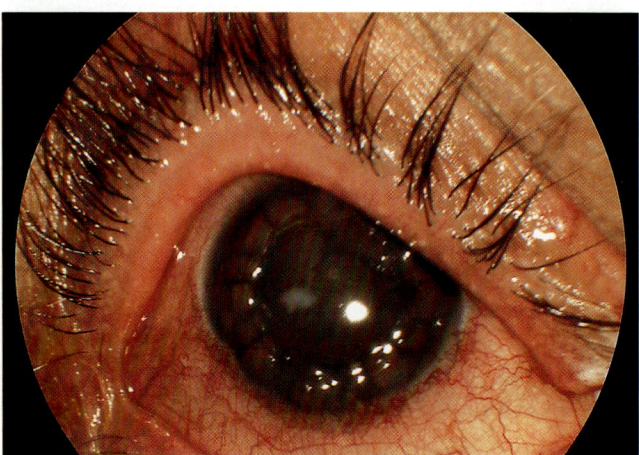

Figure 28.13 *A 50-year-old patient with bilateral keratoglobus underwent four PKPs in the left eye and subsequent phthisis in that eye. This photograph shows the right eye of this patient. The eye has central scarring from repeated attacks of corneal hydrops and has been treated by a 9.50 mm diameter planar epikeratoplasty. Best corrected spectacle visual acuity is 20/50.*

plasty than for aphakia or keratoconus. Because of the small functional optical zone that results from a concave optical onlay, a decentration of only 1.00 mm can cause significant halos and decreased quality of vision. We prefer to center the epikeratoplasty lenticule on the miotic pupil obtained by using Pilocarpine 2% before the retrobulbar block. A 3.00 mm radial keratotomy marker is then centered on the constricted pupil and the trephine centered on this 3.00 mm indentation mark.

Epithelium removal is done in the standard fashion with blunt dissection. A small amount of absolute alcohol is applied prior to application of the lenticule. A keratotomy is performed with a 7.00 mm Hessburg-Baron trephine at a depth of 0.25 mm using the technique described for aphakia. It should be emphasized that an annular keratectomy is not performed in either myopic or aphakic epikeratoplasty. The edges are undermined in a fashion similar to that for aphakia, and an 8.50 mm diameter lenticule is sutured in place with 16 interrupted sutures of 10-0 nylon. As with aphakia, all 16 interrupted sutures are placed before the lenticule is tucked into the undermined bed.

Intraoperative keratometry is quite useful in myopic epikeratoplasty and should be used at the eight-suture stage. Either a hand-held reflective keratometer or an automated keratometry device can be useful at this point. The postoperative regimen is essentially the same as for aphakic epikeratoplasty.

Epithelialization should be completed by one postoperative week and refraction and topography should be monitored starting at one week postoperatively. If the sutures are placed with excessive tension, the wing of the epikeratoplasty lenticule is pulled down, increasing the refractive power of the anterior corneal surface (and reducing the radius of curvature). To make sure the sutures are not removed too early, monitoring the postoperative spherical equivalent is critical. If at the one week visit, the spherical equivalent is still extremely myopic, half the sutures can be removed. Figure 28.14 shows the dramatic effect of suture removal in myopic epikeratoplasty. In this patient, the preoperative spherical equivalent

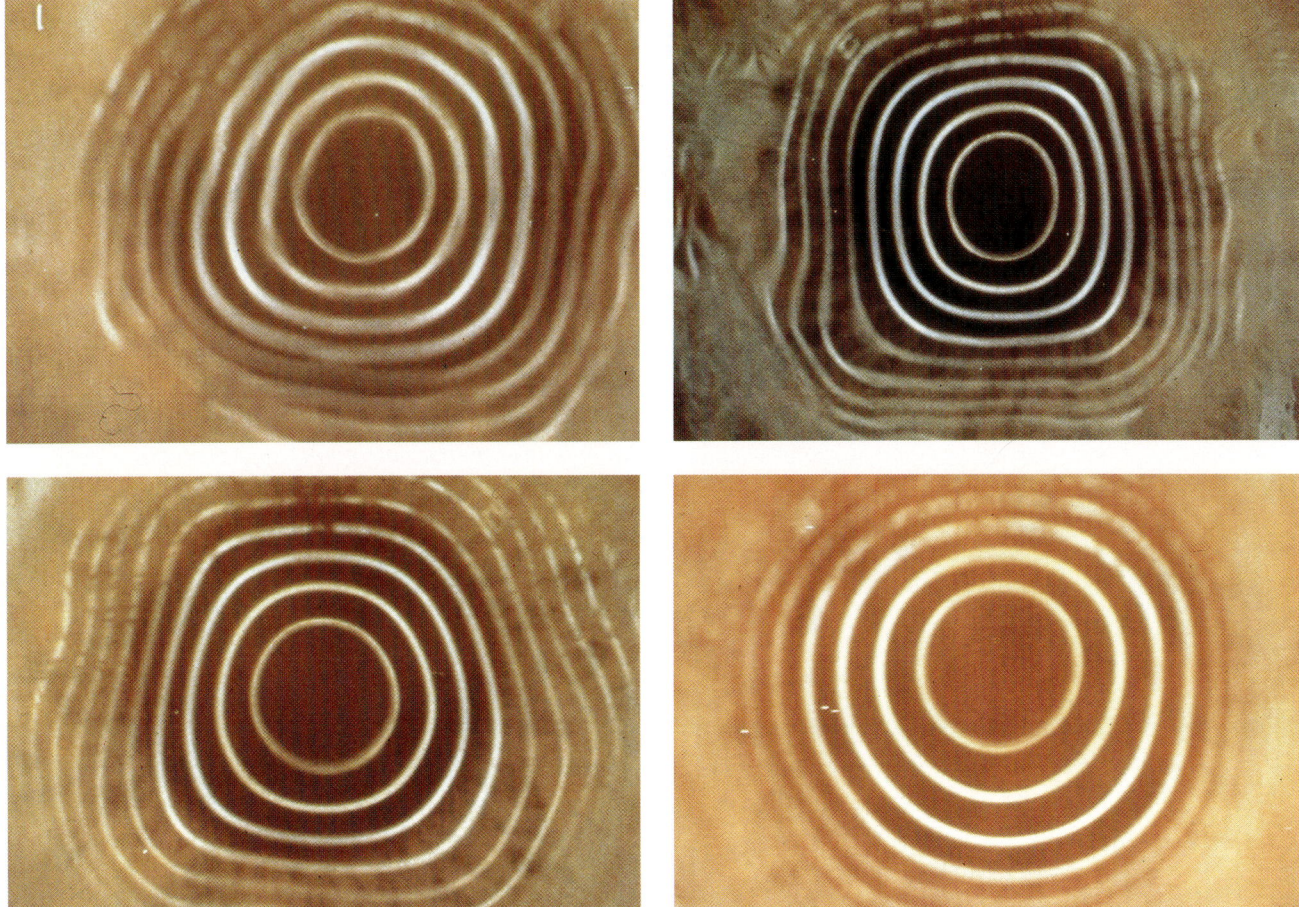

Figure 28.14 *A patient with a refractive error of −12.50 D underwent myopic epikeratoplasty.* **(Top left)** *The corneal appearance two weeks postoperatively,* **(top right)** *the same cornea after removal of four sutures,* **(bottom left)** *eight sutures, and* **(bottom right)** *all sixteen sutures.*

was –12.50 D. There was significant suture tension two weeks postoperatively and the spherical equivalent was a –10.50 D. After four sutures were removed, the spherical equivalent dropped to a –9.00 D. Four additional sutures were removed, which resulted central corneal flattening and decreased myopia to –7.00 D. All sutures were then removed, with the spherical equivalent changing to –2.00 D and the central corneal flattening obvious on the keratoscopy photograph. At the next visit, the spherical equivalent was a +1.00 D, and the one-year postoperative spherical equivalent showed a mild regression to –1.00 D.

If the spherical equivalent is close to the desired result with the sutures in, they should remain in as long as possible or a significant hyperopic shift will occur following suture removal. In children, amblyopic therapy should be instituted as soon as possible.

Clinical Results

Our clinical results support the conclusion that this procedure should only be used therapeutically. Thirty-seven procedures with two-year follow up, averaged a preoperative spherical equivalent of –13.73 D. Uncorrected acuity, best corrected visual acuity, power predictability, power stability, complications, and the need for secondary surgical intervention were evaluated.

The procedure went through two major design changes during the entry of patients into this group. The initial procedure used an 8.00 mm lenticule in a 7.50 mm trephined bed, which was designated as "old myopic lens design." The "new myopic lens design" involved an 8.50 mm lenticule in a 7.00 mm trephined bed, similar to that used for aphakia. A third design used the same trephine and lenticule diameter as the new myopic design but was done without an annular keratectomy. This was designated the "no keratectomy epikeratoplasty" or NKE technique.

In all but two cases (two patients had significant macular pathology), the uncorrected visual acuity showed definite improvement and functionally acceptable visual acuity. Best corrected visual acuity was also well preserved and the only patient losing significant best corrected visual acuity (greater than one Snellen line) was in the old myopic lens group (Fig. 28.15). Power predictability, however, was not acceptable for this level of preoperative myopia—only 73% were within 3.00 D, 50% were within 2.00 D, and 30% were within 1.00 D of emmetropia. Although there have been several reports of significant loss of power in myopic epikeratoplasty, review of our data shows acceptable stability from the one- to two-year follow up (Fig. 28.16). Five years postoperatively, stability continues to be acceptable after the one year refractive result.

A major concern with epikeratoplasty for myopia is the number of patients requiring secondary surgical intervention. Even though the number of secondary surgical interventions decreased as the procedure was refined, using the NKE technique, two of 11 procedures still required secondary surgical intervention. In total, 37 eyes required 53 surgical procedures to obtain satisfactory results. If this same data is broken

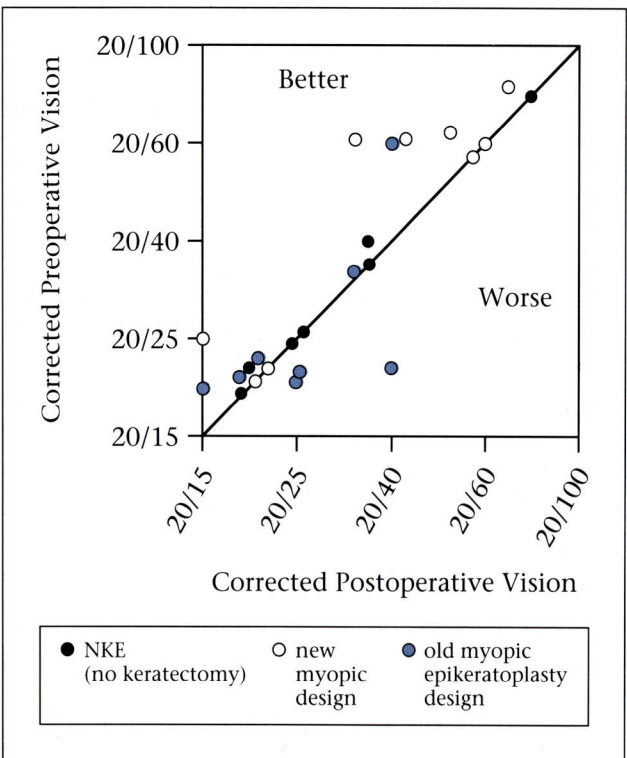

Figure 28.15 *The results of myopic epikeratoplasty using three different surgical techniques observed by the authors. (Thirty-seven patients are included in the study but only twenty-four data points appear on this graph because some data points overlap.)*

down into the indications for the procedure, the limited value of myopic epikeratoplasty as a refractive procedure can be seen.

Twenty-two procedures were performed as refractive surgery; ten eyes had significant pathology (nystagmus, macular degeneration, amblyopia, or prior retinal detachment) and six patients had the procedure because of childhood unilateral high myopia. All of the secondary surgical interventions occurred in the refractive group (Table 28.17). The difference between the refractive and therapeutic groups is due to the patients' and surgeons' expectation. The desired outcome of refractive surgery is to eliminate the need for spectacles and contact lenses by creating best corrected visual acuity and excellent optical results. When this type of procedure is performed on a therapeutic basis, however, the power predictability and final visual outcome are not evaluated as critically by the patient or surgeon.

Also, in order to correct myopia, the epikeratoplasty lenticule must create a flatter central cornea. Consequently, virtually every cornea following myopic epikeratoplasty has some degree of irregular astigmatism and reduced optical zone size due to the geometric realities of placing a concave corneal lens onto a convex cornea. Because there is no healing between Bowman's membrane of the recipient bed and the overlapping stroma of the donor, a potential tissue space without true adhesion is created. Although myopic keratomileusis enables stroma-to-stroma apposition of the central cornea, which reduces the incidence of irregular astigmatism relative to

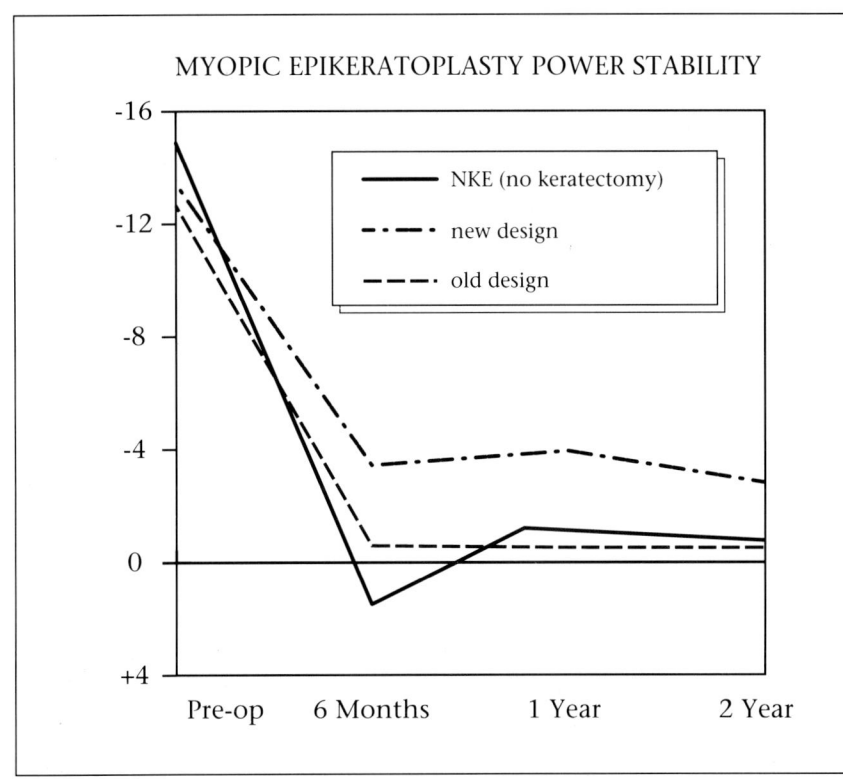

Figure 28.16 *The stability of the myopic epikeratoplasty cases described in Figure 28.14.*

Table 28.17
Refractive Myopic Epikeratoplasty:
Rate of Secondary Surgery

Type of Myopic Epikeratoplasty	Number of Cases	Number of Replaced Lenticules	Number of PKPs	Number of Relaxing Incisions	Number of Resutures	Total Number of Secondary Surgeries
Pediatric	6	0	0	0	0	0
Pathology	10	0	0	0	0	0
Refractive	22	6	2	3	5	16

22 cases of refractive myopic epikeratoplasty; 16 secondary procedures needed
16/22 = 73%

myopic epikeratoplasty, irregular astigmatism is still a significant problem.

The 22 patients described above, who underwent myopic epikeratophakia for refractive surgery, required 28 total epikeratoplasty procedures, plus ten other surgical interventions, which is unacceptable for a procedure of this type (Table 28.18). Also, the high expense of tissue onlay procedures makes secondary surgical intervention even less acceptable. Myopic epikeratoplasty, hopefully, will continue to be available for patients with unilateral high myopia, marked anisometropia, and other associated pathology, where expectations are not as great as in a purely refractive situation.

Present Status And Availability

Currently, myopic epikeratoplasty is being performed on a limited basis, and the myopic tissue epikeratophakia lenticules from AMO are available only when used in conjunction with clinical trials. Larger lenticules are being evaluated, and improved results may be possible with nonfreeze-dried lenticules. The depth of the trephined cut and its effect on the power predictability is also being evaluated. The availability of improved topographical analysis has added to our knowledge of the effect of onlay lamellar keratoplasty on the optical surface. An example of dramatic flattening is presented in Figure 28.19. This patient is five years post epikeratoplasty for –12.00 D of myopia. Topography analysis shows a well-centered lenticule and significant central flattening. The postoperative spherical equivalent has been stable at +1.00 D for four years.

Profile analysis (Fig. 28.20) shows that although the theoretical optical zone of epikeratoplasty is 6.00 mm, the functional optical zone at the desired 33.00 D is only 2.50 mm in diameter. Indeed all patients undergoing myopic epikeratoplasty have a markedly aspheric cornea, a trait common to all eyes that have undergone corneal refractive procedures (see Chapter 2). With continuing analysis of postoperative patients, improved postoperative topography with onlay procedures should be attainable.

Currently, synthetic epikeratoplasty lenticules are under study by at least two major ophthalmic companies. Although epithelialization over synthetic surfaces and an optical surface of the desired quality have yet to be obtained, recent advances in human tissue onlay procedures apply to this new technology. The significant expense inherent in tissue onlay procedures could be avoided if synthetic materials were biologically compatible and provide excellent visual function.

Moderate Hyperopia Epikeratoplasty

Although AMO, the major distributor of epikeratoplasty tissue, commenced a trial of epikeratoplasty for aphakia, it never did so for moderate to severe hyperopia (+4.00 D to +12.00 D). These hyperopic patients are not suitable candidates for hyperopic keratotomy, just as some myopes of similar severity are not suitable for radial keratotomy. Hyperopes have a strong desire for help since they are usually poor contact lens candi-

Table 28.18
Refractive Myopic Keratoplasty: Rate of Lenticule Replacement

Refractive Myopic Epikeratoplasty	Number of Cases	Number of Replaced Myopic Epilenticules
Old method (with keratectomy)	6	4
New method (larger diameter)	5	1
Non-keratectomy (NKE)	11	1
Total	22	6

22 cases of refractive myopic epikeratoplasty;
6 lenticules replaced
6/22 = 27%

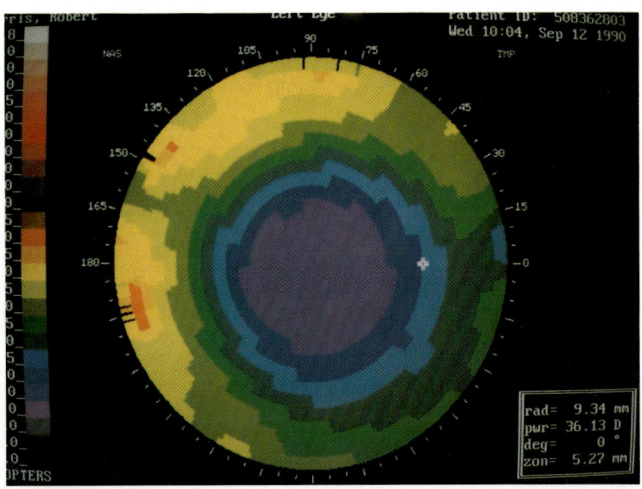

Figure 28.19 *EyeSys topographical analysis of myopic epikeratoplasty five years postoperatively. The preoperative spherical equivalent was –12.00 D and the postoperative spherical equivalent is +1.00 D.*

dates and have reduced visual acuity at distance as well as near. In response, several surgeons capable of producing NET donors use epikeratoplasty for their patients (Fig. 28.21).

Irregular astigmatism is not a major problem in hyperopic epikeratoplasty, probably because of the match between the convexity of donor and recipient. Radial keratotomy and astigmatic keratotomy have been used to modify and improve the results following hyperopic and myopic epikeratoplasty (Fig. 28.22). Contrary to original expectations, epikeratoplasty is most effectively used to treat moderate to severe hyperopia and mild keratoconus rather than myopia and aphakia.

Plano Epikeratoplasty

In addition to keratoconus, plano epikeratoplasty has been useful for patients who are significantly hyperopic or have reduced visual function from pronounced scarring and irregular astigmatism in the visual axis. A plano epikeratoplasty lenticule corrects hyperopia following RK by strengthening the paracentral knee of the cornea (Fig. 28.23). As a result of corneal flattening, the central cornea becomes steeper, thereby correcting the hyperopia. Also, epikeratoplasty is a form of lamellar corneal transplant that effectively transfers the radial keratotomy incisions into the midstroma of the cornea, reducing their effect on corneal optical function (Fig. 28.24).

Conclusion

Although the initial enthusiasm for epikeratoplasty as a refractive procedure has waned, its use as a therapeutic device has added significantly to our surgical armamentarium. More than five thousand epikeratoplasty lenticules have been provided by AMO during the past six years. Individual surgeons have continued to process their own lenticules. Advancements in tissue processing, newer materials, improved topography analysis, and the availability of wound healing agents and tissue glues may allow epikeratoplasty to become a more viable refractive surgical procedure in the future.

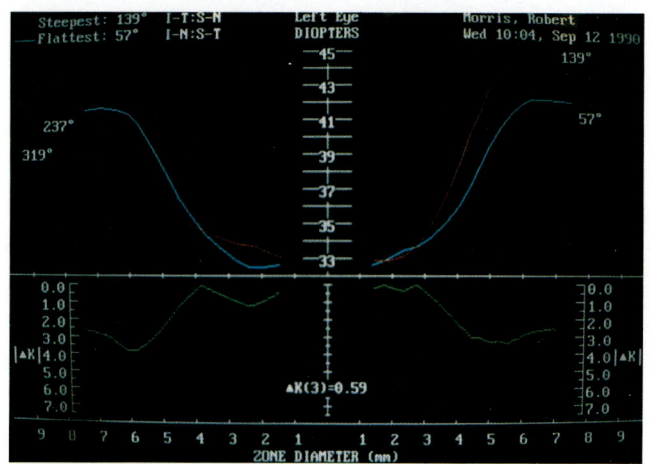

Figure 28.20 *An EyeSys profile analysis of a myopic epikeratoplasty patient demonstrates a functional optical zone of only 2.50 mm despite an optical zone of 6.00 mm created in the donor lenticule by the cryolathe.*

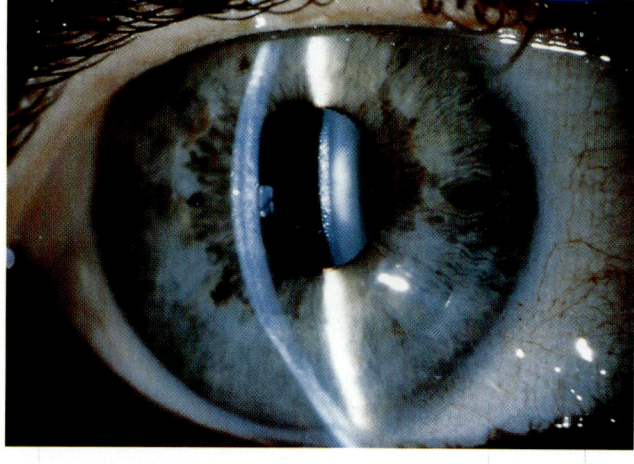

Figure 28.21 *Hyperopic epikeratoplasty. A convex collagen lens has been added to the surface of the central cornea.*

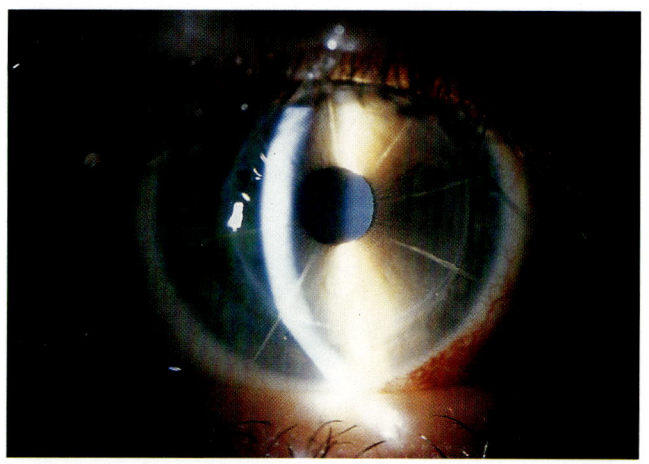

Figure 28.22 *Hyperopic epikeratoplasty with radial keratotomy to correct residual postoperative −1.50 D of myopia.*

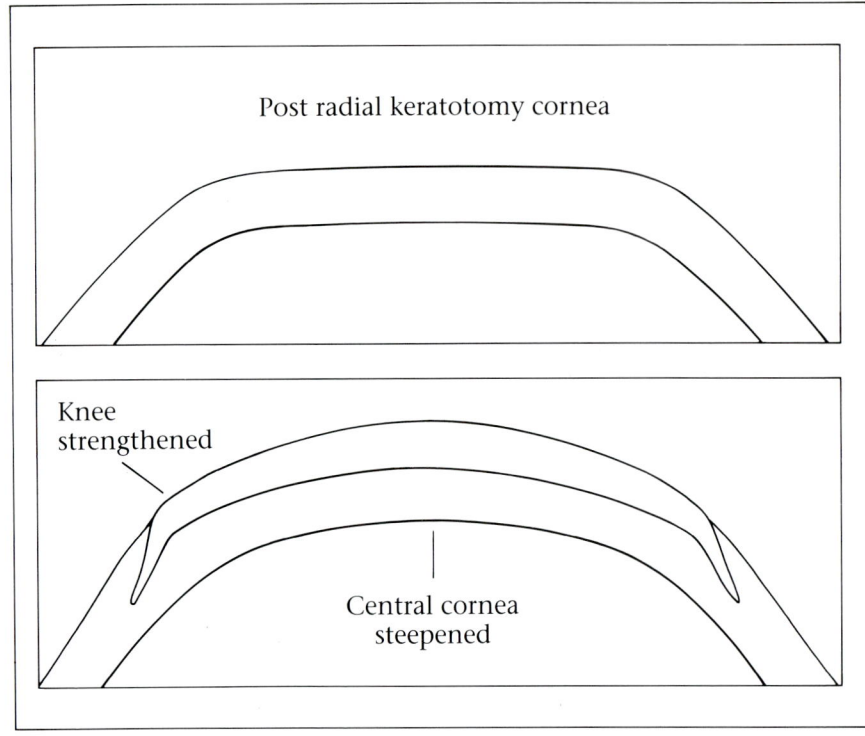
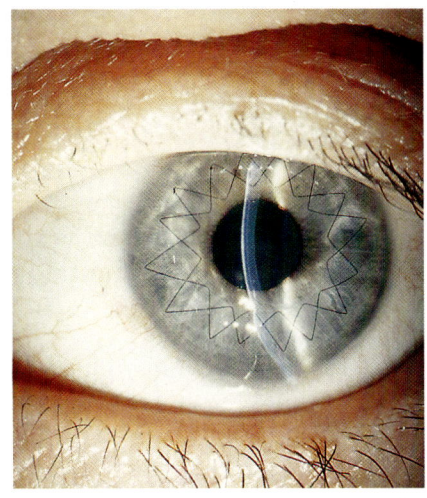

Figure 28.23 **(Left)** *Planar epikeratoplasty strengthens the corneal knee created by radial keratotomy and allows steepening of the central cornea.* **(Right)** *Planar epikeratoplasty to correct overcorrected radial keratotomy two weeks postoperatively.*

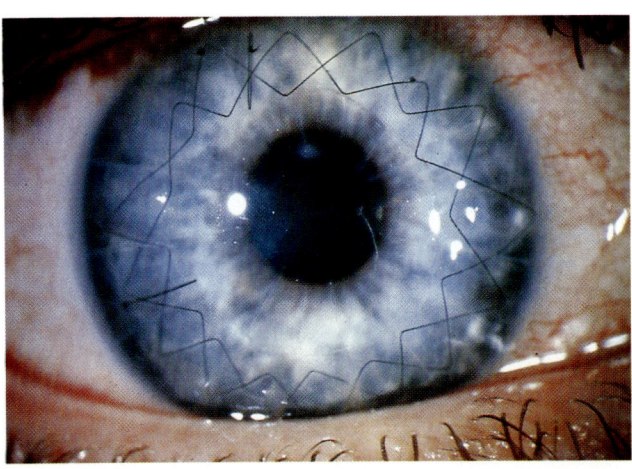
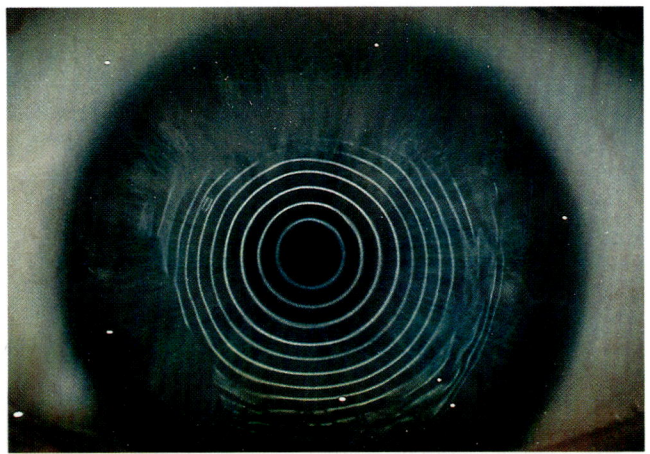

Figure 28.24 **(Left)** *Planar epikeratoplasty to improve overcorrected radial keratotomy. This –5.00 D patient became +3.00 D in one eye after 40 to 50 radial keratotomy incisions were made at two sessions, even though the other eye obtained an excellent result after the same degree of surgery. A 10-0 nylon double running suture was necessary to adequately close the wound. All sutures removed by 12 weeks postoperatively.* **(Right)** *Photokeratoscope study of the patient's cornea two years postoperatively. Uncorrected visual acuity is 20/30 and best spectacle correction yields 20/20 visual acuity.*

Clinical Points to Consider

☛ Epikeratoplasty is a form of lamellar corneal transplantation.

☛ Epikeratoplasty that corrects aphakia, moderate hyperopia, or myopia may be performed with or without a circular keratectomy of the recipient corneal tissue.

☛ Irregular astigmatism is often the limiting factor to good vision following myopic epikeratoplasty.

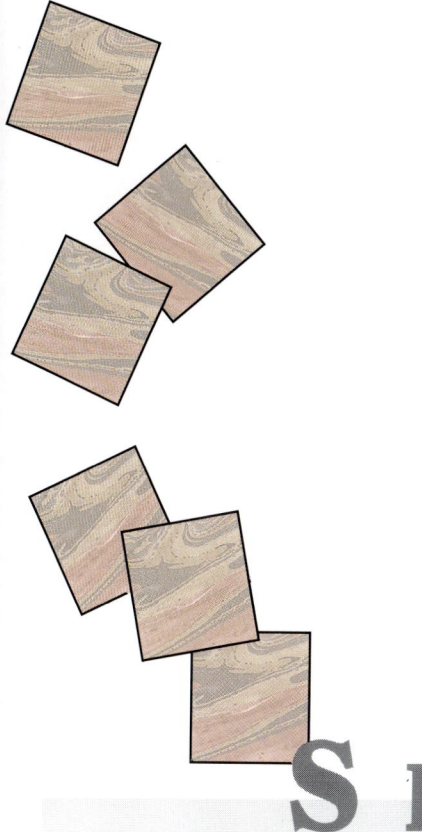

SECTION SIX
SURGERY FOR GLAUCOMA

TRABECULECTOMY

C. ERIC SHRADER, M.D.

I could make a good case for the opinion that one of the reasons why Americans with glaucoma lose their vision is because surgery is not performed soon enough! Were more surgery for glaucoma performed in the United States, patient care would probably be improved.

George Spaeth
Editorial
Ophthalmic Surgery

Glaucoma specialists are familiar with a particular type of patient referred for filtering surgery. The patient has been diagnosed and followed by a competent ophthalmologist for a number of years. Generally, the patient was treated initially with beta blockers and then miotics. Often, carbonic anhydrase inhibitors were tried and discontinued because of side effects. During the treatment's course, serial visual fields were performed, which indicated considerable variation, although if arranged sequentially, inexorable loss of visual field was evident. Eventually laser trabeculoplasty was performed. Despite reasonable intraocular pressure (IOP), usually in the low twenties, fixation was eventually lost in one eye. The referring doctor's letter usually contains a few sentences doubting the patient's compliance with the medical regimen. The referring doctor is usually a good surgeon who, without hesitation, would tackle the most complicated cataract case.

Fortunately, referral practices always bask in the comforting clarity of hindsight. Nevertheless, in a society that expends vast resources on medical care and whose physicians so often are accused of being too willing to operate, it seems odd that when effective surgical treatment is available, patients under the care of good doctors become blind.

Obviously, many ophthalmolgists believe surgical procedures for glaucoma too frequently conclude badly. In comparison with modern cataract surgery, this is certainly the case. After a filtering procedure, vision seldom is improved and frequently is worse. This can be very frustrating to a surgeon who is accustomed to restoring vision for a great majority of patients. Additionally, the glaucoma surgeon, despite excellent technique, can expect more complications than the cataract surgeon. Modern surgical techniques and sutures have all but eliminated flat chambers and hypotony after cataract surgery; many residents complete their entire training without re-forming a chamber and draining choroidal effusions. As always, lack of experience promotes anxiety, and no one enjoys learning about postoperative suprachoroidal hemorrhage on the first trabeculectomy encountered in private practice. Finally, despite the best intentions and surgical skills, often the surgeon is thwarted by fibroblasts postoperatively and watches the IOP increase daily to its preoperative level, if not higher. After one or two significant problems, an IOP of 22 mm Hg in a 20/20 patient begins to look like the lesser of two evils.

History of Filtering Surgery

Over the years, many techniques have evolved that minimize the complications of filtering surgery. The Eliot trephine gave way to the Scheie thermal sclerostomy. Shaffer developed the guarded sclerostomy, the forerunner of the modern trabeculectomy. After the development of ophthalmic microsurgery, nonfiltering approaches to the juxtacanalicular meshwork, such as trabeculotomy and sinusotomy, enjoyed brief fashion. With time it became clear that less aggressive operations resulted in fewer complications but also inadequate IOP control with disease progression. While trabeculectomy has become the most common glaucoma procedure in the world, it is frequently criticized for its inability to adequately control IOP and its late postoperative failure.

For many years, the best solution to these problems was the glaucoma shell developed in Boston by Richard Simmons, M.D., and his mentor Paul Chandler, M.D. The shell allowed the surgeon to perform an aggressive full thickness operation, yet it maintained a formed anterior chamber in the early postoperative period. Properly applied and cared for, the shell was a great advance in the history of glaucoma surgery. Unfortunately, it required a good deal of skill and experience to use it successfully and, even with skill and experience, it was costly in both time and dollars. Hospitalization of at least a week was required. Frequently, rounds were necessary two and three times a day. Improper application resulted in pain and infection. Despite the glaucoma shell's advantages, only Simmons, his associates, and his former students used it regularly.

The next advance in the effort to balance safety and results occurred in 1984. Dunbar Hoskins, M.D., and his Fellow, Carl Migliazzo, M.D., published an article outlining the management of failing filtering blebs. This method called for cutting the sutures in the scleral flap but not disrupting the conjunctiva with the argon laser and a lens of their own design. Simmons and his coworkers recognized the potential of laser suture lysis and developed an operation that began with a trabeculectomy followed by planned early conversion to a full thickness operation using the argon laser to sequentially cut the sutures in the scleral flap. The procedure outlined in this chapter is based on the operation described by Simmons and Savage but modified in order to simplify the dissection for the general ophthalmologist and minimize the potential for complications. With experience it can be done safely without hospitalization, making it cost effective despite the added expense of argon laser suture lysis.

Preoperative Considerations

The preoperative preparation of the glaucoma patient differs significantly from the cataract patient. Glaucoma patients tend to have a much higher anxiety level than cataract patients because they have lived with the threat of blindness for many months. They are having surgery only because less risky treatment has failed to halt the progress of their disease. Fortunately, the patient and surgeon have had to time to develop a trusting relationship. Before undergoing surgery, the patient should understand the nature of filtering surgery; that is, the operation is only the beginning, and the postoperative management is critical to the success of the operation. The rationale for inactivity, laser suture lysis, and digital pressure should be explained prior to the procedure so that postoperative modifications are not unexpected.

Preoperatively, the patient's medical regimen should be modified. Subconjunctival hemorrhage, an esthetic annoyance in most eye surgery, is a major contributor to the failure of glaucoma filtering operations. Aspirin, Coumadin, and other anticoagulants should be discontinued if possible. Topical epinephrine and dipivefrin (Propine) should be discontinued two weeks prior to surgery if possible. Topical steroids and prophylactic antibiotics prior to surgery should be considered. Harsh antibiotics that redden the eye (e.g., Garamycin or polymixin/neomycin/bacitracin combinations) should be avoided preperatively and postoperatively. Preoperative use of miotics on the day of surgery protects the crystalline lens and results in a more peripheral iridectomy.

Surgical Procedure

Preliminary Steps

Prepping and draping are identical to cataract surgery. Although a Jaffe speculum has certain advantages—in particular, it enables temporal access and does not cause external globe pressure—it is not necessary.

Adequate fixation is essential. I prefer a superior rectus bridal suture despite the risk of subconjunctival hemorrhage. Corneal fixation sutures, however, never result in subconjunctival hemorrhage. They can be placed on any axis so filtering surgery can be performed in any quadrant, which is useful in complicated cases where the most accessible surgical sites are scarred. Unfortunately, after the eye is decompressed, fixation sutures distort the globe, especially if tortional traction is necessary. This is troublesome in aphakic eyes, which have less structural stability and a higher risk of suprachoroidal hemorrhage.

After fixation but before the eye is opened, a beveled paracentesis incision is created. Paracentesis is necessary to the successful outcome of a filtering operation, and it is difficult to perform after the eye is opened; thus, it should be performed routinely before any other step (and not forgotten until it is time to refill the anterior chamber after the block of trabecular meshwork has been excised). The ideal instrument for this incision is a ruby knife with a puncture tip (Keeler 2744K1997). Other blades can be used, although it may be difficult to place a cannula in a flat anterior chamber if the paracentesis incision is tapered or irregular. Immediately after the paracentesis is completed, the anterior chamber should be gently irrigated until the surgeon is satisfied that the paracentesis is patent and easily accessible. Injecting BSS into the corneal stroma results in unsightly, but temporary, problems.

After paracentesis, the surgical site must be selected. Large vessels and scarred conjunctiva must be avoided; otherwise the site is a matter of individual preference. I prefer the supero-nasal quadrant because a temporal approach is then available for cataract extraction, if required. In general, filtering blebs placed nasally in the intrapalpebral fissure are more likely to cause dellen and epithelial defects and interfere with comfort than blebs covered by the superior lid. If subsequent phacoemulsification is planned and significant astigmatism exists, the glaucoma surgeon may wish to avoid the meridian of steepest corneal curvature. This allows the cataract surgeon to achieve the best uncorrected vision following cataract extraction by minimizing postoperative astigmatism.

Conjunctival Flap

Dissection of the conjunctival flap is the most critical step in the filtering operation for glaucoma. This fragile membrane must be meticulously handled; it should be grasped gingerly with toothless forceps (e.g., Gill curved iris forceps, Storz E-1475) only and manipulation should be minimal. If, as I suggest, a fornix-based flap is used, it should not be touched until after it is sutured in place. Great care should be taken not to cauterize the conjunctiva inadvertently (Figs. 29.1 and 29.2).

Arguments rage among glaucoma surgeons regarding a limbal-based flap versus a fornix-based flap for filtering surgery. As with most controversies in medicine, both approaches have important benefits as well as distinct disadvantages. The fornix-based flap will never be as watertight as the limbal flap. In fact, because the incision is close to the sclerostomy or sclerectomy and the flow in full thickness procedures is so high, the conjunctival incision may never seal. It is disconcerting, in the first few days following surgery, to watch aqueous stream down the cornea while the conjunctival flap rests against the scleral flap. If either a full thickness procedure or postoperative 5-flourouracil (5-FU) is used, the leak may persist indefinitely. Under these circumstances, the fornix-based flap should be avoided. For an initial trabeculectomy with laser suture lysis, however, the fornix-based flap offers significant advantages, the most important of which is the lessened amount of dissection. This results in shorter operating time and less postoperative inflammation. Additionally, hemostasis is easier to achieve at the operative

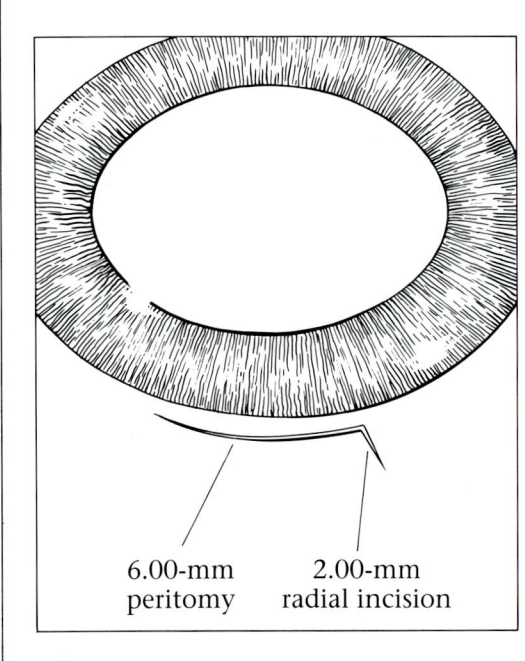
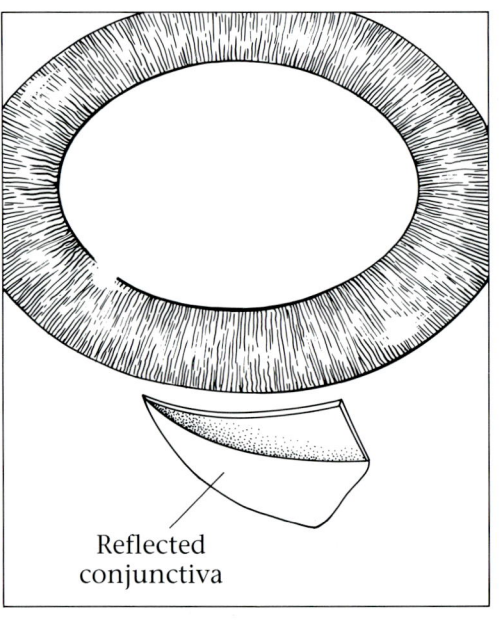

Figure 29.1 (Top and bottom) *Conjunctival incisions, one radial and one circumferential, are used to create the conjunctival flap.*

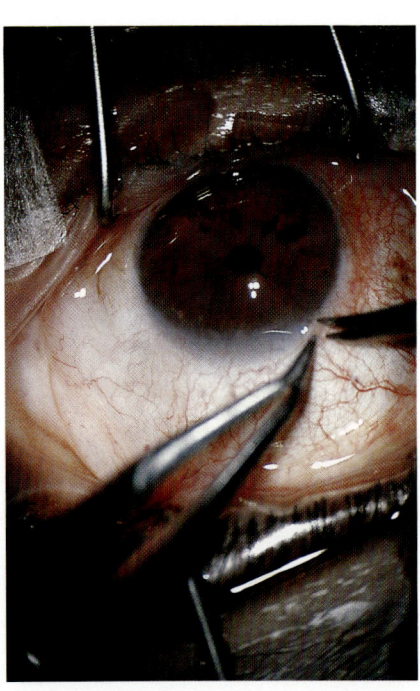

site without accidentally cauterizing the conjunctiva, button holes virtually never occur, exposure is better, and, in my experience, hypotony and chamber shallowing are less frequent.

A curved, blunt Vannas scissor is used for conjunctival dissection. A 2.00-mm radial incision is made in the conjunctiva just lateral to the planned scleral flap site, and a limbal incision is then extended from the radial incision to just past the anticipated superior border of the scleral flap. The apex of the conjunctival triangle is then grasped with Chandler forceps and reflected back on its base using the blunt Vannas scissors to release any subconjunctival attachments. Relaxing cuts are then made in the subconjunctival tissue peripheral to the triangle until adequate exposure for the scleral flap dissection is achieved. Hemostasis should be maintained meticulously throughout the conjunctival dissection. The Simmons-Savage monopolar diathermy is the preferred instrument for hemostasis. A wetfield cautery may be used, but it results in more tissue shrinkage, which leads to unwanted gaping at the edges of the scleral flap. Inadvertent damage to the conjunctival flap is also more common with the larger wetfield forceps.

Scleral Flap

When hemostasis has been achieved, the scleral flap is begun. I prefer a trapezoidal flap because it is easier to dissect than a square flap, yet it seals much better than a triangular flap (Fig. 29.3). Very anterior blebs, which interfere with tear lubrication and dissect into clear cornea, are also more common with a triangular flap.

The scleral flap is outlined with a razor blade chip. A diamond knife can be used, but I find it easier to control the depth with a slightly duller blade. The outlining incisions should be at least half thickness. More catastrophic problems occur if the flap is too thin rather than too thick, as any surgeon who has watched an assistant accidentally tear off a flap can testify. The dissection of the flap should be carried into clear cornea. In nearly every case it should be possible to see iris details through the anterior base of the scleral flap. If the iris is visible, the surgeon can be confident the sclerectomy will be anterior to the ciliary body and the chances of severe intraoperative bleeding and postoperative hyphema will be minimized. Care should be taken to identify the iris in order to avoid incising the ciliary body. The color of the two structures may be similar, but the texture of the ciliary body's surface is much more uniform—it does not have the iris's crypts and color variations. Because the excised tissue is anterior to the trabecular meshwork, this procedure is not truly a trabeculectomy, but it is far safer than working more posteriorly.

Sclerectomy

While an assistant elevates the scleral flap, the sclerectomy is performed using a diamond knife. The two radial stab incisions should be made and connected anteriorly. The rectangular keratectomy flap is then grasped with toothed forceps and excised at the base using angled Vannas scissors (Figs. 29.4 and 29.5). Without delay, a broad but very peripheral iridectomy should be made with-

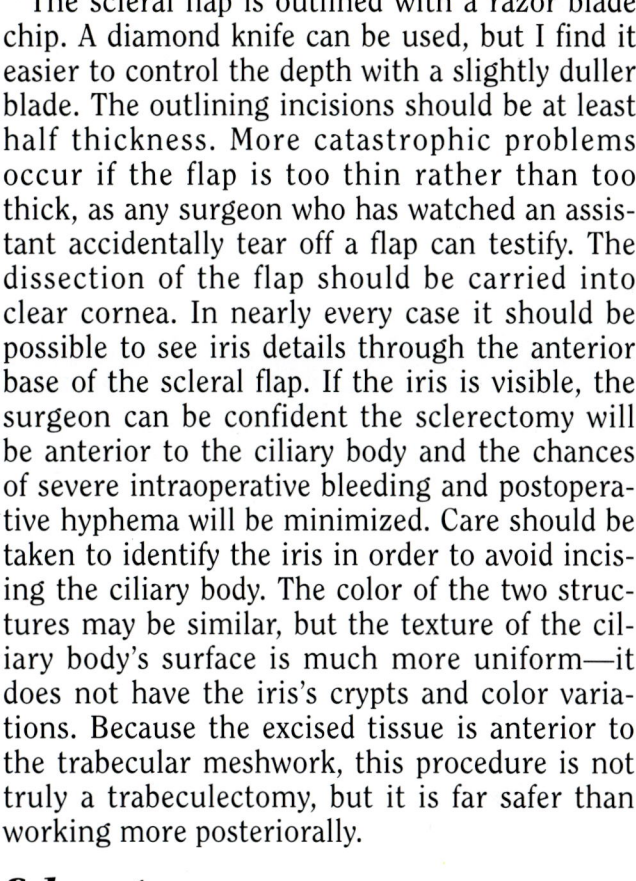

Figure 29.2 Excellent exposure to the proposed surgical site is obtained after dissection of subconjunctival tissue and reflection of the conjunctival flap.

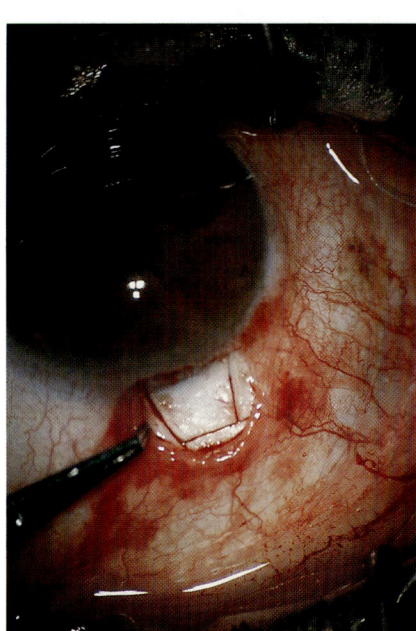

Figure 29.3 A trapezoidal, partial thickness scleral flap is fashioned.

out changing instruments. The anterior chamber is then irrigated through the paracentesis incision, washing any blood at the sclerectomy site to the exterior of the eye.

The scleral flap is then closed with two snug sutures of black 10-0 nylon at the posterior corners of the trapezoid (Fig. 29.6). Other colors or finer grades are much more difficult to sever with argon laser light. The sutures should be equally tight so as not to gape the opposite edge of the flap. The anterior chamber is then formed with BSS. At normal IOP levels, the chamber should remain formed and no fluid should leak at the edges of the scleral flap. Weck-cel pressure on the exterior edge of the flap can help judge the amount of flow or, if there is no flow, confirm the patency of the keratectomy. If there is a tendency for the chamber to shallow, additional sutures should be placed on the lateral edges of the flap. To achieve a stable chamber, two sutures are usually enough, more than four sutures is seldom necessary, and more than five sutures should never be necessary.

Flap Closure

The conjunctiva is then gently replaced in its original position with Chandler forceps. Occasionally, traction must be placed on the conjunctiva because of chemosis, shrinkage, or hemorrhage, and it will not lie loosely in its original position. If this occurs, any adhesions should be lysed with blunt dissection. The conjunctival

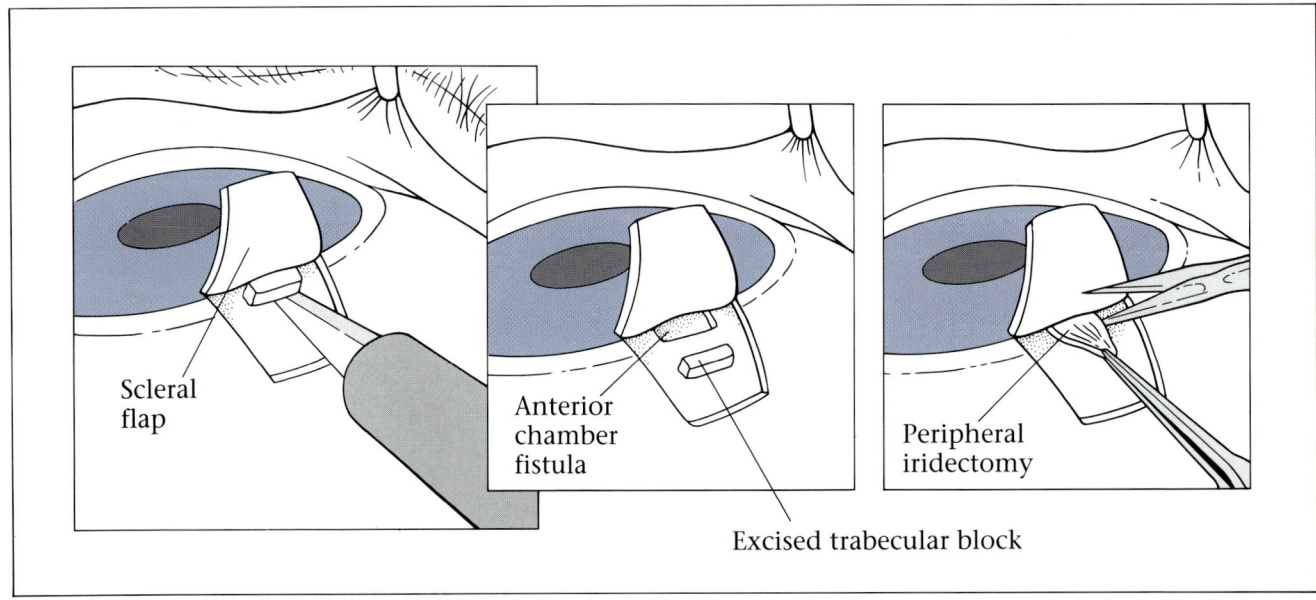

Figure 29.4 *Excision of a rectangular block of trabecular meshwork from beneath the scleral flap followed by a peripheral iridectomy. The silk superior rectus suture may be employed as necessary to orient the globe for better exposure or released, if possible, to minimize IOP during the intraocular portion of the procedure.*

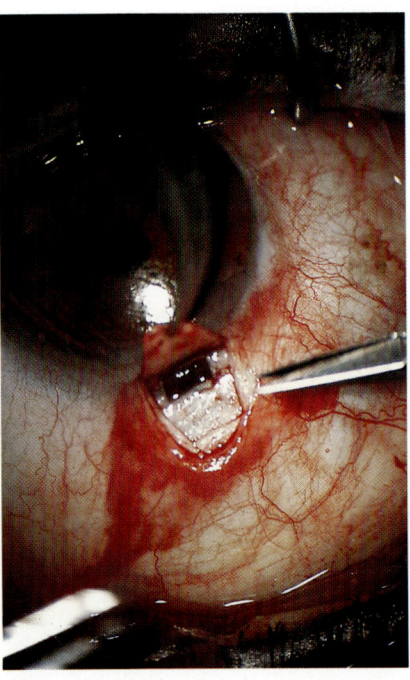

Figure 29.5 *The scleral flap is retracted to expose the trabeculectomy created by excision of the trabecular block.*

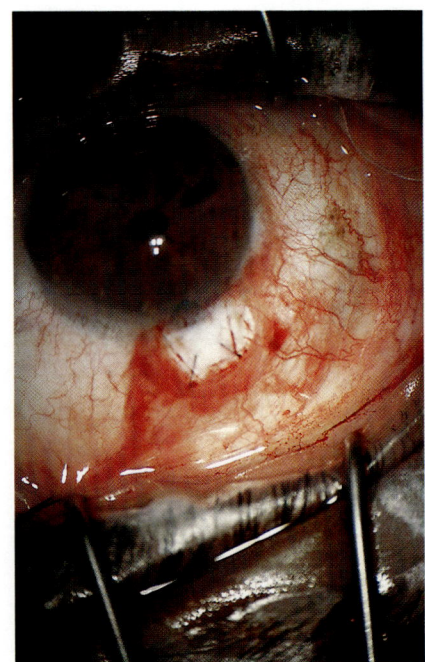

Figure 29.6 *The scleral flap is secured in place by two 10-0 nylon sutures. Postoperatively, the 10-0 nylon sutures will be lysed with the argon laser to allow aqueous to flow through the trabeculectomy site.*

flap should return easily to its original position. Using sutures that place the conjunctiva under tension will lead to "cheese-wiring" with leaking and suture failure.

The initial suture is an interrupted horizontal mattress suture placed at the limbal corner of the triangular flap (Figs. 29.7 and 29.8). It is important that the tension vector of the suture be more tangential than radial. The other end of the conjunctival-limbal incision is then closed with an identical suture (Figs. 29.9 and 29.10). The radial relaxing incision is also closed. Usually, a single interrupted or horizontal mattress suture is used. Again, 10-0 nylon suture seems to create the best balance of comfort and strength and cause minimal reactivity and cheesewiring.

The anterior chamber is filled with BSS. The bleb will probably elevate 1.00 mm to 2.00 mm before a leak develops at the limbus. The easiest way to visualize this is by placing a drop or two of

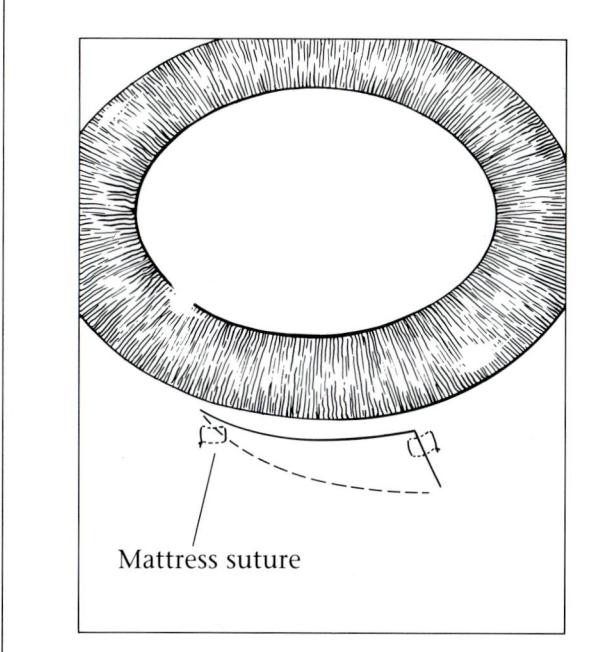

Figure 29.7 *The conjunctival flap is closed by 10-0 nylon mattress sutures anchored at the limbus. The circumferential forces of the mattress sutures are very effective in closing the conjunctival flap.*

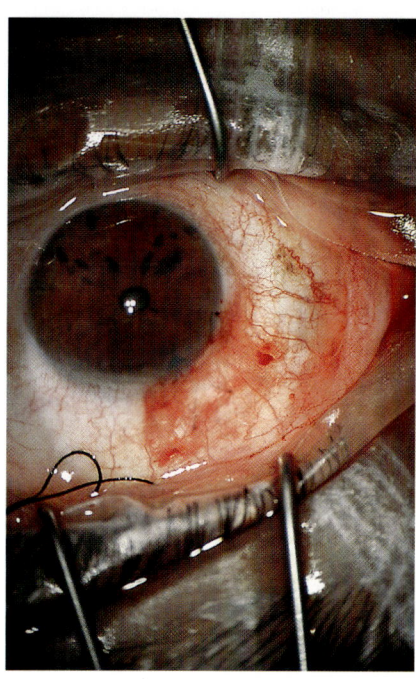

Figure 29.8 *Notice that excellent apposition of the conjunctiva and the limbus is achieved when the radial conjunctival incision is closed with only one mattress suture.*

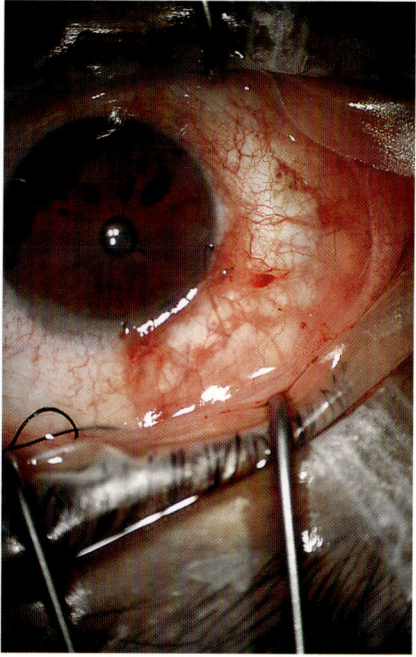

Figure 29.9 *A second mattress suture is added to further close the conjunctival flap. Individual sutures may be used, as necessary, to further close the conjunctiva.*

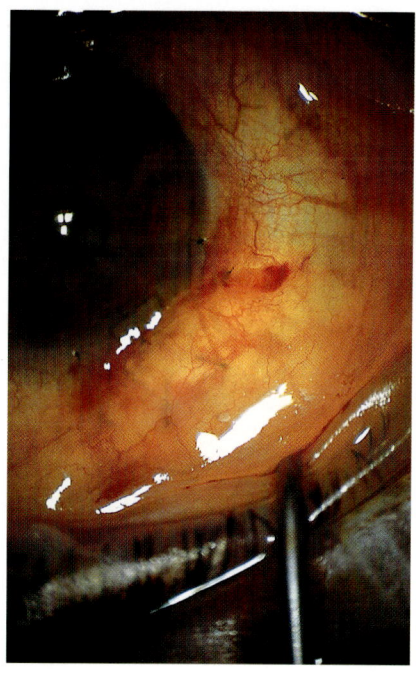

Figure 29.10 *5-FU has been injected under the conjunctival bleb and a third mattress suture has been added at the limbus to further secure the bleb.*

2% flourescein on the cornea. Additional mattress sutures can be placed at the limbus if necessary. Although it is possible to obtain a watertight closure with more sutures, this leads to more late failures in my experience. If there is still a leak ten to 14 days after surgery, another suture can be placed at that time under topical anesthesia.

At the end of the procedure, a drop of phenylephrine HCL 10%, scopolamine HBr 0.3%, and unpreserved Chloromycetin is placed on the cornea. Celestone (1 cc) is injected through the lower fornix into the sub-Tenon's space. After the speculum and the drapes are removed, the eye is inspected under the microscope to be certain the chamber is still formed. A pad and shield are placed over the eye using only enough pressure to keep the lids closed.

Postoperative Care

The surgeon's primary postoperative concern is the management of aqueous flow outward through the scleral flap. Insufficient flow causes elevated pressure, pain, and inflammation. More ominously, there is frequently apposition of the conjunctival and scleral flaps, resulting in adhesions, scarring, and bleb failure. Excessive flow results in hypotony, chamber shallowing, choroidal effusion, and accelerated cataract development.

When the scleral flap is closed in the manner described in this chapter, excessive flow is rare. If it does occur, the anterior chamber should be reformed within 48 to 72 hours. The simplest approach is to fill the chamber with a viscoelastic through the already present paracentesis incision. This rarely solves the problem unless the leakage through the scleral defect is minor. The best treatment is application of the Simmons glaucoma shell. This method is far more efficient than pressure patching because the shell vaults the external pressure over the cornea and onto the site of the excessive filtration. If these conservative methods do not solve the problem, surgical reformation with repair of external leaks and drainage of choroidal effusions must be performed.

If the scleral flap is tightly sutured, as described above, there is seldom excessive aqueous runoff. Most likely, the IOP on the first postoperative day will be between 10 mm Hg and 30 mm Hg. If the disc can tolerate the unadjusted pressure, epithelial edema is absent, and the eye is comfortable, further manipulation should be avoided. If the pressure is 30 mm Hg or above and especially if there is epithelial edema and pain, gentle digital massage should be employed. Under direct observation at the slit lamp, the patient should be instructed to rotate the eyes toward the ceiling. The surgeon then applies gentle pressure on the lower lid in a direction that leads to pressure transfer to the lower globe. Typically, the eye slowly softens, resulting in corneal clearing and pain relief.

The anterior chamber should be observed throughout the procedure. It will not shallow unless excessive digital pressure is applied. It is not uncommon for a small stream of blood to emerge from the surgical site when pressure is quickly lowered digitally. Frequently, this method results in tissue separation at the surgical site, and the elevated pressure does not recur. If it does recur, the massage procedure can be repeated in the first few days after surgery. It is preferable to avoid laser suture lysis in the initial 72 hours after surgery because, until the eye has partially recovered from surgical trauma, there is an increased risk of hypotony.

Laser Suture Lysis

Laser suture lysis (argon laser energy to cut black nylon sutures at power settings that do not disrupt the overlying conjunctival flap) and frequent follow-up visits are the keys to success. After the patient is positioned comfortably at the argon laser, topical anesthesia is applied. The patient is instructed to look straight ahead. A Zeiss or Hoskins lens is then held just above the cornea, close enough to the eye so that when the patient is instructed to look down the upper lid is held by the lens edge. Gentle pressure is then applied to blanch the conjunctiva and bring the sutures into sharp focus. If a Zeiss style lens is used, the rim around the concave posterior surface provides an excellent method of visualization and pressure application. Begin with argon laser settings of 300 mW, 100 µ, and .20 seconds. Usually, the suture will immediately divide. If not, increase the power setting. If powers above 800 mW are required, either the conjunctiva is not sufficiently blanched or there is so much fibrosis the procedure is doomed to fail. Sutures can be cut with the Nd:YAG laser but so can the conjunctiva. Because a buttonhole at this point is not desirable, the Q-switched or mode-locked Nd:YAG laser should not be used.

The trick is deciding when to cut the suture. This depends to some extent on the individual patient and the preoperative IOP goal. In a patient with low tension glaucoma, the sutures should be more aggressively cut than in a patient with a healthy disc and a preoperative IOP of 55 mm Hg. In the average patient with chronic open angle glaucoma and moderate field loss, one suture should be cut in the first seven to ten days after surgery if the IOP is over 10 mm Hg and there is no positive Seidel test. This will result in better long-term IOP control despite an adequate IOP at the time of laser suture lysis. In patients with IOPs over the desired goal, sutures should be cut until the desired goal is achieved. It is important to titrate suture lysis. After each suture is cut, the eye should be observed at the slit lamp and digital IOP applied if the IOP is still elevated and the bleb is not formed. If no change occurs after this maneuver, another suture can be cut. The patient should be observed daily during the suture lysis process.

If the IOP is consistently above the preoperative goal despite serial suture cutting, the patient should be taught how to apply digital pressure and instructed to use it at home four to six times a day. While the patient is learning, the eye should be observed and the IOP measured after each push. Most patients will not push hard enough, although occasionally a vigorous push will cause chamber shallowing and hypotony. If the patient continues to apply pressure several times a day to an eye that has a flat chamber, the results can be disastrous. Long-term digital pressure may be necessary, and it is frequently helpful years after the procedure.

Cataract and Glaucoma

Inevitably, the question of how to manage coexisting cataract and glaucoma arises. The therapeutic choices include trabeculectomy alone, cataract surgery alone, combined surgery, and staged surgery.

For the patient with mild disease, cataract surgery alone is frequently the best choice. If the rim of the optic nerve is intact and the visual field is full, the IOP may be controlled with single drug beta-blocker therapy. Routine cataract surgery is well tolerated.

For the patient with advanced glaucoma and mild cataract, trabeculectomy alone is the most reasonable approach. Too much is made of the tendency of filtering surgery to accelerate cataract development. If the chamber is not allowed to shallow and inflammation is controlled, most patients with mild to moderate senile cataract will tolerate filtering surgery with little or no progression of their lens opacity.

For the patient with severe cupping and field loss above and below the midline, the lens should be spared if at all possible. Such a patient has already lost at least 90% of the optic nerve and needs IOP control above all else. Combined operations seldom result in permanent, fully functioning filtering blebs and should never be done based on the rationale that the cataract will get worse if a filter is done.

Combined procedures are useful in patients with mild to moderate glaucoma who are marginally controlled or on multiple drug therapy. Although a truly satisfying filtering bleb rarely results, the IOP is usually well controlled during the first few weeks following surgery. If IOP elevations occur, they can be managed with digital pressure and laser suture lysis. This is especially helpful in patients with stable low or normal tension glaucoma who are particularly vulnerable to postoperative pressure spikes. In the long term, the IOP is usually somewhat lower in an eye that has undergone a combined procedure. Topical antiglaucoma medications continue to be required in the vast majority of patients who have undergone combined surgery.

Patients who have visually significant cataract and advanced glaucoma, either uncontrolled or marginally controlled, should have filtering surgery prior to cataract surgery. Occasionally, vision will improve so much following a course of atropine that cataract surgery is not necessary. Usually cataract surgery will need to be done later. A staged approach is no panacea because at least a third of the blebs will fail, but it does work better than combined procedures. Cataract surgery should be delayed at least three months and ideally six months after filtering surgery.

In theory, the smallest incision with the least manipulation of the conjunctiva is the best cataract procedure for the glaucoma patient. However, glaucoma patients tend to come with hard nuclei, posterior synechiae, small pupils, and lower endothelial cell counts. Furthermore, posterior capsular tears, vitreous loss, and anterior chamber lenses are far more troublesome in glaucomatous eyes than in normal eyes. Therefore, only surgeons with significant skill and experience in phacoemulsification should attempt cataract removal by this modality in the glaucomatous eye. The glaucoma patient is much better off with a 10.00-mm incision and an intact capsule than a 4.00-mm incision and capsular tear even if a foldable posterior chamber lens is implanted. Phacoemulsification in glaucomatous eyes should be undertaken only when the surgeon's phacoemulsification technique in difficult eyes is equal to extracapsular technique.

Additional Treatment Possibilities

Argon Laser Trabeculoplasty

Although argon laser trabeculoplasty (ALT) may seem like a fairly recent development, it has been more than a decade since Wise and Witter first described this procedure. During this time, ALT has proven to be a safe and helpful addition to the therapeutic armamentarium for chronic open angle glaucoma (COAG). Complications have largely been eliminated due to modifications, such as application of the laser energy to the anterior portion of the trabecular meshwork and divided treatment sessions. Apraclonidine (Iopidine) has improved the effectiveness of treating post-ALT IOP spikes. Concerns regarding possible long-term problems resulting from laser damage to the cells of the trabecular meshwork have essentially evaporated.

As safety has improved, the indications for ALT have changed. Initially, when maximum surgical therapy failed to control glaucoma, ALT was the last step before filtering surgery. As ophthalmologists have become more comfortable with the safety of ALT, it has replaced medical therapy in selected situations. Certainly, most ophthalmologists would rather perform ALT than subject a frail 85-year-old to Diamox (acetazolamide) or an asthmatic to Timoptic (timolol). In my practice, I have probably caused more misery with Diamox, more life-threatening situations with topical beta-blockers, and more sight-threatening problems with miotics than harm with ALT.

More recently, the results of the Glaucoma Laser Trial seem to suggest that ALT should be the initial therapy for COAG, a concept commonly advertised by the argon laser manufacturers. In my opinion, the data do not support that hypothesis. Rather, the data show that newly diagnosed COAG patients do better if they are initially treated with ALT rather than with topical medications, if both are necessary, because of the severity of their disease. The data do not show that more patients are controlled with ALT than with a single topical medication. However, the study does suggest that ALT is the equivalent of topical medications rather than a more aggressive treatment to be employed only when topical medications fail or are not tolerated.

Although, ALT appears to be an elegant, safe, comfortable, civilized therapy plan for COAG, it often does not lower a patient's IOP adequately. ALT can be very effective in patients with glaucoma associated with pseudoexfoliation and pigmentary glaucoma; it seldom causes dramatic IOP decreases in patients with routine open angle glaucoma, especially in those difficult patients who seem to be losing vision with IOP in the low twenties or high teens. Most unfortunately, ALT almost never works in the really difficult cases of inflammatory or aphakic glaucoma.

Laser Filtering Surgery
EXCIMER LASER
Obviously, ALT has limitations. As evidence mounts that very low IOP is necessary to arrest continued field loss in eyes with significant disc damage, research in filtering procedures, especially those that use lasers to create a filtering fistula, has increased. Summit Technology, which manufactures and markets an excimer laser (ExciMed 200), is currently sponsoring an FDA approved protocol to determine the safety and efficacy of partial excimer trabeculectomy (PET).

PET employs a 193-nm excimer laser to photoablate the outer layers of the trabecular meshwork and the overlying sclera. The innermost layers of the meshwork remain intact because photoablation of this tissue ceases when aqueous humor percolates into the surgical site. The proponents of PET hope that a clinical study will show that IOP is controlled with fewer complications due to maintenance of the innermost layers of the trabecular meshwork than with a standard filtering procedure employing a full thickness sclerotomy. One disadvatage of PET is that a standard conjunctival flap must be dissected, which necessitates a complete procedure at a surgical facility.

HOLMIUM LASER
Another filtering laser under clinical trial is the gLASE 210 holmium laser system. This laser uses a longer wavelength than excimer to photoablate an external, full thickness sclerostomy. The laser energy is delivered through a 26-gauge fiber-optic probe that can be inserted subconjunctivally through a conjunctival puncture wound. This capability obviates the need for the surgical creation of a conjunctival flap and, potentially, allows this procedure to be performed routinely in the office.

As experience with holmium filtering procedures accumulates, it will become clear if long-term success equals or betters conventional filtering surgery, if the absence of a peripheral iridectomy is a problem, and if the rate of flat chamber is acceptable with this new variation of filtering surgery.

Wound Healing Inhibition
Hopefully, laser techniques will make filtering surgery safer and simpler. However, filtering surgery often fails because of cellular response to injury. This response may be minimized using lasers instead of knives, but it will not be eliminated. Pharmacologic manipulation of wound healing holds the greatest promise of improving our success rate in routine and difficult cases.

A tremendous addition to the postoperative management of filtering surgery has been 5-FU. It is probably the greatest treatment method since topical steroids were introduced. However, 5-FU is uncomfortable for the patient and inconvenient to deliver. Corneal complications occur frequently, although they are usually self-limiting. Better delivery systems for newer antimetabolites and biologic agents should increase our ability to keep filtering fistulas open, whether or not we create them with lasers or trephines.

Shunts

When filtering surgery with adjunctive 5-FU fails, the only options remaining are shunts and cyclodestructive procedures. Since the majority of eyes that undergo cyclocryotherapy are doomed to severe sight-threatening complications, shunts make the most sense for eyes with central vision. Early hypotony, with its attendant complications of intraocular hemorrhage and choroidal effusion, has been noted frequently during the initial studies of shunt use.

Early glaucoma shunts functioned by transporting aqueous from the anterior chamber to a reservoir from which the aqueous percolated into the sub-Tenon's space. Some newer designs have replaced the reservoir with a plate (or band) that creates a sub-Tenon's space for the aqueous transported by the shunt tube from the anterior chamber. The plate has no reservoir capability and does not collect aqueous.

A variety of glaucoma shunts have been developed, each with its own potential advantages and disadvantages.

White Shunt. The White shunt has a reservoir that occupies two quadrants of the globe under Tenon's capsule behind the rectus muscle insertions and a flutter valve that controls the flow of aqueous from the anterior chamber to the reservoir. If the IOP remains low, however, this flutter valve may seal, rendering the shunt inoperable. Also, Tenon's capsule may occlude the aqueous release ports of the reservoir.

Shocket and Joseph Shunts. These shunts are essentially silicone tubes that encircle the globe under Tenon's capsule incorporating a shunt that leads into the anterior chamber. These tubes are intended to create a sub-Tenon's space for the aqueous, which is transported by the shunt from the anterior chamber. Implantation necessitates surgical exposure in all four quadrants.

Krupin Shunt. The Krupin shunt employs a slit valve to control aqueous flow. Time will tell whether this type of valve is susceptable to occlusion in the presence of prolonged low IOP with minimal aqueous flow.

Molteno Shunt. The Molteno shunt has a narrow shunt tube that controls aqueous flow by capillary action. The rather hard plate is made of polypropylene and has a tendency to extrude from beneath Tenon's capsule with time. The plate forms a sub-Tenon's space for the aqueous.

Baerveldt Shunt. The Baerveldt shunt, constructed entirely of silicone, is essentially a modification of the Molteno shunt. The soft pliable plate is available in several sizes to create blebs of different dimensions depending on preoperative IOP and other pre-existing pathology (i.e., retinal detachment). These plates can be implanted under Tenon's capsule in only one quadrant, and the control of aqueous flow by capillary action rather than a flow valve make this shunt worthy of further trial (Figs. 29.11 to 29.14).

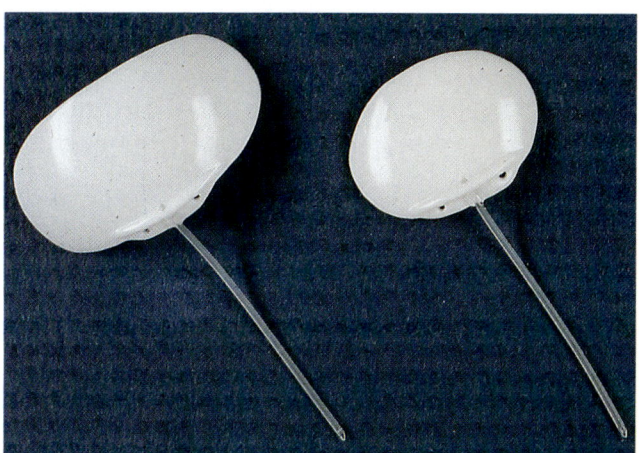

Figure 29.11 *The Baerveldt glaucoma shunt, with two different sized plates.*

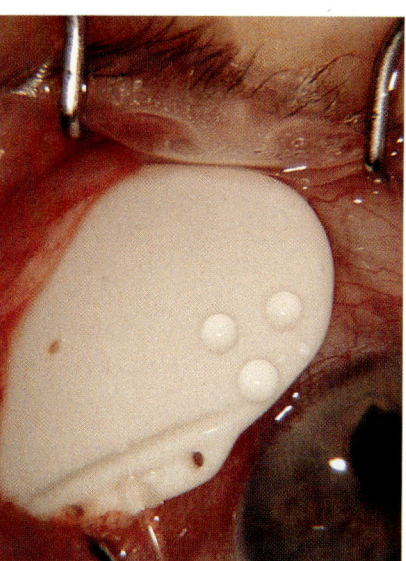

Figure 29.12 *The plate of the Baerveldt glaucoma shunt being inserted beneath Tenon's capsule.*

Conclusion

Measuring success in filtering surgery is more complex than counting attached retinas or clear grafts. Most publications consider an IOP of 22 mm Hg, even with topical glaucoma medications, a success. Others consider the operation a failure unless progression of the disease is arrested. In private practice, most ophthalmologists hope to achieve an appropriate IOP level and avoid surgical complications, thus limiting further loss of visual field and acuity. The technique described in this chapter is designed to achieve these goals.

The necessary elements are few: a fornix-based flap that is dissected easily in minimal time with minimal trauma, meticulous hemostasis with underwater diathermy, a trapezoidal scleral flap of adequate thickness to achieve a good seal and posterior flow, an anterior sclerectomy to minimize bleeding, and laser suture lysis with supplementary digital pressure to titrate aqueous flow. With these techniques and careful postoperative follow-up, success with glaucoma surgery can be achieved at a rate approximating that of cataract surgery.

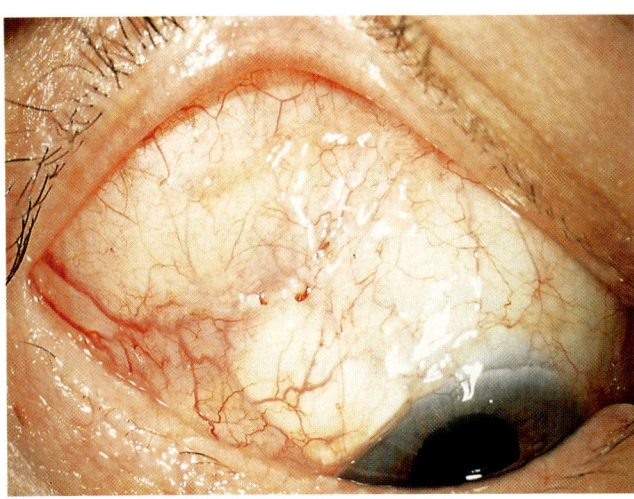

Figure 29.13 *The Baerveldt glaucoma shunt covered by Tenon's capsule and conjunctiva after implantation.*

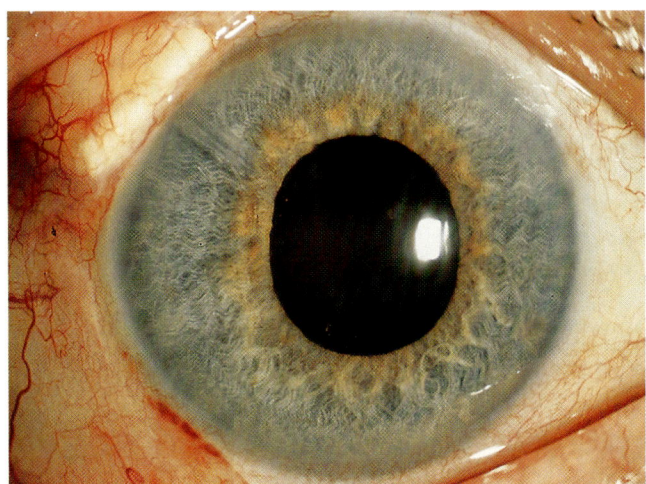

Figure 29.14 *The shunt tube of the Baerveldt glaucoma shunt is visible entering the anterior chamber at 10:00 o'clock.*

Clinical Points to Consider

☞ The incidence of complications following trabeculectomy is much higher than for cataract/IOL surgery, but a filtering procedure may be the only method of saving a patient's vision.

☞ The long term-success of a filtering procedure probably depends less on the method of creating the sclerectomy than on maintaining a patent scleral flap.

☞ Glaucoma shunts may be used in desperate cases, but infection, extrusion, and blockage remain areas of critical concern and investigation.

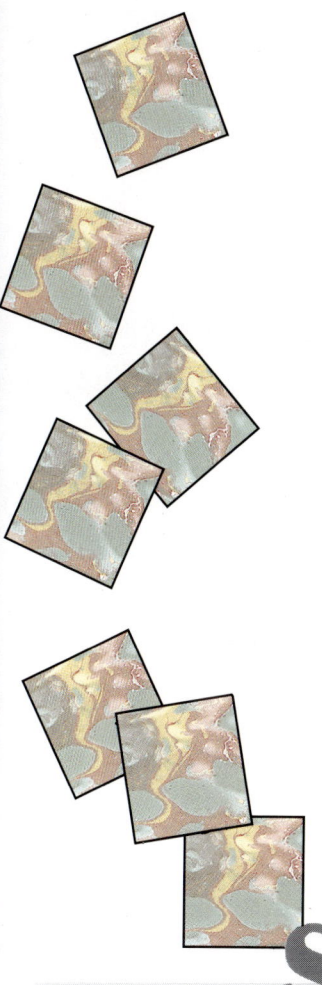

SECTION SEVEN
SURGERY FOR PTERYGIUM

PTERYGIUM EXCISION

LEE T. NORDAN, M.D.

Pterygium is a common ocular affliction that is usually correctable by surgical excision. Although environmental factors such as wind and sun are thought to cause this condition—the severest occurrences and recurrences are found in the sun-rich portions of the world—genetic predisposition also seems to be an important factor. Measuring and documenting the exact influence of these factors, however, is difficult because socioeconomic factors, for example, affect the speed with which an individual seeks medical attention and, consequently, the stage at which the condition is diagnosed. Furthermore, although one might think that a disease process exacerbated by sun and wind would be more prevalent in the left eye (which is exposed to the elements while driving), pterygia most commonly presents bilaterally, with neither eye having a predilection for severity. Recurrent pterygia can lead to visual impairment and necessitate advanced corneal and conjunctival surgery (Fig. 30.1). This chapter will present a plan for dealing with primary and recurrent pterygia.

Pathophysiology

Pterygium is thought to be a reaction to a chronic, low-grade inflammation at the nasal limbus. A similar histologic change is noted in pingueculum formation, which, in essence, is a pterygium that has not yet crossed the limbus to cover the cornea. The extreme predilection for pterygium to occur on the nasal side of the limbus is not known—one would expect greater chronic irritation at the less protected temporal side of the limbus.

A pterygium is a subconjunctival fibrovascular stalk that crosses the limbus and adheres to Bowman's membrane (Fig. 30.2). The pterygium adheres to the corneal surface from the limbus to the tip but does not adhere to the sclera. Recurrent pterygia or traumatic pannus adhere to the corneal surface, although there may be skip areas (i.e., areas of nonadherence) along their course. The larger blood vessels of a pterygium may course from the inferocentral aspect of the inner canthus to the tip of the pterygium, creating a slightly oblique orientation to the conjunctival aspect of the pterygium.

Clinical Significance

A pterygium or its excision may adversely affect vision in several ways:

    1. Occlusion of the visual axis by the pterygium

    2. Irregular astigmatism in the visual axis adjacent to the advancing head of the pterygium

    3. Limitation of duction of the globe by subconjunctival scarring with resultant diplopia after primary resection of the pterygium

    4. Inadvertent disinsertion of the medial rectus muscle or scleral perforation during pterygium excision

    5. Corneal irregularity in the visual axis secondary to deep stromal excision of the pterygium

Differential Diagnosis

The clinical diagnosis of pterygium is relatively straightforward, although the list of lesions in the differential diagnosis is quite extensive and includes papilloma, corneal dermoid, phlyctenule, and squamous cell carcinoma of the conjunctiva. Squamous cell carcinoma of the conjunctiva, like pterygia, has sun exposure as a causative factor (and occurs with equal frequency in both eyes), but it occurs most commonly at the inferotemporal aspect of the limbus and must be differentiated from the rare temporal pterygium that tends to extend horizontally.

Surgical techniques for the primary excision of a pterygium can easily be applied to squamous cell carcinoma. Deep stromal incision is contraindicated. As with a pterygium, excision should be as superficial as possible, leaving Bowman's membrane intact. This lessens the chance of intraocular invasion by the carcinoma, which can spread into the anterior chamber through the limbal vessels but not through an intact Bowman's membrane. (The surgeon should request pathologic confirmation that the conjunctival surgical margins are free of the carcinoma.)

Surgical Planning

Surgical excision of a pterygium is usually contemplated for one of three reasons:

    1. Decrease in vision (a 2.50-mm pterygium may cause a 3.00-mm corneal scar)

    2. Cosmesis (a pterygium may be very noticeable)

    3. Foreign body sensation (secondary to associated dellen) caused by the raised head of the pterygium; contact lens intolerance

Approximately 75% to 85% of pterygia can be cured by primary excision. For recurrent pterygium cases, however, more aggressive surgical techniques must be used. The placement of a conjunctival flap in the area of the excised pterygium is thought to inhibit recurrence because the vertical direction of the blood supply of this flap is perpendicular to the growth of the pterygium. I suggest the following plan:

Primary pterygium excision: bare sclera approach
Recurrent pterygium × 1: pedicle conjunctival graft
Recurrent pterygium × 2: "bucket-handle" conjunctival graft
Recurrent pterygium × 3: localized lamellar corneal transplant with conjunctivoplasty

I do not use radiation and cytotoxic agents, except in rare instances, because a conjunctivoplasty, if

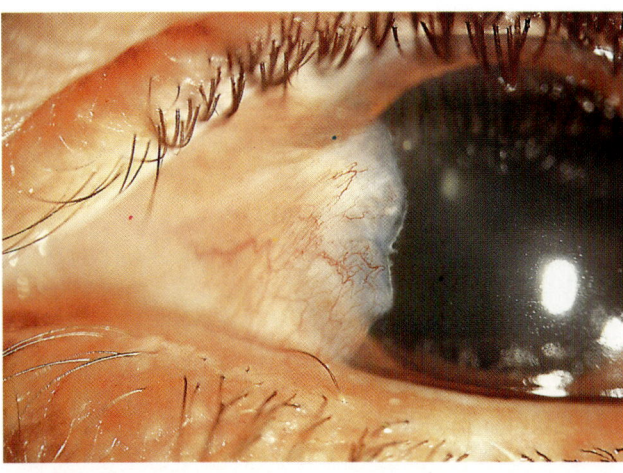

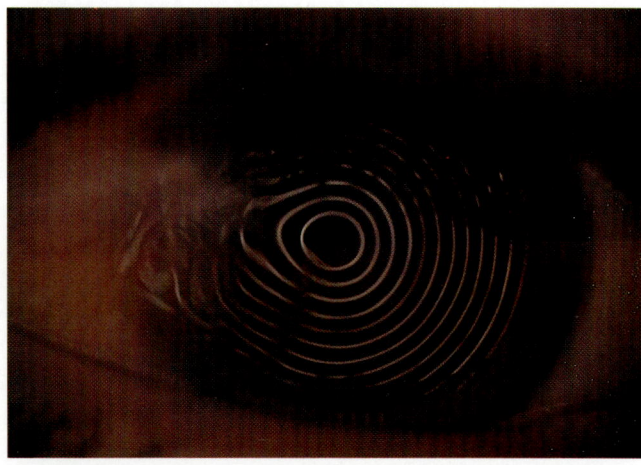

Figure 30.1 (Left) *A primary pterygium that is encroaching on the visual axis.* **(Right)** *Distorted photo-keratoscope mires demonstrate an irregular corneal surface in the visual axis adjacent to the tip of the pterygium.*

necessary afterwards, will be more difficult due to increased conjunctival friability. Also, the true efficacy of these agents is difficult to assess since well-controlled clinical studies are very difficult to design and evaluate.

Special attention should be paid to the limbal area after primary pterygium excision since irregularities in this area are thought to contribute to minor irritation and recurrence. A smooth limbal area is insured by scraping with a blade edge or motorized diamond burr.

After primary pterygium excision, it is best to leave the remaining nasal conjunctiva in its normal anatomic location and bare sclera near the limbus. Attempting to affix this conjunctiva to the limbal edge can limit abduction of the globe and result in diplopia as well as obliteration of the semilunar fold.

Surgical Procedure

Excision of Primary Pterygium

1. Preoperative considerations:
   Pilocarpine 1%
   Anesthesia:
      Topical proparacaine 0.50% and/or tetracaine
      Subconjunctival, peribulbar, or retrobulbar if problem with patient cooperation
      Pupillary occluder
2. Wire lid speculum
3. Instruct patient to look temporally.
4. Perform radial conjunctival incisions of 3.00 mm, starting at the limbus and proceeding nasally, above and below pterygium (Fig. 30.3).

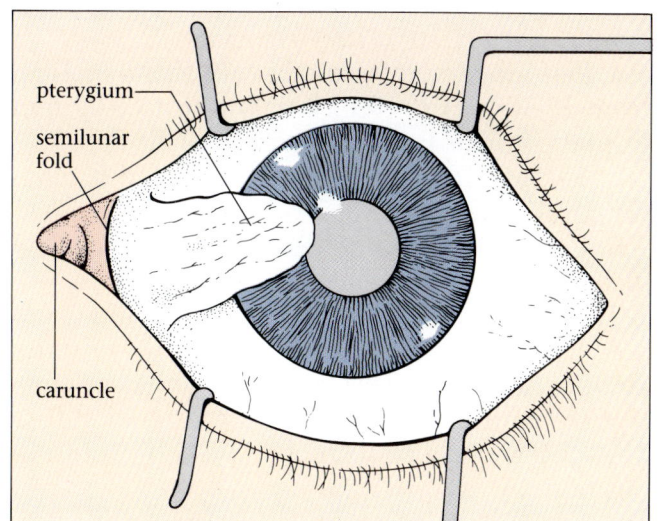

Figure 30.2 *Primary pterygium. The normal semilunar fold and caruncle are normal.*

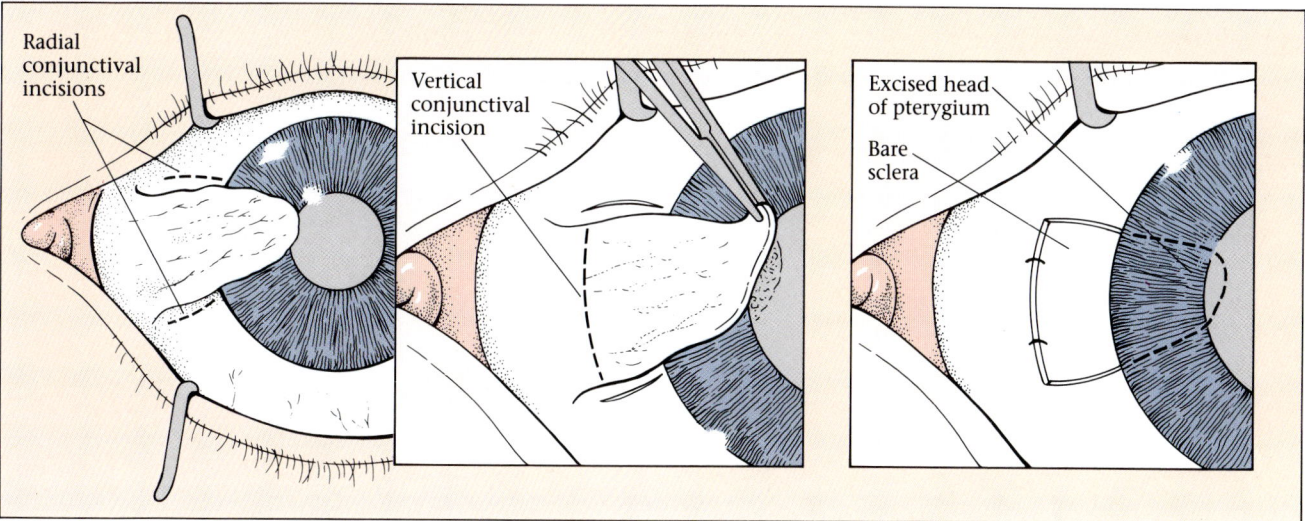

Figure 30.3 *Excision of a primary pterygium using a bare sclera technique.*

5. Sharply dissect head of pterygium toward limbus with No. 69 Beaver blade, Alcon crescent blade, or an equivalent; grasp head of pterygium with Colibri forceps and put it on stretch.

6. Clear nonadherent zone encountered at limbus.

7. Connect nasal aspects of radial conjunctival incisions with vertical conjunctival incision.

8. Control localized bleeding of sclera with wetfield cautery.

9. Suture nasal conjunctival edge to sclera in front of medial rectus muscle.

10. Meticulously smooth limbal region and area from which head of pterygium was excised.

11. Apply antibiotic/cortisone ointment and semipressure dressing.

12. Postoperative treatment: patch until nasal cornea is epithelialized (one to three days, depending on size of excised pterygium).

Excision of Recurrent Pterygium

The various surgical techniques for treating recurrent pterygia include many of the steps already set forth. Therefore, the recurrent pterygia surgery outlines refer to steps in previous outlines.

EXCISION WITH PEDICLE CONJUNCTIVOPLASTY (LEFT EYE)

1. Perform steps 1 to 5 of excision of primary ptergyium.

2. Excise lesion at limbus; allow temporal edge of pterygium to retract nasally, thereby recreating the semilunar fold (Fig. 30.4).

3. Use wetfield cautery as necessary to control bleeding.

4. Scrape nasal cornea, as necessary, with edge of blade to remove residual pterygium from cornea.

5. Perform limbal and corneal smoothing.

6. Perform limbal peritomy and concentric conjunctival incisions, 5.00-mm width, from 10 o'clock to 1 o'clock at the limbus and 11 to 1 o'clock in the conjunctiva.

7. Swing conjunctival flap, which is hinged superonasally (Fig. 30.5).

8. Use 10-0 nylon suture to join conjunctiva at the limbus; use absorbable nylon suture to join conjunctiva to conjunctiva nasally and superiorly and to episclera temporally.

9. Apply semipressure patch with cortisone/antibiotic ointment until cornea is epithelialized.

EXCISION WITH BUCKET-HANDLE CONJUNCTIVOPLASTY (LEFT EYE)

1. Perform steps 1 to 7 of excision of primary pterygium under retrobulbar anesthesia.

2. Remove conjunctiva from 7:30 to 11:30 o'clock.

3. Perform limbal peritomy of remaining limbal conjunctiva (11:30 to 7:30 o'clock).

4. Perform circumferential conjunctival incision from 12:30 to 5:30 o'clock 6.00 mm to 8.00 mm from the limbus to create bucket-handle flap.

5. Remove Tenon's capsule from potential conjunctival flap.

6. Use wetfield cautery as necessary to control bleeding.

7. Slide bucket-handle nasally (Fig. 30.6).

8. Use absorbable suture temporally to unite conjunctiva to episclera, nasally to unite conjunctiva to conjunctiva, and with occasional suture bites that include episclera to hold conjunctiva in position.

9. Use 10-0 nylon suture to secure conjunctiva at the limbus.

10. Apply semipressure patch with cortisone/antibiotic ointment for 48 hours.

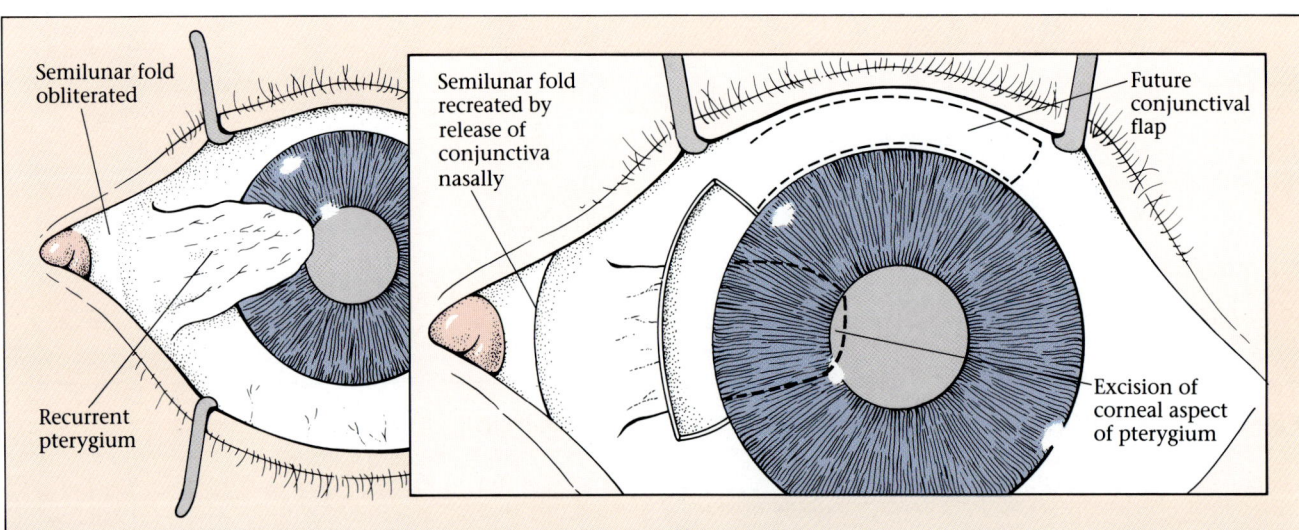

Figure 30.4 *Excision of a recurrent pterygium using a pedicle conjunctivoplasty. The semilunar fold has been recreated by allowing the conjunctiva adherent to the limbus to fall back nasally to its normal anatomic position.*

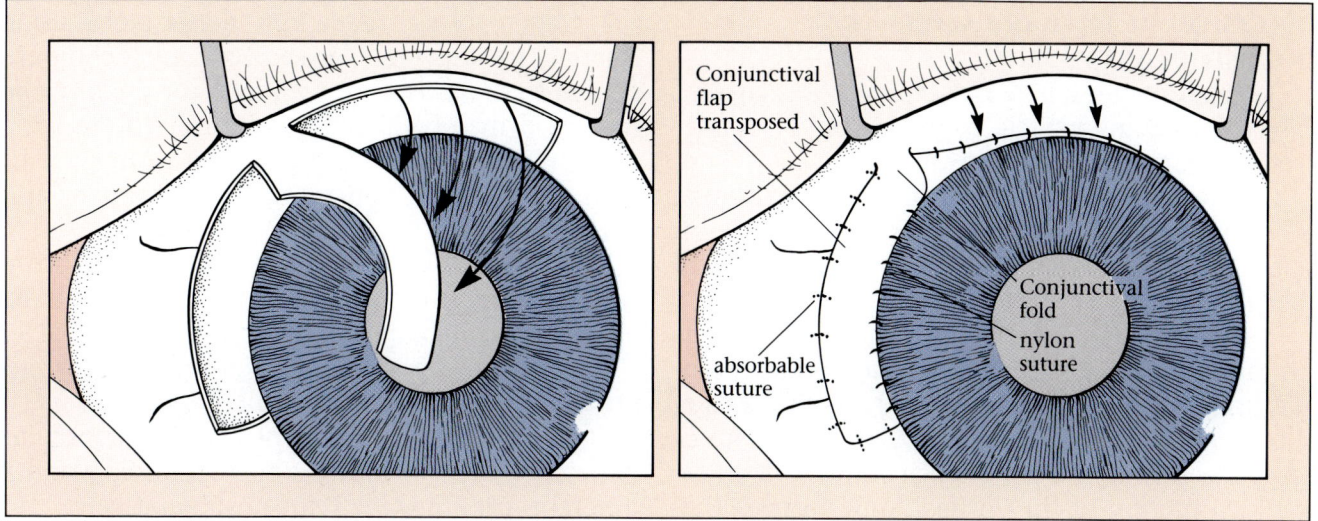

Figure 30.5 *The bare sclera nasal to the limbus has been covered by the conjunctival pedicle, which is hinged under the nasal aspect of the upper lid.*

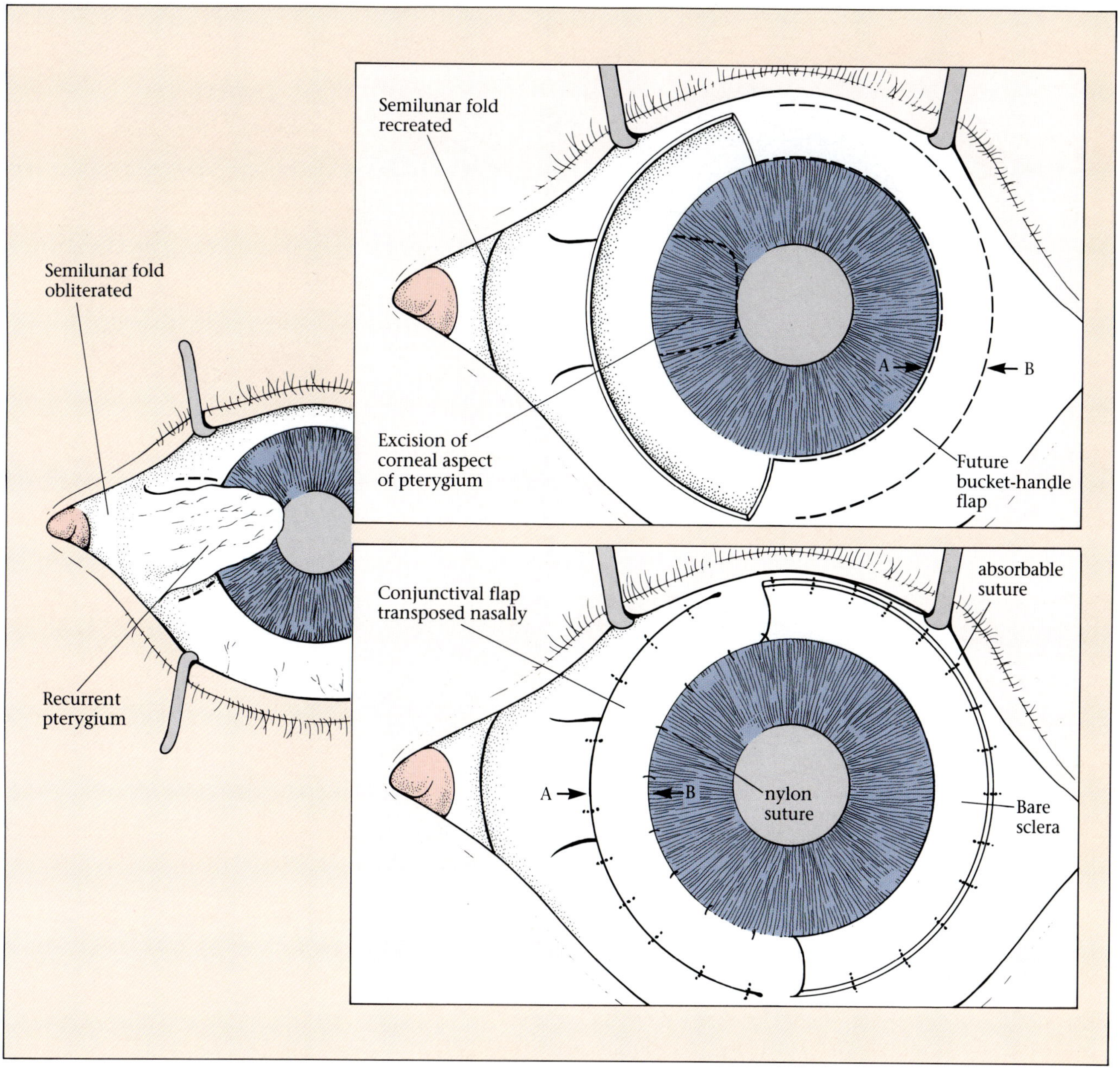

Figure 30.6 *A bucket-handle conjunctivoplasty involves sliding a temporal "bucket handle" of conjunctiva across the cornea and anchoring it in position nasally.*

EXCISION OF LIMBAL LAMELLAR KERATOPLASTY

1. Perform steps 1 to 3 of excision of recurrent pterygium using pedicle conjunctivoplasty under retrobulbar anesthesia (Fig. 30.7).
2. Use corneal trephine of appropriate size (7.00-mm to 9.00-mm diameter) to create semicircular corneolimbal incision to about one-third corneal depth.
3. Begin lamellar keratectomy with a razor blade at the appropriate level of the cornea, then continue using a corneal knife within the boundaries of the trephination, removing the semicircular piece of corneoscleral tissue; a circular rather than a to-and-fro motion of the corneal knife insures that the knife remains in the same corneal plane.
4. Obtain corneal tissue from donor globe, using trephination and lamellar keratectomy techniques similar to those used for recipient; the donor globe may be firmed by injecting air through the optic nerve (which is then clamped) and wrapped with gauze, facilitating control of the slippery scleral surface.
5. Place donor tissue into position and suture with a running 10-0 nylon suture along the curved portion and interrupted sutures at the limbal edge.
6. Perform steps 7 to 9 of excision of recurrent pterygium with pedicle conjunctivoplasty.

Figure 30.7 shows a patient who had a circular lamellar graft two months postoperatively and a different patient three years postoperatively.

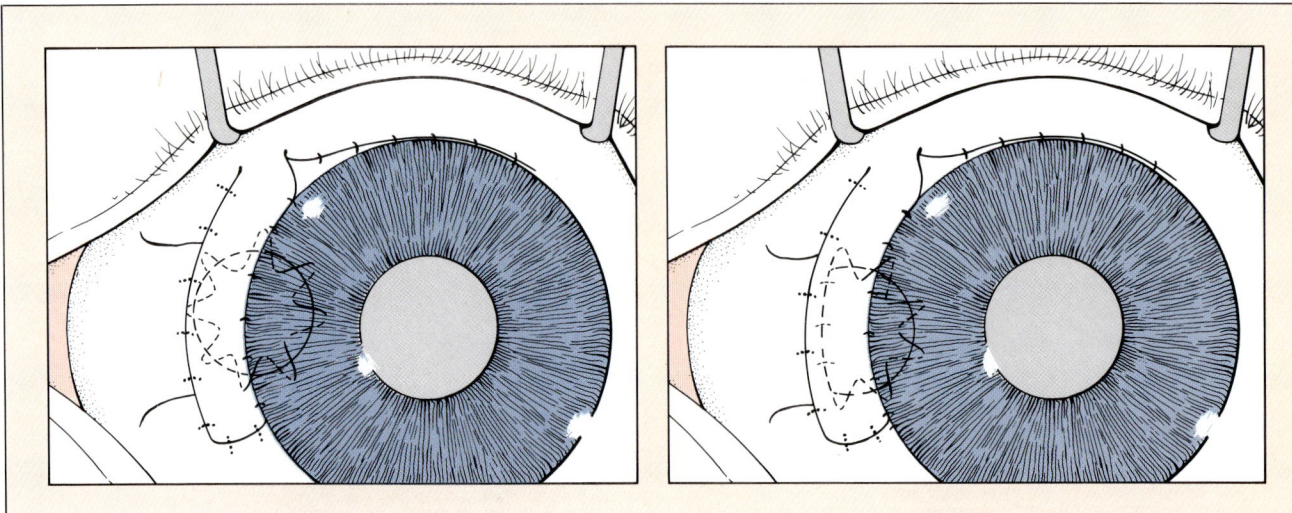

Figure 30.7 (Left) *Recent lamellar graft for treatment of recurrent pterygium. In order to expose bare sclera nasally and reconstitute the semilunar fold, the initial steps of excision by pedicle conjunctivoplasty are performed.* (Right) *A semicircular or circular graft may be used and the graft may be covered by a conjunctivoplasty, if desired.*

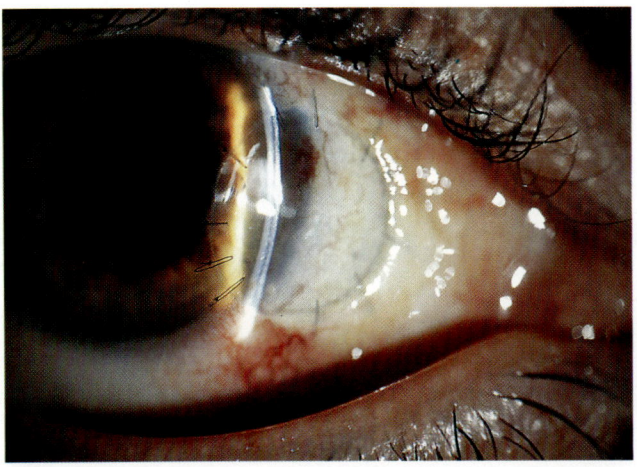
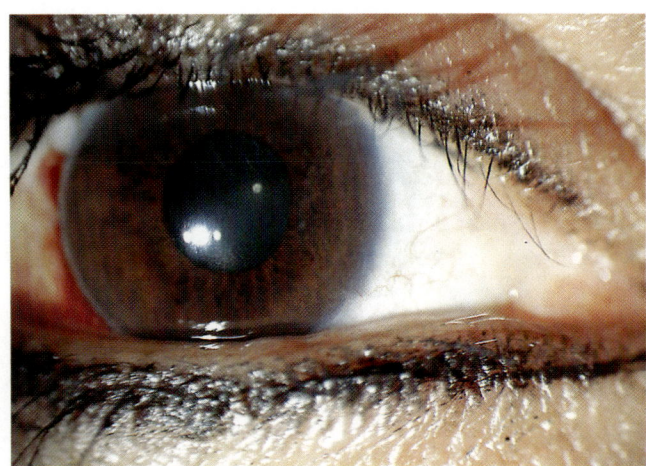

Figure 30.8 *Circular lamellar graft for the treatment of recurrent pterygium, two months postoperatively* (**left**) *and three years postoperatively* (**right**).

Conclusion

Pterygia are common ocular lesions, usually cured by primary excision. The surgeon should remain aware that relatively simple pterygium cases, if allowed to progress, can impair vision. When a pterygium recurs, more sophisticated surgery is necessary. Excellent microsurgical technique for the initial and secondary treatment of pterygium should keep these deleterious consequences to a minimum.

Clinical Points to Consider

- A good surgical technique for removal of recurrent pterygium should reconstitute the semilunar fold.

- A bucket-handle conjunctivoplasty, which takes about 45 minutes, should be performed under retrobulbar or peribulbar anesthesia.

- A limbal lamellar keratoplasty may be an excellent way to perfect lamellar keratoplasty skills.

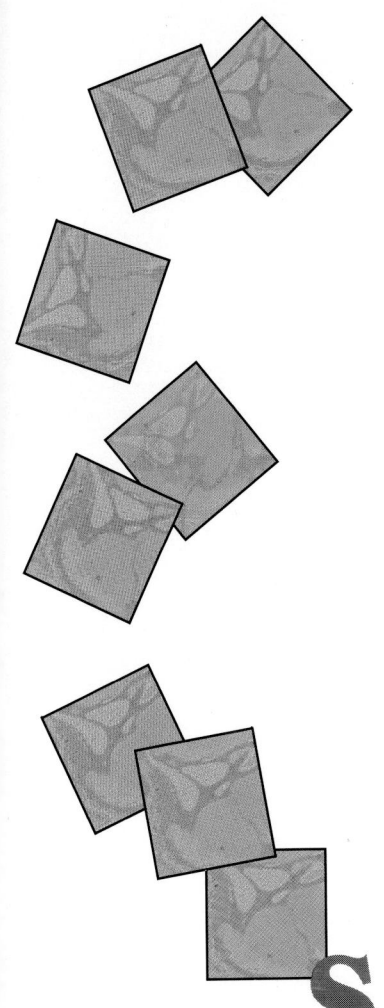

Section Eight
Surgery of the Lids

Acquired Ptosis

NORMAN SHORR, M.D. MARC S. COHEN, M.D.

Ptosis is a condition in which the upper eyelid margin is lower than normal. The upper lid should cross the cornea at 2.00 mm or less below the superior limbus, i.e., the lid should be about 2.00 mm above the superior pupillary border (assuming a 4.00 mm pupil) or 4.00 mm above the central corneal light reflex. Usually, ptosis is measured by determining the distance of the lid margin from either the pupillary border or from the corneal light reflex (Fig. 31.1). The cornea is 12.00 mm in diameter; thus, an eyelid 1.00 mm above the pupillary border, or 3.00 from the light reflex, has 1.00 mm of ptosis. An eyelid that just touches the upper pupillary border, or is 2.00 mm from the light reflex, has 2.00 mm of ptosis. An eyelid that obstructs the upper 25% of the pupil, or is 1.00 mm from the light reflex, has 3.00 mm of ptosis.

Anatomy

A thorough understanding of eyelid anatomy is necessary in order to choose the appropriate surgical approach. A detailed description of eyelid anatomy is beyond the scope of this text; however, a basic overview follows (Fig. 31.2).

The anterior-most portion of the upper lid is formed by skin and orbicularis oculi. The orbicularis is the sphincter of the eyelid and is divided into an orbital part and a palpebral part, which has both a pretarsal and a preseptal portion. The orbicularis is extremely vascular and accounts for most intraoperative bleeding. Deep to the orbicularis is the orbital septum, a fibrous sheet that separates the lid from the orbit. It is formed at the orbital rim as the arcus marginalis, which is a thickening of the periostium. In non-Asians the orbital septum inserts into the levator aponeurosis 3.00 mm to 4.00 mm superior to the superior tarsal border. In Asians it inserts into the levator aponeurosis anterior to the tarsus.

Posterior to the orbital septum is a layer of preaponeurotic fat, which is partially removed during blepharoplasty. This fat layer is an important landmark in upper eyelid surgery because the levator aponeurosis lies posterior to it. There are generally two fat pads in the upper eyelid—the central and the nasal. The nasal pad tends to be paler than the central pad. Temporally, care must be taken to distinguish the lacrimal gland from orbital fat. Posterior to the fat is the levator aponeurosis. The levator muscle becomes aponeurotic about 10.00 mm superior to the tarsal border. The aponeurosis inserts over the anterior surface of the tarsus. Müller's muscle, which arises from the posterior surface of the levator muscle approximately 10.00 mm to 15.00 mm superior to the tarsal margin, inserts into the superior tarsal margin and is sympathetically innervated. The conjunctiva lines the posterior aspect of the upper eyelid.

The upper eyelid crease represents the most superior point of attachment between the skin and the levator aponeurosis. This occurs inferior to the insertion of the orbital septum on the levator aponeurosis.

Evaluation of the Acquired Ptosis Patient

When evaluating patients with acquired ptosis, it is necessary to determine if there is any underlying systemic disorder. Thus, all patients should undergo a thorough medical history as well as ophthalmic and neuro-ophthalmic examinations. In particular, the physician should look for a history or signs of myasthenia gravis, ophthalmopathy, or cranial neuropathies. Tear function, corneal sensation, and any ocular surface disease must be evaluated. Surgery to correct ptosis will often exacerbate underlying ocular problems, and this must be taken into account when developing a surgical plan. Finally, millimeters of ptosis and levator function should be measured.

Ptosis Following Cataract Extraction

Although the cause of ptosis following cataract surgery is not known, ptosis is a well-documented condition, with a reported incidence of up to 13% following cataract extraction. Levator aponeurosis disinsertion following cataract surgery has been described. In addition, it has been reported that the incidence of ptosis increases significantly following cataract extraction performed under local anesthesia compared to the incidence under general anesthesia; the use of a Nadbath facial nerve block is less likely to result in postoperative ptosis than use of a Van lint lid block; and superior rectus bridla sutures are more likely to cause ptosis than episcleral bridle sutures. While the data are controversial, it appears likely that postoperative ptosis results from damage to the levator-superior rectus muscle complex. Interesting, ptosis is very rare following radial keratotomy performed under topical anesthesia, yet using a large lid speculum (e.g., Lancaster). Perhaps, the retained tonus of the levator complex minimizes passive trauma as may occur following retrobulbar anesthesia.

We feel that the majority of patients who develop postsurgical ptosis have levator dehiscence. Most of these patients probably had preoperative weakness of the levator aponeurosis and thus were predisposed to postoperative ptosis. While minimal trauma to the levator complex may cause predisposed patients to develop ptosis, studies suggest that the incidence of postsurgical levator ptosis is minimized by not directly manipulating the superior rectus and levator complex.

Surgical Procedure

In the majority of patients with acquired ptosis, the condition can be corrected by one of three methods: Müller's muscle resection (Müllerectomy), levator resection (anterior approach), or the Fasanella-Servat procedure.

During the initial evaluation, one drop of 2.5% Neo-Synephrine should be applied to the eye with the ptotic lid. After about five minutes lid position should be remeasured. Because Neo-Synephrine constricts Müller's muscle, the lid may elevate to a normal or higher than normal position during this time (Fig. 31.3). If one drop of 2.5% Neo-Synephrine results in an ideal upper eyelid margin position, a 9.00 mm Müller's muscle resection is indicated. If the eyelid margin actually rises too high from the drop of Neo-Synephrine, calculate the number of millimeters of resection: 4:00 mm of resection will elevate the eyelid 1.00 mm, or subtract 4.00 mm from 9.00 mm for every millimeter the eyelid was higher than the goal. A Müller's muscle resection is the procedure of choice in patients who respond to 2.5% Neo-Synephrine because it offers significant advantages over other methods; i.e., it is easy to perform, has highly predictable results, and does not destroy the normal architecture of the lid, which allows for a second operation in the rare event that one is needed. Müller's muscle resection should not be performed for ptosis greater than 2.50 mm to 3.00 mm.

In patients who do not respond to 2.5% Neo-Synephrine or have ptosis of 3.00 mm or greater, the procedure of choice is anterior levator resection, which corrects severe ptosis in an anatomically logical way and allows for correction of eyelid contour abnormalities Anterior levator resection is considerably more difficult to perform than a Müllerectomy. It requires significant patient cooperation compared to that required for other procedures. Unless the surgeon very familiar with eyelid anatomy and is experienced in this technique, results are unpredictable.

The Fasanella-Servat procedure (tarsoconjunctival Müllerectomy) removes part of the tarsus and may be performed in any patient with up to 3.00 mm of ptosis. While it is an easy procedure and familiar to most ophthalmologists, it is the least desirable; because the tarsus is the eyelid's skeleton, its removal leads to eyelid contour abnormalities and, in the event of unsatisfactory results, reoperation is difficult. For this reason, the Fasanella-Servat procedure is not advised as a primary operation; it is reserved as a reliable and forgiving touch-up operation for the last one or two millimeters of ptosis when Müller's muscle resection or anterior levator resection has undercorrected.

Müller's Muscle–Conjunctival Resection (Müllerectomy)

1. This procedure requires approximately 2.00 cc of local infiltrative anaesthesia per lid, using

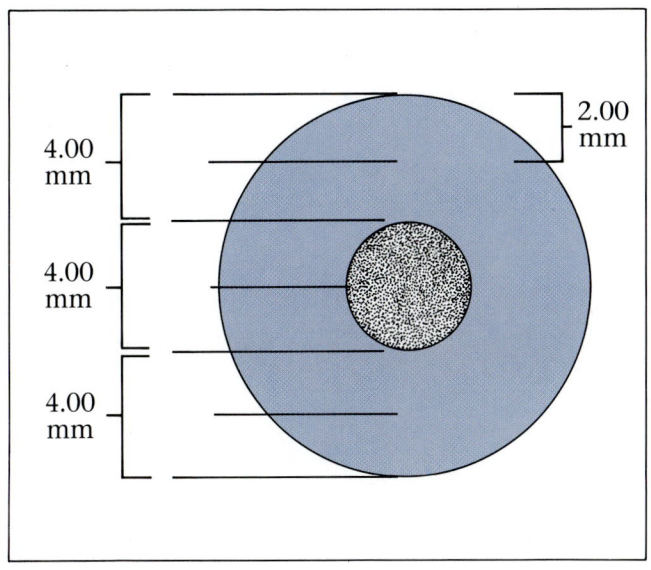

Figure 31.1 *The degree of ptosis is determined by measuring the distance of the lid margin from the pupillary border or central corneal light reflex.*

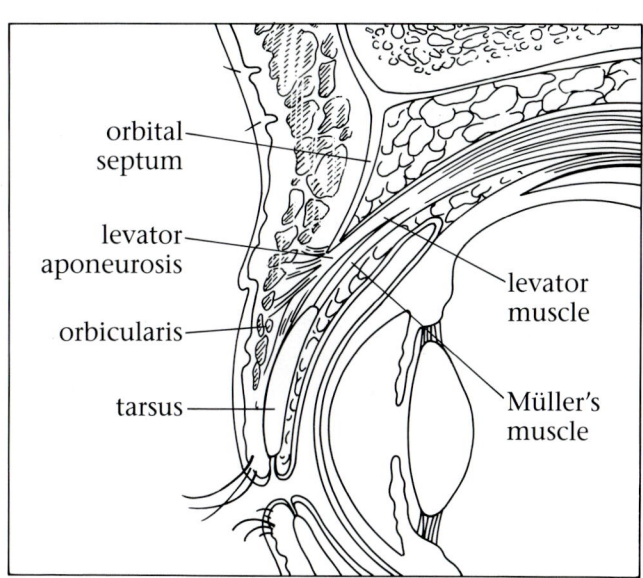

Figure 31.2 *Upper eyelid anatomy.*

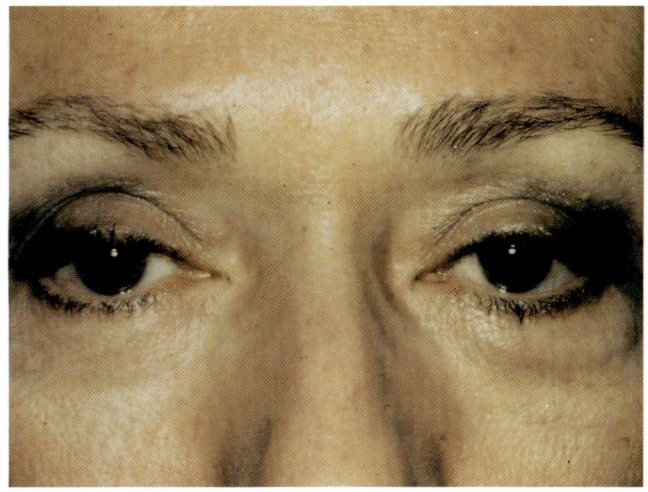

Figure 31.3 (Left) *Patient with 3.00 mm of bilateral acquired ptosis.* **(Right)** *The same patient five minutes*

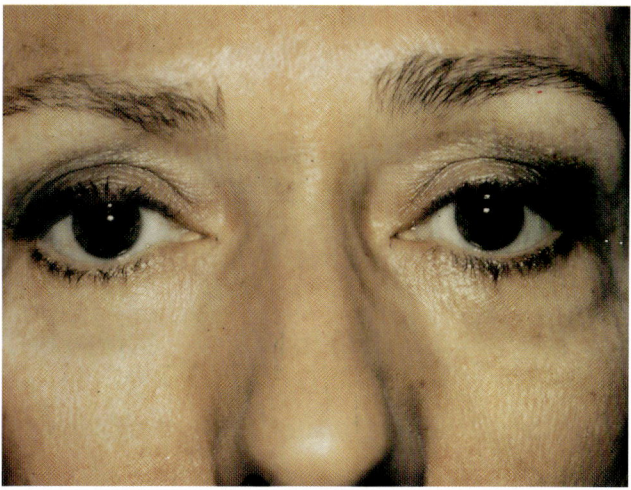

after injection of 2.5% Neo-Synephrine in each eye. Note "resolution" of ptosis.

2% Xylocaine with 1:100,000 epinephrine and Wydase, if medically acceptable. The block is placed transconjunctivally just superior to the superior tarsal border (Fig. 31.4).

2. The eyelid is everted over a Desmarres rectractor. Toothed forceps are used to grasp conjunctiva and Müller's muscle 3.00 mm to 4.00 mm superior to the tarsus. Because Müller's muscle adheres to the conjunctiva, grasping the conjunctiva and lifting it away from the underlying tissue results in a separation of Müller's muscle from the levator aponeurosis. A caliper is used to make a mark 9.00 mm (or a smaller amount, determined by the above formula) above the superior tarsal border, and a cautery or marking pen is used to mark the conjunctiva medially, centrally, and laterally (Fig. 31.5).

3. The surgeon grasps the conjunctiva and Müller's muscle centrally 4.50 mm above the superior tarsal border (halfway between the mark and the tarsal border) with toothed forceps. The surgical assistant grasps the conjunctiva and Müller's muscle at 4.50 mm above the superior tarsal border 12.00 mm medially and 12.00 mm laterally from the surgeon's forceps. These three forceps are lifted in unison in a plane perpendicular to the lid. The Desmarres retractor is removed (Fig. 31.6).

4. A specially designed clamp (Karl Ilg) is used to grasp the conjunctiva and Müller's muscle that are to be excised. The clamp is placed adjacent to the tarsus, with care taken not to incorporate the tarsus in the clamp (Fig. 31.7).

5. A 6-0 Prolene serpentine suture is woven back and forth through the "sandwich" of conjunctiva, Müller's muscle, and conjunctiva. The suture is externalized at each end. A running suture is started at the skin surface 3.00 mm superior to the tarsus at the lateral aspect of the eyelid, ending at the medial aspect of the lid, at

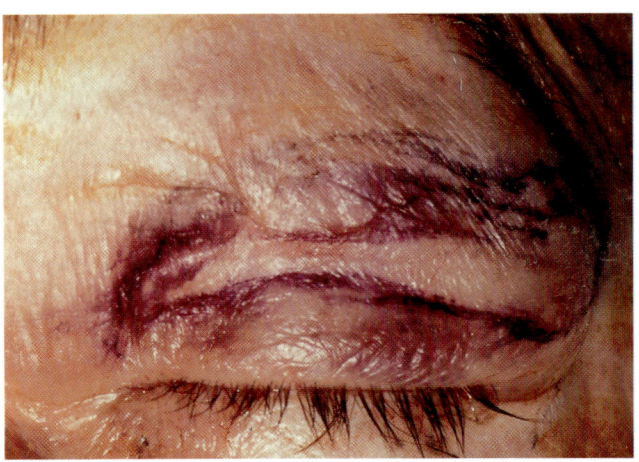

Figure 31.4 *Preoperatively, the eyelid is marked for a Müller's muscle resection followed by an upper eyelid blepharoplasty.*

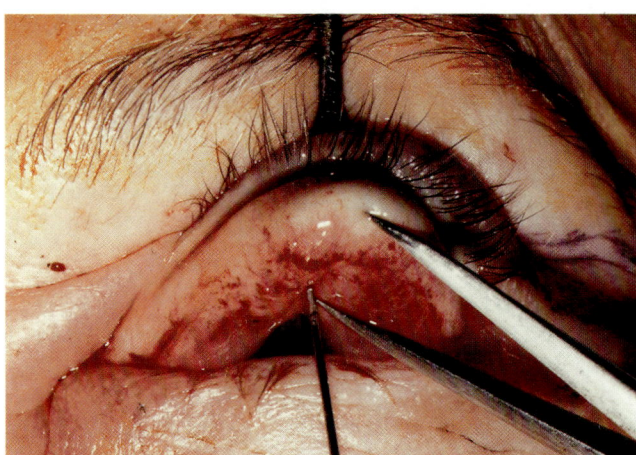

Figure 31.5 *A caliper is used to mark the amount of conjunctiva and underlying Müller's muscle to be removed.*

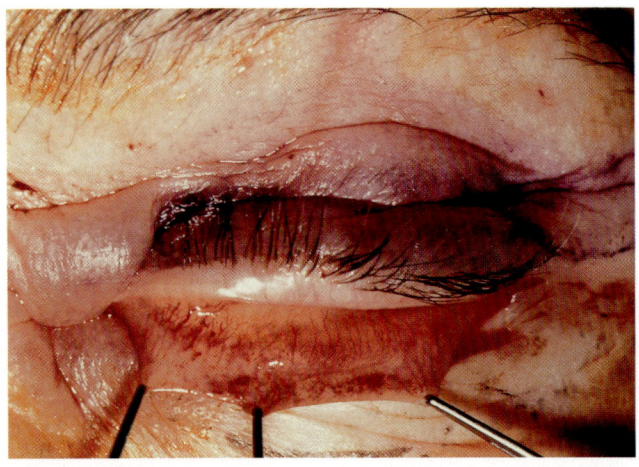

Figure 31.6 *Conjunctiva and Müller's muscle are lifted with three forceps.*

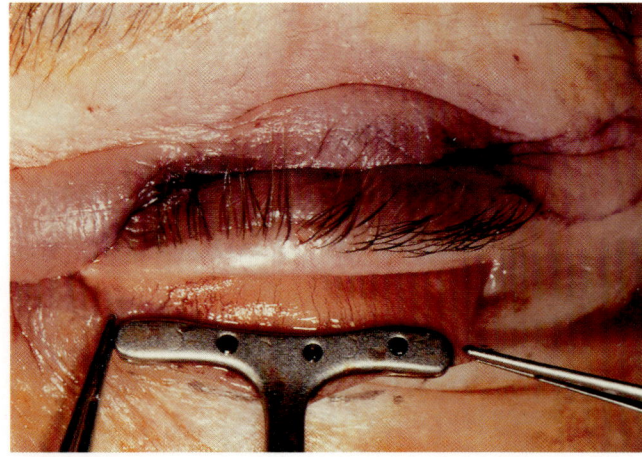

Figure 31.7 *Müller's muscle and conjunctiva are grasped in a specially designed clamp.*

which point the suture is externalized. The suture is then passed back through the skin adjacent to the externalizing pass. A small piece of suture is tied around the loop so that it is not lost. The suture is then woven back across the lid between the previously placed sutures. When the lateral aspect of the lid is reached, the suture is externalized adjacent to the original pass and tied to itself (Fig. 31.8). About five bites are necessary to cover the entire length of the lid.

A No. 15 Bard Parker blade is used to excise the conjunctiva and Müller's muscle held in the

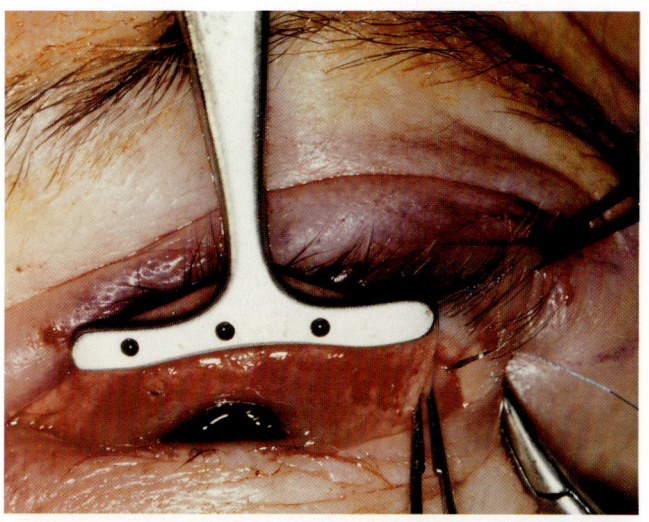
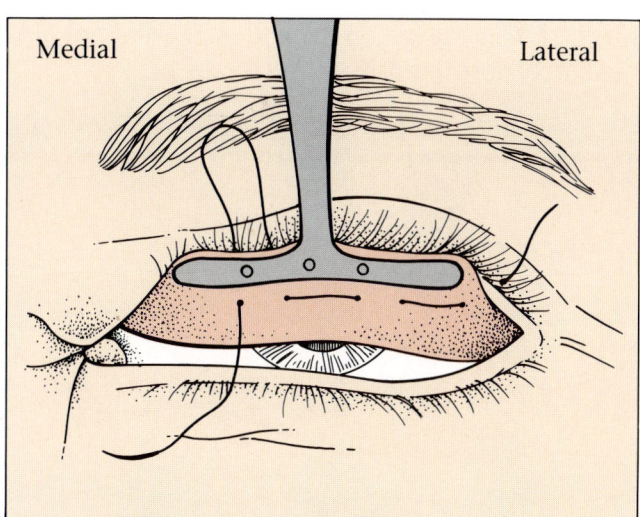
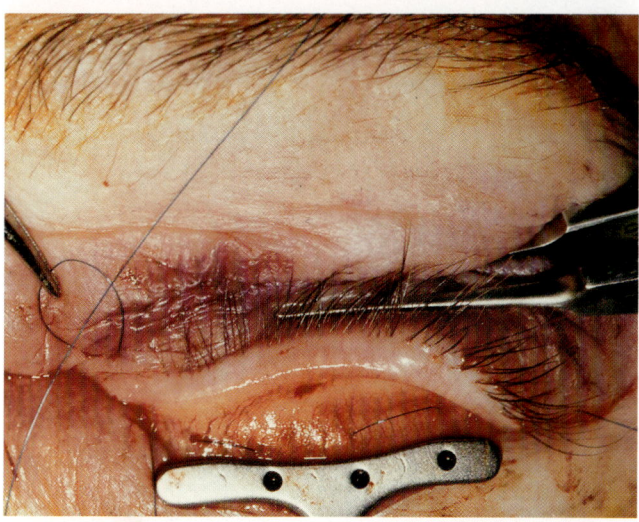
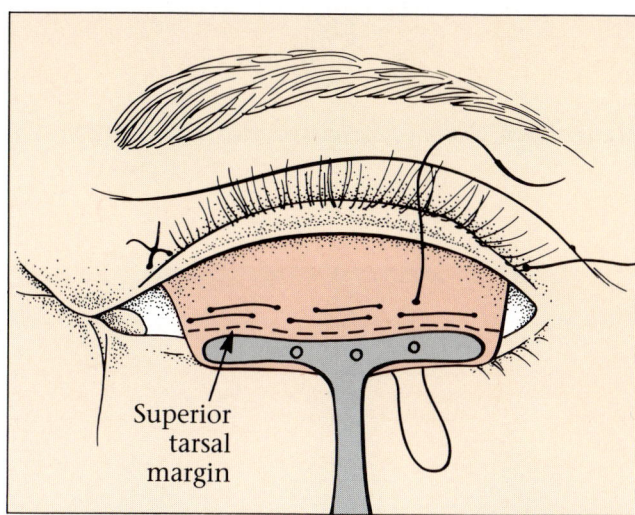
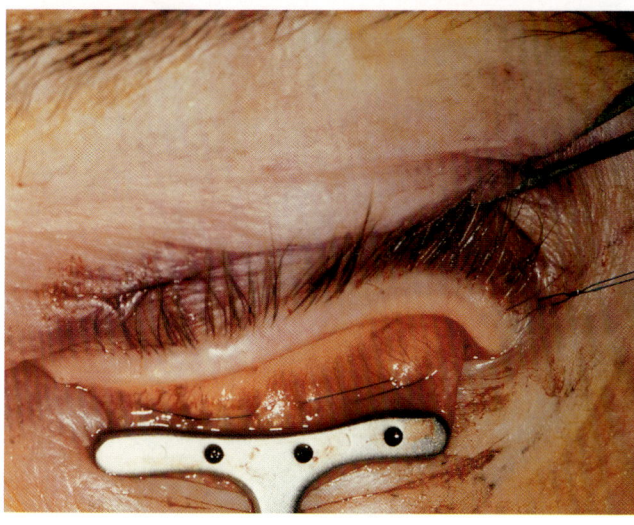
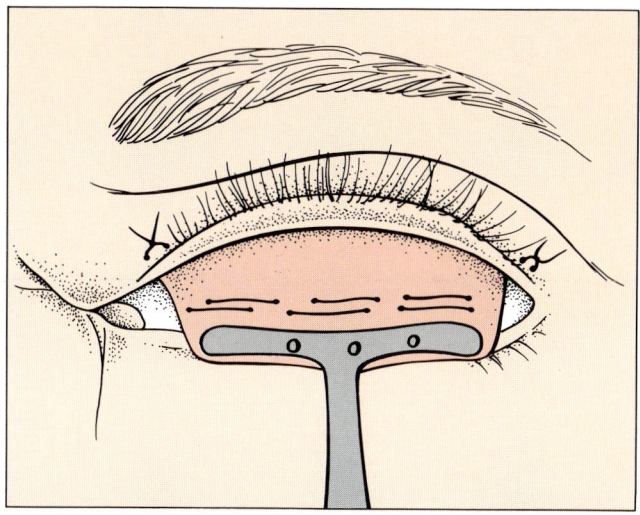

Figure 31.8 *Externalized serpentine sutures are placed. Suture is introduced laterally* **(top left)** *run lateral to medial* **(top right)** *externalized* **(middle left)**. *Suture is run medial to lateral* **(middle right)** *externalized, and tied on itself* **(bottom left)**. *Suturing is complete* **(bottom right)**.

clamp (Fig. 31.9). During this incision the blade should hug the clamp and care should be taken not to cut the serpentine sutures (Fig. 31.10).

The eyelid is returned to the anatomic position. A scalpel handle is passed over the tarsal conjunctival surface to help reapproximate the wound edges.

At this time, excess upper eyelid skin should be removed in a standard blepharoplasty fashion (Fig. 31.11). Figure 31.12 shows the patient immediately postoperatively.

Fasanella-Servat Procedure (Tarsoconjunctival Müllerectomy)

1. This procedure requires approximately 3.00 cc of local infiltrative anaesthesia per lid, using 2% Xylocaine with 1:100,000 epinephrine and Wydase, if medically acceptable. The block is placed transconjunctivally just superior to the superior tarsal border (Fig. 31.13).

2. The eyelid is everted over a Desmarres retractor (Fig. 31.14). The superior tarsal border is iden-

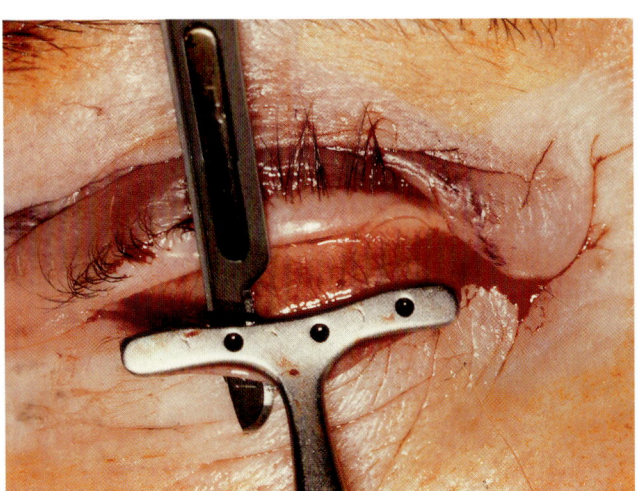

Figure 31.9 *Clamped tissue is excised with a scalpel.*

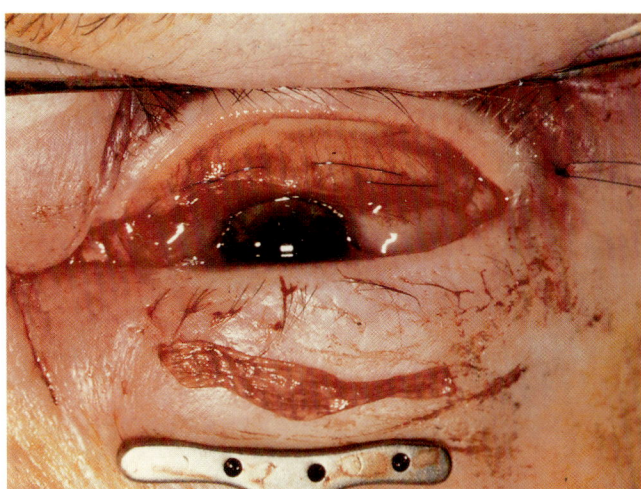

Figure 31.10 *The serpentine sutures should not be cut.*

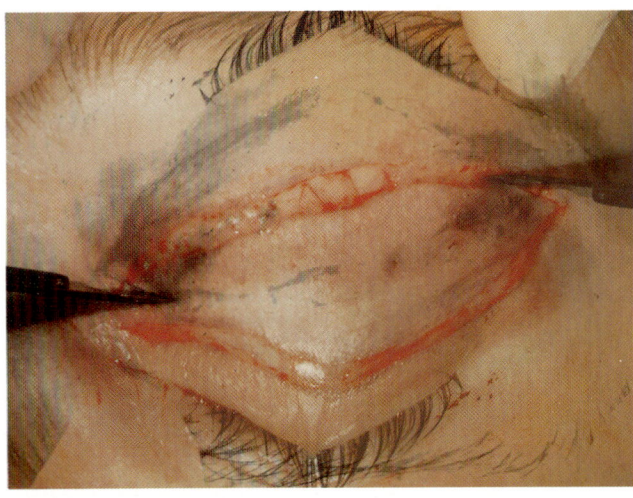

Figure 31.11 *Excess skin is excised in a standard blepharoplasty fashion.*

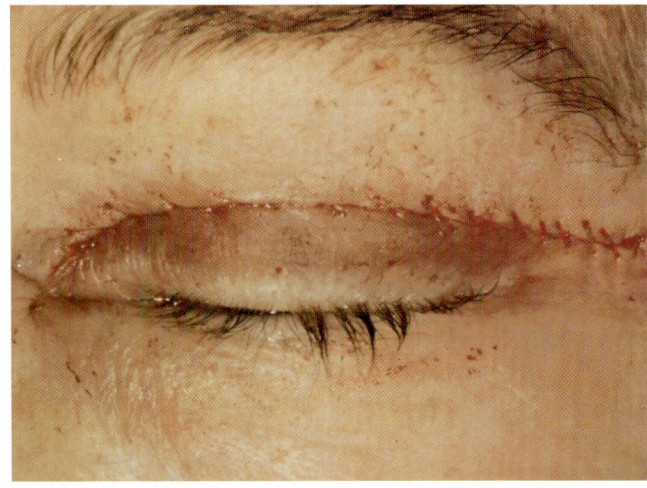

Figure 31.12 *Immediate postoperative appearance of eye following Müller's muscle resection and excision of upper eyelid skin.*

tified. The skin and underlying levator complex are grasped and pulled anteriorly with forceps (Fig. 31.15). Hemostats should engage tarsus, Müller's muscle, and conjunctiva; however, it is important that they not incorporate the levator.

3. Two hemostats are applied with the everted superior tarsal margin held (see Fig. 31.13) after the Desmarres retractor has been removed. The tarsus, Müller's muscle, and the overlying conjunctiva are clamped. Care must be taken to orient the hemostats properly, i.e., their tips should point away from the eyelid margin. This guarantees that the remaining piece of tarsus is vertically higher centrally rather than laterally, thus maintaining the proper contour. It is important to place the hemostats properly before they are tightly clamped because they are difficult to move once the tarsus is crushed (Fig. 31.16).

4. A 6-0 Prolene suture is woven through conjunctiva, tarsus, Müller's muscle, and conjuncti-

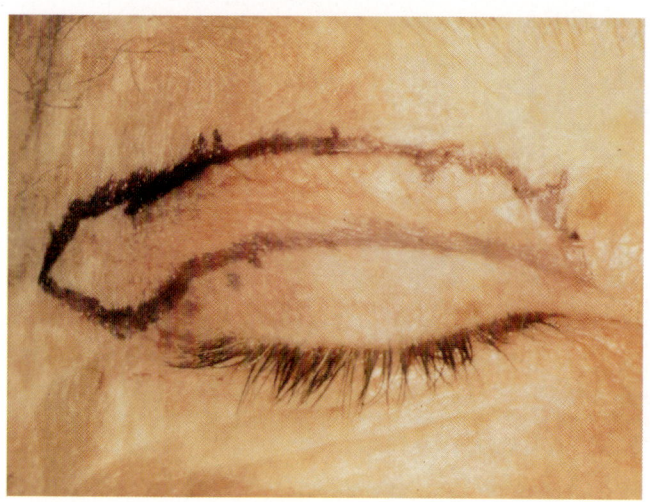

Figure 31.13 *Preoperatively, the eyelid is marked for a Fasanella-Servat procedure followed by an upper eyelid blepharoplasty.*

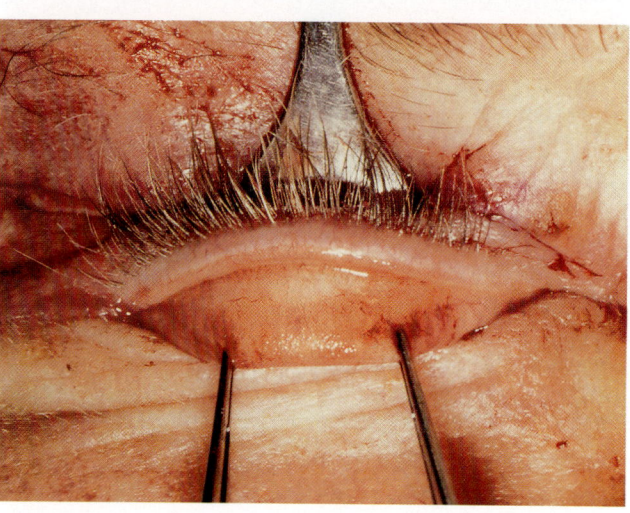

Figure 31.14 *The eyelid is everted and the superior tarsal border identified.*

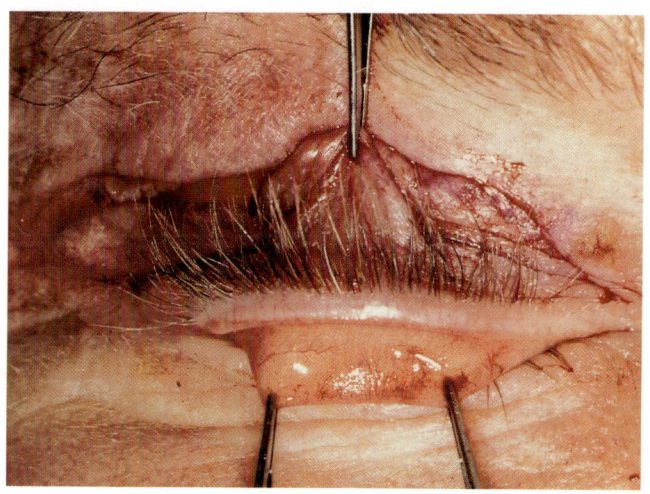

Figure 31.15 *Skin and levator muscle are grasped and pulled anteriorly so that in subsequent steps the levator will not be incorporated in the hemostats.*

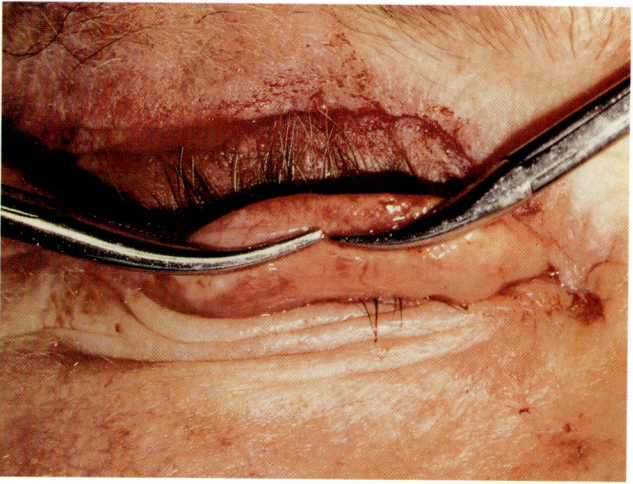

Figure 31.16 *Proper placement of hemostats on tarsus. Note that the tips of the clamps point away from eyelid margin.*

va and externalized at each end (Fig. 31.17). Some surgeons use a 6-0 plain gut, nonexternalized suture. We use the externalized Prolene because it can be easily removed at any time for overcorrection.

5. The hemostats are removed. The tarsus, Müller's muscle, and the overlying conjunctiva immediately adjacent to hemostats are removed by cutting in the crush mark made by the hemostats (Fig. 31.18).

6. The eyelid is returned to the anatomic position. A scalpel handle is passed over the tarsal conjunctival surface to help reapproximate and smooth the wound edges.

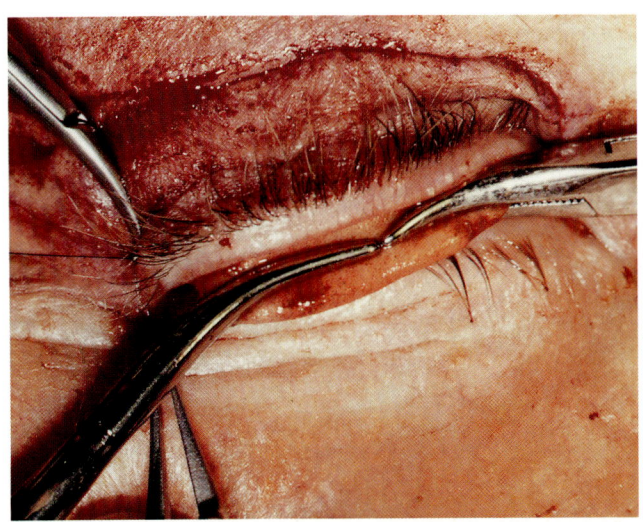
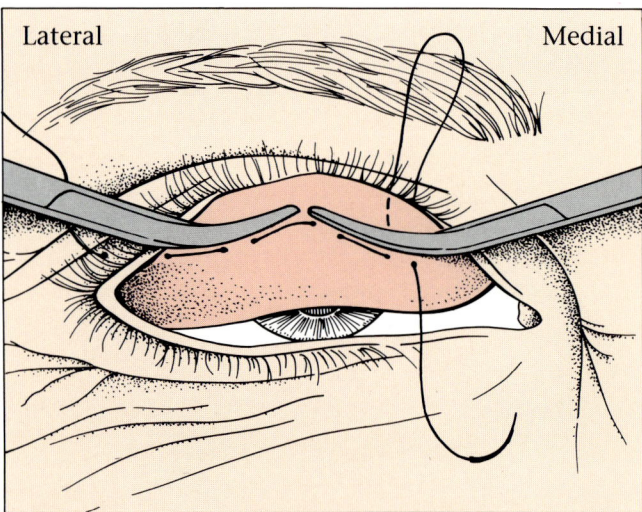
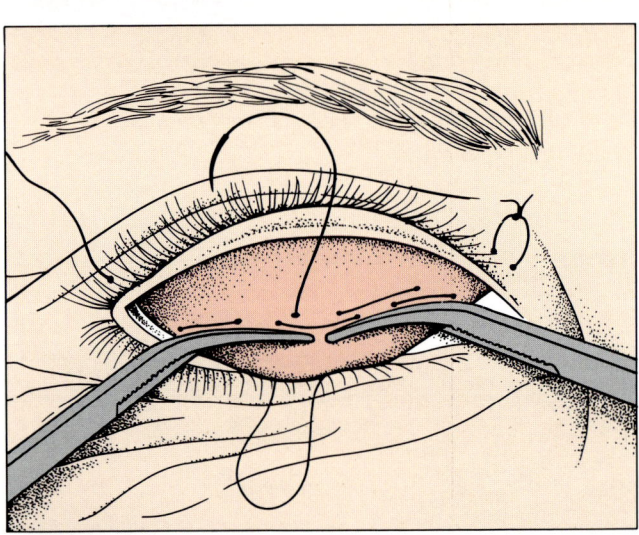
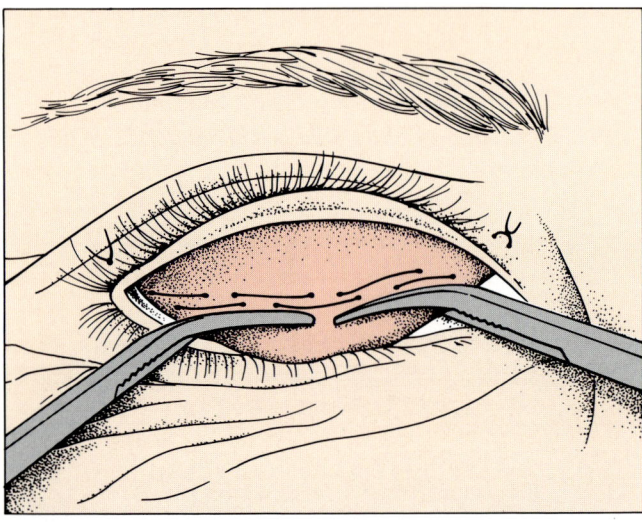
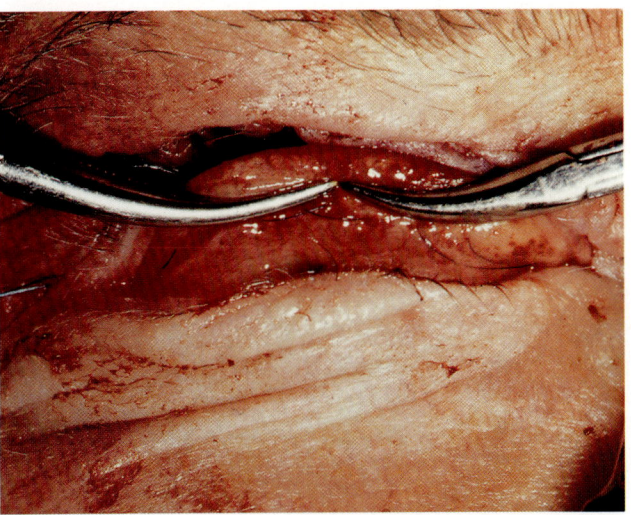

Figure 31.17 *Externalized serpentine sutures are placed.* **(Top left)** *Suture is introduced through skin laterally.* **(Top right)** *Suture is passed lateral to medial immediately adjacent to the clamps (sutures drawn slightly away from the hemostats for clarity).* **(Middle left)** *After externalization, suture is run medial to lateral.* **(Middle right)** *Suture is externalized laterally and tied on itself.* **(Bottom left)** *Suturing is complete; the surgeon should prepare to remove the nasal hemostat.*

7. Eyelid skin is often removed in a standard blepharoplasty fashion at this point (Fig. 31.19) because excess eyelid skin is frequently present and this procedure tends to cause the upper eyelid skin to bunch together. Figure 31.20 shows the patient immediately postoperatively.

Levator Resection (Anterior Approach)

1. This procedure requires 1.00 cc to 2.00 cc of local infiltrative anesthesia per lid, using 2% Lidocaine with 1:100,000 epinephrine and Wydase, if medically acceptable. While the patient

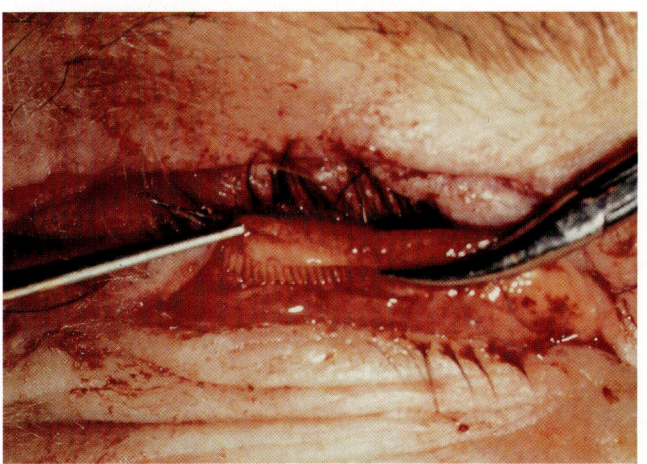

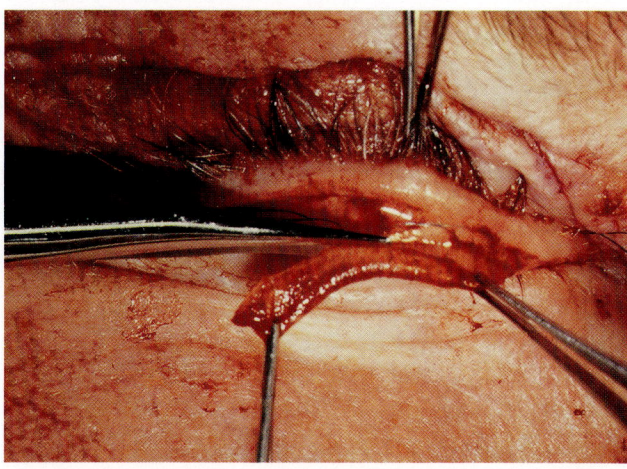

Figure 31.18 (Top left) *The hemostats are removed.* **(Top right and bottom left)** *The excision of tarsus, Müller's muscle, and conjunctiva is made by scissors in the crush mark so the suture is not cut.*

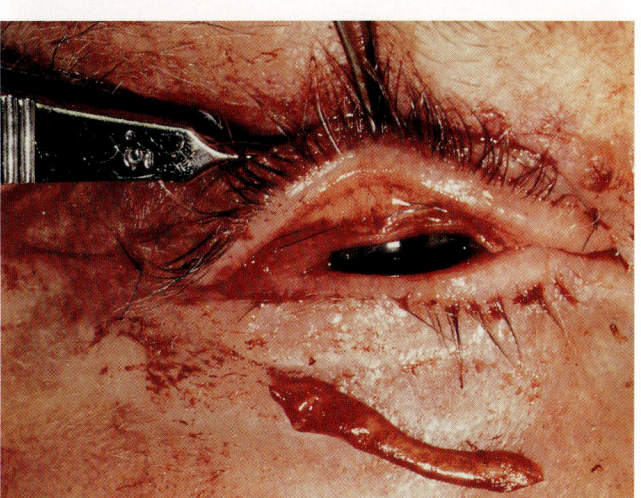

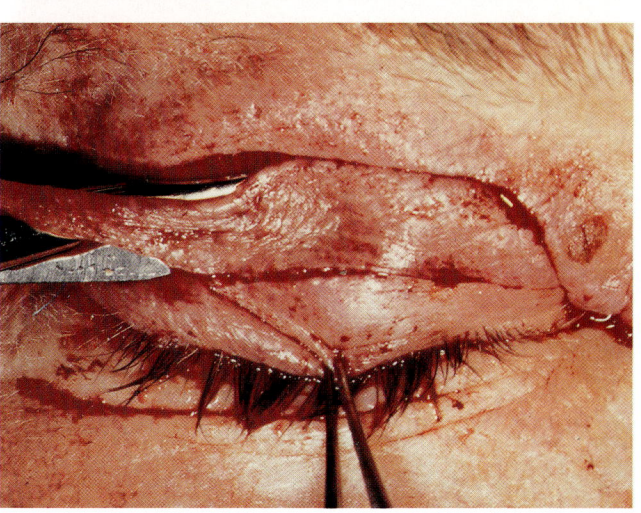

Figure 31.19 *Excess skin is excised in a standard blepharoplasty fashion.*

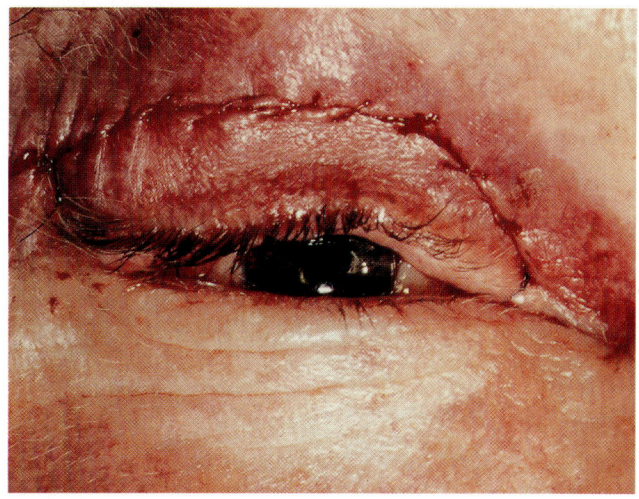

Figure 31.20 *Immediate postoperative appearance of eye following a Fasanella-Servat procedure/tarsoconjunctival-Müllerectomy and excision of upper eyelid skin.*

must be comfortable, it is essential that levator function remain intact. Both conditions can be achieved by injecting the block subcutaneously just anterior to the tarsus (31.21).

2. During anterior levator resection, excess upper eyelid skin is excised in a standard blepharoplasty fashion. A standard blepharoplasty incision line is drawn using a marking pen. The assistant, using Castroviejo forceps, stretches the eyelid by grasping skin just superior to the lash line so the lid is pulled inferiorly and slightly posteriorly. Putting the levator on stretch causes the preaponeurotic fat to prolapse forward, which helps the surgeon avoid inadvertently cutting the levator. Using a No. 15 Bard Parker blade, an incision is made through skin and orbicularis. With the lid stretched, the skin and orbicularis within the marks are excised, using Wescott scissors, so that the orbital septum is exposed (Fig. 31.22). Mobility helps differentiate the levator aponeurosis from the septum. While the levator aponeurosis can be moved freely upon inferior traction, the septum, because it is firmly attached to the orbital rim, is immobile. The surgeon can have the patient look up so it can be observed if the tissue moves. The septum is opened horizontally along the entire length of the wound. The levator complex can now be identified just posterior to preaponeurotic fat (Fig. 31.23).

3. The levator aponeurosis must be disinserted from the anterior aspect of the tarsus and dissected from the underlying Müller's muscle and conjunctiva. Although this can be done with scissors, we have found that using a disposable hot blue cautery (Concept 4200) (Fig. 31.24) helps maintain hemostasis while working in this highly vascularized plane. Because the globe lies just posterior to Müller's muscle and the conjunctiva, a protective shield over the eye is necessary during this maneuver.

4. Three 6-0 double-armed nonabsorbable sutures are used to attach the levator aponeurosis to the anterior aspect of the tarsus (Fig. 31.25). Proper lid contour is dependent on the proper placement of the sutures in the tarsus. The central suture is placed first. With a toothed forceps, the surgeon grasps the center part of the superior tarsus directly above the pupil, about 4.00 mm inferior to the superior tarsal border. If the sutures are placed lower than this, the patient may develop postoperative upper eyelid ectropion.

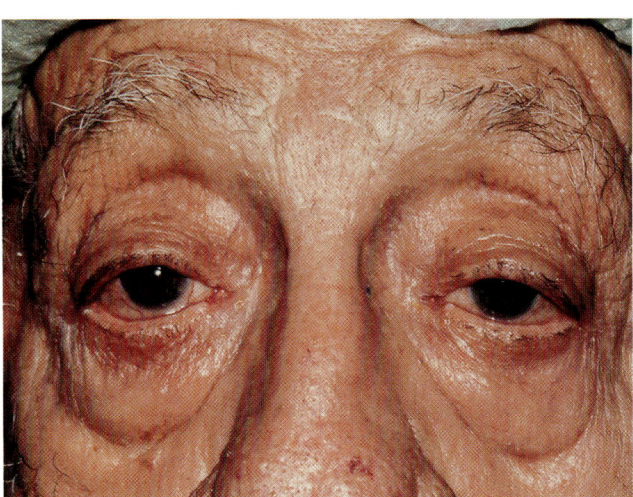

Figure 31.21 *Preoperative appearance of patient with 3.00 mm of bilateral blepharoptosis.*

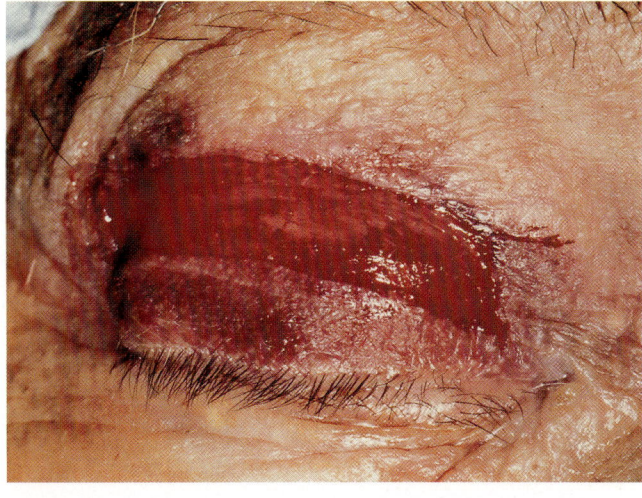

Figure 31.22 *Skin and orbicularis are excised in a standard blepharoplasty fashion.*

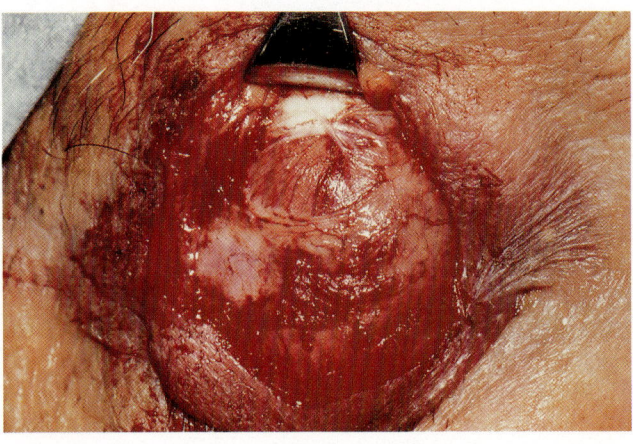

Figure 31.23 *The septum is opened and the levator complex is identified.*

When the proper position is found, the surgeon can elevate the lid without distortion of the normal eyelid contour and without the lid pulling away from the globe. At this point the suture is placed, using a partial thickness tarsal bite in a horizontal fashion. Each end of the suture is passed through the levator complex, posteriorly to anteriorly, about 12.00 mm above the original insertion. The same procedure is carried out for the medial and lateral sutures. The sutures are then tied with slip knots.

5. The patient is asked to sit upright so that lid position and contour can be assessed (Fig. 31.26). The protective eye shield should be removed. At

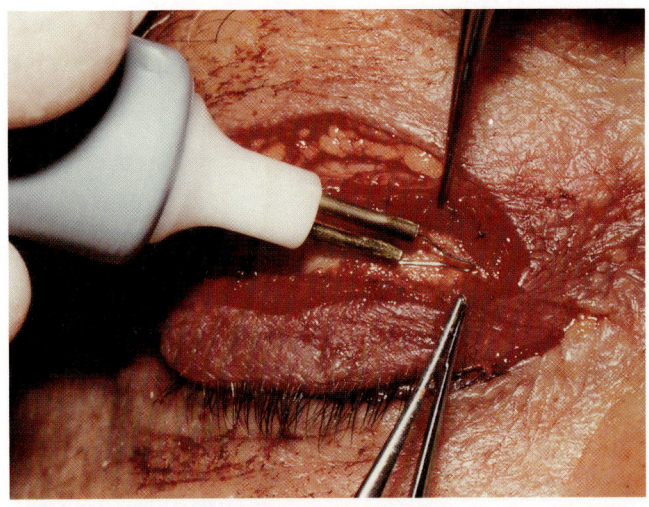
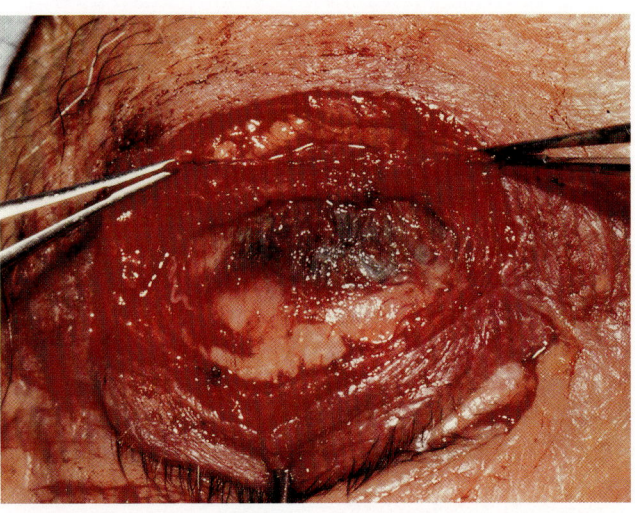

Figure 31.24 *The levator complex dissected from anterior tarsus and underlying Müller's muscle and conjunctiva using a hot blue cautery* **(left).** *The levator is freed from Müller's muscle* **(right).** *Note the thin layer of tissue between the surgical plane and the globe.*

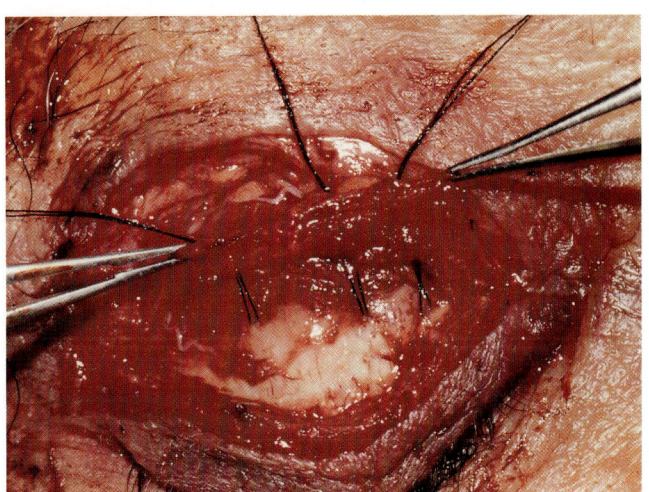

Figure 31.25 *Three double-armed permanent sutures reattach the levator to the tarsus.*

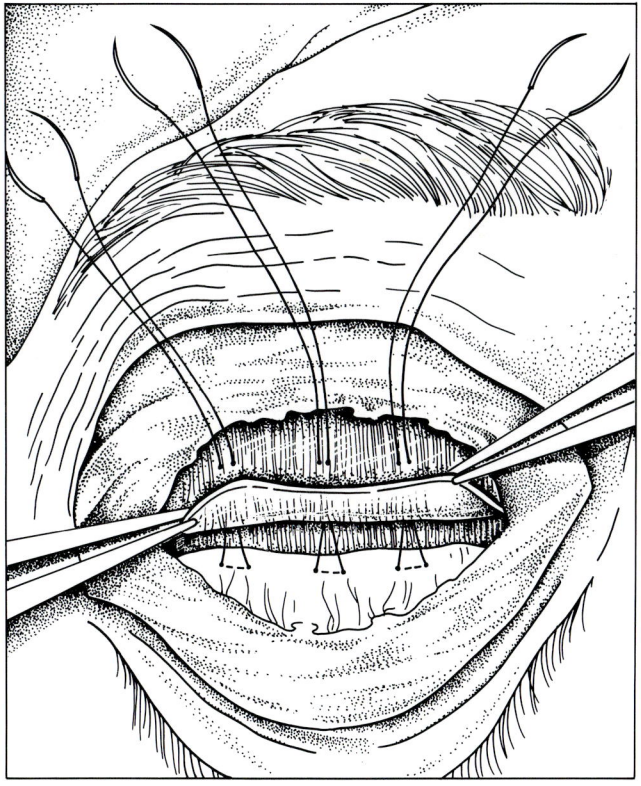

this point the eyelid should be in the desired postoperative position. However, the surgeon must take into account the many factors that affect intraoperative lid position (e.g., Xylocaine-induced orbicularis weakness, levator weakness, and swelling) and, therefore, the final result. This is the most challenging aspect of levator surgery. If the lid is not in the desired position, the sutures can be replaced. Once the desired position is obtained, the sutures are permanently tied and the excess levator complex is excised with scissors (Fig. 31.27).

6. The blepharoplasty skin incision is closed using 6-0 fast absorbing chromic sutures in a running fashion (Fig. 31.28). Figure 31.29 shows the patient in figure 31.21 following bilateral levator resection.

Postoperative Care

After undergoing one of the above procedures, patients are instructed to use cold compresses four times a day for three days and then warm

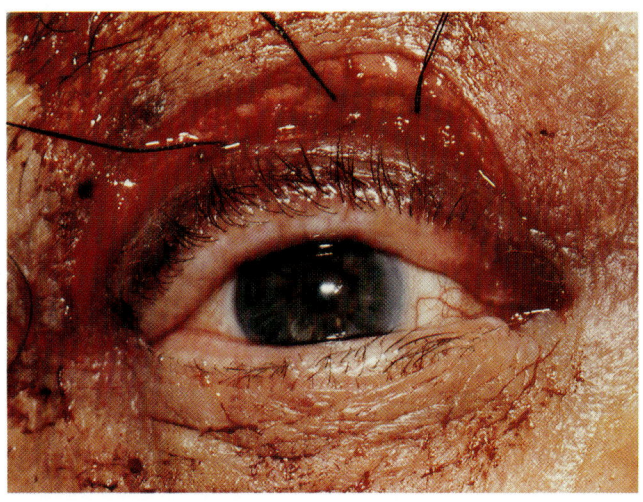

Figure 31.26 *The patient sits in an upright position. Note the proper position and lid contour.*

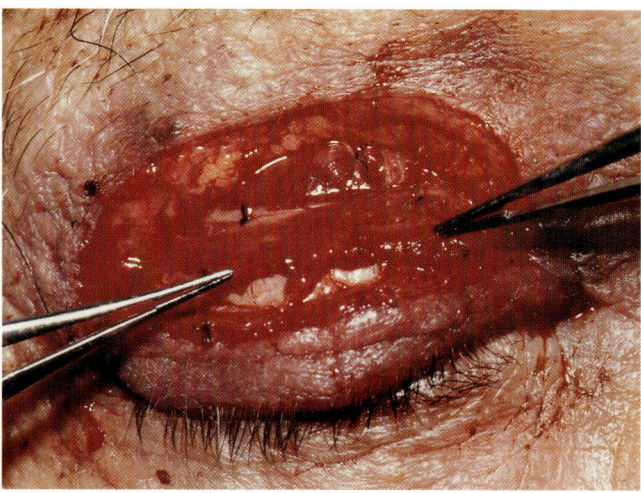

Figure 31.27 *The three double-armed permanent sutures are tied and excess levator aponeurosis is excised.*

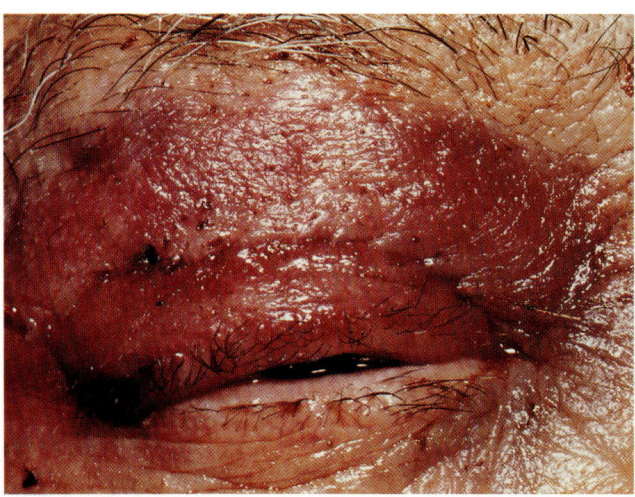

Figure 31.28 *Skin is sutured in a running fashion.*

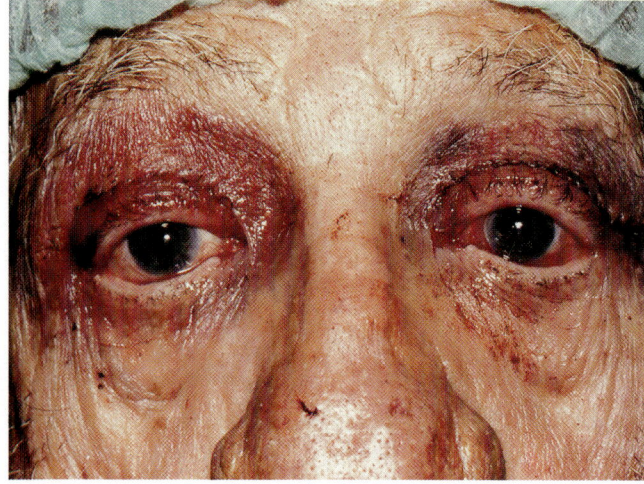

Figure 31.29 *Immediate postoperative appearance of patient in Fig. 31.21 following bilateral levator resection.*

compresses four times a day until the swelling and ecchymosis have resolved. The patient should apply steroid antibiotic ointment twice daily for one week and then at bedtime until the swelling has resolved. In addition, patients are instructed to use artificial tears at least six times a day for two weeks. Usually, pain can be managed with extra strength acetaminophen and, occasionally, acetaminophen with codeine.

For Müller's muscle resection or the Fasanella-Servat procedure, the externalized serpentine Prolene suture is removed five to seven days postoperatively. Often, the knot retracts beneath the skin. If this occurs, lift the free ends of the suture and cut off both ends beneath the knot. The opposite end of the suture is then grasped and the suture is removed with a gentle but steady pull. In the rare event of an overcorrection, the sutures may be removed earlier.

Clinical Points to Consider

☛ A thorough understanding of eyelid anatomy is essential for the ptosis surgeon.

☛ Episcleral fixation sutures with small spatula needles instead of rectus sutures with large needles may reduce the incidence of post-cataract surgery ptosis.

☛ The suturing patterns for the Fasanella-Servat procedure and the Müllerectomy are similar, although different tissues are included in the suture bites.

☛ A levator resection (anterior approach) can help restore normal lid position and function only if some levator muscle function is present.

☛ A trial of topical Neo-Synephrine 2.5% can help to differentiate between the need for a Müller's muscle resection and an anterior levator resection procedure.

☛ Reserve Fasanella-Servat procedure for re-operations.

REFERENCES

CHAPTER 2

Beuerman RW, Crosson CE, Kaufman HE. Alteration of corneal topography by refractive keratoplasty, healing prcesses in the cornea. Lin DTC, Wilson SE, Klyce SD, eds. The Woodlands, Tx: Portfolio Publishing Company of Texas; 1989: 183–193.

Holladay JT, et al. The relationship of visual acuity, refractive error, and pupil size after radial keratotomy. *Arch Ophthalmol.* 1991;109:70–76.

Nordan LT, Grene RB. The importance of corneal asphericity and irregular astigmatism in refractive surgery. *Refractive and Corneal Surgery.* 1990;6:200-204.

Ogle KN. *Optics—An Introduction for Ophthalmologists.* Springfield, Ill: Charles C Thomas Publisher; 1971.

Wittenberg S, Ludlam W. Planar reflected imagery in photokeratoscopy. *J Opt Soc Am.* 1970;60:981–985.

CHAPTER 3

Balazs EA. Ultrapure hyaluronic acid and the use thereof. U.S. Patent No. 4.141.973, 1979.

Balazs EA, Freeman MI, Kolti R, Meyer-Schwickerath G, Regnault FL, Sweney DB. Hyaluronic acid and replacement of vitreous in aqueous humor. *Mod Probl Ophthalmol.* 1972;10:3–21.

Balazs E, Hultsch E. Replacement of the vitreous with hyaluronic acid collagen and other polymers. In: Irvine AR, O'Malley C, eds. *Advances in Vitreous Surgery.* Springfield, Ill: Charles C Thomas Publisher; 1976;57:601–623.

Benedetto DA. Viscoelastic Agents, Clinical Effects -Physical Properties. Presented at the American Society of Cataract and Refractive Surgery Annual Meeting; 1987; Orlando, Fla.

Benedetto DA, Sharma MK, Shah DO. Surface properties of viscoelastic materials and intraocular lenses. In: Rosen ES, ed. *Viscoelastic Materials.* Elmsford, NY: Pergamon Press Inc; 1989.

Bothner H, Wik O. Rheology of intraocular solutions. In: Rosen ES, ed. *Viscoelastic Materials.* Elmsford, NY: Pergamon Press Inc; 1986.

Denlanger JL, El-Mofty AAA, Balazs EA. Replacement of the liquid vitreous with sodium hyaluronate in monkeys, II: long-term evaluation *Exp Eye Res.* 1980;30:101–117.

Eisner G (ed). *Ophthalmic Viscosurgery.* Montreal, Canada: Medicopea; 1986.

Edelhauser HF, Hanneken A, Pederson HJ, VanHorn DL. Osmotic tolerance of rabbit and human corneal endothelium. *Arch Ophthalmol.* 1981;99:1281–1287.

Gonnering R, Edelhauser HF, VanHorn DL, Durant W. The pH tolerance of rabbit and human corneal endothelium. *Invest Ophthalmol Vis Sci.* 1979;18:373–390.

Hruby K. Weitere erfahrungen mit: hyaluronsaure als glasskorperensatz bei netzhautblosung. *Mod Probl Ophthalmol.* 1966;4:228.

Larson RS, Lindstrom LL, Skelnik DL. Viscoelastic agents. *CLAO J.* 1989;15:151–160.

Liesegang T. Viscoelastic substances in ophthalmology. *Surv Ophthalmol.* 1990;34:268-293.

Madsen K, Schenholm M, Jahnke G, Tenbald A. Hyaluronate binding to intact corneas and cultured endothelial cells. *Invest Ophthalmol Vis Sci.* 1989;30:2132–2137.

McGilvery RW. *Biochemistry: A Functional Approach.* 2nd. ed Philadelphia, Pa: WB Saunders Co;1979:166–190.

Miller D, O'Connor P, Williams J. Use of sodium hyaluronate during intraocular lens implantation in rabbits. *Ophthalmic Surg.* 1977;7:8–58.

Miller D, Stegmann R. *The use of Healon in intraocular lens implantation.* Boston, Mass: Little, Brown & Co; 1980.

Miller D, Stegmann R. Use of sodium hyaluronate in human intraocular lens implantation. *Ann Ophthalmol.* 1981;13:811–815.

Miller D, Stegmann R, eds. *Healon (Sodium Hyaluronate): A Guide to Its Use in Ophthalmic Surgery.* New York, NY: John Wiley & Sons Inc; 1983.

Polack FM. Healon (Na hyaluronate) a review of the literature. *Cornea.* 1986;5:81–93.

Schroder H, Sperling S. Polysaccharide coating of human corneal endothelium. *Acta Ophthalmol (Copenh).* VCH Pub Inc. 1977;55:819–826.

Silver F, Doillon C. Biocompatibility, interactions of biological & implantable materials. *Polymer* New York, NY:VCH Pub Inc.;1989:1.

CHAPTER 6

Emory JM, McIntyre DJ. *Extracapsular Cataract Surgery.* St. Louis, Mo: CV Mosby; 1983:62–67.

Hughes WL. The evolution of ophthalmic sutures. *Ann Plast Surg.* 1981;6:48–51.

CHAPTER 8

Evans DW, Ginsburg AP. Contrast sensitivity predicts age-related differences in highway-sign discriminability. *Human Factors.* 1985;27:639-642.

Holladay JT, et al. Optical performance of multifocal intraocular lenses. *J Cataract Refract Surg.* 1990;16:413–422.

Jindra LF, Zemon V. Contrast sensitivity testing: a more complete assessment of vision. *J Cataract Refract Surg.* 1990;15:141–148.

Maxwell WA, Nordan LT, eds. *Current Concepts of Multifocal Intraocular Lenses.* Thorofare, NJ: Slack Inc; 1991.

Neumann AC, et al. The relationship between cataract type and glare disability as measured by the Miller–Nadler glare tester. *J Cataract Refract Surg.* 1988;14:40–45.

Regan Low Contrast Acuity Charts. Lower Sackville, Nova Scotia: Paragon Services.

Shimizu H. Intraoperative and postoperative complications with a posterior chamber lens with five-degree angulated loops. *J Cataract Refract Surg.* 1988;14:281–285.

CHAPTER 9

Apple DJ, Park SB, Merkely KH, et al. Posterior chamber intraocular lenses in a series of 75 autopsy eyes, I: loop location. *J Cataract Refract Surg.* 1986;12:358–362.

Apple DJ, Kincaid MC, Mamalis N, Olson RJ. *Intraocular Lenses. Evolution, Designs, Complications, and Pathology.* Baltimore, Md; Williams & Wilkins, 1989.

Apple DJ, Lims ES, Morgan RE, et al. Preparation and study of human eyes obtained postmortem with the Miyake posterior photographic technique. *Ophthalmology.* 1990;97:810–816.

Blumenthal M, et al. Lens anatomical principles and their technical implications in cataract surgery; part 1: the lens capsule. *J Cataract Refract Surg.* 1991;17:205–210.

Brems RN, Apple DJ, Pfeffer BR, Park SB, Piest KL, Isenberg RA. Posterior chamber intraocular lenses in a series of 75 autopsy eyes, III: correlation of positioning holes and optic edges with the pupillary aperture and visual axis. *J Cataract Refract Surg.* 1986;12:367–371.

Davison JA. Analysis of capsular bag defects and intraocular lens position for consistent centration. *J Cataract Refract Surg.* 1986;12:124–129.

Davison JA. Minimal lift-multiple rotation technique for capsular bag phacoemulsifcation and intraocular lens fixation. *J Cataract Refract Surg.* 1988;14:25–34.

Davison JA. A short haptic diameter modified J-loop intraocular lens for improved capsular bag performance. *J Cataract Refract Surg.* 1988;14:161–166.

Davison JA. Capsular bag distention after endophacoemulsification and posterior chamber intraocular lens implantation. *J Cataract Refract Surg.* 1990;16:99–108.

Davison, JA. Silicone IOL insertion spares optic decentration. *Ocular Surgery News.* Nov. 15, 1990:44–45.

Fercho C. Welsh Cataract Congress; Houston, Tx:1986.

Gimbel HV, Neuhann, T. Development, advantages, and methods of the continuous circular capsulorhexis technique. *J Cataract Refract Surg.* 1990;16:31–37.

Graether J. Continuous circular anterior capsulotomy under Healon. Presented at the 1986 Welsh Cataract Congress. *Ocular Surgery News.* July 1, 1986:30–31.

Koch P, Davison JA, eds: *Textbook of Advanced Phacoemulsification Techniques.* Thorofare, NJ: Slack Inc; 1991:56–75.

Hansen SO, Tetz MR, Solomon KD, et al. Decentration of flexible loop posterior chamber intraocular lenses in a series of 222 postmortem eyes. *Ophthalmology.* 1988;95:344–349.

McDonnell PJ, Champion R, Green WR. Location and composition of haptics of posterior chamber intraocular lenses: histological study of postmortem eyes. *Ophthalmology.* 1987;94:136–142.

Neuhann T. Theorie and operationstechnik der kapsulorrhexis. *Klin Monatsbl Augenheilkd.* 1987;190:542–545.

Smiddy WE, et al. Implantation of scleral-fixated posterior chamber intraocular lenses. *J Cataract Refract Surg.* 1990;16:691–696.

CHAPTER 11

Buratto L. *Extracapsular Cataract Microsurgery and Posterior Chamber Intraocular Lenses.* Milano, Italy: Centro Ambrosiano, Microchirurgia Ocular; 1989.

Devine T, Banko W. *Pharcoemulsification Surgery.* New York, NY: Pergamon Press; 1990.

CHAPTER 13

Alfano G. Pretercapsular cataract extraction with capsular enclosed implant. *Am Intra-Ocular Implant Soc J.* 1984;10:203.

Apple DJ, Park SB, Merkley KH, et al. Posterior chamber intraocular lenses in a series of 75 autopsy eyes, I: loop location. *J Cataract Refract Surg.* 1986;12:358–362.

Baikoff G. Insertion of the Simcoe posterior chamber lens into the capsular bag. *Am Intra-Ocular Implant Soc J.* 1981;7:267–269.

Brems RN, Apple DJ, Pfeffer BR, Park SB, Piest KL, Isenberg RA. Posterior chamber intraocular lenses in a series of 75 autopsy eyes, III: correlation of positioning holes and optic edges with the pupillary aperture and visual axis. *J Cataract Refract Surg.* 1986;12:367–371.

Colvard DM, Kratz RP, Mazzocco TR, Davidson B. Endothelial cell loss following phacoemulsification in the pupillary plane. *Am Intra-Ocular Implant Soc J.* 1981;7:334–336.

Davison JA. Bimodal capsular bag phacoemulsification: a serial cutting and suction ultrasonic nuclear dissection technique. *J Cataract Refract Surg.* 1989;15:272–282.

Davison JA. Analysis of capsular bag defects and intraocular lens positions for consistent centration. *J Cataract Refract Surg.* 1986;12:124–129.

Davison JA. Minimal-lift multiple rotation technique for capsular bag phacoemulsification and intraocular lens fixation. *J Cataract Refract Surg.* 1988;14:25–34.

Fukaya V, Hara T, Hara T, Iwata S. Effect of freezing on lens epithelial cell growth. *J Cataract Refract Surg.* 1988;14:309–311.

Galand A. A simple method of implantation within the capsular bag. *Am Intra-Ocular Implant Soc J.* 1983;9:330–332.

Gindi JJ, Wan WL, Schanzlin DJ. Endocapsular cataract surgery, I: surgical technique. *Cataract.* 1985;2:6–10.

Girard LJ. Pars plana vs. the limbal approach to intraocular surgery. *Ophthalmic Surg.* 1981;12:317.

Gimbel HV. Capsulotomy method eases in the bag posterior chamber lens implantation. *Ocular Surgery News.* July 1,1985:20.

Hara T, Hara T. Clinical results of endocapsular phacoemulsification and complete in-the-bag intraocular lens fixation. *J Cataract Refract Surg.* 1987;13:279–286.

Hara T, Hara T. Roundel phacoemulsification technique for in-the-bag intraocular lens fixation. *J Cataract Refract Surg.* 1987;13:441–446.

Hara T, Hara T. Fate of the capsular bag in endocapsular phacoemulsification and complete in-the-bag intraocular lens fixation. *J Cataract Refract Surg.* 1986;12: 408–412.

Hara T, Hara T. Recent advance in intracapsular phacoemulsification and complete in-the-bag intraocular lens fixation. *J Cataract Refract Surg.* 1985;13:279–286.

Hara T, Hara T. Subcapsular phacoemulsification and aspiration. *Am Intra-Ocular Implant Soc J.* 1984;10:333–337.

Hara T, Hara T. Subcapsular phacoemulsification and aspiration. *Ganka.* 1982;24:1203–1207.

Hansen SO, Tetz MR, Solomon KD, et al. Decentration of flexible loop posterior chamber intraocular lenses in a series of 222 postmortem eyes. *Ophthalmology.* 1988;95:344–349.

Graether JM. Continuous circular anterior capsulotomy under Healon. *Ocular Surgery News.* July 1, 1986:30–31.

Kelman CD. Phacoemulsification and aspiration. *Am J Ophthalmol.* 1967;64: 23–35.

Masket S. Deep versus appositional suturing of the scleral pocket incision for astigmatic control in cataract surgery. *J Cataract Refract Surg.* 1987;13:131–135.

Michelson MA. Endocapsular phacoemulsification: the storm within the calm. *Ocular Surgery News.* September 15, 1989:60–61.

Neuhann T. Theorie and Operationstechnik der Kapsulorhexis. *Klin Monatsbl Augenheilkd.* 1987;190:542–545.

Nishi O. Removal of lens epithelial cells by ultrasound in endocapsular cataract surgery. *Ophthalmic Surg.* 1987;18:577–580.

Park SB, Brems RN, Parsons MR, et al. Posterior chamber intraocular lenses in a series of 75 autopsy eyes, II: postimplantation loop configuration. *J Cataract Refract Surg.* 1986;12:363–366.

Patel J. One-handed technique of endocapsular phacoemulsification. *Ocular Surgery News.* January 1, 1987:24.

Patel J, Apple DJ, Hansen SO, et al. Protective effect of the anterior lens capsule during extracapsular cataract extraction, II: preliminary results of clinical study. *Ophthalmology.* 1989;96:598–602.

Personal correction of a phacoemulsification machine problem. *J Cataract Refract Surg.* 1988;14:456–458. Letter to the Editor.

Shepherd JR. Induced astigmatism in small incision cataract surgery. *J Cataract Refract Surg.* 1989;15:85–88.

Shepherd JR. "In situ fracture phaco method" interview. *Phaco and Foldables.* 1989;1:8.

Wan WL, Gindi JJ, Schanzlin DJ. Endocapsular cataract surgery, II: effects on the corneal endothelium. *Cataract.* 1985;2:1–14.

Wilson DL. Parel J-M, Phacoexcavation as an alternative pars plana technique for lens removal. *Am J Ophthalmol.* 1985;100:528–533.

CHAPTER 14

Brems RN, Apple DJ, Pfeffer BR, et al. Posterior chamber intraocular lenses in a series of 75 autopsy eyes, III: correlation of positioning holes and optic edges with the pupillary aperture and visual axis. *J Cataract Refract Surg.* 1986;12:367–371.

Masket S. Reversal of glare disability after cataract surgery. *J Cataract Refract Surg.* 1989;15:165–168.

CHAPTER 15

Barrett GD, Constable IJ. Corneal endothelial loss with new intraocular lenses. *Am J Ophthalmol.* 1984; 98:157–165.

Barrett GD, Constable IJ, Stewart AD. Clinical results of hydrogel lens implantation. *J Cataract Refract Surg.* 1986;12:623–631.

Brint SF, de Faller JM, Rosenthal AL, Houchens VM, Disbrow DT. Early visual rehabilitation following small incision implantation of a hydrogel (IOGEL model 1103) intraocular lens. Presented at the European Intraocular Implant Council Meeting; August 28, 1989; Zurich, Switzerland.

Brint SF, Ostrick DM, Bryan JE. Keratometric cylinder and visual performance following phacoemulsification and implantation with silicone small-incision or PMMA intraocular lenses. *J Cataract Refract Surg.* In press.

Epstein E. Insertion techniques and clinical experience with HEMA lenses. In: Mazzocco TR, Rajacich GM, Epstein E, eds. *Soft Implant Lenses in Cataract Surgery.* Thorofare, NJ: Slack Inc; 1986:143–150.

Faulkner GD. Early experience with STAAR^{TM} *silicone elastic lens implants. J Cataract Refract Surg.* 1986;12:36–39.

Faulkner GD. Folding and inserting silicone intraocular lens implants. *J Cataract Refract Surg.* 1987;13:678–681.

Fine IH. Initial experience with the AMO PC28LB (Phacofit) small incision implant: a preliminary report. *J Cataract Refract Surg.* 1989;15:327–332.

Fyodorov SN, Puchkov SG. Chemical and mechanical influence of intraocular lenses on rabbit eye tissue. *Ann Ophthalmol.* 1981;13:1259–1264.

Gimbel HV, Neuhann T. Development, advantages, and methods of the continuous circular capsulorhexis technique. *J Cataract Refract Surg.* 1990;16:31–37.

Grabow HB. Results of 800 Staar silicone lenses. Presented at the Symposium on Cataract, IOL and Refractive Surgery; March 5, 1990; Los Angeles, Calif.

Kassar BS, Varnell ED. Effect of PMMA and silicone lens material on normal rabbit corneal endothelium: an in vitro study. *J Am Intra-Ocular Implant Soc.* 1980; 6:344–346.

Martin SS. The Iogel intraocular lens implant: a report on the national experience and our personal experience, II: complications: lens dislocation. Presented at the Symposium on Cataract, IOL and Refractive Surgery; March 7, 1990; Los Angeles, Calif.

Mazzocco TR. Silicone implant lens. *Cataract.* 1985; 2:31.

Mehta KR, Sathe SN, Karyekar DS: The new soft intraocular lens implant *J Am Intra-Ocular Implant Soc.* 1978;4:200–205.

Neumann AC, Cobb G. Advantages and limitations of current soft intraocular lenses. *J Cataract Refract Surg.* 1988;15:257–263.

Neumann AC, McCarty GR, Osher RH. Complications associated with Staar silicone intraocular lens implants. *J Cataract Refract Surg.* 1987;13:653–656.

Nordan LT. Quantifiable astigmatism correction: concepts and suggestions. *J Cataract Refract Surg.* 1986;12:507–518.

Ridley H. Intra-ocular acrylic lenses: a recent development in the surgery of cataract. *Br J Ophthalmol.* 1952;36:113–122.

Shepherd JR. Induced astigmatism in small incision cataract surgery. *J Cataract Refract Surg.* 1989;15:448–450.

Shepherd JR. Capsular opacification associated with silicone implants. *J Cataract Refract Surg.* 1989;15:448–450.

Shepherd JR. Correction of pre-existing astigmatism at the time of small incision cataract surgery. *J Cataract Refract Surg.* 1989;25:55–57.

Shepherd JR. Induced astigmatism in small incision cataract surgery — a two year follow-up of the single stitch horizontal closures. Presented at the Symposium on Cataract, IOL and Refractive Surgery; March 5, 1990; Los Angeles, Calif.

Watt RH. Pigment dispersion syndrome associated with silicone posterior chamber intraocular lenses. *J Cataract Refract Surg.* 1988;14:431–433.

Yalon M, Blumenthal M, Goldberg EP. Preliminary study of hydrophilic hydrogel intraocular lens implants in cats. *J Am Intra-Ocular Implant Soc.* 1984;10:315–317.

Zhou KY. 50 cases with IOL transparent silicone anterior chamber suture type implantation. *Chin J Ophthalmol.* 1981;17:21–22.

CHAPTER 20
Shepherd JR. Increased astigmatism in small incision surgery. *J Cataract Refract Surg.* 1989;15:85–88.

CHAPTER 21
Ashrafzadeh MT, Schepens CL, Elzeneiny IH, et al. Aphakic and phakic retinal detachment. *Arch Ophthalmol.* 1973;89:476.

Baikoff G, Joly P, Colin J, et al. Clinical results with anterior chamber myopic lenses in phakic eyes: survey of the French multicenter study. Presented at Refractive Corneal Surgery Symposium, March 16–17, 1990; Singapore.

Clayman HM, Jaffe NS, Light DS. Intraocular lenses, axial length, and retinal detachment. *Am J Ophthalmol.* 1981;92:778.

Colvard DM, Kratz RP, Mazzocco TR, Davidson B. Endothelial cell loss following phacoemulsification in the pupillary plane. *J Am Intraocular Implant Soc.* 1981;7:334–336.

Coonan P, Fung WE, Webster RG, et al. The incidence of retinal detachment following extracapsular cataract extraction: a ten-year study. *Ophthalmology.* 1985;92:1096.

Curtin BJ. The Myopias: Basic Science and Clinical Management. Philadelphia, Pa; Harper & Row; 1985.

Dardenne MU, Gerten GJ, Kolkas K, Kermani O. Retrospective study of retinal detachment following neodymium:YAG laser posterior capsulotomy. *J Cataract Refract Surg.* 1989;15:676–680.

Gimbel HV, Neuhann T. Development, advantage and methods of the continuous circular capsulorhexis technique *J Cataract Refract Surg.* 1990;16:31–37.

Goldberg M. Clear lens extraction for axial myopia: an appraisal. *Ophthalmology.* 1987;94:571–582.

Holladay JT, Prager TC, Chandler TY, et al. A three part system for refining intraocular lens power calculation. *J Cataract Refract Surg.* 1988;14:17–14

Hyams SW, Bialik M, Neumann E. Myopia-aphakia, I: prevalence of retinal detachment. *Br J Ophthalmol.* 1975;59:480–482.

Hyams SW, Neumann E, Friedman Z. Myopia-aphakia, II: vitreous and peripheral retina. *Br J Ophthalmol.* 1975;59:483–485.

Kreiger A. Retinal detachment. In: Thompson FB, ed. *Myopia Surgery.* New York, NY: Macmillan Publishing Co; 1990:239.

Livernois R, Sinskey RM. Low power intraocular lenses. *J Am Intra-Ocular Implant Soc.* 1983;9:321–323.

Neumann AC, McCarty GR. Lensectomy for the treatment of myopia. In: Thompson FB, ed. *Myopia Surgery.* New York, NY: Macmillan Publishing Co; 1990:101.

Percival SPB, Anand V, Das SK. Prevalence of aphakic retinal detachment. *Br J Ophthalmol.* 1983;67:43.

Perkins ES. Morbidity from myopia. *Sightsav Rev.* 1979;49:11–19.

Ruben M, Rajpurohit P. Distribution of myopia in aphakic retinal detachments. *Br J Ophthalmol.* 1976;60:517.

Sanders DR, Retzleff J, Kraff MC. Comparison of the SRK II formula and other second generation formulas. *J Cataract Refract Surg.* 1988;14:136–141.

Schepens CL, Marden BA. Data on the natural history of retinal detachment: further characterization of certain unilateral non-traumatic cases. *Am J Ophthalmol.* 1966;61:213–226.

Seward HC, Doran RML. Posterior capsulotomy and retinal detachment following extracapsular lens surgery. *Br J Opthalmol.* 1984;68:379.

Smith PW, Stark WJ, Maumenee AE, et al. Retinal detachment after extracapsular cataract extraction with posterior chamber intraocular lens. *Ophthalmology.* 1987;94:495.

Verezella F. Refractive microsurgery of the lens myopia: the risk-benefit ratio. *J Cataract Refract Surg.* 1988;4:27–28.

CHAPTER 22
Jaffe NS. *Atlas of Ophthalmic Surgery.* Philadelphia, Pa: JB Lippincott; 1990.

Kremer FV, Marks RG. Radial keratotomy: prospective evaluation of safety and efficacy. *Ophthalmic Surg.* 1983;14:925–930.

Sawelson HR, Marks RG. Three year results of radial keratotomy. *Arch Ophthalmol.* 1987;105:81–85.

Waring GO, et al. Results of the prospective evaluation of radial keratotomy (PERK) study 1 year after surgery. *Ophthalmology.* 1985;92:177–198.

CHAPTER 23
Astigmatism. *J Cataract Refract Surg.* 1989;15:1-124.

Nordan LT. Quantifiable astigmatism correction: concepts and suggestions. *J Cataract Refract Surg.* 1986;12:507–518.

Steinert RF, et al. Astigmatism after small incision cataract surgery: a prospective, randomized, multicenter comparison of 4 and 6.5. mm incisions. *Ophthalmology.* 1991;98:417–424.

CHAPTER 26
Excimer laser corneal surgery. *Refractive and Corneal Surgery.* 1990;6(special issue):305-388.

Macaulay D. *The Way Things Work.* Boston, Mass: Houghton Mifflin; 1988.

Maguire LJ. Topography and raytracing analysis of patients with excellent visual acuity 3 months after excimer laser photorefractive keratectomy for myopia. *Refractive and Corneal Surgery.* 1991;7:122–128.

Taylor DM, et al. Experimental corneal studies with the excimer laser. *J Cataract Refract Surg.* 1989;15:384–389.

Trokel S. Evolution of excimer laser corneal surgery. *J Cataract Refract Surg.* 1989;15:373–383.

Sher NA, et al. Clinical use of the 193-nm excimer laser in the treatment of corneal scars. *Arch Ophthalmol.* 1991;109:491–498.

CHAPTER 27
Alfonso E, Mandelbaum S, Fox MJ, Forster RK. Ulcerative keratitis associated with contact lens wear. *Am J Ophthalmol.* 1986; 101:429.

Aquavella JV, Barraquer J, Gullapalli NR, Ruiz LA. Morphological variations in corneal endothelium following keratophakia and keratomileusis. *Ophthalmology.* 1981;88:721–723.

Barraquer JI. Long-term results of myopic keratomileusis—1982. *Arch Soc Ame Oftal Optom.* 1983;17:137–148.

Barraquer JI. Results of hypermetropic keratomileusis, 1980–1981. In: Binder PS, ed *Refractive corneal surgery: the correction of aphakia, hyperopia, and myopia. Int Ophthalmol Clinics.* 1983;23:25–44.

Barraquer JI. Keratomileusis for the correction of myopia. *Arc Soc Amer Oftal Optom.* 1982;16:221-232.

Barraquer JI. Keratomileusis for myopia and aphakia. *Ophthalmology.* 1981;88:701-708.

Barraquer JI. Queratomileusis y queratofaquia. Bogota, Colombia: Litografia Arco; 1980:430–434.

Barraquer JI. Keratomileusis for the correction of aphakia, In: *Symposium on Medical and Surgical Diseases of the Corneal Transactions of the New Orleans Academy of Ophthalmology.* St. Louis, Mo: CV Mosby; 1980;450–479.

Barraquer JI. Keratophakia. *Jpn J Ophthalmol.* 1974;18:199–212.

Barraquer JI. Keratophakia. *Trans Ophthalmol Soc UK.* 1972;92:499–16.

Barraquer JI. Keratomileusis. *Int Surg.* 1967;48:103–117.

Barraquer JI. Keratomileusis for the correction of myopia. *Ann Inst Barraquer.* 1964;5:209–229.

Barraquer JI, Viteri E. Results of myopic keratomileusis. *J Caract Refract Surg.* 1987;3:98–101.

Duran JA, Refojo MF, Gipson IK, Kenyon KR. Psuedomonas attachment to new hydrogel contact lenses. *Arch Ophthalmol.* 1987;105:106–109.

El-Maghraby MA, Vitero E, Ruiz L. Keratomileusis in situ to correct high myopia. *Ophthalmology.* 1988;95(Suppl):145.

Friedlander MH, Werblin TP, Kaufman HE, Granet NS. Clinical results of keratophakia and keratomileusis. *Ophthalmology.* 1981;88:716–720.

Galentine PG, Cohen EJ, Laibson PR, Adams CP, Michaud R, Arentsen JJ. Corneal ulcers associated with contact lens wear. *Arch Ophthalmol.* 1986;104:79.

Krumeich JH. Indications, techniques, and complications of myopic keratomileusis. In: Binder PS, ed. Refractive corneal surgery: the correction of aphakia, hyperopia, and myopia. *Int Ophthalmol Clinic.* 1983;23:75–92.

Krumeich JH, Swinger CA. Non-freeze epikeratophakia for the correction of myopia. *Am J Ophthalmol.* 1987;103:397–403.

Maxwell WA, Nordan LT. Myopic keratomileusis: early experience. *J Cataract Refract Surg.* 1985;1:99.

Neumann AC, McCarty G, Sander DR. Delayed regression of effect in myopic epikeratophakia vs myopic keratomileusis for high myopia. *Refractive & Corneal Surgery.* 1989;5:161–166.

Nordan LT, Havins WE. Undercorrected radial keratotomy treated with myopic keratomileusis. *J Refractive Surg.* 1985;1:56–58.

Swinger CA, Barker BA. Myopic keratomileusis following radial keratotomy. *J Refractive Surg.* 1985;1:53–55.

Swinger CA, Barraquer JI. Keratophakia and keratomileusis. *Ophthalmology.* 1981;88:709–715.

Swinger CA, Villasenor RA. Homoplastic keratomileusis for the correction of myopia. *J Refractive Surg.* 1985;1:219–223.

Troutman RC, Swinger C. Refractive keratoplasty: keratophakia and keratomileusis. *Trans Am Ophthalmol Soc.* 1978;76:329–339.

Villasenor RA, Jester JV, Siaz J, et al. Preliminary study of keratomileusis in primates (Macaca speciosa). *Ophthalmology.* 1981;88:724–728.

CHAPTER 28

American Academy of Ophthalmology. Epikeratoplasty: ophthalmic procedures assessment. *Ophthalmology.* 1990;97:1225–1232.

Deitz TR, Durrie DS. Indications and treatment of keratoconus using epikeratophakia. *Ophthalmology.* 1988;95:236–246.

Durrie DS, Habrich DL, Dietz TR. Secondary intraocular lens implantation vs epikeratophakia for the treatment of aphakia. *Am J Ophthalmol.* 1987;103:384–391.

Goosey JD, Prager TC, Goosey CB, Martin DI. One year follow-up of epikeratoplasty for myopia. *J Cataract Refract Surg.* 1990;16:21–30.

Goosey JD, Prager, TC, Marvelli TL, Allison ME, Hook SR, Carlson KA. Epikeratophakia without annular keratectomy. *Ann Ophthalmol.* 1987;19:388–391.

Kaufman, HE. The correction of aphakia. *Am J Ophthalmol.* 1980;89:1–10.

Kaufman HE, Werblin, TP. Epikeratophakia for the treatment of keratoconus. *Am J Ophthalmol.* 1982;93:342–347.

Kelley, CG, Keates, RH, Lembach, RG. Epikeratophakia for pediatric aphakia. *Arch Ophthalmol.* 1986;104:680–682.

Maguire LJ, Klyce SD, Singer DE, McDonald MB, Kauffman HE. Corneal topography in myopic patients undergoing epikeratophakia. *Am J Ophthalmol.* 1987;103:404–416.

McDonald MB, Kaufman HE, Aquavella JV, Durrie DS, et al. The nationwide study of epikeratophakia in adults. *Am J Ophthalmol.* 1987;103:358–365.

McDonald MB, Kaufman HE, Durrie DS, Keates RH, et al. The nationwide study of epikeratophakia for keratoconus. *Arch Ophthalmol.* 1986;104:1294–1300.

McDonald MB, Morgan KS. Epikeratophakia for aphakia and myopia. In: Kaufman HE, Baron BA, McDonald MB, Naltman SR, eds. *The Cornea.* New York, NY: Churchill Livingstone Inc; 1988;823–847.

McDonnell PJ, Deitze T, Durrie DS, Schanzlin DJ. Surgical correction of aphakia: intraocular lens implantation and epikeratophakia. *J Refract Surg.* 1987;3:209–214.

Morgan KS, et al. Epikeratophakia in children. *Opthalmology.* 1984;91:780–784.

Werblin TB, Kaufman HE, Friedlander MH, Granet N. Epikeratophakia and the surgical correction of aphakia, III. Preliminary results of a prospective clinical trial. *Arch Ophthalmol.* 1981;99:1957–1960.

Price, FW, Binder PS. Scarring of a recipient cornea following epikeratoplasty. *Arch Ophthalmol.* 1987;105:1556–1560.

Schlichtemeier WR, Arbegast KD. Long-term loss of effect of myopic epikeratophakia. *Refract Surg.* 1987;3:46–69.

Steinert RF, Grene RB. Postoperative management of epikeratoplasty. *J Cataract Refract Surg.* 1988;14:255–264.

Steinert RF, Wagoner MD. Long-term comparison of epikeratoplasty and penetrating keratoplasty for keratoconus. *Arch Ophthalmol.* 1988;106:493–496.

U.S. Food and Drug Administration, Ophthalmic Devices Advisory Panel, 60th Meeting, January 21, 1988; Washington D.C.

Uusitalo RJ, Lethosalo J. Epikeratophakia in aphakic children. *Am J Ophthalmol.* 1987;103:465–466.

Woodhams TJ. Regression of myopic epikeratophakia effects. *J Cataract Refract Surg.* 1987;13:343–344.

CHAPTER 29

Beebe WE, et al. The use of molteno implant and anterior chamber tube shunt to encircling band for the treatment of glaucoma in keratoplasty patients. *Ophthalmology.* 1990; 97:1414–1422.

The Glaucoma Laser Trial Group. The glaucoma laser trial (GLT), II. results of argon laser trabeculoplasty versus topical medications. *Ophthalmology.* 1990;97:1403–1413.

CHAPTER 30

Apple DJ, Rabb MF. *Clinicopathologic Correlation of Ocular Disease.* St. Louis, Mo: CV Mosby; 1974.

Duke Elder S, Leigh AG. *System of Ophthalmology, VIII: Diseases of the Outer Eye—Cornea and Sclera.* St. Louis, Mo: CV Mosby; 1965.

CHAPTER 31

Alpar JJ. Aquired ptosis following cataract and glaucoma surgery. *Glaucoma.* 1982;4:66–8.

Kaplan LJ, Jaffe NS, Clayman, HM. Ptosis and cataract surgery. *Ophthalmology.* 1985;92:237–242.

Paris GL, Quickert MH. Disinsertion of the aponeurosis of the levator palpebrae superioris muscle after cataract extraction. *Am J Ophthalmol.* 1976;81:337–340.

CREDITS

Many individuals and companies have provided the editors and authors of *The Surgical Rehabilitation of Vision* with important photographs and diagram information. We acknowledge and deeply appreciate this material, which has helped us compile a more realistic and comprehensive presentation of anterior segment surgery.

FOREWORD
Fig. 1 *Innovation: The Attacker's Advantage* by Richard N. Foster. Copyright © 1986 by McKinsey & Co Inc. Reprinted by permission of Summit Books, a division of Simon & Schuster Inc.

CHAPTER 2
2.9 (bottom left) Linda Villanueva and Perry Binder, MD; 2.11, 2.14 Henry D'Souza, EyeSys Inc; 2.12, 2.13, 2.15, 2.16 Computed Anatomy Inc; 2.17, 2.18 Leo Bores, MD, Kerametrics Inc.

CHAPTER 3
Redrawn with permission from Bothner J, Wic O. The rheology of intraocular solutions. In: Rosen ES, ed. *Viscoelastic Material*. July 7, 1986.

CHAPTER 6
6.1–6.7, 6.9–6.11, 6.13, 6.17, 6.20–6.23 Storz Instrument Co; 6.18 ASICO Inc; 6.19 Visitec Inc.

CHAPTER 7
7.1–7.9, 7.11–7.13, 7.25, 7.27 Ethicon Inc; 7.17–7.21, 7.23 Alcon Surgical Inc.

CHAPTER 8
8.1, 8.5 (left), 8.7 (top left and right), 8.11 (middle, right), 8.27, 8.45, 8.47 Ioptex Research Inc; 8.4 Ehud I. Assia, MD, Storm Eye Center, University of South Carolina; 8.5 (right), 8.7 (bottom left), 8.11 (left), 8.34, 8.41 American Medical Optics Inc; 8.8, 8.40 3M Company; 8.10, 8.12–8.20, 8.22–8.25 James A. Davison, MD, Pharmacia Inc; 8.21 Philippe Crozafon, MD, Pharmacia Inc; 8.26 Lance Alworth; 8.35, 8.36, 8.45 Jack Holladay, MD; 8.37 Iolab Inc; 8.7 (bottom right), 8.38 Pharmacia Inc; 8.42–8.44 Wright Medical Inc.

CHAPTER 11
11.1, 11.9, 11.10, 11.14, 11.16, 11.18 Alcon Surgical Inc; 11.20 Optical Micro Systems Inc.

CHAPTER 12
12.10, 12.11 Philippe Crozafon, MD.

CHAPTER 13
13.1 Thomas Neuhann, MD; 13.2 John Graether, MD; 13.5 Charles Kelman, MD; 13.11, 13.14 T. Hara, MD; 13.22–13.24 Marc Michelson, MD; 13.82 David Dillman, MD; 13.132 Laboratory of Intraocular Lens Research, Charleston, SC.

CHAPTER 21
21.3 George Baikoff, MD.

CHAPTER 22
22.10 Chiron Ophthalmics Inc.

CHAPTER 23
23.13–23.15 Reichert Instrument Co; 23.18 William Steen, MD; 23.40 Hi-Line Inc.

CHAPTER 25
25.5, 25.23–25.25 American Medical Optics Inc; 25.26 Bernie McCarey, PhD, Emory School of Medicine; 25.27 Surgidev Inc.

CHAPTER 26
26.1 Modified from Macaulay D. *The Way Things Work*. Boston, Mass: Houghton Mifflin; 1988:206 26.2, 26.6, 26.7 Intelligent Laser Systems Inc; 26.4 Michael Gordon, MD; 26.5 Daniel S. Durrie, MD.

CHAPTER 27
26.13 Allergan Medical Optics Inc; 26.15 Luis Ruiz, MD.

CHAPTER 29
29.11–29.14 Wright Medical Inc.

CHAPTER 30
30.1, 30.2 John Bokowsky, MD.